Therapeutic Electrophysical Agents

Evidence Behind Practice

EDITION 2

Therapeutic Electrophysical Agents

Evidence Behind Practice

EDITION 2

ALAIN-YVAN BÉLANGER, BSc, MSc, PhD, PT

Professor
Department of Rehabilitation
Faculty of Medicine
Laval University
Quebec City, Canada

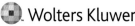 Wolters Kluwer | Lippincott Williams & Wilkins
Health

Philadelphia • Baltimore • New York • London
Buenos Aires • Hong Kong • Sydney • Tokyo

Acquisitions Editor: Emily Lupash
Managing Editor: Meredith Brittain
Marketing Manager: Allison Noplock
Senior Production Editor: Sandra Cherrey Scheinin
Designer: Teresa Mallon
Compositor: Spearhead Global Inc.

Second Edition

351 West Camden Street   530 Walnut Street
Baltimore, MD 21201   Philadelphia, PA 19106

Printed in China

9 8 7 6 5 4 3 2 1

Library of Congress Cataloging-in-Publication Data
Bélanger, Alain.
  Therapeutic electrophysical agents : evidence behind practice / Alain-Yvan Bélanger. — 2nd ed.
    p. ; cm.
  Rev ed. of: Evidence-based guide to therapeutic physical agents, c2002.
  Includes bibliographical references and index.
  ISBN-13: 978-0-7817-7001-9
  ISBN-10: 0-7817-7001-7
 1. Physical therapy—Handbooks, manuals, etc. 2. Medicine, Physical—Handbooks, manuals, etc.
I. Bélanger, Alain. Evidence-based guide to therapeutic physical agents. II. Title.
    [DNLM: 1. Therapeutics—Handbooks. 2. Therapeutics—Outlines. 3. Evidence-Based Medicine—Handbooks. 4. Evidence-Based Medicine—Outlines. 5. Physical Medicine—Handbooks. 6. Physical Medicine—Outlines. WB 39 B4266t 2010]
  RM701.B45 2010
  615.8′2—dc22
                                                        2009002847

Care has been taken to confirm the accuracy of the information present and to describe generally accepted practices. However, the authors, editors, and publisher are not responsible for errors or omissions or for any consequences from application of the information in this book and make no warranty, expressed or implied, with respect to the currency, completeness, or accuracy of the contents of the publication. Application of this information in a particular situation remains the professional responsibility of the practitioner; the clinical treatments described and recommended may not be considered absolute and universal recommendations.

The authors, editors, and publisher have exerted every effort to ensure that drug selection and dosage set forth in this text are in accordance with the current recommendations and practice at the time of publication. However, in view of ongoing research, changes in government regulations, and the constant flow of information relating to drug therapy and drug reactions, the reader is urged to check the package insert for each drug for any change in indications and dosage and for added warnings and precautions. This is particularly important when the recommended agent is a new or infrequently employed drug.

Some drugs and medical devices presented in this publication have Food and Drug Administration (FDA) clearance for limited use in restricted research settings. It is the responsibility of the health care provider to ascertain the FDA status of each drug or device planned for use in their clinical practice.

To purchase additional copies of this book, call our customer service department at **(800) 638-3030** or fax orders to **(301) 223-2320**. International customers should call **(301) 223-2300**.

Visit Lippincott Williams & Wilkins on the Internet: http://www.lww.com. Lippincott Williams & Wilkins customer service representatives are available from 8:30 am to 6:00 pm, EST.

CCS0904

To my wife, Susanne, and to my three children, Mark, Julie, and Kimberly.

To all of you, present and future evidence-based practitioners, who, through your relentless efforts to seek the best evidence, will assure the survival of therapeutic electrophysical agents for years to come.

Whoever ceases to be a student has never been a student.
—Georges Iles

It is impossible for a man to learn what he thinks he already knows.
—Epictetus

The worth of a book is to be measured by what you can carry from it.
—James Bryce

The possession of facts is knowledge; the use of them is wisdom.
—Thomas Jefferson

The whole of science is nothing more than a refinement of everyday thinking.
—Albert Einstein

Whoever ceases to be a student has never been a student.
—Georges Iles

It is impossible for a man to learn what he thinks he already knows.
—Epictetus

The worth of a book is to be measured by what you can carry from it.
—James Bryce

The possession of facts is knowledge; the use of them is wisdom.
—Thomas Jefferson

The whole of science is nothing more than a refinement of everyday thinking.
—Albert Einstein

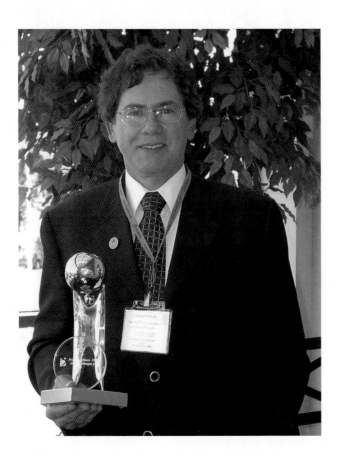

Alain Yvan Bélanger, BSc, MSc, PhD, PT is Professor, Department of Rehabilitation, Physiotherapy program, Faculty of Medicine, Laval University, Quebec City, Canada. Dr. Bélanger holds a bachelor's degree in physiotherapy from University of Montreal, a master's of science degree in kinesiology from Simon Fraser University, and a doctoral degree in neurosciences from McMaster University. He has more than 30 years of experience as a teacher, researcher, and author in the field of human neuromuscular physiology and therapeutic electrophysical agents.

Dr. Bélanger has an extensive list of communications and publications. He is a member of the Canadian Physiotherapy Association (CPA), and has held the positions of Scientific Editor of the journal *Physiotherapy Canada* and President of CPA. In addition, he served as Associate Editor of the journals *Physiotherapy Canada, Physiotherapy Theory and Practice,* and *Journal of Occupational Rehabilitation*. He is the sole author of the first edition of this book, titled *Evidence-Based Guide to Therapeutic Physical Agents,* for which he won the Prize for Excellence from the Quebec Physiotherapy Licensing Board in 2005. Always in motion and passionate about sports, Dr. Bélanger has recently traded his marathon shoes for golf shoes.

Therapeutic Electrophysical Agents: Evidence Behind Practice, Second Edition is much more than an update of *Evidence-Based Guide to Therapeutic Physical Agents*, published in 2002. In addition to the title change, the second edition features significant additional material that make this textbook one of the most comprehensive ever written on the topic of therapeutic electrophysical agents (EPAs).

My goals in writing the first edition were to provide faculty, researchers, students, practitioners, and manufacturers with an easy-to-consult, portable, evidence-based guide to the practice of therapy with EPAs. For the first time, readers were provided with a pocket-sized EPA text, which was written in outline format and based on the scientific evidence available at the time.

Since the publication of the first edition, my publisher and I have gathered feedback from readers. Two elements were unanimously appreciated: The focused nature of the content (evidence-based) and the format (outline). However, readers differed on whether they preferred the pocket size or would prefer a more traditional textbook. This second edition reflects their remarks and suggestions in an attempt to develop and deliver the most comprehensive and practical evidence-based EPA textbook for college and university courses at the bachelor's, master's, and doctoral degree levels.

This second edition expands on the content of the first by including foundation material, such as tissue healing and pain, as well as additional EPAs, while retaining the original outline format. In addition, the pedagogical approach has been enhanced by the addition of learning objectives, critical thinking questions, and case studies.

CONTENT CHANGES

This second edition contains 27 chapters divided into three parts, plus two appendices. The five new chapters in Part I lay the foundation for the use of therapeutic EPAs. Readers first learn about the use of EPA in health care and are then provided with material related to all the important concepts of soft-tissue injury, healing, and pain. Part I goes on to introduce the spectrum of EPAs

and wraps up with a comprehensive illustrated glossary of electrophysical terminology.

Part II (Chapters 6 through 23) covers the spectrum of EPAs currently in use worldwide. These chapters present the major sources of energy underlying the practice of therapeutic EPAs, namely electrical, electromagnetic, thermal, and mechanical. Four new chapters (on ultraviolet, spinal traction, intermittent pneumatic compression, and continuous passive motion therapy) have been added to the original fourteen chapters in the first edition that were devoted to EPAs. The structure of each of these chapters now includes an introductory section covering the rationale of usage as well as a section dedicated to the presentation of evidenced-based case studies.

Part III (Chapters 24 thorough 27) presents practical clinical guidelines designed to facilitate the practice of therapy with EPAs. Readers learn about the purchase of EPAs and testing thermal sensory skin discrimination, measuring thermal gradients using a portable noncontact thermometer, and practicing safety aspects through the concepts of electrical shock and maintenance of therapeutic electrophysical devices and accessories.

The two appendices provide equivalency of units of measurement between the metric and the U.S. systems and between the Celsius and Fahrenheit temperature units.

PRESENTATION CHANGES

The two most striking changes in this edition are the title and the textbook size. The new title reflects the true nature of this textbook, which is to present scientific evidence behind the practice of therapeutic EPAs. The change of trim size was motivated by the fact that the addition of a significant amount of material would make the original pocket size less practical and attractive to users. This larger format presents several advantages. In addition to being easier to read, there is now room to include many photographs of EPA devices and accessories. Additional tables, boxes, and figures have also been incorporated to further enhance learning, with a clearer distinction made between risks, precautions, and recommendations.

PEDAGOGICAL CHANGES

Educators often overfeed students with endless content to remember, thus emphasising the development of their rote memorization skills. Too often we also fail to present our material in a way that encourages students to use their higher cognitive skills and to ask thought-provoking questions, which would serve to develop their thinking skills. Most students, unfortunately, ask few of these types of questions about course material. If a question does arise, it is often simply to ask whether the material will be part of an exam.

I believe it is our main responsibility to turn our students into generators of questions and answers as opposed to recipients of material. We must stop being seen by students as simple purveyors of answers. We must stimulate them to ask questions and to answer them. To do so we must guide their learning process by laying down sound learning objectives and asking them deep questions about the material we teach, because thinking and learning are fostered by questions, not by knowledge and rote memorization. This second edition uses a pedagogical approach aimed at helping educators meet this responsibility.

LEARNING OBJECTIVES

Each chapter now begins with a series of learning objectives based on Bloom's classic taxonomy of learning, which touches on our lower and higher levels of cognition or brain power. Objectives related to the domains of knowledge, comprehension, and application address students' lower brain capacity, while those related to the domains of analysis, synthesis, and evaluation call on their higher brain power. As stated by Bloom, learning objectives indicate what we educators want students to learn; they are explicit formulations of the ways in which students are expected to be transformed by the educative process (Bloom et al., 1956). In order to meet these objectives and be transformed by the learning process, students will have to engage both their lower and higher cognitive skills. In each chapter, an objective is presented for each of Bloom's six levels of learning, which are defined as follows:

- *Knowledge* is the ability to recall, to retrieve, or to recognize knowledge from our short- and long-term memory.
- *Comprehension* is the ability to grasp or construct meaning from instructional messages, including oral, written, and graphic communication, in order to interpret, exemplify, classify, summarize, compare, or explain.
- *Application* is the ability to carry out, or use, a procedure or technique in a given situation in order to execute or implement.
- *Analysis* is the ability to break material into its constituent parts and determine how the parts relate to one another and to the overall structure and purpose in order to differentiate, organize, or attribute.
- *Synthesis* is the ability to put elements together to form a coherent or functional whole; it is to reorganize elements into a new pattern or structure in order to generate, plan, or produce something.
- *Evaluation* is the ability to make judgment based on criteria and standards in order to check or critique.

CRITICAL THINKING QUESTIONS

Each chapter now ends with a series of critical thinking questions to stimulate students' critical thinking skills. The term *critical thinking* derives its roots from the Greek word *kritico*, meaning discerning judgment. To discern is to perceive clearly, and to perceive clearly requires deep thinking. To think critically is simply to engage the brain to ask deep questions that analyze and evaluate the truth about the material we are reading (Paul, 1990; Paul et al., 2002, 2006; Jackson et al., 2004). Socrates is recognized as one of the world's greatest teachers. His main technique was to ask his pupils questions rather than by giving answers.

The purpose of these questions is to challenge students' thinking, using Socratic questioning prompts listed by Richard Paul (1990), as follows:

- Questions of *clarification* force students to improve their answers by providing additional information and clarification.
- Questions of *assumption* force students to examine what they are taking for granted, or their beliefs about answers.
- Questions of *reason* and *evidence* force students to seek the reason and evidence behind their answer.
- Questions of *viewpoint* and *perspective* force students to examine the point of view and perspective underlying their own answer while considering those of others.
- Questions of *implication* and *consequence* force students to consider the implication and consequence related to their answers.
- *Questions about the question* force students to realize the importance or relevance of the question just asked.

Together these questions examine students' critical thinking answers for clarity, accuracy, relevance, depth, logic, and significance. The questions found in each chapter are presented as examples for educators and students to use. Students are strongly encouraged to formulate more questions to further develop their critical thinking skills and deep understanding of the material.

Traditional thinkers preserve the status quo and accept knowledge as presented, while critical thinkers question the status quo and seek the truth about it. *Critical thinkers* question what they know and what they do for the purpose of making a decision, or taking action, which will consequently be less biased, more informed, and closest to the truth.

The critical thinking questions presented at the end of each chapter, therefore, are much more than the traditional summary or review questions found in most textbooks, which ensure that students have covered all the material. The purpose of critical thinking questions is to challenge students on the accuracy and completeness of their thinking about their answers and material.

Critical Thinking Questioning in the Classroom

How can educators and students make use of critical thinking questioning in the classroom? Presented below are tips that should make critical thinking questioning sessions part of the overall EPA course structure and learning process. There is a consensus that this teaching approach is best suited for small group seminars (10 to 15 students), or case study resolution sessions, which usually follow theoretical and laboratory teaching sessions.

TIPS FOR EDUCATORS

- Use a quiet, bright, and well-ventilated room.
- Sit students in a circle, with you at the front with a flip chart and a pen.
- Write the question under consideration on the flip chart; use any of the questions provided in this textbook, or any other probing type question you may have, to open the session.
- Allow or disallow the use of the course or textbook material.
- Limit the duration of the dialectic session to 2 hours to prevent mental fatigue.
- Act as a facilitator, not as the expert.
- Lead as opposed to directing the exchanges between students.
- Remain impartial and protect slow thinkers by allowing them more time to express themselves.
- Encourage full participation, but realize that a student has the right to remain silent.
- Inform silent students that you will work with them privately during the week so that their answers are heard during the next dialectic session.
- Ensure that the students maintain focus on the question under consideration, but allow them to ask other questions related to it.
- Ensure fruitful, open, and respectful student exchanges.
- Make sure each student has time to express himself or herself clearly.
- Articulate any unease or concerns students may have.
- Work to obtain a consensus on each answer, but realize that a question may remain open-ended, meaning no consensus was reached.
- Make sure that each student is building on the answer by making use of what was said previously by you and the other students.
- A few minutes before ending the session, ask two or three students how they felt during the critical thinking session and how this method of teaching has im-

proved their ability to think more critically about their textbook's or course's material.

TIPS FOR STUDENTS

- Come prepared by reading and thinking about the questions listed at the end of each chapter.
- Come to the session with an open mind.
- Be prepared to answer and ask deep questions.
- Be critical of what you say and hear.
- Be open to critique of your answers by others.
- Participate by volunteering or wait for the facilitator to call on you.
- Speak slowly, loudly, and clearly.
- Listen carefully and respectfully to what your peers and the facilitator are saying.
- Do not simply repeat what you heard, but use your turn to further expand your answer by building on valuable elements raised previously by your peers and the facilitator.
- Stick to the question under consideration.
- Avoid inappropriate language and hostile exchanges.
- Do not hesitate to ask the facilitator to clear up confusion.

Keep in mind that the goal of these dialectic sessions is to further enhance your ability to think deeper about questions and answers; to help you forge a discerning or critical judgment about what you read, say, and hear; and to help you critique your thinking and that of your peers in order to come up with the best answer you can possibly formulate.

CASE STUDIES

A new feature in this second edition is the presentation of cases studies for each of the 18 EPAs covered in Part II. The evidence-based approach to their resolution in the context of the Disablement Model proposed by Nagi sets the cases in this textbook apart from those found in other texts. Readers are presented with the basic steps toward the resolution of the case based on the best available evidence. Clinical effectiveness resulting from usage of the best available evidence is demonstrated on the basis of the Disablement Model, which takes into account three important dimensions related to any disease or trauma: impairment, functional limitation, and disability. The therapeutic impact of each EPA in each case study is illustrated based on this model. Any given EPA may have a therapeutic impact on the patient's condition that goes beyond the traditional impairment (cellular level) by improving his or her functional limitation (personal level) and disability (society level). For example, the therapeutic effectiveness of transcutaneous electrical nerve stimulation (TENS) for a chronic pain syndrome may be demonstrated by a combination of decreased pain intensity (impairment), increased sleeping time (functional limitation), and return to work (disability).

ADDITIONAL RESOURCES

Therapeutic Electrophysical Agents: Evidence Behind Practice, Second Edition includes additional resources for purchasers that are available on the book's companion website at thepoint.lww.com/Belanger2e. Approved adopting educators will be given access to an image bank and a Brownstone test generator. In addition, purchasers of the text can access the searchable Full Text On-line by going to the book's companion website at thepoint. lww.com/Belanger2e. See the inside front cover of this text for more details, including the passcode you will need to gain access to the website.

SUMMARY

Users of the first edition will quickly discover that the second edition goes well beyond the expected revisions and updates of the original material. This new edition contains nine new chapters, of which five are dedicated to the foundations underlying the practice of therapy with EPAs. It features a comprehensive and innovative pedagogical approach that should benefit educators as well as students. This comprehensive textbook focuses more than ever on the evidence behind the practice of therapeutic EPAs by incorporating case studies that are resolved based on scientific evidence and on the disablement model. This textbook is designed to be an evidence-based core course textbook for adoption by faculty, researchers, instructors, and students as well as a reference text for clinicians and government regulators, third-party payers, and corporate staff associated with this field of practice.

I hope you enjoy this second edition. Please feel free to contact me at alain-yvan.belanger@rea.ulaval.ca. I look forward to your feedback!

References

Bloom BS (Ed), Engelhart MD, Furst EJ, Hill W, Krathwolh DR (1956) Taxonomy of Educational Objectives: Handbook I: Cognitive Domain. David McKay, New York

Jackson M, Ignatavicius DD, Case B (2004) Conversations in Critical Thinking and Clinical Judgement. Pohl Publishing, Pensacola

Paul R (1990) Critical Thinking: What Every Person Needs to Survive in a Rapidly Changing World. Center for Critical Thinking and Morale Critique, Rohnert Park.

Paul R, Elder L (2002) Critical Thinking: Tools for Taking Care of Professional and Personal Life. Pearson Education, Upper Saddle River

Paul R, Elder L (2006) The Art of Socratic Questioning. Foundation for Critical Thinking, Dillon Beach.

Julia Chevan, PT, PhD, MPH, OCS
Professor of Physical Therapy
Department of Physical Therapy
Springfield College
Springfield, MA

L. Vince Lepak, PT, DPT, MPH, CWS
Assistant Professor
Department of Physical Therapy
Oklahoma University Health Sciences Center
Tulsa, OK

David Levine, PT, PhD, DPT, OCS, CCRP
Walter M. Cline Chair of Excellence in Physical Therapy
Department of Physical Therapy
The University of Tennessee at Chattanooga
Chattanooga, TN

Steve Pfister, PT, MS, OCS
Assistant Professor
Department of Physical Therapy
Nova Southeastern University
Ft. Lauderdale, FL

Keith G. Rau, DC, CCEP, CCSP
Associate Professor
Sport Health Science
Life University
Marietta, GA

Joanne Rivard, PT, DPT, MS, OCS
Instructor
Program in Physical Therapy
School of Health Sciences
Simmons College Boston, MA

ACKNOWLEDGMENTS

The second edition of this textbook would have been only a dream of mine if it were not for all of the educators, students, and clinicians who purchased the first edition.

It would also have been an unfinished project without the commitment of my publisher Lippincott Williams & Wilkins.

Thanks to Pete Sabatini and Emily Lupash, Acquisition Editors, for their support and guidance. Special thanks to Meredith Brittain, Editorial Manager, for her commitment and exemplary work.

To all of you, I will always be grateful.

Alain-Yvan Bélanger

CONTENTS

PART III PRACTICAL CLINICAL GUIDELINES

PART I

Foundations

Therapeutic Electrophysical Agents in Health Care

Learning Objectives

Knowledge: List the electrophysical agents (EPAs) by types of therapy and energy delivered.

Comprehension: Define and distinguish between the terms pathology, impairment, functional limitation, and disability.

Application: Show how the use of therapeutic EPAs is related to Nagi's disablement model.

Analysis: Explain why the use of EPAs fits Nagi's disablement model.

Synthesis: Formulate the EPA impact concept model.

Evaluation: Discuss the therapeutic role of EPAs in relation to the overall management of soft-tissue pathology.

I. OVERVIEW OF USAGE

A. STUDY AND USAGE

The study and use of therapeutic electrophysical agents, referred to by the acronym EPAs, are widespread in the fields of physical rehabilitation, physical medicine, and sports therapy as evidenced by several recently published textbooks on the subject (e.g., Hayes, 2000; Kahn, 2000; Low et al., 2000; Nalty, 2001; Belanger, 2002; Horodyski et al., 2004; Starkey, 2004; Hecox et al., 2005; Michlovitz et al., 2005; Prentice, 2005; Behrens et al., 2006; Robertson et al., 2006; Fox et al., 2007; Cameron, 2008; Knight et al., 2008; Robinson et al., 2008; Watson, 2008) and by the findings of numerous studies on EPA practices conducted in countries such as the United States, Canada, Australia, England, the Netherlands, and Ireland (Robinson et al., 1988; Ter Haar et al., 1988; Lindsay et al., 1990, 1995; Taylor et al., 1991; Pope et al., 1995; Robertson et al., 1998; Roebroeck et al., 1998; Shields et al., 2001; Shields et al., 2004; Nussbaum et al., 2007).

B. COMPLEMENTARY ROLE

The body of literature on EPAs indicates that their main role is to treat human soft-tissue pathologies by dealing with the impairments, functional limitations, and disabilities associated with such pathologies. Because EPAs are used to manage a broad variety of pathologies, their role in the global therapeutic spectrum is to complement other physical, medical, and surgical therapeutic interventions. As a result, EPAs seldom are the sole therapeutic intervention in any given clinical case. After a thorough assessment of the clinical case under study, it is the responsibility of the practitioner to determine and implement an optimal combination of EPAs that would best match the set of physical, medical, or surgical interventions that together will lead to optimal therapeutic outcomes for the patient.

C. THERAPEUTIC APPROACHES

The treatment of human soft-tissue pathology rests with three basic treatment approaches: pharmacological, surgical, and conservative. Contrary to the pharmacological and surgical approaches, which are invasive in nature and often associated with major side effects, the conservative approach to treatment is noninvasive and characterized by minimal side effects. The use of EPAs covered in this textbook falls within the conservative approach to the treatment of soft-tissue pathology.

II. DEFINITION AND CLASSIFICATION

A. DEFINITION

The word *electrophysical* is a generic term that refers to a broad group of therapeutic agents used to supply various forms of energy to the body. This word is defined on the basis of its makeup or form of energy supplied.

1. Makeup
EPAs are made of various electrically powered devices (hence the prefix "electro-"), such as ultrasound and transcutaneous electrical nerve stimulation devices, and of various materials (hence the stem "physical") such as packs and paraffin immersed in thermal tubs or baths.

2. Energy
EPAs may also be defined on the basis of the form of energy supplied to the tissues, such as electric or electromagnetic energy (hence "electro-") and physical energy—for example, thermal or mechanical (hence "physical").

B. CLASSIFICATION

EPAs are typically classified on the basis of the type of therapy delivered or form of energy supplied to pathological tissues. **Table 1-1** classifies all the EPAs covered in this textbook.

III. SCOPE OF THERAPEUTIC APPLICATION

A. PHYSICAL REHABILITATION

The use of EPAs falls within the scope of physical rehabilitation of persons affected by pathologies. Physical rehabilitation can be defined as the art and science of promoting the functional independence and well-being of those persons affected by pathologies, through the use of a broad set of therapeutic interventions, such as EPAs, medication, and surgery.

B. THE DISABLEMENT CONCEPT

The American Physical Therapy Association (APTA), in the second edition of their *Guide to Physical Therapy Practice*, refers to the concept of *disablement* as "various impact(s) of chronic and acute conditions ... on the functioning of specific body systems, *on basic human* performance, and on people's functioning in necessary, usual, expected, and personally desired roles in society" (APTA, 2001).

C. DISABLEMENT MODELS

A number of disablement models have emerged in the literature over the past 30 years. Essentially, these disablement models are attempts to better delineate the interrelationship among pathologies, impairments, functional limitations, disabilities, and handicaps (Lee Kirby, 1998; APTA, 2001; Jette, 2006).

TABLE 1-1	CLASSIFICATION OF THERAPEUTIC ELECTROPHYSICAL AGENTS

THERAPY	ENERGY SPECTRUM	AGENT
Thermotherapy	Infrared	Chapter 6: Hot pack and paraffin bath therapy
		Chapter 7: Fluidotherapy
		Chapter 8: Cryotherapy
		Chapter 9: Hydrotherapy
	Shortwave	Chapter 10: Shortwave diathermy therapy
Phototherapy	Visible and infrared	Chapter 11: Low-level laser therapy
	Ultraviolet	Chapter 12: Ultraviolet therapy
Electrotherapy	Electric	Chapter 13: Iontophoresis therapy
		Chapter 14: TENS therapy
		Chapter 15: Microcurrent therapy
		Chapter 16: High-voltage pulsed current therapy
		Chapter 17: Russian current therapy
		Chapter 18: Interferential current therapy
		Chapter 19: Diadynamic current therapy
Ultrasonotherapy	Mechanical	Chapter 20: Ultrasound therapy
Mecanotherapy	Mechanical	Chapter 21: Spinal traction therapy
		Chapter 22: Intermittent pneumatic compression therapy
		Chapter 23: Continuous passive motion therapy

D. NAGI'S DISABLEMENT MODEL

Nagi's disablement model takes into account the interrelationship between a pathology caused by disease or injury and its related impairments, functional limitations, and disabilities (Nagi, 1991). The terminology selected by APTA in their *Guide to Physical Therapy Practice* is based on Nagi's disablement model (APTA, 2001). This textbook is also based on Nagi's model and terminology.

1. Pathology

The term pathology is used as a generic term for injury, disease, disorder, or condition, and refers to an ongoing pathological state usually evidenced by a series of signs and symptoms (Lee Kirby, 1998; APTA, 2001). It implies the dysfunction of a tissue, organ, or system and is related to the level of the human body. For example, a cerebral vascular accident, or stroke, is brain pathology, as evidenced by a state of body hemiparalysis.

2. Impairments

Impairments are the consequences of pathologies and are defined as abnormalities of structures and functions (Lee Kirby, 1998; APTA, 2001). They are related to the cellular level. For example, abnormal muscle tone is a common impairment related to a stroke.

3. Functional Limitations

Functional limitations result when impairments restrict a person's ability to perform regular physical tasks, activities, or

functions, in a normal and competent manner, in his or her own physical environment (Lee Kirby, 1998; APTA, 2001). They are related to the level of one's ability to function as a person. The inability to dress or to bathe, for example, is a functional limitation often associated with a stroke.

4. Disabilities

When impairments or functional limitations restrict a person's ability to perform tasks, activities, or functions in his or her own working and sociocultural context, these limitations are known as disabilities (Lee Kirby, 1998; APTA, 2001). These are related to the level of one's ability to live a normal societal life. For example, the inability to drive a car or to swim is a disability often associated with a stroke.

E. THE IMPACT CONCEPT

The therapeutic application of EPAs in the field of physical rehabilitation fits nicely in Nagi's disablement model. **Figure 1-1** is a conceptual representation of how EPAs can impact the four key elements of Nagi's model, namely, the pathology and its related impairment, functional limitation, and disability. This impact concept model will be used in this textbook to illustrate how any given EPA affects the impairment, functional limitation, and disability associated with a given pathology.

1. Soft-Tissue Pathologies

EPAs can address, as illustrated in **Figure 1-1**, a large number of soft-tissue pathologies, caused by either dis-

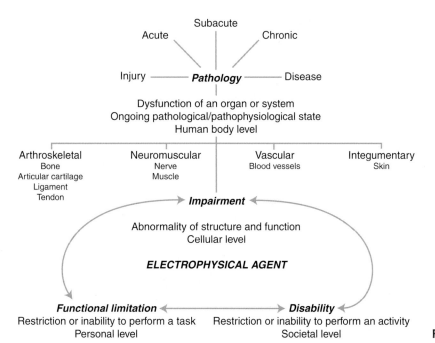

FIGURE 1-1 The EPA impact concept model.

ease or injury, in their acute, subacute, or chronic state. These pathologies may concern the following four systems and related tissues: (1) arthroskeletal, (2) neuromuscular, (3) vascular, and (4) integumentary.

2. Levels of Impact

As shown in **Figure 1-1**, the use of EPAs can impact the patient's pathology at the cellular level (impairment), personal level (functional limitation), and societal level (disability). For example, the use of an EPA, or set of EPAs, may ameliorate a pathological condition by promoting tis-

sue healing (impairment), which in turn may minimize the functional limitations and disabilities normally associated with such a pathology, if left untreated.

3. Impact Concept Example

Figure 1-2 illustrates the impact concept model presented in the earlier figure, using, as a case example, a post-immobilization, subacute bone fracture resulting from injury. This case example, which relates to the arthroskeletal system, shows that the application of three EPAs (continuous passive motion [see Chapter 23], transcutaneous

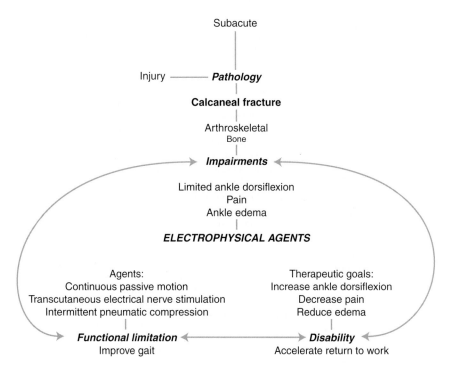

FIGURE 1-2 An example illustrating the EPA impact concept.

electrical nerve stimulation [see Chapter 14], and intermittent pneumatic compression [see Chapter 22]) worked upon the impairments (decrease pain, decrease edema, increase ankle ROM) and related functional limitation (improved gait) and disability (accelerated return to work). This conceptual representation emphasizes the importance of using outcome measures related not only to impairments but also functional limitations and disabilities in the assessment of global therapeutic effectiveness of EPAs.

F. LIMITED THERAPEUTIC SCOPE

The scope of therapeutic EPAs, as with all therapeutics used in health care, is limited. For example, EPAs are not designed to replace therapeutic exercises, in the same way that surgical procedures are not designed to replace medications—*they complement each other*. This textbook will show that the evidence-based use of EPAs to treat soft-tissue pathologies, applied as a complementary treatment to other physical, medical, and surgical therapeutic interventions, can promote healing while minimizing the functional limitations and disabilities associated with such pathologies.

CRITICAL THINKING QUESTIONS

Clarification: What is meant by therapeutic electrophysical agents (EPAs)?

Assumptions: You assume that the use of EPAs impacts on Nagi's model of disablement. How do you justify that assumption?

Reasons and evidence: Therapeutic EPAs are classified according to the form of energy supplied or type of therapy delivered. Why does it make sense to use such classifications?

Viewpoints or perspectives: You agree with the consensus that EPAs should be used in conjunction with, or as a complement to, other therapeutic interventions. What would say to a colleague who disagrees with you?

Implications and consequences: You state that therapeutic EPAs can be used for the management of soft-tissue pathologies related to the arthroskeletal, neuromuscular, vascular, and integumentary systems. What are you implying by that?

About the question: Why are EPAs valuable complements to medical or surgical interventions for the treatment for soft-tissue pathology? Why do you think I ask this question?

References

Articles

American Physical Therapy Association (2001) Guide to Physical Therapy Practice. Phys Ther, 81: 27–34; 105–138

Jette AM (2006) Toward a common language for function, disability, and health. Phys Ther, 86, 726–734

Lindsay DM, Dearness J, McGinley CC (1995) Electrotherapy usage trends in private physiotherapy practice in Alberta. Physiother Can, 47: 30–34

Lindsay DM, Dearness J, Richardson C (1990) A survey of electromodality usage in private physiotherapy practices. Aust J Physiother, 36: 249–256

Nussbaum EL, Burke S, Johnstone L, Lahiffe G, Robitaille E, Yoshida K (2007) Use of electrophysical agents: Findings and implications of survey of practice in Metro Toronto. Physiother Can, 59: 118–131

Pope GD, Mockett SP, Wright JP (1995) A survey of electrotherapeutic modalities: Ownership and use in the NHS in England. Physiotherapy, 81: 82–91

Robertson VJ, Spurritt D (1998) Electrophysical agents: Implications of their availability and use in undergraduate clinical placements. Physiotherapy, 84: 335–334

Robinson AJ, Snyder-Mackler L (1988) Clinical application of electrotherapeutic modalities. Phys Ther, 68: 1235–1238

Roebroeck ME, Dekker J, Ostendorp RA (1998) The use of therapeutic ultrasound by physical therapists in Dutch primary health care. Phys Ther, 78: 470–478

Shields N, Gormley J, O'Hare N (2001) A survey into the availability of shortwave diathermy equipment in Irish hospitals and private practices. Br J Ther Rehab, 8: 331–339

Shields N, O'Hare N, Gormley (2004) Contra-indications to shortwave diathermy: Survey of Irish physiotherapists. Physiotherapy, 90: 42–53

Taylor E, Humphry R (1991) Survey of physical agent modality use. Am J Occup Ther, 45: 924–931

Ter Haar G, Dyson M, Oakley S (1988) Ultrasound in physiotherapy in the United Kingdom: Results of a questionnaire. Physiother Pract, 4: 69–72

Chapters of Textbooks

Lee Kirby R (1998) Impairment, disability and handicap. In: Rehabilitation Medicine: Principles and Practice, 3rd ed. Delisa JA, Gans BM (Eds). Lippincott-Raven Publishers, Philadelphia, pp 55–60

Nagi S (1991) Disability concepts revisited. Implications for prevention. In: Disability in America: Towards a National Agenda for Prevention. Pope AM, Tarlov AR (Eds). National Academy Press, Washington, pp 309–327

Textbooks

Behrens BJ, Michlovitz SL (2006) Physical Agents: Theory and Practice, 2nd ed. FA Davis, Philadelphia

Belanger AY (2002) Evidence-Based Guide to Therapeutic Physical Agents. Lippincott Williams & Wilkins, Philadelphia

Cameron MH (2008) Physical Agents in Rehabilitation: From Research to Practice, 3nd ed. Saunders, St-Louis

Fox JE, Sharp TN (2007) Practical Electrotherapy: A Guide to Safe Application. Churchill Livingstone, London

Hayes KW (2000) Manual for Physical Agents, 5th ed. Prentice-Hall Health, Upper Saddle River, New York

Hecox B, Weisberg J, Mehreteab TA, Sanko J (2005) Integrating Physical Agents in Rehabilitation, 2nd ed. Prentice Hall, New York

Horodyski M, Starkey C (2004) Laboratory Activities for Therapeutic Modalities, 3rd ed. FA Davis, Philadelphia

Khan J (2000) Principles and Practice of Electrotherapy, 4th ed. Churchill Livingstone, New York

Knight KL, Draper DO (2008) Therapeutic Modalities: The Art and Science. Lippincott Williams & Wilkins, Philadelphia

Low J, Reed A (2000) Electrotherapy Explained: Principles and Practice, 3rd ed. Butterworth Heinemann, Oxford

Michlovitz SL, Nolan TP (2005) Modalities for Therapeutic Intervention, 4th ed. FA Davis, Philadelphia.

Nalty T (2001) Electrotherapy: Clinical Procedures Manual. McGraw-Hill, New York.

Prentice WE (2005) Therapeutic Modalities in Rehabilitation, 3rd ed. McGraw-Hill Medical, New York

Robertson V, Ward A, Low J, Reed A (2006) Electrotherapy Explained: Principles and Practice, 3rd ed. Butterworth-Heinemann, Oxford

Robinson AJ, Snyder-Mackler L (2008) Electrophysiology: Electrotherapy and Electrophysiologic Testing, 3rd ed. Lippincott Williams & Wilkins, Philadelphia

Starkey C (2004) Therapeutic Modalities, 3rd ed. FA Davis, Philadelphia

Watson T (2008) Electrotherapy: Evidence-Based Practice, 12th ed. Churchill Livingstone, London

2 CHAPTER

Soft-Tissue Pathology and the Healing Process

Chapter Outline

Learning Objectives

Knowledge: List the main anatomical components of skin, tendon, ligament, articular cartilage, bone, skeletal muscle, peripheral nerve, artery, and vein.

Comprehension: Compare the healing process, with regard to the quality of healing commonly obtained, for each of the soft tissues discussed.

Application: Explain why skin, bone, and skeletal muscle have a better healing capacity than ligament, tendon, and articular cartilage.

Analysis: Outline the types of injury sustained by soft tissues.

Synthesis: Formulate the relationship between each of the four basic phases of soft-tissue healing.

Evaluation: Discuss the characteristics of the hemostatic, inflammatory, proliferative, and remodeling/maturation phases of soft-tissue healing.

I. SOFT TISSUES

A. PATHOLOGY

In the course of our lifetime, most of us will see our soft tissues affected by pathologies caused by disease or injury, each with their share of impairments, functional limitations, and disabilities (see Chapter 1). Although many of these pathologies will heal naturally, without the therapeutic intervention of health practitioners, a fair number will require specialized therapeutic interventions such as medication, surgery, and electrophysical agents (EPAs).

B. TARGET TISSUES

The human body is composed of a variety of tissues regrouped into different systems. The tissues and systems (see Chapter 1) most likely to benefit from the application of therapeutic EPAs are the skin (the integumentary system), tendon, ligament, articular cartilage, bone (the arthroskeletal system), skeletal muscle and peripheral nerve (the neuromuscular system), and artery and vein (the vascular system). The purpose of this chapter is threefold: (1) to present an overview of the anatomical components related to each of these soft tissues, (2) to list the most common types of pathologies or injuries sustained by these tissues, and (3) to present an overview of the healing process associated with each of them.

II. ANATOMICAL COMPONENTS

A. SKIN

The integumentary system is made up of the skin and its appendages—hair and nail tissues. The skin is the largest tissue in the body and has a number of important and interrelated functions. Its major functions are to (1) provide protection from the outside environment, (2) afford the sensation of mechanical, thermal, and nociceptive stimuli, and (3) allow the secretion of fluids (sebum, sweat) for regulation of body temperature (Harvey, 2005; Johnstone et al., 2005; Whitney, 2005).

1. Hierarchical Structures

Shown in **Figure 2-1** is a cross-sectional view of the skin, revealing its layers and appendages. The epidermis has important protective functions against injury to subcutaneous tissues and excessive water loss. The dermis, on the other hand, provides nutrition through its vascular system and neural functions through its multiple neural receptors. The subcutaneous layer, made of adipose tissue, acts as a cushion for the skin while contributing to body heat regulation.

2. Appendages

The skin contains numerous appendages such as blood vessels, nerves, and glands, as well as thermal, mechanical, and nociceptive receptors.

B. TENDON

The arthroskeletal system is made up of four tissues: tendon, ligament, bone, and articular cartilage. A tendon is a fibrous, cord-like structure of collagenous tissue by which muscle is attached to bone. The major function of tendons is to transmit forces generated by muscles to bones, resulting in joint movements (Clancy, 1990; Herzog et al., 1994; Almekinders et al., 1998; Khan et al., 1999; Sevier et al., 2000; Woo et al., 2000; Sharma et al., 2005).

1. Hierarchical Structures

Shown in **Figure 2-2** is a schematic cross-sectional representation of a tendon. The tendon splits into smaller entities called fascicles. Each fascicle then splits into fibers, which split further into fibrils, subfibrils, microfibrils, and, ultimately, into tropocollagen filaments. Tropocollagen is the fundamental unit of collagen (Herzog et al., 1994). These filaments or molecules group together to form a microfibril, which agregates to form a subfibril. The tendon is composed of many fascicles that are made of several fibers and fibrils. Fibrils are the basic tensile load-bearing units of the tendon (Herzog et at., 1994).

2. Connective-Tissue Sheaths

The tendon is made up of three connective-tissue sheaths, which play important physiological and mechanical roles (Sharma et al., 2005).

a. Paratenon

The paratenon is a loose areolar connective-tissue sheath, consisting of type I and type II collagen fibrils. Because it is the most superficial, it surrounds the tendon's epitenon sheath.

b. Epitenon

The epitenon is a loose connective-tissue sheath containing the vascular, lymphatic, and nerve supply to the tendon. This sheath surrounds all the fascicles within the tendon.

c. Endotenon

The endotenon is a thin reticular network of connective tissue surrounding each fascicle.

C. LIGAMENT

The word ligament is derived from the Latin word *ligare*, meaning to bind. Ligaments, which are part of the arthroskeletal system, consist of collagen and elastin fibers. The major function of ligaments is to attach articulating bones together to provide joint stability and to guide joint

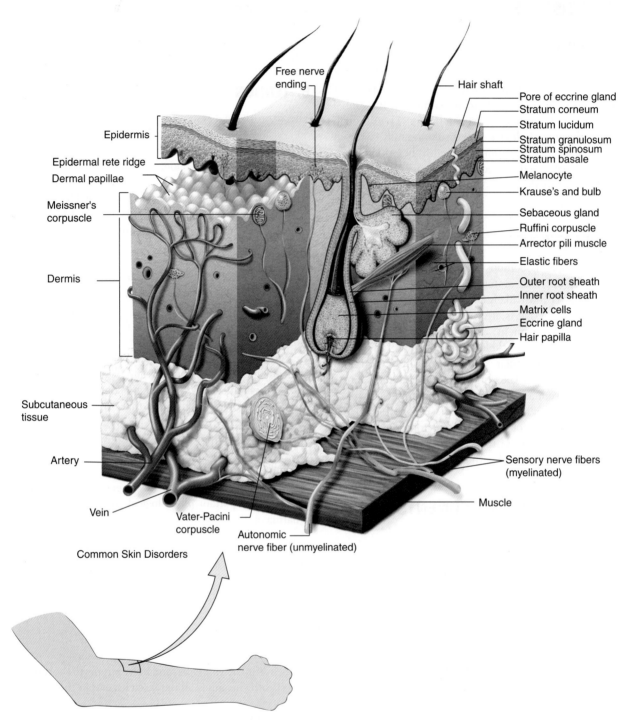

Free nerve ending

Hair shaft

Pore of eccrine gland
Stratum corneum
Stratum lucidum
Stratum granulosum
Stratum spinosum
Stratum basale

Epidermis

Epidermal rete ridge
Dermal papillae

Melanocyte
Krause's and bulb

Meissner's corpuscle

Sebaceous gland
Ruffini corpuscle
Arrector pili muscle
Elastic fibers

Dermis

Outer root sheath
Inner root sheath
Matrix cells
Eccrine gland
Hair papilla

Subcutaneous tissue

Artery

Sensory nerve fibers (myelinated)

Vein
Vater-Pacini corpuscle
Autonomic nerve fiber (unmyelinated)

Muscle

Common Skin Disorders

FIGURE 2-1 The structural hierarchy of the skin. (Used with permission from the Anatomical Chart Co.)

movement (Frank et al., 1994; Woo et al., 2000; Frank, 2004).

1. Hierarchical Structures

Shown in **Figure 2-3** is a cross-sectional view of a typical ligament. These structures very much resemble those of a tendon, as illustrated in **Figure 2-2**, with its fascicles, fibers, fibrils, subfibrils, microfibrils, and tropocollagen filaments.

2. Epiligament Sheath

This connective-tissue structure encloses the blood vessels and nerves necessary for ligament survival and function.

3. Fibrils

Just as for the tendon, fibrils are the tensile load-bearing units of ligaments.

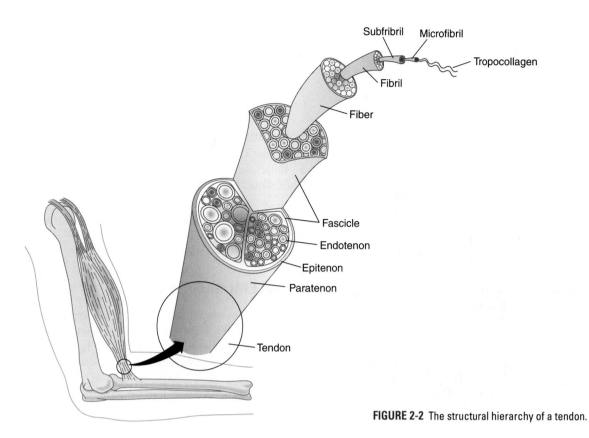

FIGURE 2-2 The structural hierarchy of a tendon.

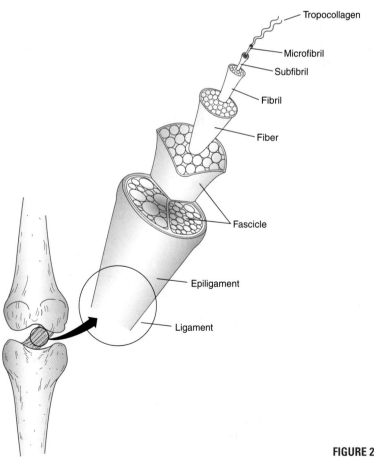

FIGURE 2-3 The structural hierarchy of a ligament.

D. ARTICULAR CARTILAGE

This tissue, which is also part of the arthroskeletal system, consists of a thin fibrous connective tissue on the articular surface of bones in synovial joints. The articular or hyaline cartilage differs from the white and yellow fibrocartilages found in the intervertebral disks and the ears and larynx, respectively (Shrive et al., 1994; Chen et al., 1999a,b; Farmer et al., 2001; Hayes et al., 2001; Buckwalter, 2002; Buckwalter et al., 2004; Mandelbaum et al., 2005). The major function of articular cartilage is to dampen the load imposed on the articular surfaces by distributing it within the subchondral bone and the cartilage itself. It also provides joint movement through its extremely low surface coefficient of friction.

1. Hierarchical Structures

Figure 2-4 shows a cross-sectional view of a synovial articulation, revealing the articular cartilage on the surface of the calcified cartilage layer on top of the subchondral bone.

2. Avascular Aspect

A very important anatomical consideration is the fact that articular cartilage, in comparison with all the other soft tissues considered in this chapter, is avascular in nature. This aspect is crucial in relation to the articular cartilage's capacity to repair itself or heal after injury or disease.

E. BONE

Bone, the fourth and last tissue making up the arthroskeletal system, is the hardest of all the soft tissues considered in this chapter. Its connective tissue is made of organic, inorganic, and mineral elements (Nigg et al., 1994;

Childs, 2003; La Stayo et al., 2003; Phillips, 2005). Bones have two important physiological roles: to form blood cells (hematopoiesis) and to store calcium (mineral homeostasis). Bones also provide protection for vital internal organs, support the body against the force of gravity, and act as a lever system for muscles during joint movements.

1. Hierarchical Structures

The major components of a bone are shown in **Figure 2-5**. Bones are made of compact (cortical) and spongy (cancellous) bone material.

2. Diaphysis and Epiphyses

The proximal and distal epiphyses are made of spongy bone and the diaphysis of compact bone.

F. SKELETAL MUSCLE

The neuromuscular system, as its name implies, is made up of two tissues: nerve and muscle. Skeletal muscle is a type of tissue composed of contractile cells, called muscle fibers, which cause movement of the skeleton (Herzog, 1994; Ehrhardt et al., 2005; Jarvinen et al., 2005). The basic function of skeletal muscles is to develop the force necessary to overcome gravity and to move the body through space.

1. Hierarchical Structures

Shown in **Figure 2-6** is a cross-sectional view of a skeletal muscle. Each skeletal muscle splits into fascicles; fascicles split into muscle fibers, and muscle fibers into myofibrils. Each myofibril contains myosin (thick) and actin (thin) filaments that interact with each other, causing the muscle to contract.

2. Connective-Tissue Sheaths

Three connective-tissue sheaths cover a skeletal muscle: epimysium, perimysium, and endomysium.

a. Epimysium

This sheath covers the outside of the muscle and plays a vital role in the transfer of muscular tension to the bone.

b. Perimysium

A dense connective-tissue sheath, the perimysium provides a pathway for nerve fibers and blood vessels and surrounds each fascicle.

c. Endomysium

Endomysium is a fine sheath covering each fiber. It carries the capillaries and the nerves that nourish and innervate each muscle fiber.

3. Sarcolemma

The sarcolemma is a delicate plasma membrane, located directly underneath the endomysium, which covers or envelops every muscle fiber. It is through the sarcolemma

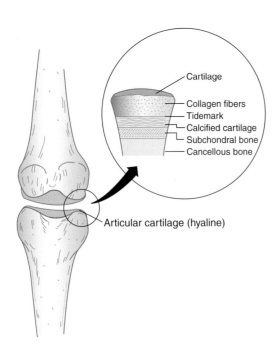

FIGURE 2-4 The structural hierarchy of an articular cartilage.

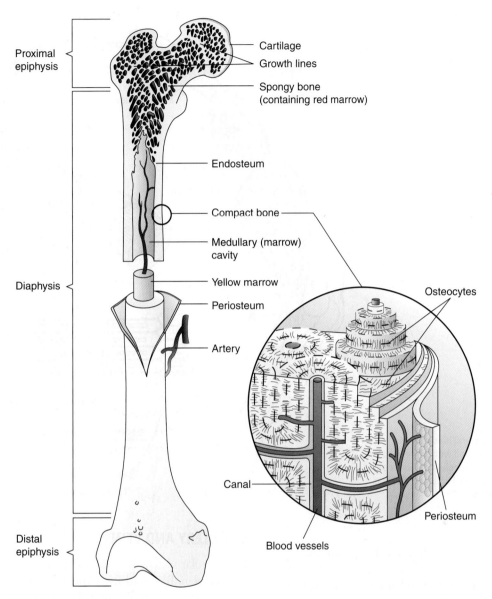

FIGURE 2-5 The structural hierarchy of a bone. (Reprinted with permission from Smetltzer SC, Bare BG (2000) Textbook of Medical-Surgical Nursing, 9th ed. Lippincott Williams & Wilkins, Philadelphia.)

that nerve impulses eventually reach each individual contractile unit.

4. Sarcomere

The sarcomere is the contractile unit of each skeletal muscle; it represents a band of thick (myosin) and thin (actin) filaments.

G. PERIPHERAL NERVE

This structure, the second component of the neuromuscular system, arises from the spinal cord by rootlets, which converge to form a spinal, or peripheral, nerve (Burnett et al., 2004; Rummler et al., 2004; Wernig et al., 2005). Its role is to convey neural impulses from the central nervous system to tissues and organs (efferent nerves), and from

organs and tissues back to the central nervous system (afferent nerves).

1. Hierarchical Structures

Shown in **Figure 2-7** is a cross-sectional view of a peripheral nerve. Similar to skeletal muscle, tendon, and ligament, a peripheral nerve also splits into fascicles, which further split into nerve fibers. Each nerve fiber is made up of an axon and its covering, the myelin sheath (some nerve fibers are unmyelinated).

2. Connective-Tissue Sheaths

Peripheral nerves are strong and resilient structures as a result of the support and protection they receive from their three connective-tissue sheaths: epineurium, perineurium, and endoneurium.

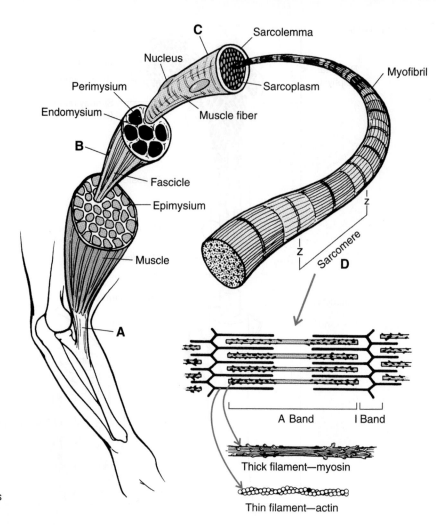

FIGURE 2-6 The structural hierarchy of a skeletal muscle. (Reprinted with permission from Hamill J (2008) Biomechanical Basis of Human Movement, 3rd ed. Lippincott Williams & Wilkins, Philadelphia.)

a. Epineurium

The epineurium is a thick sheath of loose connective tissue that surrounds all nerve fascicles forming the outermost covering of the peripheral nerve. This sheath encloses blood and lymphatic vessels.

b. Perineurium

This sheath encloses each nerve fascicle, providing an efficient barrier against penetration of the nerve fibers by foreign substances.

c. Endoneurium

This is a delicate connective sheath that surrounds the axon and its myelin sheath.

3. Axon

This structure is the fundamental unit of a peripheral nerve. Nerve impulses are generated as a result of axon depolarization.

4. Myelin Sheath

This sheath is formed by the neurolemma, or Schwann, cells. It wraps isolated parts of the axon, playing a fundamental role in the process (speed) of nerve conduction velocity.

H. ARTERY AND VEIN

The vascular system is made up of two basic tissues: artery and vein. Blood, which carries nutrients, oxygen, and waste products to and from cells, circulates in our body through our arteries and veins. Adequate blood supply is critical to all living tissues.

1. Hierarchical Structures

Shown in **Figure 2-8** are the structures of an artery and vein, which interact, one with the other, via the capillary bed.

a. Artery

Arteries carry blood from the heart to the capillaries, where it is distributed to the target tissue. Each artery is made of three coats, or tunicae, named adventitia, media, and intima (Moore et al., 1999). A large part of the tunica media is made of smooth muscle, which, under the influence of the autonomic nervous system, either constrict or dilate the arterial walls, thus narrowing or enlarging its lumen. The endothelium layer, within the tunica intima, plays a major role in the process of vascular repair. It is through the activation of endothelial cells that the growth or repair of blood vessels is initiated.

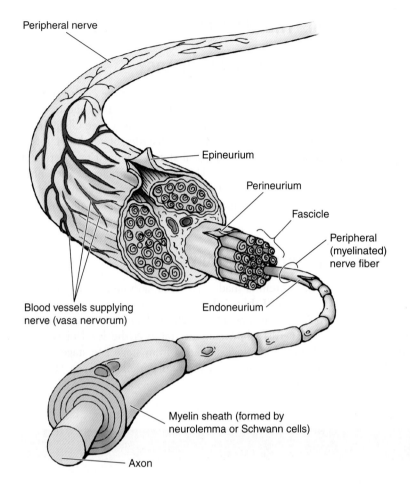

Peripheral nerve

Epineurium

Perineurium

Fascicle

Peripheral (myelinated) nerve fiber

Endoneurium

Blood vessels supplying nerve (vasa nervorum)

Myelin sheath (formed by neurolemma or Schwann cells)

Axon

FIGURE 2-7 The structural hierarchy of a peripheral nerve. (Reprinted with permission from Moore KL (1999) Clinically Oriented Anatomy, 4th ed. Lippincott Williams & Wilkins, Philadelphia.)

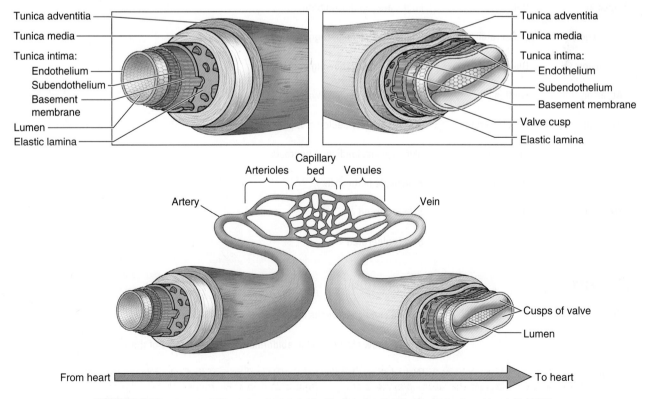

Tunica adventitia

Tunica media

Tunica intima:
  Endothelium
  Subendothelium
  Basement membrane

Lumen

Elastic lamina

Tunica adventitia

Tunica media

Tunica intima:
  Endothelium
  Subendothelium
  Basement membrane

Valve cusp

Elastic lamina

Arterioles

Capillary bed

Venules

Artery

Vein

Cusps of valve

Lumen

From heart

To heart

FIGURE 2-8 The structural hierarchy of artery and vein. (Reprinted with permission from Moore KL (1999) Clinically Oriented Anatomy, 4th ed. Lippincott Williams & Wilkins, Philadelphia.)

b. Vein

Veins return blood from the capillary beds to the heart. Like arteries, veins are also made of three coats, or tunicae, bearing identical names (**Figure 2-8**). Unlike arteries, veins are not wrapped with smooth muscle. Instead, they are filled with cuspid valves, which allow the blood to flow toward the heart.

c. Capillary Bed

It is at the level of the capillary bed that the interchange of oxygen, nutrients, waste products, and other substances occurs. It is the junction between the arterioles and the venules.

2. Vascular System

Following injury and disease to a soft tissue, part of its vascular components (i.e., artery, veins, and capillaries) is damaged or destroyed, which leads to bleeding. For soft-tissue healing to occur, new blood vessels will need to grow back at the wound site and invade the newly formed repair tissue. Endothelial cells, which form the lining of the endothelium layer of both arteries and veins (**Figure 2-8**), play a key role as organizers and regulators of vascular healing (see Section K, Artery and Vein Healing).

III. THE SPECTRUM OF PATHOLOGY

A. SOFT-TISSUE PATHOLOGY

A large majority of individuals, during the course of their lives, will suffer from pathologies affecting one or more of their soft tissues. The term pathology (see Chapter 1), also known as injury, disease, disorder, or condition, refers to an ongoing pathological state evidenced by a series of signs and symptoms. The types of pathologies presented below are the most common disorders affecting the integumentary, arthroskeletal, neuromuscular, and vascular systems.

B. INTEGUMENTARY SYSTEM

This system is made up of the skin and its appendages. Listed in **Table 2-1** are common types of skin pathologies (Johnstone et al., 2005; Harvey, 2005; Whitney, 2005). Also shown in this table is the level of severity of these pathologies, graded from stage I to stage IV. For a detailed discussion on skin pathologies, see Harvey's article (2005).

TABLE 2-1	SKIN PATHOLOGY	
TYPE	**CAUSE**	**DESCRIPTION**
Incision	Cut	Edges are regular, smooth
Laceration	Cut/scratch	Edges are irregular, ragged
Contusion	Blow	Skin is bruised, showing ecchymoses
Abrasion	Friction	Skin is lightly peeled away
Avulsion	Severe scratch	Skin is severely peeled away
Ulcer	Pressure	Skin hypoxia, leading to necrosis
Penetrating	Puncture	Hole made in the skin
Thermal	Heat	Skin is burned
Systemic	Disease	Skin is ulcerated

SEVERITY	DESCRIPTION
Stage I	Wound shows no breaks in the skin
Stage II	Wound shows breaks in the epidermal and dermal layers of the skin
Stage III	Wound shows breaks in the epidermal, dermal, and subcutaneous tissues
Stage IV	Wound shows breaks in full-thickness skin tissue, including surrounding tissues

C. ARTHROSKELETAL SYSTEM

This system comprises four tissues: tendon, ligament, articular cartilage, and bone.

1. Tendon

Listed in **Table 2-2** are the most common types of pathology affecting tendons. Also shown are the newest and oldest terminologies used to differentiate, for example, between tendinitis and tendinosis. Tendon pathology falls under the generic name of *strain* injuries (Clancy, 1990; Herzog et al., 1994; Almekinders et al., 1998; Khan et al., 1999; Sevier et al., 2000; Woo et al., 2000; Sharma et al., 2005). For details on tendon pathology, see Clancy (1990) and Leadbetter (2001).

2. Ligament

Pathologies caused to ligaments fall under the generic name of *sprain*, as described in **Table 2-3**, and range in severity from grade I to grade III (Frank et al., 1994; Woo et al., 2000; Frank, 2004).

3. Articular Cartilage

Table 2-4 shows that pathology to articular cartilage can result from impact or shearing force as well as overuse, causing damage to the cartilage matrix and chondral surfaces (Shrive et al., 1994; Chen et al., 1999a,b; Hayes et al., 2001; Farmer et al., 2001; Buckwalter, 2002; Buckwalter et al., 2004; Mandelbaum et al., 2005). There is no standardized categorization with regard to the grading of severity; this textbook proposes a grading system ranging from grade I to grade III.

4. Bone

Pathology to bone falls within the generic term of fracture. There are several types of bone fractures, as presented in **Table 2-5**, and each requires a particular conservative or surgical intervention (Nigg et al., 1994; Childs, 2003; La Stayo et al., 2003; Phillips, 2005). There is no standardized categorization with regard to the severity of bone fracture. The type, the location, and the damage caused by the fractured bone will dictate its severity.

TABLE 2-2	TENDON PATHOLOGY	
TYPE	**CAUSE**	**DESCRIPTION**
Tendinitis	Strain/tear	Inflammatory intratendinous degeneration
		Older terminology: tendon strain or tear
Tendinosis	Overuse/aging	Noninflammatory intratendinous degeneration
		Older terminology: tendinitis
Paratenonitis	Strain/overuse	Inflammation of the paratenon sheath, either lined by synovium or not
		Older terminology: tenosynovitis, tenovaginitis, patendinitis
Paratenonitis with tendinosis	Strain/overuse	Inflammation of paratenon sheath with intratendinous degeneration
		Older terminology: tendinitis
Tendon rupture	Strain	Complete rupture of tendon due to excessive tensile force
SEVERITY		**DESCRIPTION**
Grade I		Paratenosis
Grade II		Paratenonitis with tendinosis
Grade III		Tendinitis
Grade IV		Tendinosis
Grade V		Tendon rupture

TABLE 2-3   LIGAMENT PATHOLOGY

TYPE	CAUSE	DESCRIPTION
Sprain	Sprain/tear	Stretching/tearing of ligament

SEVERITY	CAUSE	DESCRIPTION
Grade I	Mild stretch	Minor lesion, no joint instability
Grade II	Moderate/severe stretch	Moderate/severe lesion, moderate joint instability
Grade III	Tear	Complete rupture lesion, complete joint instability

TABLE 2-4   ARTICULAR CARTILAGE PATHOLOGY

TYPE	CAUSE	DESCRIPTION
Microdamages to the cartilage matrix and cells	Impact/shearing; overuse	Microdamages to cartilage matrix; no damage to chondral surfaces
Microdamages to the superficial/partial-thickness of the chondral surfaces	Impact/shearing; overuse	Microdisruption of the articular surface without violation of the subchondral plates
Damages to the deep/full-thickness osteochondral surfaces	Impact/shearing; overuse	Damages to articulate surface, including the osteo chondral bone surface

SEVERITY	DESCRIPTION
Grade I	Microdamages to cartilage matrix
Grade II	Microdamages to superficial/partial chondral surfaces
Grade III	Damages to deep/full chondral surfaces

TABLE 2-5   BONE PATHOLOGY

TYPE	CAUSE	DESCRIPTION
Simple	Impact	Bone broken in one place, skin intact
Compound	Impact	Bone broken in one or more places, skin opened
Transverse	Impact	Fracture at angle to the long axis of bone
Greenstick	Impact	Fracture at only one side of bone
Comminuted	Impact	Part of the bone broken into many small pieces
Avulsion	Tear	Fracture resulting from tendon pull, following a powerful muscle contraction
Compression	Compression	Fracture resulting from two bones forced against each other (e.g., vertebrae)

(Continued)

TABLE 2-5	CONTINUED
SEVERITY	**DESCRIPTION**
Grade I	Simple fracture
Grade II	Compound fracture
Grade III	Communited fracture

This textbook proposes a grading system, from I to III, according to the complexity of the fracture.

D. NEUROMUSCULAR SYSTEM

This system, as its name implies, comprises both skeletal muscle and peripheral nerve.

1. Skeletal Muscle

As shown in **Table 2-6**, two main types of pathologies affect skeletal muscles: strain and contusion (Leadbetter, 2001). Delayed-onset muscle soreness after vigorous exercise is more a transient, temporary syndrome than a disease. Myositis ossificans traumatica, on the other hand, is a pathological condition resulting from inadequate healing of a previous injury, such as a contusion. Muscle contusion is graded according to severity as mild, moderate, or severe. Muscle strain injury, on the other hand, is graded as first, second, or third degree, depending on severity (Herzog et al., 1994; Ehrhardt et al., 2005; Jarvinen et al., 2005).

2. Peripheral Nerve

Shown in **Table 2-7** are the three types of pathology a peripheral nerve can suffer (Burnett et al., 2004). Neurapraxia is a functional injury, whereas axonotmesis and neurotmesis are both anatomical and functional types of

TABLE 2-6	SKELETAL MUSCLE PATHOLOGY	
TYPE	**CAUSE**	**DESCRIPTION**
Strain	Stretch	Muscle fiber tear
Contusion	Blow	Muscle is bruised, showing bleeding
Delayed-onset	Stretch	Muscle tenderness, stiffness, and soreness
Myositis ossificans traumatica	Blow	Muscle ossification
SEVERITY OF CONTUSION		**DESCRIPTION**
Mild		Light muscle tenderness, normal function
Moderate		Moderate muscle tenderness, swollen injured area, moderate functional loss
Severe		Marked tenderness and swollen, severe functional loss
SEVERITY OF STRAIN		**DESCRIPTION**
First degree		Minimal tissue damage, minimal bleeding, rapid healing
Second degree		Moderate tissue damage, significant bleeding, partial tear most often at the myotendinous junction, some functional loss
Third degree		Severe tissue damage, massive bleeding, severe tear to rupture, severe functional loss

TABLE 2-7	PERIPHERAL NERVE PATHOLOGY	
TYPE	**CAUSE**	**DESCRIPTION**
Neurapraxia	Compression	Axon and myelin intact; epineurium, perineurium, and endoneurium sheaths intact; damage to the myelin sheath; full functional recovery expected
Axonotmesis	Compression	Axon and myelin disrupted; epineurium, perineurium, and endoneurium sheaths intact; axon and myelin degeneration cause denervation; full to partial functional recovery expected
Neurotmesis	Cut	Axon and myelin disrupted; endoneurium sheath damaged; axon and myelin degeneration causing denervation; partial functional recovery expected depending on the extent of damage to the endomysium

SEVERITY		DESCRIPTION
Grade I		Neuropraxia
Grade II		Axonotmesis
Grade III		Neurotmesis

injuries. Nerve injuries are categorized on the basis of two classification systems. In Seddon's classification, peripheral nerve injuries are classified as neurapraxia, axonotmesis, and neurotmesis. In Sunderland's classification, these are classified as first, second, third, fourth, and fifth degree injuries (Burnett et al., 2004; Rummler et al., 2004; Wernig et al., 2005). Severity ranges from neuropraxia (least severe) to neurotmesis (most severe).

E. VASCULAR SYSTEM

Damages to soft tissues mentioned previously imply damages to their vascular system, since all these tissues are well vascularized, with the exception of one, the articular cartilage. Shown in **Table 2-8** are common types of pathology affecting peripheral arteries and veins. This textbook is concerned with vascular damages resulting primarily from trauma to soft tissues. Generally speaking, the extent of vascular damages to arteries, veins, and capillary beds is proportional to the severity and size of the wound.

IV. THE HEALING PROCESS

A. TISSUE'S INNATE CAPACITY TO HEAL

There is ample evidence in our daily experiences and in the literature to demonstrate that our body tissues,

TABLE 2-8	VASCULAR PATHOLOGY	
TYPE	**CAUSE**	**DESCRIPTION**
Laceration	Tensile/shearing force	Tearing of vessels
Contusion	Blunt force trauma	Bruising/crushing of vessels
Puncture	Needle, knife	Hole in vessels
Transection	Major trauma, knife	Cutting of vessels

SEVERITY		
Severity of vascular injury is directly related to the amount of damaged tissues at the wound site. Transection of blood vessels is the most severe type of injury.		

after injury and disease, immediately and automatically respond by triggering their own healing processes with the aim of restoring their lost structural integrity and function (Leadbetter, 1990; Salter, 1999; Leadbetter, 2001; Norris, 2004; Woo et al., 2004; Hess, 2005; Hildebrand et al., 2005). This innate capacity of our body to heal itself is remarkable but, unfortunately, often *limited* and *imperfect*.

B. NEED FOR THERAPEUTIC INTERVENTION

When the nature and severity of soft-tissue pathology are such that the person's own capacity to heal the wound fails, therapeutic interventions are needed to promote healing (Denegar, 2000; Leadbetter, 2001; Delforge, 2002a,b,c,d; Prentice, 2002; Pride, 2003; Starkey, 2004; Hess, 2005; Ruberton et al., 2005; Behrens, 2006).

C. PREREQUISITE FOR THERAPY

The goal of most therapeutic interventions is to minimize the adverse effects of tissue pathology (i.e., functional limitation and disability) while promoting tissue repair, thereby expediting a more rapid and effective return to activity and performance. To accomplish this goal, health practitioners must be familiar with a key prerequisite: *the human wound-healing process*.

D. DEFINITION OF HEALING

Tissue healing has been defined as the natural response to pathology through which dead or lost tissue is replaced by living tissue (Delforge, 2002a). The purpose of this healing process is to restore the structural and functional continuity of body tissues that have been disrupted by pathological processes (Martinez-Hernandez et al., 1990).

E. HEALING MECHANISMS

Research has shown that injured tissues heal through one of two primary mechanisms: *regeneration* and *repair* (Martinez-Hernandez, 1994).

1. Regeneration
This mechanism refers to the restoration of tissue that is identical in structure and function to the tissue that has been destroyed.

2. Repair
This mechanism involves fibrous scar formation, which alters the normal structure and functional properties of the affected tissues.

3. Combined Mechanisms
Soft-tissue healing occurs, in most cases, through a combination of regeneration and repair mechanisms.

F. QUALITY OF HEALING

Qualities of wound healing have been defined as *ideal*, *acceptable*, *minimal*, and *failed* (Leadbetter, 2001). Regardless of the therapeutic interventions used, tissue pathology rarely yields ideal healing; minimal-to-acceptable healing is most often the final outcome in case of moderate-to-severe tissue injury.

1. Ideal
The healed wound shows normal structure, function, and appearance. The new tissue is identical to the original one.

2. Acceptable
The healed wound shows almost normal structure and appearance and less-than-optimal function.

3. Minimal
The healed wound shows minimal normal structure and appearance and partial function.

4. Failed
The healed wound shows abnormal structure, appearance, and function.

G. HEALING PROCESS

Soft-tissue healing by means of regeneration or repair is characterized by a process, illustrated in **Figure 2-9**, involving four successive key physiological *phases*, all of which overlap one another over time (Denegar, 2000; Leadbetter, 2001; Delforge, 2002a–d; Prentice, 2002; Pride, 2003; Starkey, 2004; Hildebrand et al., 2005; Ruberton et al., 2005).

1. Hemostasis Phase
The first phase of healing, called *hemostasis*, is characterized by the arrest of bleeding at the wound site. This phase usually lasts a few seconds or, in case of moderate-to-severe pathologies that involve multiple well-vascularized tissues, up to several minutes. It involves the process of blood clotting and subsequent dissolution of the clot (Delforge, 2002a). The hemostatic response to injury is a complex series of regulatory events that require the interaction of both cellular elements and blood plasma proteins. The initial hemostatic mechanisms that occur within seconds after the blood vessel trauma include vasoconstriction and the development of a temporary hemostatic plug in the damaged vessels. Coagulation, or blood clotting, is the secondary hemostatic mechanism through which the initial platelet plug in the damaged vessels is reinforced (Delforge, 2002a). The presence of a blood mass outside the blood vessels is called a hematoma. The hemostasis phase is the body's own emergency response to pathology, which prevents hemorrhaging.

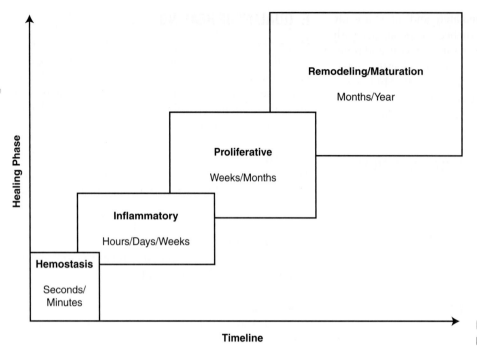

FIGURE 2-9 Soft-tissue healing process.

2. Inflammatory Phase

The second phase, called the *inflammatory* phase, is related to inflammation, the aim of which is to clean the wound of its cellular debris, preparing it for the deposition of new, repaired, or regenerated tissues. Inflammation, from the Latin word *inflammare*, which means to set on fire, is a localized tissue response initiated by pathology. It is a time-dependent, evolving process characterized by vascular, chemical, and cellular events that lead to the proliferative phase of healing. This phase may last hours, days, or weeks depending on the severity of the pathology. It is the crucial phase of healing because without it no tissue healing is possible.

3. Proliferative Phase

The third, the *proliferative* phase deals with the formation and proliferation of new, immature repair tissues to replace the damaged tissues. *Fibroplasia* and *angiogenesis* are key processes during this phase. Angiogenesis is the process of growing new blood vessels. Because this process is common to all vascularized soft tissues and relates to the vascular system, it is described in Section K, Artery and Vein Healing. Angiogenesis is concomitant with all the other cellular responses during this phase of healing. The proliferative phase lasts for weeks or sometimes months, depending on the severity of pathology and the type of soft tissue affected.

4. Remodeling/Maturation Phase

The fourth and final phase of healing is the *remodeling* (fiber alignment) and *maturation* (increase of mechanical strength) of immature tissue to form the most structurally functional tissue at the wound site. This phase usually lasts for months, sometimes more than a year, depending,

again, on the severity of the pathology and the type of tissue affected.

5. Timeline

Generally speaking, as illustrated in **Figure 2-9**, the hemostasis phase is of the shortest duration (seconds/minutes), followed by the inflammatory phase, which may last for hours, days, or weeks. The longest healing phases are the proliferative phase, lasting weeks to months, followed by the remodeling/maturation phase, which may take several months, sometimes more than a year, to run its course.

H. SKIN HEALING

Described in **Table 2-9** is an overview of the healing process that takes place following skin pathology (Harvey, 2005; Johnstone et al., 2005; Whitney, 2005). The final common outcome in most moderate-to-severe cases is the formation of weaker, less elastic but functional cutaneous repair tissue. Because the skin is a well-vascularized tissue, its quality of healing usually ranges from acceptable to ideal.

I. TENDON, LIGAMENT, ARTICULAR CARTILAGE, AND BONE HEALING

Presented in **Tables 2-10** to **2-13** is an overview of the healing processes taking place in tendon, ligament, articular cartilage, and bone (Sevier et al., 2000; Woo et al., 2000; Sharma et al., 2005)

1. Tendon and Ligament

These two tissues are relatively well vascularized via their respective epitenon and epiligament sheets, which bring blood vessels to them. As shown in **Tables 2-10** and **2-11**, their healing processes and final outcomes are very

TABLE 2-9	SKIN HEALING PROCESS	
PHASE	**CELLULAR RESPONSES**	**TIMELINE**
PHASE I	**HEMOSTASIS**	**SECONDS/MINUTES**

- Blood-clotting cascade leads to the arrest of bleeding by coagulation
- Blood clotting results in the release of pro-inflammatory molecules
- Fibrin clot establishes a provisional extracellular matrix, which will serve as a platform for the subsequent crucial inflammatory phase

PHASE II	**INFLAMMATORY**	**HOURS/DAYS/WEEKS**

- Inflammatory cells enter the site of injury
- Phagocytosis of necrotic material
- Release of growth factors to stimulate and regulate the functions of these migrating cells
- Wound is prepared for the subsequent proliferative phase of healing

PHASE III	**PROLIFERATIVE**	**WEEKS/MONTHS**

- Deposition in the wound of repair tissue
- Fibroblasts migrate to the wounded area and proliferate (fibroplasia)
- Granulation tissue, which will mature into scar tissue, forms
- Budding and growing of capillaries surrounding the repair zone (angiogenesis)
- The wound site fills up with new collagen fibers, which are weak and randomly oriented

PHASE IV	**REMODELING/MATURATION**	**MONTHS/YEAR**

- Maturation of new collagen from type III to type I
- Maturity and remodeling add strength to new collagen fibers and promote the normal orientation of collagen fibers

FINAL COMMON OUTCOME

- *Repair tissue:* Weaker and less elastic but functional. The structural, biomechanical, and functional properties of the healed skin often match those of intact skin.
- *Quality of healing:* Acceptable to ideal

TABLE 2-10	TENDON HEALING PROCESS	
PHASE	**CELLULAR RESPONSES**	**TIMELINE**
PHASE I	**HEMOSTASIS**	**SECONDS/MINUTES**

- Blood-clotting cascade leads to the arrest of bleeding by coagulation
- Blood clotting results in the release of pro-inflammatory molecules
- Fibrin clot establishes a provisional extracellular matrix, which will serve as a platform for the subsequent crucial inflammatory phase

PHASE II	**INFLAMMATORY**	**HOURS/DAYS/WEEKS**

- Inflammatory cells enter the site of injury
- Phagocytosis of necrotic material
- Tenocytes migrate to the injury site
- Type III collagen synthesis is initiated

(Continued)

TABLE 2-10	CONTINUED	
PHASE III	**PROLIFERATIVE**	**WEEKS/MONTHS**

- Deposition in the wound of repair tissue
- Fibroblasts migrate to the wounded area and proliferate (fibroplasia)
- Granulation tissue, which will mature into scar tissue, forms
- Budding and growing of capillaries surrounding the repair zone (angiogenesis)
- The wound site fills up with new type III collagen fibers, which are weak and randomly oriented

PHASE IV	**REMODELING/MATURATION**	**MONTHS/YEAR**

- Consolidation stage: Repair tissue changes from cellular to fibrous
- Tenocytes and collagen fibers align in the direction of stress
- Type I collagen synthesis occurs
- Maturation stage: Fibrous tissue changes to scar-like tendon tissue

FINAL COMMON OUTCOME

- *Repair tissue:* Weaker and less elastic but functional. The structural, biomechanical, and functional properties of the healed tendons never match those of intact tendons.
- *Quality of healing:* Minimal to acceptable

TABLE 2-11	LIGAMENT HEALING PROCESS	
PHASE	**CELLULAR RESPONSES**	**TIMELINE**
PHASE I	**HEMOSTASIS/INFLAMMATORY**	**MINUTES/HOURS/DAYS**

- Retraction of disrupted ligament ends
- Blood clot formation
- Increased vascularity and blood flow in the gap between the ligament ends

PHASE II	**PROLIFERATIVE**	**DAYS/WEEKS**

- Granulation tissue, which will mature into scar tissue, forms
- Budding and growing of capillaries surrounding the repair zone (angiogenesis)
- Production of scar tissue by hypertrophic fibroblastic cells (fibroplasia)
- Scar tissue becomes less disorganized as collagen fibers align with the long axis of the ligament
- Collagen content abnormal (more type III in relation to type I, and more type V than normal)

PHASE III	**REMODELING/MATURATION**	**MONTHS/YEAR**

- Scar tissue matures to become more ligament-like, although major differences in composition, architecture, and function remain

FINAL COMMON OUTCOME

- *Repair tissue:* Weaker and less elastic but functional. The structural, biomechanical, and functional properties of the healed ligaments never match those of intact ligaments.
- *Quality of healing:* Minimal to acceptable

similar (Woo et al., 2000, 2004; Frank, 2004; Sharma et al., 2005). Following most pathologies, a tendinous, or ligamentous, repair tissue forms, whose structural, mechanical, and physiological properties never match those of an intact tendon or ligament (Woo et al., 2000, 2004; Frank, 2004). Because tendons and ligaments are relatively well-vascularized tissues, their quality of healing is usually minimal to acceptable.

2. Articular Cartilage

Because of the *avascular* nature of this tissue, the healing process of articular cartilage differs according to the type of pathology sustained (Chen et al., 1999a,b; Buckwalter, 2002; Buckwalter et al., 2004). As shown in **Table 2-12**, pathology-causing microdamages to the cartilage matrix (grade I) or to the superficial partial thickness of the chondral bone (grade II) fail to heal because of the absence of the two initial phases: hemostatic and inflammatory. No inflammatory response can be initiated unless the wound bleeds. A full manifestation of the four classic healing phases will occur only if the pathology is severe enough (grade III) to damage both the articular cartilage and the underlying deep full thickness of the osteochondral. The final common outcome in such severe cases is nonetheless disappointing because the repaired articular cartilage is made of a mixture of two cartilages (hyaline cartilage and fibrocartilage). This repaired cartilage, unfortunately, can only approximate the structural and mechanical properties of intact articular cartilage and, as a result, is very likely to be damaged again with normal activity.

3. Bone

This tissue, because of its excellent vascularization, is the tissue that presents, with the skin, the best potential for healing, as shown in **Table 2-13**. In most cases of fracture in relatively healthy individuals, the injured bone will repair itself with identical bone material, thus providing original structural, mechanical, and functional bone properties (Delforge, 2002d; Childs, 2003; La Stayo et al., 2003; Phillips, 2005). Its quality of healing is usually ideal.

J. SKELETAL MUSCLE AND PERIPHERAL NERVE HEALING

Presented in **Tables 2-14** and **2-15** is an overview of the healing processes taking place in the skeletal muscle and peripheral nerve, respectively (Burnett et al., 2004; Wernig et al., 2005).

TABLE 2-12	ARTICULAR CARTILAGE HEALING PROCESS	
GRADE I: MICRODAMAGES TO THE CARTILAGE MATRIX AND CELLS		
PHASE	**CELLULAR RESPONSES**	**TIMELINE**
PHASE I	**HEMOSTASIS/INFLAMMATORY**	**ABSENT**
■ Chondrocytes necrosis with no hemorrhagic response ■ No hemostasis ■ No hemostasis, thus no inflammation		
PHASE II	**PROLIFERATIVE**	**ABSENT**
■ No proliferative response		
PHASE III	**REMODELING/MATURATION**	**ABSENT**
■ Repair response insufficient to maintain a normal and functioning articular surface due to lack of blood supply to cartilage, which leads to a largely absent inflammatory phase vital for tissue repair ■ The limited capability of chondrocytes to restore lost matrix components is overcome by the rate of loss of compressive and tensile stiffness properties of cartilage, resulting in irreversible articular degeneration		
FINAL COMMON OUTCOME		
■ *Repair tissue:* Absent ■ *Quality of healing:* Failed		

(Continued)

TABLE 2-12	CONTINUED

GRADE II: SUPERFICIAL/PARTIAL-THICKNESS CHONDRAL SURFACES

PHASE	CELLULAR RESPONSES	TIMELINE
PHASE I	HEMOSTASIS/INFLAMMATORY	ABSENT

- Chondrocytes necrosis with no hemorrhagic response
- No hemostasis
- No hemostasis, thus no inflammation

PHASE II	PROLIFERATIVE	ABSENT

- No proliferative response

PHASE III	REMODELING/MATURATION	ABSENT

- Limited increase in metabolic and mitotic activities of surviving chondrocytes that border the defect or injury site
- Newly synthesized matrix remains on periphery and does not fill the lesion

FINAL COMMON OUTCOME

- *Repair tissue:* Absent
- *Quality of healing:* Failed

GRADE III: DEEP/FULL-THICKNESS OSTEOCHONDRAL PATHOLOGY

PHASE	CELLULAR RESPONSES	TIMELINE
PHASE I	HEMOSTASIS/INFLAMMATORY	SECONDS/MINUTES

- Articular damages important enough to initiate the classic healing phases observed in vascularized tissues
- Arrest of bleeding at wound site
- Recruitment and proliferation of chondrocyte-like cells begins

PHASE II	PROLIFERATIVE	WEEKS/MONTHS

- Chondrocyte-like cells progressively differentiate into chondroblasts, chondrocytes, and osteoblasts, which synthesize cartilage and bone matrices
- Limited angiogenesis

PHASE III	REMODELING/MATURATION	MONTHS/YEAR

- Osteochondral ossification occurs to heal the subchondral bone defect (several months)
- Unfortunately, subsequent degenerative changes occur within 6 months, including the fissuring of the articular surface

FINAL COMMON OUTCOME

- *Repair tissue:* Mixture of hyaline and fibrocartilage tissues at the wound site. Repair cartilage does not approximate the structure and function of intact articular cartilage
- *Quality of healing:* Minimal to failed

TABLE 2-13	BONE HEALING PROCESS

PHASE	CELLULAR RESPONSES	TIMELINE
PHASE I	**HEMOSTASIS/INFLAMMATORY**	**SECONDS/MINUTES**

- Arrest of bleeding by the formation of a hematoma
- Hematoma provides an environment for the proliferation of osteogenic cells and granulation formation necessary for collagen synthesis and new bone formation

PHASE II	**PROLIFERATIVE**	**HOURS/DAYS/WEEKS**

- Angiogenesis
- Development of fibrocartilaginous callus and formation of bone matrix at the fracture site
- Process of ossification is underway with the mineralization of the bone matrix

PHASE III	**REMODELING/MATURATION**	**WEEKS/MONTHS**

- Restoration of stability at the fracture site
- Resorption of existing bone by osteoclasts
- Deposition of new bone by osteoblasts (callus)
- The fractured bone resumes its normal structure, size, and shape

FINAL COMMON OUTCOME

- *Repair tissue:* Identical to intact bone
- *Quality of healing:* Ideal

TABLE 2-14	SKELETAL MUSCLE HEALING PROCESS

PHASE	CELLULAR RESPONSES	TIMELINE
PHASE I	**HEMOSTASIS**	**SECONDS\MINUTES**

- Blood clotting cascade leads the arrest of bleeding by coagulation
- Blood clotting results in the release of proinflammatory molecules
- Fibrin clot establishes a provisional extracellular matrix, which will serve as a platform for the subsequent crucial inflammatory phase

PHASE II	**INFLAMMATORY**	**DAYS/WEEKS**

- Macrophages engage in proteolysis and phagocytosis of necrotic material
- Rupture and necrosis of myofibers
- Tear of sarcoplasmic membrane
- Contraction band seals off the membrane defect, forming a protective barrier so the torn membrane can be repaired
- Angiogenesis
- Blood-borne inflammatory cells access the site of injury
- Satellite cells begin the formation of new myofibers

PHASE III	**PROLIFERATIVE/REMODELING**	**WEEKS/MONTHS**

- Concomitant activation of two supportive processes: regeneration of the disrupted myofiber and formation of connective-tissue scar
- A balanced progression of both of these processes is necessary for optimal healing and recovery

(Continued)

TABLE 2-14	CONTINUED

Regeneration process
- Satellite cells begin to proliferate, then differentiate into myoblasts to finally join together to form myotubes
- Myotubes then fuse with part of the myofibers that survived the injury
- Regenerating parts of the myofibers grow to maturity
- Good vascularization of the injured muscle and successful regeneration of the intramuscular nerves are vital to this process

Connective-tissue scar process
- Blood-derived fibrin and fibroblasts fill the gap between ruptured myofibers with connective tissue, forming a functionally disabling fibrous scar
- Large majority of muscle lesions heal without the formation of such a fibrous scar

FINAL COMMON OUTCOME

- *Repair tissue:* Mixture of regenerative and repair muscle fibers; partial to normal function
- *Quality of healing:* Acceptable to ideal

TABLE 2-15	PERIPHERAL NERVE HEALING PROCESS	
GRADE I	**NEURAPRAXIA**	
PHASE	**CELLULAR RESPONSES**	**TIMELINE**
PHASE I	**FOCAL REMYELINATION**	**DAYS/WEEKS**

- Focal demyelination caused by compression or stretch
- Transient disrupted focal nerve conduction
- Intact axons initiate remyelination through Schwann cell activity

FINAL COMMON OUTCOME

- *Repaired tissue:* Identical to intact nerve
- *Quality of healing:* Ideal

GRADE II AND III	**AXONOTMESIS AND NEUROTMESIS**	
PHASE	**CELLULAR RESPONSES**	**TIMELINE**
PHASE I	**WALLERIAN DEGENERATION**	**MONTHS**

- Degeneration process distal to the injured axon
- Removal of degenerated axonal/myelin debris within the endoneurial tubes
- Endoneurial tubes empty; ready to receive regenerating axons

PHASE II	**AXONAL REGENERATION/COLLATERAL REGENERATION**	**MONTHS/YEAR**

Axonal regeneration
- Regrowth of axons into empty endoneurial tubes

Collateral regeneration
- Sprouting of empty endoneurial tubes into which new axons can grow
- All growing axons move toward their targets attempting to reestablish neural contact and functional re-innervation
- Rate of axonal regeneration estimated to be 1 mm/day but may vary significantly according to the severity of the nerve injury
- Axonal and collateral regeneration is not synonymous with functional recovery

(Continued)

TABLE 2-15	**CONTINUED**

FINAL COMMON OUTCOME

- *Repair tissue*—Neuropraxia: Focal remyelination leads to comple repair and full functional recovery
- *Repair tissue*—Axonotmesis: New tissue will be functional if adequate neural connection is made with target tissue
- *Repair tissue*—Neurotmesis: New tissue may be functional if there is proper neurosurgical intervention and adequate neural connection made by new axons with target tissue
- *Quality of healing:* Acceptable to minimal to failed

1. Skeletal Muscle

In addition to skin and bone, skeletal muscle tissue, which is also well vascularized, presents the third-best potential for healing, as shown in **Table 2-14**. The final common outcome in most cases is a repaired muscle tissue that has structural, physiological, and mechanical properties very similar to intact skeletal muscle. Its quality of healing is usually acceptable to ideal.

2. Peripheral Nerve

The healing process of peripheral nerves differs significantly from all the other soft tissues, as illustrated in **Table 2-15**, in that none of the classic four phases of healing are present. In case of neurapraxia, the myelin sheath is damaged as a result of compression, and the axon remains intact. This type of nerve injury heals through a process of remyelination of the axon, which leads to full functional recovery. In case of axonotmesis and neurotmesis injuries, where the axon is damaged, healing occurs through the process of Wallerian degeneration, followed by a combination of axonal regeneration and collateral regeneration. The final common outcome in case of axonotmesis is the formation of a repaired nerve, which may become functional if the nerve makes adequate connections with the target organ. In case of neurotmesis, the nerve may not heal unless expert neurosurgical intervention is available and adequate connection is established with its target tissue.

K. ARTERY AND VEIN HEALING

Because some arterial, venous, and capillary damage occurs with soft-tissue pathology, new blood vessels (i.e., neovascularization) must grow into the wound space and eventually within the newly formed repair tissue to help it survive and function normally. The process of vascular repair, therefore, is concomitant with, and not independent of, the basic four healing phases of integumentary, arthroskeletal, and neuromuscular tissues described earlier. Research has shown that neovascularization occurs via two processes: angiogenesis and vasculogenesis (Tonnesen et al., 2000; Li et al., 2003; Bauer et al., 2005; Li et al., 2005; Walsh, 2007).

1. Angiogenesis

This process is defined as the growth of new blood vessels from preexisting ones (Walsh et al., 2007). It occurs when endothelial cells sprout from preexisting blood vessels, then migrate, and proliferate to form a cordlike structure (Bauer et al., 2005; Li et al., 2005). In other words, it is the process by which resident endothelial cells of the wound's adjacent mature vascular network proliferate, migrate, and remodel into neovessels, which grow into the initially vascular wound. Angiogenesis also occurs by intususceptive microvascular growth, also known as splitting angiogenesis, whereby a mature vessel divides, or splits, to form two vessels.

2. Vasculogenesis

This process refers to *de novo* formation of blood vessels as a result of the differentiation of bone marrow-derived precursor cells (Bauer et al., 2005). Initially believed to occur only during fetal development, there is recent but limited evidence to suggest that vasculogenesis may occur also in adults and contribute to the neovascularization process following soft-tissue injury and disease.

3. Vascular Repair

Illustrated in **Table 2-16** is an overview of the different steps associated with the phenomenon of neovascularization following soft-tissue injury (Bauer et al., 2005; Li et al., 2005). These steps are related to the process of angiogenesis, which is well established in the literature. Until more evidence is presented to support the role of vasculogenesis in the process of neovascularization, this textbook recognizes the role of angiogenesis as the key process.

a. Endothelial Cells

These cells, housed in the endothelial sheath of endothelium (**Figure 2-8**), play a key role, as shown in **Table 2-16**, in the process of angiogenesis.

b. Angiogenesis Cycle

Angiogenesis is at its peak during the proliferation phase of healing, bringing more-than-adequate oxygen and nutrients

TABLE 2-16	VASCULAR HEALING PROCESS	
STEP	**CELLULAR RESPONSE**	**TIMELINE**
1[a]	Initiation of angiogenesis through the release of angiogenic cytokines and growth factors such as VEGF, from platelets, monocytes, fibroblasts, and ruptured cells	HOURS/DAYS
2[a]	Activation of endothelial cells and disruption of the extracellular matrix (ECM)	
3[b]	Proliferation and budding of activated endothelial cells outward through the vascular basement membrane—full angiogenesis Capillary sprouts orient and migrate directionally toward the source of growth stimuli—the wound bed Vascular tubes and loops are formed, making immature arteriovenous tubules Formation of granulation tissue at wound site	DAYS
4[b]	Maturation of new tubules with recruitment of smooth muscle cells to form a covering around the newly formed capillary Formation of matured vascular network (capillary, arterioles, and venules at the wound site) Blood flows to these newly formed vessels to irrigate the newly formed or repaired tissue Large majority of newly formed vessels atrophy and eventually disappear	

FINAL COMMON OUTCOME

- *Repair tissue:* Normal blood vessels
- *Quality of healing:* Ideal

[a]Steps 1 and 2 occur during the hemostatic and inflammatory phases of tissue healing.
[b]Steps 3 and 4 occur during the proliferative and maturation phases of tissue healing.

to the granulation tissue. With the remodeling and maturation phase, angiogenesis ceases, with most of the new vessels going through atrophy and becoming nonfunctional. A few of these new vessels will form into arterioles, veinules, and capillaries within the newly formed repair tissue, ensuring adequate blood supply.

L. FACTORS INFLUENCING TISSUE HEALING

Research and practice have shown that factors other than therapeutic interventions can influence soft-tissue healing. Listed in **Table 2-17** are some of the factors that can either maximize or impede the healing process. Health

TABLE 2-17	FACTORS IMPEDING AND MAXIMIZING THE SOFT-TISSUE HEALING PROCESS
MAXIMIZING FACTORS	**IMPEDING FACTORS**
Good general health status	Poor general health status
No comorbidity	Comorbidities
Younger age	Older age
Proper nutrition	Malnutrition
Active lifestyle	Sedentary lifestyle
Good compliance with treatment	Poor compliance with treatment

practitioners must take these factors as well as others into consideration when determining the potential healing outcome of any given soft-tissue injury.

M. HEALING OF ACUTE, SUBACUTE, AND CHRONIC PATHOLOGY

The timeline of the healing process described is characteristic of acute and subacute soft-tissue pathologies. Chronic pathology occurs when one or many of the phases (inflammatory, proliferative, remodeling, or maturation) of the healing process is incomplete, delayed, or absent. Therefore, management of chronic wounds with EPAs aims at completing or enhancing the healing process by targeting the faulty phases of repair.

CRITICAL THINKING QUESTIONS

Clarification: What is meant by soft-tissue pathology and tissue healing?

Assumptions: You assume that soft-tissue healing occurs primarily through repair, rather than by regeneration. How do you justify making that assumption?

Reasons and evidence: The consensus is that the natural process of soft-tissue healing involves four distinctive, successive, and overlapping phases. What led you to believe that?

Viewpoints or perspectives: You believe that, although the quality of healing of soft-tissue pathology is rarely ideal, it is nonetheless beneficial to patients. How can you answer an objection to this viewpoint?

Implications and consequences: The various connective-tissue sheaths found in many soft tissues, such as tendon, skeletal muscle, and peripheral nerves, play important roles in the healing process. What is implied by that statement?

About the question: Is there a close relationship between the vascularity of a soft tissue and its capacity of healing? Why do you think I ask this question?

References

Review Articles

Almekinders LC, Temple JD (1998) Etiology, diagnosis, and treatment of tendonitis: An analysis of the literature. Med Sci Sports Exerc, 30: 1183–1190

Bauer SM, Bauer RJ, Valazquez OC (2005) Angiogenesis, vasculogenesis, and induction of healing in chronic wounds. Vasc Endovascular Surg, 39: 293–306

Buckwalter JA (2002) Articular cartilage injuries. Clin Orthop Rel Res, 402: 21–37

Buckwalter JA, Brown TD (2004) Joint injury, repair and remodeling: Roles in post-traumatic osteoarthritis. Clin Orthop Rel Res, 423: 7–16

Burnett MG, Zager EL (2004) Pathophysiology and peripheral nerve injury: A brief review. Neurosurg Focus, 16: 1–7

Chen FS, Frenkel SR, Di Cesare PE (1999a) Repair of articular cartilage defects: Part I. Basic science of cartilage healing. Am J Orthop, 28: 31–33

Chen FS, Frenkel SR, Di Cesare PE (1999b) Repair of articular cartilage defects: Pat II. Treatment options. Am J Orthop, 28: 88–96

Childs SG (2003) Stimulators of bone healing. Orthop Nurs, 22: 421–428

Ehrhardt J, Morgan J (2005) Regenerative capacity of skeletal muscle. Curr Opin Neurol, 548–553

Farmer JM, Martin DF, Boles CA, Curl WW (2001) Chondral endosteochondral injuries: Diagnosis and management. Clin Sports Med, 20: 299–320

Frank CB (2004) Ligament structure, physiology and function. J Musculoskel Neuron Interact, 42: 199–201

Hayes DW, Brower RL, John KJ (2001) Articular cartilage. Anatomy, injury and repair. Clin Podiatr Med Surg, 18: 35–53

Harvey C (2005) Wound healing. Orthop Nurs, 24: 143–159

Hildebrand KA, Gallant-Behm CL, Kydd AS, Hart DA (2005) The basics of soft-tissue healing and general factors that influence such healing. Sports Med Arthrosc Rev, 13: 136–144

Jarvinen TAH, Jarvinen TLN, Kaariainen M, Kalimo H, Jarvinen M (2005) Muscle injury: Biology and treatment. Am J Sports Med, 33: 745–764

Johnstone CC, Farley A (2005) The physiological basics of wound healing. Nurs Stand, 19: 59–65

Khan KM, Cook JL, Bonar F, Harcourt P, Astrom M (1999) Histopathology of common tendinopathies: Update and implications for clinical management. Sports Med, 27: 393–406

La Stayo PC, Winters KM, Hardy M (2003) Fracture healing: Bone healing, fracture, management, and current concept to the hand. J Hand Ther, 16: 81–93

Li J, Zhang YP, Kirsner RS (2003) Angiogenesis in wound repair: Angiogenic growth factors and the extracellular matrix. Micros Res Tech, 60: 107–114

Li WW, Talcott KE, Zhai AW, Kriger EA, Li, VW (2005) The role of therapeutic angiogenesis in tissue repair and regeneration. Adv Skin Wound Care, 18: 491–500

Mandelbaum B, Waddell D (2005) Etiology and pathophysiology of osteoarthritis. Orthop, 28: S207–S214

Phillips AM (2005) Overview of the fracture healing cascade. Int J Care Inj, 365: S5–S7

Rummler LS, Gupta R (2004) Peripheral nerve repair: A review. Curr Opin Orthop, 15: 215–219

Sevier TL, Wilson JK, Helfst RH, Stover SA (2000) Tendinitis: A critical review. Crit Rev Phys Med Rehab Med, 12: 119–130

Sharma P, Maffulli N (2005) Tendon injury and tendinopathy: Healing and repair. J Bone Joint Surg (Am), 87: 187–202

Tonnesen MG, Feng X, Clark RA (2000) Angiogenesis in wound healing. J Investig Dermatol Symp Proc, 5: 40–46

Walsh DA (2007) Pathophysiological mechanisms of angiogenesis. Adv Clin Chem, 44: 187–221

Wernig A, Schafer R, Knauf U, Mundegar RR, Zweyer M, Hogemeier O, Martens UM, Zimmermann S (2005) On the regenerative capacity of human skeletal muscle. Artif Org, 29: 192–198

Whitney JD (2005) Overview: Acute and chronic wound. Nurs Clin North Am, 40: 191–205

Woo SLY, Debski RE, Zeminski J, Abramowitch SD, Chan Saw, SS, Fenwick JA (2000) Injury and repair of ligaments and tendons. Annu Rev Biomed Eng, 2: 83–118

Woo SLY, Thomas M, Chan Saw SS (2004) Contribution of biomechanics, orthopaedics and rehabilitation: The past, present and future. Surg J R Coll Surg Edinb Irel, 2: 125–136

Chapters of Textbooks

Behrens BJ (2006) Tissue response to injury. In: Physical Agents: Theory and Practice, 2nd ed. Behrens BJ, Michlovitz SL (Eds). FA Davis Co., Philadelphia, pp 3–21

Clancy WG (1990) Tendon trauma and overuse injuries. In: Sports-Induced inflammation: Clinical and Basic Science Concepts. Leadbetter WB, Buckwalter JA, Gordon SL (Eds). American Academy of Orthopaedic Surgeons, Park Ridge, pp 609–618

Delforge G (2002a) Hemorrhage and hemostasis. In: Musculoskeletal Trauma: Implications for Sports Injury Management. Human Kinetics, Champaign, pp 21–26

Delforge G (2002b) Soft connective tissue repair. In: Musculoskeletal Trauma: Implications for Sports Injury Management. Human Kinetics, Champaign, pp 29–52

Delforge G (2002c) Therapeutic implications: Scar formation and maturation. In: Musculoskeletal Trauma: Implications for Sports Injury Management. Human Kinetics, Champaign, pp 87–14

Delforge G (2002d) Fracture healing. In: Musculoskeletal Trauma: Implications for Sports Injury Management. Human Kinetics, Champaign, pp 117–131

Denegar CR (2000) Tissue injury, inflammation and repair. In: Therapeutic Modalities for Athletic Injuries. Human Kinetics, Champaign, pp 28–45

Frank CB, Shrive NG (1994) Ligament. In: Biomechanics of the Musculoskeletal System. Nigg BM, Herzog W (Eds). John Wiley & Sons, New York, pp 106–132

Herzog W (1994) Muscle. In: Biomechanics of the Musculoskeletal System. Nigg BM, Herzog W (Eds). John Wiley & Sons, New York, pp 154–190

Herzog W, Loitz B (1994) Tendon. In: Biomechanics of the Musculoskeletal System. Nigg BM, Herzog W (Eds). John Wiley & Sons, New York, pp 133–153

Leadbetter WB (2001) Soft-tissue athletic injury. In: Sports Injury: Mechanisms, Prevention and Treatment, 2nd ed. Fu FH, Stone DA (Eds). Lippincott Williams & Wilkins, Philadelphia, pp 839–888

Martinez-Hernandez A (1994) Repair, regeneration, and fibrosis. In: Pathology, 2nd ed. Rubin E, Farber JL (Eds). Lippincott Williams & Wilkins, Philadelphia, pp 31–64

Martinez-Hernandez A, Amenta PS (1990) Basic concepts in wound healing. In: Sports-Induced Inflammation. Leadbetter WB, Buckwalter JA, Gordon SL (Eds). American Academy of Orthopaedic Surgeons, Park Ridge, pp 132–178

Nigg BM, Grimson SK (1994). Bone. In. Biomechanics of the Musculoskeletal System. Nigg BM, Herzog W (Eds). John Wiley & Sons, New York, pp 48–78

Norris C (2004) Healing. In: Sports Injuries: Diagnosis and Management, 3rd ed. Norris C (ed). Butterworth-Heinemann, Edinburg, pp 29–60

Prentice WE (2002) The healing process and guidelines for using therapeutic modalities. In: Therapeutic Modalities for Physical Therapists, 2nd ed. McGraw-Hill, New York, pp 14–27

Pride JA (2003) Inflammation and tissue repair. In: Physical Agents in Rehabilitation: From Research to Practice, 2nd ed. Cameron MH (ed). Saunders, New York, pp 13–40

Ruberton JA, Barbe M (2005) Wound healing and pain. In: Modalities for Therapeutic Intervention, 4th ed. Michlovitz SL, Nolan TP (Eds). FA Davis co, Philadelphia, pp 15–40

Shrive NG, Frank CB (1994) Articular cartilage. In: Biomechanics of the Musculoskeletal System. Nigg BM, Herzog W (Eds). John Wiley & Sons, New York, pp 79–105

Starkey C (2004) The injury response process. Starkey C (ed). In: Therapeutic Modalities, 3rd ed. FA Davis Co., pp 2–28

Textbooks

Hess CT (2005) Clinical Guide: Wound Care, 5th ed. Lippincott Williams & Wilkins, Philadelphia

Leadbetter WB, Buckwalter JA, Gordon SL (1990) Sports-Induced Inflammation. American Academy of Orthopaedic Surgeons, Park Ridge, IL

Salter RB (1999) Textbook of Disorders and Injuries of the Musculoskeletal System, 3rd ed. Lippincott Williams & Wilkins, Baltimore

CHAPTER 3

Pain Following Soft-Tissue Pathology

Chapter Outline

Learning Objectives

Knowledge: List the categories of pain.

Comprehension: Compare the categories of pain and the various pain assessment tools.

Application: Explain how the use of pain assessment tools can help in the diagnosis and therapy of painful soft-tissue pathology.

Analysis: Outline the different phases related to the perception of nociceptive pain.

Synthesis: Formulate the relationship between the different categories of pain and the various pain therapies available.

Evaluation: Discuss the peripheral and central mechanisms of pain modulation.

I. NATURE AND TYPES OF PAIN

A. EARLY CONCEPTS

The concept of pain as a form of punishment for sinful activity is as old as humankind. Christians believed that pain during childbirth was a consequence of Eve's sin that was transferred to women directly by God (Parris, 2003). As far back as the first century, many people endured suffering in order to identify with Christ's suffering on the cross during his crucifixion (Parris, 2003).

1. Pain and Patient
The word *pain* comes from the Latin word *poena*, meaning punishment. The word *patient* comes from the Latin word *patior*, meaning to endure suffering or pain (Parris, 2003).

2. Descartes
Although Plato believed the brain was the destination of all peripheral stimulation, Aristotle advanced the theory that the heart was the processing center for pain. As anatomy became better understood, Descartes' description of pain conduction from the site of peripheral tissue damage through nerves to the brain led to the first plausible pain theory, called the specificity theory (Parris, 2003).

B. DEFINITION

Pain is undoubtedly the main reason why people seek treatment from health professionals (Turk et al., 2001). The International Association for the Study of Pain (IASP) defines *pain* as "an unpleasant sensory and emotional experience associated with actual or potential tissue damage, or described in terms of such damages" (Merskey et al., 1994).

1. Duality of Pain
This definition highlights the duality of pain as a physiological and psychological experience. Pain is a physiological event within the body that depends on its subjective recognition or perception by the individual, or on the person's psychological awareness of it, in order to exist. It also highlights the fact that pain can arise from both actual and perceived tissue damage, meaning that pain can occur in the absence of tissue damage, even though the experience may be described as if the damage had occurred.

2. Unique Sensation
Although no one likes pain, this unique sensation is nonetheless essential to our survival, serving as our body's final line of self-awareness and protection against pathology and harmful environments (Strong, 2002; Sikes, 2004). Pain usually helps tissue healing by preventing us from further aggravating our pathological and painful conditions.

3. Perception Versus Tolerance Threshold
It is important to distinguish between the *pain perception threshold*, which is relatively constant, and the *pain tolerance threshold*, which is the maximum amount of pain that we are willing to tolerate. The pain tolerance threshold is the most important in the patient's perception and attitude toward pain, and thus influences the decision about whether to seek treatment.

C. ACUTE AND CHRONIC PAIN

Humans present with two major types of pain: acute and chronic. Distinguishing between acute and chronic pain has important implications for therapeutic interventions. Acute pain practically always signals tissue damage, whereas chronic pain may or may not be associated with tissue damage. **Box 3-1** presents key characteristics that distinguish acute from chronic pain. Acute pain serves a crucial biologic purpose: to protect the patient from further aggravating his or her pathology. Chronic pain, on the other hand, not only serves no biologic purpose but very often imposes several psychological, emotional, and socioeconomic stresses on the patient, his or her family, and society in general (i.e., through the patient's lack of productivity). Acute pain, if not properly diagnosed, treated, and managed, can become chronic pain. Chronic pain, unfortunately, is prevalent and very often difficult to treat and manage.

II. DIMENSIONS AND CATEGORIES OF PAIN

A. DIMENSIONS

Pain is one of the most complex phenomena to study in the field of health care because of its strong subjective aspect. Nonetheless, there is a consensus among researchers and clinicians that pain is essentially a three-dimensional phenomenon, consisting of evaluative (i.e., its intensity), sensory, and affective dimensions [see McMahon and Koltzenburg's (2006) recent edition of Wall and Melzack's classic, *Textbook of Pain*, first published in 1982, for a thorough review on the topic of pain].

1. Evaluative
The first dimension of pain relates to its evaluative aspect, or its intensity, that is, how much it hurts (e.g., a little, a lot). Intensity is the dimension of pain most assessed by clinicians. There is a linear relationship between the level of pain intensity, treatment delivery, and discharge: the more intense the pain, the more aggressive the treatment delivery and the less rapid the discharge. Inversely, the lesser the pain, the less aggressive the treatment and the more rapid the patient's discharge.

Box 3-1	Key Characteristics Distinguishing Acute from Chronic Pain

ACUTE	CHRONIC
Sudden	Gradual
Localized	Diffuse and/or referred
Related to tissue damages	Poorly related to tissue damages[a]
Serves biological purpose (self-protection)	Serves no biologic purpose
Lasts days to weeks	Lasts months to years
Limited to physical signs and symptoms	Often associated with psychological, emotional, or social distress
Normal use of therapy	Often abusive use of therapy
Normal pain behavior	Often abnormal pain behavior
No pain-compounding factors	Pain response may be compounded by economic or legal problems
Good response to treatment	Poor/limited response to treatment
Monodisciplinary approach	Multidisciplinary approach required
Good prognosis	Poor prognosis

[a]There are cases in which chronic pain is directly related to tissue damage, as evidenced by most degenerative diseases such as arthritis and multiple sclerosis. Thus, it is important to determine whether the cause is biologic and, if so, whether it is significant enough to explain the chronic pain pattern displayed by the patient.

2. Sensory

The second dimension of pain is the sensory aspect, that is, how it feels to the patient (e.g., burning, itching, etc.). This dimension is very informative in determining the cause or nature of the pain. Sensory manifestation of pain is often related to nociceptive and neuropathic pain.

3. Affective

The third and final dimension of pain concerns its affective aspect, that is, how it affects the suffering patient emotionally (e.g., sickening, punishing feeling). This dimension is also very important to the clinician in determining the extent to which the patient is emotionally affected by his or her pain condition. This information can help the clinician to make a better choice of pain therapy—a psychological versus somatic approach, for example.

4. Objective Assessment

Although pain is a highly personal and subjective phenomenon, it can be assessed objectively with various standardized scales or tools for patients of all ages [see Turk and Melzack's (2001) *Handbook of Pain Assessment* for a

comprehensive review of the subject of pain assessment, as well as Section V, Pain Assessment and Scoring].

B. CATEGORIES

Before addressing the anatomical and physiological aspect of pain, it is important to identify and briefly describe the major categories of pain in humans. **Box 3-2** lists the categories of pain recognized by the IASP and commonly seen in practice (Derasari, 2003). Pain is categorized as nociceptive (either somatic or visceral), neuropathic (either peripheral or central), psychogenic, and carcinogenic.

1. Nociceptive Pain

This first category of nociceptive pain includes somatic and visceral pain. The term nociceptive implies that pain is caused by the activation of nociceptors.

a. Somatic

This subcategory of pain stems from the activation of nociceptors found in most body tissues, with the

Box 3-2   Categories of Human Pain

Nociceptive

Somatic

All tissues except neural tissue
Caused by nociceptor activity
Examples: tendinitis, arthritis, bursitis
Use of EPAs: frequent

Visceral

Visceral tissue only
Caused by nociceptor activity
Examples: angina, pancreatitis, cholecystisis
Use of EPAs: rare

Neuropathic

Peripheral

Tissue related to the peripheral nervous system only
Caused by malfunctioning of the system
Examples: neuropathy, herpes zoster, causalgia
Use of EPAs: frequent

Central

Tissue related to the central nervous system only
Caused by malfunctioning of the system
Examples: stroke, multiple sclerosis
Use of EPAs: rare

Psychogenic

Within the psychological and psychiatric domain
Caused by nonorganic sources
Examples: depression, anxiety, schizophrenia
Use of EPAs: never

Carcinogenic

All cancerous tissues
Caused by a tumor
Examples: lung cancer, bone cancer
Use of EPAs: never

---

exception of neural tissue, which has none. Nociceptors, labeled as pain receptors, are mainly present in tissues belonging to the integumentary system (skin) and arthro-musculoskeletal system (muscle, tendon, ligament, and bone). Somatic pain is the most prevalent category of pain and results primarily from pathologies caused by injuries, chronic diseases, and surgical interventions (i.e., postoperative pain).

i. Normal pain. Somatic pain is commonly described as normal pain because the sensation felt (pain) usually matches the noxious nature of the stimulus. For example, if one touches a very hot source or surface with a finger, a severe burning pain is perceived. This is a classic example of somatic pain.

ii. Use of electrophysical agents. Somatic pain is the subcategory of nociceptive pain most frequently treated with electrophysical agents (EPAs).

b. Visceral
Visceral pain is also a subcategory of nociceptive pain, resulting from the activation of nociceptors found in our viscera (Derasari, 2003; Bielefeldt et al., 2006). Disease, rather than injury, is the most common cause of such pain. Visceral pain, as illustrated in **Figure 3-1**, is frequently perceived as referred pain, meaning that pain is perceived at some distance from the site of the affected organ.

i. Referred. The neural basis for referred visceral pain rests on a phenomenon called *viscerosomatic convergence* (Galea, 2002, Bielefeld et al., 2006). The reason for this convergence is the lack of a dedicated sensory pathway to the brain for information concerning the internal organs. It is proposed that the sensory neurons from the viscera connect to the brain via a sensory pathway that carries information from the skin and muscles. As a result, the brain interprets the nociceptive input that originates from the diseased organs as also coming from these soft tissues. Angina is a perfect example of referred pain. Angina, a pain originating from the heart due to poor oxygen supply, is very often perceived as a pain in the left part of the chest and sometimes in the left arm and hand, which corresponds to the cutaneous segments supplied between the third cervical level (C3) and the fifth thoracic level (T5). Cardiac pain is thus referred to this cutaneous zone because the heart is derived from the mesoderm in the neck and upper thoracic area, with the result that nociceptive afferents from the heart enter the spinal cord through the dorsal roots C3–T5, rather than lower down (Galea, 2002).

ii. Distinctive nature. Visceral pain differs significantly from somatic pain in that it is a referred, diffuse, and poorly localized type of pain, often associated with strong psychological and emotional responses (Bielefeldt et al., 2006).

iii. Specificity. Not all viscera are sensitive to pain. For example, many diseases of the lungs, kidneys, and liver are painless until abnormal functioning becomes severe, whereas a relatively minor lesion in viscera such as the bladder, the stomach, or the ureters can produce excruciating pain.

iv. Nociceptors. Visceral nociceptors are similar to those associated with somatic pain, in that they respond to mechanical (overstretching, distension) and chemical (inflammation) stimuli.

v. Locations. Illustrated in **Figure 3-1** are pain locations commonly associated with several human viscera. This figure clearly shows the true referred nature of pain in many viscera—for example, heart pain felt in the left arm.

vi. Use of EPAs. Therapeutic EPAs are rarely used to modulate visceral pain.

2. Neuropathic Pain

This second category of pain includes peripheral and central pain. The term *neurogenic* implies that pain is caused by malfunctioning of the neural system. Neuropathic pain is often characterized, especially when it has become chronic, by an array of abnormal painful sensations such as allodynia, pain due to a stimulus that does not normally provoke pain, and hyperalgesia—an increased response to a stimulus that is normally painful (see Devor, 2006 for details).

a. Peripheral

This subcategory of neuropathic pain results from the pathological functioning of the peripheral nervous system (PNS), namely, sensory and motor nerves (Derasari, 2003; Devor, 2006). Injury and disease to peripheral nerves are common causes of such pain.

b. Central

This other subcategory relates to the pathological functioning of the central nervous system, namely, the spinal cord, the medulla, the brainstem, and the brain (Derasari, 2003; Boivie, 2006). Disease is the common cause of such pain. Central pain may start almost immediately after occurrence of the malfunction, or it may be delayed for up to several years, as seen in many cases of stroke, multiple sclerosis, and Parkinson's disease.

c. Use of EPAs

Therapeutic EPAs are frequently used to modulate peripheral pain. They are, however, seldom used to modulate central pain.

3. Psychogenic Pain

As its name implies, this third category of pain, listed in **Box 3-1**, originates from nonorganic psychological sources (Flor et al., 2006). For example, when the pain reported by the patient cannot be objectively confirmed, is judged to be disproportionate to objectively determined pathology, or is unresponsive to appropriate treatment, then such pain is assumed to be of psychogenic origin (Flor et al., 2006).

a. Complexity

Psychogenic pain is complex in that it is frequently associated with emotional, cognitive, and behavioral responses (Flor et al., 2006).

b. Use of EPAs

Psychogenic pain is managed with therapeutic interventions other than EPAs because it is caused by sources other than organic pathology. Its management is therefore beyond the scope of this textbook.

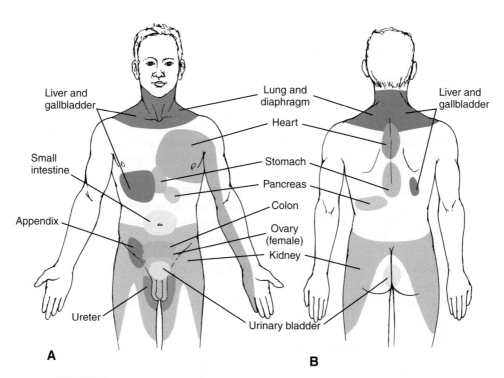

FIGURE 3-1 Visceral pain: anterior (**A**) and posterior (**B**) views of pain referred from viscera.

4. Carcinogenic Pain

This fourth and last category of pain is caused by the presence of cancerous pathology (nonmalignant or malignant tumor) anywhere in the body (Mantyh, 2006).

a. Severity

This pain is unique in that in addition to its being often severe, the pathology underlying this pain may also have a significant impact on both the quality of life and the survival of the patient (Mantyh, 2006).

b. Use of EPAs

Carcinogenic pain is also beyond the scope of this textbook because it is practically never treated using EPAs. When EPAs are used, it is more than often in the context of palliative care. Because of its severity, the effective management of carcinogenic pain requires the use of powerful pharmacological (narcotic) pain killers delivered orally, or by means of patches or implanted pumps, in addition to radiotherapy and oncologic surgery.

III. THE EXPERIENCE OF PAIN

A. EXPERIENCING PAIN

How do we experience or feel pain from soft-tissue pathology resulting from an injury, a surgical incision, or disease? The experience of pain can be described as the process of five distinct and successive physiological phases: transduction, peripheral transmission, modulation, central transmission, and, finally, perception (Dahl et al., 2006). The first phase, transduction, originates at the level of the nociceptors (for nociceptive and carcinogenic pain) or at the level of the malfunction (neurogenic pain), or from other nonorganic sources (psychogenic pain). The last phase, perception, takes place at the level of the cerebral cortex or brain. The five phases leading to the experience of pain are illustrated in **Figure 3-2.**

1. Nociceptors

Before considering each of these phases it is important to characterize the nociceptors, because nociceptive and carcinogenic pain begins with their activation. The term nociceptor is derived from the Latin word *nocere*, meaning to harm. There is a consensus in the scientific literature to designate free nerve endings as pain receptors or nociceptors (McMahon et al., 2006).

2. High Activation Threshold

Most nociceptors have a high stimulation or activation threshold and, as a result do not respond to everyday stimuli (Mense et al., 2001; Mense, 2003). This means, for example, that the nociceptors in our skin are not activated when we are sitting (compression of the gluteal skin area) or that muscle nociceptors are not activated when we are

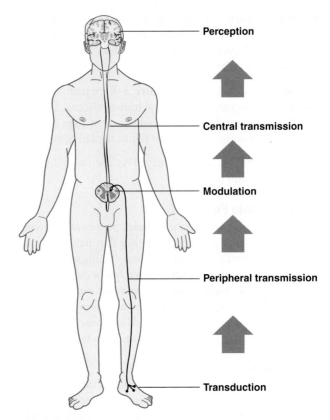

FIGURE 3-2 Physiological phases leading to the experience of nociceptive pain.

walking (muscle fiber contraction and elongation). Only when their activation threshold is exceeded is a noxious stimulus message generated.

3. Noxious Stimuli

Nociceptors respond to intense mechanical, thermal, and chemical stimuli capable of damaging the tissues surrounding them. Stimuli that activate nociceptors are called noxious stimuli.

a. Mechanoception

Cutaneous mechanoreceptors, such as Meissner and Pacinian corpuscles and Merkel tactile disks, provide us with the senses of touch, pressure, and vibration.

b. Thermoception

Cutaneous thermoreceptors provide our thermal sense for detecting heat (Ruffini corpuscles) and cold (Krause end bulbs).

c. Pain Threshold Versus Tolerance

Pain threshold is the level of noxious stimulus required to alert the individual to a potential threat to tissue. Pain tolerance, on the other hand, is a measure of how much pain a person can or will withstand (Sikes, 2004). Both pain threshold and pain tolerance can vary greatly between individuals.

B. PHASES OF NOCICEPTIVE PAIN PERCEPTION

As stated previously and shown in **Figure 3-2**, there are five physiological phases in the experience or perception of pain. Nociceptive pain is the most prevalent category of pain in health-care practice, and the following paragraphs focus on describing its five phases, which begin with nociceptive activity.

1. Transduction

Transduction is the phase of converting mechanical energy (i.e., of mechanical, thermal, and chemical forms) affecting nociceptors at the site and around the wound into electrical energy, which generates action potentials that lead to the production of nerve impulses. As stated previously, pain initially develops in nociceptors, the specialized nerve endings that are activated by strong mechanical and thermal stimuli and by chemical substances produced and released (inflammatory response) in the tissue at the wound site. Readers should note that in cases of neurogenic pain, transduction originates from the overall dysfunction of the peripheral or central system, not from the activation of nociceptors. Also, it must be remembered that, in cases of psychogenic pain, transduction arises from nonorganic sources or sites acting in the regulation of psychological and emotional states.

a. Process

This transduction, or conversion, of energy results from a change in the nociceptor's structural confirmation with the formation of pores (ionic channels) within its cell membrane. Ion exchanges in and out of the nociceptor cell membrane generate action potentials leading to the production of nerve impulses, which will later be transmitted along specialized sensory afferent fibers toward the spinal cord.

b. Quantum of Energy

For transduction to occur, the quantum of physical energy available at the tissue injury site must be large enough, or intense enough, to exceed the nociceptor's membrane threshold of activation, because most nociceptors are dormant—that is, they do not respond to light and moderate stimuli.

2. Peripheral Transmission Phase

This second phase includes the propagation or transmission of nerve impulses generated as a result of transduction from the nociceptors to the spinal cord. The terminal ends of the nociceptors, that is, the free nerve endings, connect with the spinal cord through two distinct afferent sensory nerve fibers: A delta and C fibers (Weisberg et al., 2006; Wright, 2002).

a. Process

The noxious message, now coded in nerve impulses, is transmitted to the dorsal horn of the spinal cord along these two afferent sensory fibers, whose cell body (neuron) resides in the dorsal root ganglia. Impulse transmission in the A delta fibers occurs more rapidly than in the C fibers (approximately 15 m/s versus 1 m/s) because the axons of the former are lightly myelinated (larger in diameter), whereas those of the latter are unmyelinated (smaller in diameter).

b. A-delta and C Fibers

A-delta fibers conduct mechanical as well as thermal noxious stimuli. C fibers, on the other hand, conduct mechanical, thermal, and chemical noxious stimuli. These nerve fibers are sustained by *first-order neurons* located in the dorsal root ganglia.

3. Modulation

Modulation, as illustrated in **Figure 3-2**, is the third phase leading to the experience of pain. This phase is characterized by a diminution, suppression, or amplification of pain (hence the word modulation). Research has shown that pain modulation occurs as a result of the action of nociceptive nerve impulses on the spinal gating system located in the dorsal horn of the spinal cord (McMahon et al., 2006). Because pain modulation reflects the action of our own thoughts and emotions, it is logical that the two remaining phases, central transmission (fourth phase) and perception (fifth phase), are addressed before the modulation phase which is described in detail later in the chapter.

4. Central Transmission

This is the phase that encompasses the ascending transmission, or projection, of nociceptive nerve impulses, generated by the spinal pain-transmitting neurons, also called T neurons, along the spinal cord and through the anterolateral system (ALS) and the lower brain and cortex areas (Dostrovsky et al., 2006).

a. Pain-Transmitting Neurons

There are two types of T neurons: nociceptive-specific (NS) and wide dynamic range (WDR), both located in the dorsal horn of the spinal cord (Rubertone et al., 2005). Both NS and WDR neurons are referred to as *second-order neurons*.

b. Anterolateral System

Nerve impulses are first transmitted centrally, i.e., from the spinal cord and up to the medulla, pons, and midbrain, along the axons of the anterior and lateral portions (or bundles) of the anterolateral system (ALS). They are then transmitted through the ALS to various subcortical areas directly involved in the detection and modulation of pain, such as the thalamus, the reticular formation, the limbic system, the nucleus raphe magnus (NRM), and the periaquaductal gray matter (PAG) (see Galea, 2002; Dostrovsky et al., 2006).

i. Pathways. The ALS is composed of several specific pathways or tracts: the spinothalamic tract, the spinoreticular tract, the spinomesencephalic tract, and the spinohypothalamic-limbic tract (Rubertone et al., 2005). These pathways serve different functions. The *spinothalamic tract* is the primary nociceptive pathway within the ALS, carrying discriminative aspects of pain such as type and location (Rubertone et al., 2005). The *spinoreticular tract* is linked to the motivational, emotional, and unpleasant aspects of pain (Rubertone et al., 2005). The *spinomesencephalic tract* is associated with the sensorimotor integration of pain, which includes motor reflex responses to pain (Rubertone et al., 2005). Finally, the *spinohypothalamic-limbic tract* is involved in the tissue autonomic responses following pain (Rubertone et al., 2005).

ii. Ascending function. The nociceptive message ascends along the ALS tracts, from the spinal cord, ipsilaterally and contralaterally, to a number of subcortical sites, bilaterally (Rubertone et al., 2005).

c. Subcortical and Cortical Neurons

After the long axons in the ALS system have made their synaptic contact with the subcortical neurons (*third-order neurons*), a new set of nerve impulses is then generated by those neurons along their own axons. These nerve impulses, carrying the nociceptive message from the subcortical areas, are finally transmitted to the cortical neurons (*fourth-order neurons*) for pain perception to finally occur. There is an enduring notion in the field of pain-related studies that the lateral thalamus is involved in discriminative pain (i.e., location and intensity), whereas the medial thalamus is linked to its motivational and emotional aspects (Dostrovsky et al., 2006).

5. Perception

This fifth and final phase relates first to the detection of pain and subsequently to the determination of its meaning and relevance (Bushnell et al., 2006). It is during this crucial phase that nociception (the organic aspect) finally becomes pain (the cognitive aspect). It is also during this phase that pain is processed.

a. Cortical Regions

There is evidence from brain imaging and electrophysiological studies that different cortical regions (**Figure 3-2**) may be preferentially involved in different aspects of the complex experience of pain (Bushnell et al., 2006). Most evidence suggests that the somatosensory cortex is more important for the perception of spatial and temporal features, such as the location and duration of pain, whereas the limbic and paralimbic regions are more important for

the emotional and motivational aspects of pain (Bushnell et al., 2006).

b. Modulation

As soon as we perceive pain, we try to modulate it downward; that is, we attempt to diminish or suppress it by acting on it ourselves or by seeking the help of health practitioners. Unfortunately, pain can also be modulated up, or amplified, through a cascade of biological mechanisms and cognitive/emotional responses. Therefore, we discuss in the following section the third and key phase of modulation, shown in **Figures 3-2** and **3-3**, which leads to the experience of nociceptive pain.

IV. PAIN MODULATION

A. THE SPINAL GATING SYSTEM

According to the literature, the modulation of pain requires peripheral or central interventions on the classic spinal pain gating system. This theory was originally proposed by Wall and Melzack (1965) and further revised, subsequently, by both authors (Melzack et al., 1982). According to the gate control theory, pain is perceived only if the spinal gate is open. It thus follows that, to suppress pain, we need interventions to *close* this gate. **Figure 3-3** is a schematic representation of the revised gate control theory (Melzack et al., 1982).

1. Dorsal Horn

Illustrated in **Figure 3-3** is a simplified cross-sectional view of the *spinal cord*, showing its dorsal and ventral horns made of gray matter and surrounded by white matter. The gating system is located in the dorsal horn, more precisely within Rexed anatomical laminae II and V. The gating effect (open or closed) occurs after physiological interaction between the inhibitory neurons located in the substantia gelatinosa (SG) and the pain-transmitting neurons [T cells made of nociceptive-specific (NS) and wide dynamic range (WDR) T neurons] located deeper in the dorsal horns.

2. A and C Afferent Nerve Fibers

Also illustrated in **Figure 3-3** is a schematic representation of the neurological connections between the gating system located in the spinal cord and the peripheral tissues containing nociceptors. Shown are nociceptors attached to the large-diameter A-beta (A-b mechanoceptors) fibers, the small-diameter A-delta (A-d), and smaller-diameter C fibers. These three afferent sensory fibers, whose cell bodies or neurons (first-order neurons) are located in the dorsal root ganglia, are shown making their excitatory (+) and inhibitory (−) synaptic contacts with the inhibitory neurons of the substantia gelatinosa (SG) and the T neurons, respectively.

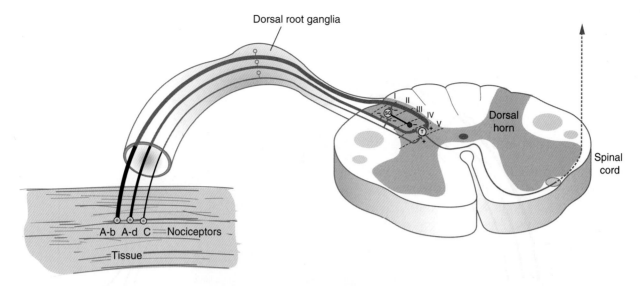

FIGURE 3-3 Schematic representation of the spinal gate control theory of pain. This gating system occurs at the level of the pain-transmitting neurons (T neurons) and is under the powerful inhibitory action trigger by the neurons contained in the substantial gelatinosa (SG). Nociceptors buried in tissues are connected to the spinal cord through the larger A-beta (A-b) and A-delta (A-d) and smaller C afferent sensory fibers, whose neurons (first-order) are located in the dorsal root ganglia. These three fibers make synaptic contact with both the inhibitory neurons located in the SG and T neurons (second-order) located deeper in the dorsal horn of the spinal cord.

B. PERIPHERAL MODULATING INTERVENTIONS

On the basis of the spinal gating mechanism, it logically follows that to close the gate (to suppress pain), a greater neural activity must be present in the *larger* A-beta mechanosensitive afferent fibers, as opposed to the neural activity in the *smaller* A-delta and C fibers. A greater neural activity along the A-beta fibers will activate or excite (+) the inhibitory neurons within the SG. Those neurons then will induce a net and powerful inhibitory effect (–) on the pain-transmitting (T) neurons, causing the gate to close, thus suppressing pain. How can the suffering patient or the treating clinician provoke such a large neural activation along the A-beta fibers by acting on the periphery, that is, at the injury site and surrounding areas?

1. Mechanical Modulation

The patient can decrease some of his or her pain, as shown in **Figure 3-4A**, simply by rubbing or massaging the skin area over and around the site of the lesion. This action preferentially activates the mechanoreceptors attached to A-beta fibers, as illustrated by the larger number of nerve impulses (squiggles) along the nerve fiber, which leads to pain modulation. A common intervention by humans when experiencing relatively intense nociceptive pain immediately after trauma is to rub or massage the painful body area.

2. Electrical Modulation

Practitioners can also activate these mechanoceptors using a transcutaneous electrical nerve stimulator (S), as shown in **Figure 3-4B**. The purpose of this intervention

is to electrically yet *preferentially* activate the A-beta fibers using a pair of electrodes positioned over or around the painful area. The use of electrical stimulation to suppress pain falls into the broad field of electroanalgesia or TENS therapy (see Chapter 14) and represents one of the many therapeutic EPAs covered in this textbook.

C. CENTRAL MODULATING SYSTEMS AND INTERVENTIONS

Research has shown that the brain not only senses pain but can also exert a powerful suppressing or amplifying modulating effect on it. Two supraspinal, or central pain-modulating, systems are described in the scientific literature (McMahon et al., 2006): the descending endogenous opiate system (DEOS) and the cortical system (CS). **Figure 3-5** is a simplified schematic representation of these two modulating systems.

1. Descending Endogenous Opiate System (DEOS)

The DEOS system (**Figure 3-5A**), as its name implies, exerts a *descending* (from central to spinal level) inhibitory effect (closing the gate) on the spinal pain-transmitting neurons (T neurons) by releasing *endogenous* opiate morphine-like substances known as endorphins into the bloodstream and cerebrospinal fluid The powerful pain-relieving effect of opioids (from the term opium, the juice extracted from the poppy seeds of the *Papaver somniferum* plant) has been known for centuries in medicine. Of all the opioid drugs available, morphine is still the gold standard for opioid pain therapy (Schug et al., 2006). Scientific evidence supporting the existence of

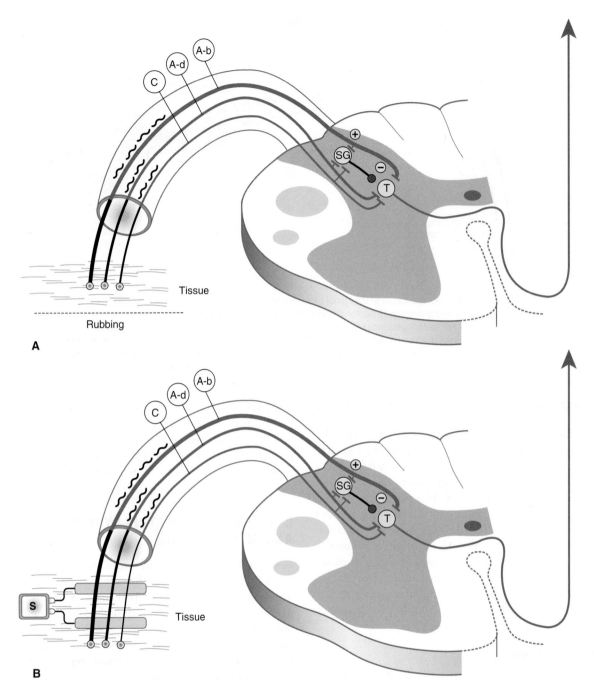

FIGURE 3-4 Schematic representation of two peripheral interventions resulting in the closing of the spinal gate, or pain suppression, through T neuron inhibition. Shown are the mechanical activation of A-beta (A-b) nerve fibers by rubbing the skin **(A)** and electrical activation of the same nerve fibers with an electrical stimulator (S) connected to a pair of surface electrodes **(B)**.

this endogenous opiate system in humans is found in the results of studies using naloxone, a powerful morphine antagonist (Fields et al., 2006).

a. DEOS Pain Mechanism

The DEOS originates primarily from neurons located in the PAG and the NRM areas, both located in the midbrain. Theoretically, pain can only be perceived if the spinal gate is open, that is, if T cells are activated. As shown in **Figure 3-5A**, these pain-transmitting neurons (T) send their axons (see arrows) to the DEOS via the ALS. The

arrival of these peripheral nociceptive nerve impulses activates the DEOS, which in turn attempt to close the gate (or decrease pain) by releasing endorphins. These will inhibit T cells, thus closing the gate. This pain inhibitory response occurs through a negative feedback loop, which dictates a larger nociceptive input, leads to a larger DEOS response, and, subsequently, a larger pain inhibitory effect (see Chapter 14). How can practitioners further activate the DEOS, thus decreasing their patients' pain? How can the patients themselves further activate their own DEOS, also for the purpose of decreasing their pain?

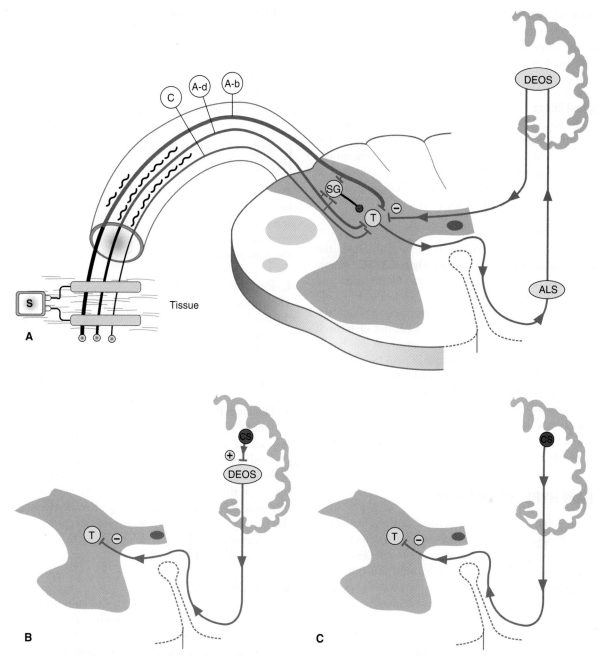

FIGURE 3-5 Schematic representation of the descending endogenous pain system (DEOS) and cognitive system (CS) with peripheral and central interventions causing their activation. Preferential electrical stimulation (S) of A-delta (A-d) and C fibers (C) opens the gate and triggers the activation of the DEOS, which then exerts its inhibitory action over the pain-transmitting neurons (T). Pain suppression is caused by the activation of the negative feedback loop system **(A).** Activation of the DEOS by the cognitive system (CS) results in pain suppression **(B).** Direct inhibitory action exerted by the CS over the T neurons **(C).**

b. Electrical Activation

Research has shown that the DEOS can be activated by a peripheral intervention very similar to the one described previously (electrical stimulation) to close the gate. In this case, however, the practitioner's intervention, as shown in **Figure 3-5A,** is to electrically trigger a *preferential and larger* activation in the A-delta and C fibers as illustrated by the larger number of nerve impulses (squiggles) along those fibers, in comparison to the A-beta fibers, so as to fully open the gate, thus temporarily increasing the patient's pain.

c. Negative Feedback Loop

The resulting effect of this induced and increased pain message is to trigger the DEOS, which in turn responds by gradually suppressing pain through a negative feedback loop (see arrows). In the present context, this negative feedback loop is synonymous with inputting more pain into the system, to eventually inhibit T neurons, thus decreasing pain. This peripheral intervention corresponds to the application of the brief intense mode during pain therapy with the help of TENS (see Chapter 14).

2. Cortical System (CS)

The CS refers to the patient's cognitive (thoughts) and emotional responses to painful events and situations. As its name implies, this system is located in the brain cortex, above the DEOS, as illustrated in **Figure 3-5B**.

a. Spinal Effect

Research has shown that the CS can express its inhibitory action on the spinal gate by directly activating (+) the DEOS, which then inhibits (–) pain by acting on the T neurons (**Figure 3-5B**). In other words, activation of the CS triggers the excitation of the DEOS, which then closes the gate, thus suppressing pain.

b. Cortical Effect

Research also suggests that the CS can also inhibit the spinal gating system, as shown in **Figure 3-5C**, simply with positive modification of the patient's thoughts and emotional response to pain (Sikes, 2004; Fields et al., 2006). In other words, events and situations in which the patient is distracted (thoughts), takes control of himself or herself, or feels reassured that the pain is not that harmful (emotions) can lead to a decrease of pain (Sikes, 2004; Fields et al., 2006). Practitioners should always remember that patients who focus on and worry about their pain too much (cognitive) or who express excessive anger, anxiety, frustration, and hopelessness about it (emotional) will inhibit their CS, which may further amplify their pain (Sikes, 2004; Fields et al., 2006, Craig, 2006).

D. PAIN HYPERSENSITIVITY

The pain perception system described, with its five physiological phases, must be sensitive enough to detect harmful or nociceptive stimuli, thus warning us early enough so that we can protect ourselves from harmful situations. But what happens when our nociceptive pain system becomes hypersensitive to pain after injury and disease?

1. Examples

A common clinical example is the increased perception of pain in the hours and days after the injury (acute pain) from non-noxious stimuli (such as a light pressure) applied over and around the tissue injury site. Another example is this same increase in pain, this time months after the injury has occurred (chronic pain), with the application of the same non-noxious stimuli at the site of injury. Research has shown that this hypersensitivity arises because our pain system has increased its sensitivity to noxious stimuli when it relays pain messages to the brain (Mense, 2003; Meyer et al., 2006).

2. Allodynia and Hyperalgesia

Pain hypersensitivity takes two forms. First, pain thresholds are lowered so that stimuli that would normally not produce pain are now perceived as painful; this is known as allodynia. Second, pain responsiveness is increased so that noxious stimuli now produce an exaggerated pain; this is known as hyperalgesia.

3. Adaptive Response

Pain hypersensitivity is an adaptive response that helps the healing process by ensuring minimal contact with, and minimal use of, the injured tissues until healing is complete. Pain hypersensitivity is thus present in acute pain after tissue injury and disease, and plays a useful role, although we may experience more pain as a result of it.

E. MECHANISMS BEHIND PAIN HYPERSENSITIVITY

Two mechanisms are proposed in the scientific literature to explain pain hypersensitivity: peripheral and central sensitization. Sensitization is defined as an increase in the excitability of peripheral and central neurons involved in the pain process (Mense, 2003; Meyer et al., 2006).

1. Peripheral Sensitization

This process takes place at the peripheral level, that is, at the level of the nociceptors buried in the tissues. It is characterized by a reduction in pain thresholds, and an increase in responsiveness, of the nociceptors (Mense, 2003). Peripheral sensitization is very closely associated with the presence of tissue inflammation, as discussed later.

a. Chemical Release

Peripheral or nociceptor sensitization arises primarily from the action of chemicals released (sensitizing chemical cocktail) by the damaged cells within and around the site of the lesion during the postinjury inflammatory phase. The release of these inflammatory chemicals, such as bradykinin, prostaglandins, substance P, and other chemicals, in the vicinity of the nociceptors triggers the process of pain transduction, the first physiological phase in the experience of pain (see **Figure 3-2**).

b. Example: Acute Pain

Peripheral sensitization contributes to pain hypersensitivity found in both acute and chronic pain. For example, pain hypersensitivity to heat stimuli after sunburn, when the normally warm water from the shower feels burning hot over the sunburned area, is an example of acute pain hypersensitivity. In such a case, inflammatory chemicals directly activate the nociceptors until the damaged tissue has been repaired. Once the tissue has healed, acute pain theoretically ends. Because the duration of healing varies, the duration of acute pain will also vary, but the presence or absence of pain is usually tightly linked to the healing process.

c. Example: Chronic Pain

An example of peripheral sensitization in chronic pain is the presence of an ongoing degenerative disease that continually activates or sensitizes nociceptors, as in the case of arthritis, when chronic inflammation (rheumatoid arthritis) or increasing tissue damage (osteoarthritis) results in severe chronic pain when the affected joints are moved.

2. Central Sensitization

Central sensitization is one of the first steps in the transition from acute to chronic muscle pain (Mense, 2003). Sometimes pain persists long after the biological healing process is completed or the amount of pain perceived by the patient is much greater than the detectable tissue damage would seem to suggest. This is chronic pain that extends beyond the normal course of injury or illness. This type of chronic pain may be explained by a mechanism called central sensitization, which is characterized by an increase in the excitability of neurons within the spinal cord. An example may be pain hypersensitivity to mechanical stimuli (such as gently bending forward), felt for months after a mild episode of back pain, for which the patient has received appropriate and timely treatments.

a. Neuroplasticity

Central sensitization is believed to be a manifestation of abnormal sensory processing within the central nervous system (i.e., neural plasticity affecting synaptic organization). It is as if the pain system has increased its gain (i.e., becomes more sensitive) such that a previously normal innocuous stimulus is now perceived as a noxious stimulus despite the absence of tissue damage and peripheral sensitization. Neuroplastic changes (neuroplasticity), such as sprouting of spinal afferent fibers and the formation of new synaptic contacts within the dorsal horns, have to be considered important steps in the transition from acute to chronic pain (Mense, 2003).

b. Manifestation

Central sensitization is responsible for tactile allodynia (when light brushing of the skin causes pain) and for the enlargement of the painful area (when pain extends to adjacent nonoriginally damaged tissues or areas), both responses often observed in cases of chronic pain.

3. Clinical Importance of Sensitization

Peripheral and central sensitizations are observed in somatic, neuropathic, and visceral pain. The main conclusion reached by Mense (2003) on the topic of sensitization is the importance of abolishing acute pain as early and effectively as possible to prevent central nervous alterations (central sensitization). If a patient has already developed alterations in the nociceptive system, treatment will be difficult and long lasting because these alterations resolve very slowly.

V. PAIN ASSESSMENT AND SCORING

A. PAIN: THE FIFTH VITAL SIGN

Because pain is the *primary symptom* leading most people to seek the attention of a health care provider, it is now considered by many clinicians as the fifth vital sign, together with heart rate, respiration rate, blood pressure, and body temperature.

1. Dual Physiological Phenomenon

Like all sensations, pain is both a physiological and a psychological phenomenon. Like all the other vital signs, it must be assessed so that adequate therapeutic interventions can be used to reduce or alleviate it.

2. Importance of Assessment

If the study of pain in people is to have a scientific foundation, it is essential to assess it. The measurement of pain is important (1) to determine pain intensity, quality, and duration; (2) to aid in diagnosis; (3) to decide on appropriate therapy; and (4) to evaluate the relative effectiveness of different therapies (Katz et al., 1999; Melzack et al., 2006).

3. Clinical Tools

Despite the subjective nature of pain, researchers and clinicians have several standardized and valid tools to assess pain in patients of all ages. Readers are directed to Turk et al. (2001) for a thorough review of pain assessment.

B. ASSESSMENT TOOLS

The essence of pain assessment is to *quantify* pain. **Box 3-3** lists the most common pain assessment tools used by researchers and clinicians to assess pain in infants, children, adolescents, adults, and the elderly. These tools are grouped under age category: infants (up to 3 years); children (4–12 years); adolescents, adults, and the elderly (13 years and older).

C. TOOLS FOR INFANTS

Several tools are described in the literature to assess pain in infants, which category includes newborns and preverbal children—those up to 3 years old. Readers are directed to Duhn et al. (2004) and McGrath et al. (2006) for a complete review of the subject. There is a consensus among experts that the best way to assess pain in infants is to assess their behavioral responses to pain, such as vocalization, facial expressions, and body movements. Because EPAs are rarely used to treat infants, only a brief description of two of those pain assessment tools is given here: the Neonatal Facial Coding System (NFCS) and the Postoperative Pain Measures for Parents (PPMP). Readers interested in the subject of infant pain assessment may refer to Duhn et al. (2004) and McGrath et al. (2006).

1. Neonatal Facial Coding System

In this tool, practitioners observe the face of the infant experiencing pain and compare and code his or her responses against a set of ten standard facial actions or expressions. Coding may be done live at the infant's bedside or later in the office after videotaping the infant's face (Grunau et al., 1987, 1998). The videotaping technique may be time-consuming. Proper training of practitioners is necessary before using the live or bedside technique.

Box 3-3   **Tools Commonly Used to Assess Human Pain**

CATEGORIES	TOOLS
Infants: up to 3 years	■ Neonatal Facial Coding System (NFCS) ■ Postoperative Pain Measure for Parents (PPMP)
Children: 4 to 12 years	■ Oucher Pain Scale (OPS) ■ Faces Pain Scale–Revised (FPS–R)
Adolescents, adults, and elderly: 13 years and older	■ Visual Analog Scale (VAS) ■ 101-point Numerical Rating Scale (NRS-101) ■ 5-point Verbal Rating Scale (VRS-5) ■ Short Form McGill Pain Questionnaire (SF-MPQ) ■ Pain Disability Index (PDI)

2. Postoperative Pain Measures for Parents

This tool is a checklist of 15 behavioral actions the suffering infant may or may not display when visually observed for a given period of time (Chambers et al., 1996, 2003). Parents and practitioners can use this tool at the infant's bedside. The PPMP is easy to use and score and provides both parents and the treating clinicians with a valid assessment of the infant's pain.

3. Infant's Overall Pain Response

These two pain assessment tools measure the infant's overall response to pain as perceived by the practitioner or parents. They do not measure, as shown later in this chapter, each of the three dimensions of pain (evaluative, affective, and sensory) separately.

D. TOOLS FOR CHILDREN

Measuring pain in children between 4 and 12 years of age presents a major challenge to practitioners (McGrath et al., 2006). Although verbal self-report has been considered the gold standard in human pain assessment, all self-reported measures, however, have intrinsic limitations. According to McGrath et al. (2006), reliable and valid behavioral scales should be used instead of verbal self-reports to assess pain in children.

1. Common Tools

The most common tools to assess pain in children, as listed in **Box 3-3**, are the Oucher Pain Scale (OPS) and the Faces Pain Scale-Revised (FPS–R). These two tools make use of face-type scales because they are easy to understand by children, regardless of their cognitive and verbal development. Facial expressions are important, as they are relatively free of learning biases and represent the child's response to invasive and noxious events.

2. Oucher Pain Scale

Shown in **Table 3-1**, the OPS is a variant of the many face scales described in the literature and is designed to measure pain intensity in children aged 4–12 years (Beyer, 1992; Beyer et al., 1998, 2005). The scale is displayed in a poster format and consists of a vertical numerical scale (0–100) on the left and six photographs of children in varying degrees of pain positioned vertically to the right. Variants of the Caucasian OPS version presented in this figure have been designed and validated for African American and Hispanic children (Beyer et al., 1998). The young child is asked to point, with a finger, to the face that best matches how much he or she is hurting now. The older child is asked to put an X on the line, beside the number, that best represents how much he or she is hurting now.

3. The Faces Pain Scale–Revised

Shown in **Table 3-1**, the FPS–R also assesses the intensity of children's pain (Bieri et al., 1990). This tool consists of six faces expressing different levels of pain intensity, ranging from no pain to the worst pain (Hicks et al., 2001). The child is ask to point, with his or her finger, to the picture that best describes his or her current level of pain.

E. TOOLS FOR ADOLESCENTS, ADULTS, AND THE ELDERLY

Listed in **Box 3-3** are five pain assessment tools commonly used with adolescents, adults, and the elderly. The Visual Analog Scale (VAS), the 101-point Numerical Rating Scale (NRS-101), and the 5-point Verbal Rating Scale (VRS-5) tools are widely used. They are known as one-dimensional tools because they asses only one dimension or component of pain, that is, its intensity. The well-known Short-Form McGill Pain Questionnaire (SF-MPQ) is a

TABLE 3-1	SCORING THE OUCHER PAIN SCALE AND THE FACES PAIN SCALE–REVISED[a]

OUCHER PAIN SCALE

PHOTOGRAPHIC SCALE—SCORE: X/5

The first (bottom) photograph is scored 0 (not hurt).
The second photograph is scored 1 (a little bit of hurt).
The third photograph is scored 2 (a little more hurt).
The fourth photograph is scored 3 (even more hurt).
The fifth photograph is scored 4 (a lot of hurt).
The sixth photograph is scored 5 (the biggest hurt you could ever have).

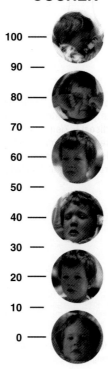

Oucher Pain Scale

Directives: The Oucher pain scale consists of two separate vertical scales; a numerical scale for older children and a photographic scale for younger children. *For younger children only.* Point to the face that shows how much you hurt now. *For older children only.* Put an X on the line beside the number that best represents how much you hurt now.

OUCHER

The Oucher Pain Scale. (From the Caucasian version of the Oucher, developed and copyrighted by Judith E. Beyer, PhD, RN. With permission.)

(Continued)

TABLE 3-1	CONTINUED

NUMERIC SCALE FOR OUCHER PAIN SCALE—SCORE: X/100

0 means no hurt.
10 to 30 means minimal hurt.
40 to 60 means moderate hurt.
70 to 90 means big hurt.
100 means the biggest hurt you could ever have.

THE FACES PAIN SCALE–REVISED

The Faces Pain Scale Revised

Directives: These faces show how much something can hurt. This face *(point to leftmost face)* shows <u>no pain</u>. The faces show more and more pain *(point to each from left to right)* up to this one *(point to the rightmost face)* – it shows <u>very much pain</u>. Please point to the face that shows how much you hurt *(right now)*.

The Faces Pain Scale–Revised (From Hicks CL, von Baever CL. Soafford P. van Koriaar I, Goodenough B. The Faces Pain Scale-Revised; Toward a common metric in pediatric pain measurement. Pain 2001; 93:173–183; scale adapted from Bieri D, Reeve R, Champion GD, Addicoat L, Ziegter J. The Faces Pain Scale for the self-assessment of the severity of pain experienced by children: Development, initial validation and preliminary investigation for ratio scale properties. Pain 1990:41:139–150. Used by permission of the International Association for the Study of Pain and the Pain Research Unit. Sydney Children's Hospital, Randwick, NSW 2031, Australia.)

NUMERIC SCALE—SCORE: X/10

The first (on the left) photograph is scored 0.
The second photograph is scored 2.
The third photograph is scored 4.
The fourth photograph is scored 6.
The fifth photograph is scored 8.
The sixth photograph is scored 10.

[a]*Note:* The examiner scores these tools by scoring the photograph identified by the suffering child (photographic scale—OPS and FPS–R) or by taking down the number (numeric scale—OPS), also identified by the suffering child.

multidimensional tool because it measures all three dimensions (intensity, sensory, and affective) of pain. The fifth tool, the Pain Disability Index (PDI), assesses multiple factors related to the patient's own level of disability resulting from his or her pain.

1. Visual Analog Scale

The VAS, illustrated in **Figure 3-6**, is one of the most common and reliable pain intensity assessment tools (Turk et al., 2001). It is a self-reported measurement consisting of a horizontal line with extreme anchors of no pain to the

Visual Analog Scale (VAS)

Directives: Using the vertical line, please mark on the line below your current level of pain.

No pain _____ Pain as bad as it could be

The 101-point Numerical Rating Scale (NRS – 101)

Directives: Please indicate on the line below the number between 0 and 100 that best describes your pain now. A zero (0) means no pain, and a one hundred (100) means pain as bad as it could be. Please write only one number.

_____

The 5-point Verbal Rating Scale (VRS – 5)

Directives: Please place an X beside the pain adjective below that best describes your current level of pain.

(_____) Mild

(_____) Discomforting

(_____) Distressing

(_____) Horrible

(_____) Excruciating

FIGURE 3-6 The Visual Analog Scale, the 101-point Numerical Rating Scale, and the 5-point Verbal Rating Scale. (Adapted from Jensen MP, Karoly P, Braver S (1986). The measurement of clinical pain intensity: A comparison of six methods. Pain, 27: 117–126. With permission.)

worst pain. The horizontal line represents a continuum of pain intensity and is 10 cm long. The patient is asked to mark on the line his current level of pain. Caution is advised when using the VAS with elderly patients because increasing age has been associated with a higher frequency of incomplete or unscorable responses (Bird, 2005; Gagliese et al., 2006). Compared with younger adults, elderly people may be more reluctant to report painful stimuli. Moreover, pathological conditions that are painful to young adults may, in the elderly, produce only behavioral changes such as confusion, restlessness, aggression, anorexia, and fatigue (Gagliese et al., 2006).

2. The 101-point Numeric Rating Scale
Presented in **Figure 3-6**, the NRS-101 is a numerical variant of the VAS and uses numbers from 0 to 100 (thus 101 numbers to choose from) to rate the pain. The patient is asked to write a number which best represents his current level of pain.

3. The 5-point Verbal Rating Scale
Also illustrated in **Figure 3-6**, the VRS-5 is a verbal variant of both the VAS and the NRS-101 tools. It uses five adjectives describing pain, and each adjective is assigned a blank bracket. The patient is asked to select which of the five adjectives best represents his or her current level of pain by putting an X in its corresponding bracket. Practitioners can choose to verbalize these adjectives out loud to the patient, or ask the patient to read them off the sheet of paper, before making the selection.

4. Short-Form McGill Pain Questionnaire

The SF-MPQ, illustrated in **Figure 3-7**, is a shorter version (Melzack, 1987) of the original McGill Pain Questionnaire (MPQ) developed by Ronald Melzack (1975). Melzack developed his short form in an attempt to make his multidimensional tool more attractive to practitioners and patients who did not have the time to use the original MPQ version. This version takes approximately 10 minutes to administer after instructions are given to the patient. This self-report contains 11 sensory and 4 affective descriptors rated on an intensity scale of 0 to 3. It also contains the VAS and the Present Pain Index (PPI). The SF-MPQ has been shown to have high correlations (correlation coefficients vary from 0.67 to 0.90) with the original MPQ. The SF-MPQ is not intended to replace the original MPQ, but simply to provide an alternative when time is a concern. The patient is asked to fill the questionnaire by following the directives, described in **Figure 3-7**, with regard to each section of the questionnaire. The questionnaire may be filled by the patient independently or with the practitioner's assistance.

5. Pain Disability Index

Shown in **Figure 3-8**, the PDI assesses another important aspect of pain: the level of disability caused by it (Tait et al., 1987; Jerome et al., 1991). The PDI was developed to be a brief measure of the degree to which pain interferes with normal functioning (Tait et al., 1987) and has been used to measure function disability in a wide range of chronically painful conditions. The PDI assesses perceived disability related to seven dimensions of life: family and home responsibilities, recreation, social activity, occupation, sexual behavior, self-care (e.g., taking a shower, getting dressed, driving), and life-support activity (e.g., eating, sleeping, breathing). Each dimension is rated by the patient on an 11-point scale (from 0, no disability, to 10, total disability),

F. ASSESSING PAIN LOCATION

Assessing pain location is important in helping clinicians to better locate and diagnose the cause of pain, and can aid in visualizing pain when it is felt at multiple sites on the body. Shown in **Figure 3-9** are four body diagrams (**A**: front and left-side views; **B**: back and right-side views) that can be used by practitioners and patients to assess the location of pain.

G. SCORING PAIN ASSESSMENT TOOLS

As Ronald Melzack has stated, to make the topic of pain a science, we must not only assess it but also measure or score it (Melzack et al., 2006).

1. OPS, FPS–R, VAS, NRS-101, VRS-5 Tools

Table 3-1 shows practitioners how to score the OPS and the FPS–R tools. For the OPS, the maximum score with

the photographic scale is 5; it is 100 if the numeric scale is used. **Table 3-2** shows how to score the VAS, the 101-point Numeric Rating Scale (NRS-101), and the 5-point Verbal Rating Scale (VRS-5). The maximum score for the VAS is 10; it is 100 for the NRC-101 and 4 for the VRS-5. The larger the scores on these pain assessment tools, the more severe the pain.

2. SF-MPQ and PDI Tools

Tables 3-3 and **3-4** show practitioners how to score the SF-MPQ and the PDI tools, respectively. These tools may be filled out by the patient independently or with the practitioner's assistance.

a. SF-MPQ

This powerful assessment tool indicates which pain dimension is dominant in the patient, thus helping clinicians to determine the best type of pain therapy to use. For example, a pain profile with a high intensity score (VAS = 8.5), a high sensory score (30/33), and a low affective score (3/12) is indicative of a pathology likely to benefit more from physical therapeutic interventions, such as the use of drugs, EPAs, and possibly surgery. Inversely, a pain profile revealing a high affective score (11/12), a low sensory score (8/33), and a moderate intensity score (VAS = 5) will guide the clinician toward using a cognitive/psychological type of intervention instead of a physical intervention. Moreover, the patient's pain intensity score (VAS) and present pain intensity (PPI) score, if known, would further help practitioners in gauging the acuity of pain and the potency of his or her therapeutic interventions. This textbook highly recommends the use of this tool particularly in cases of chronic pain.

b. PDI

As explained above, this tool assesses the level of disability related to pain. The patient's overall score provides the treating clinician additional insight into what activities are more disabling to the patient because of his or her pain. This tool provides the patient's total disability index (total PDI score) and apprises the clinician of the nature of activities that most disable the patient (i.e. physical, self-care, or life supporting).

VI.   OVERVIEW OF PAIN THERAPY

A. PAIN MANAGEMENT: AN OBLIGATION

Health-care systems, as well as all caregivers, have an obligation to provide comfort, and thus adequate pain management, to all suffering human beings. This is why pain is now considered as the fifth vital sign, requiring the same level of attention caregivers provide when facing dysfunctions of the other classic vital signs (body

Short Form McGill Pain Questionnaire (SF-MPQ)

Directives: *For the sensory and affective dimension only.* From the set of pain descriptors or words below, please select the words that best describe your pain now and for each of these words, rate the intensity of that particular quality of pain by putting a circle around the appropriate number. If a word does not correspond to your pain, please circle the number 0. *For the intensity dimension only.* VAS; Visual Analog Scale: Using a vertical line please mark, on the line below, your current level of pain. PPI; Present Pain Index: Please place an X beside the pain adjective below that best describes your current level of pain.

	None	Mild	Moderate	Severe
Sensory dimension:				
Throbbing	0	1	2	3
Shooting	0	1	2	3
Stabbing	0	1	2	3
Sharp	0	1	2	3
Cramping	0	1	2	3
Gnawing	0	1	2	3
Hot-Burning	0	1	2	3
Aching	0	1	2	3
Heavy	0	1	2	3
Tender	0	1	2	3
Splitting	0	1	2	3
Affective dimension:				
Tiring-Exhausting	0	1	2	3
Sickening	0	1	2	3
Fearful	0	1	2	3
Punishing-Cruel	0	1	2	3

Intensity dimension:

VAS   No pain _____ Worst possible pain

PPI   No pain   0   _____
            Mild   1   _____
            Discomforting 2   _____
            Distressing   3   _____
            Horrible   4   _____
            Excruciating   5   _____

FIGURE 3-7 The Short-Form McGill Pain Questionnaire. (From Melzack R (1987) The Short-Form McGill Pain Questionnaire. Pain, 30: 191–197. With permission.)

Pain Disability Index

Directives: The rating scales below are designed to measure the degree to which several aspects of your life are presently disrupted by pain. In other words, we would like to know how much your pain is preventing you from doing what you would normally do, or from doing it as well as you normally would. Respond to each category by indicating the overall impact of pain in your life, not just when the pain is at its worst. For each of the seven categories of live activity listed, please circle the number on the scale, which describes the level of disability you typically experience. A score of 0 means no disability at all, and a score of 10 signifies that all of the activities in which you would normally be involved have been totally disrupted or prevented by your pain.

1. Family/Home Responsibilities. This category refers to activities related to the home or family. It includes chores and duties performed around the house (i.e., yard work) and errands or favors for other family members (i.e., driving the children to school).

0	1	2	3	4	5	6	7	8	9	10

No
disability

Total
disability

2. Recreation. This category includes hobbies, sports, and other similar leisure time activites.

0	1	2	3	4	5	6	7	8	9	10

No
disability

Total
disability

3. Social Activity. This category refers to activities, which involve participation with friends and acquaintances other than family members. It includes parties, theater, concerts, dining out, and other social functions.

0	1	2	3	4	5	6	7	8	9	10

No
disability

Total
disability

4. Occupation. This category refers to activities that are part of or directly related to one's job. This includes non-paying jobs as well, such as that of a housewife or volunteer worker.

0	1	2	3	4	5	6	7	8	9	10

No
disability

Total
disability

5. Sexual Behavior. This category refers to the frequency and quality of one's sex life.

0	1	2	3	4	5	6	7	8	9	10

No
disability

Total
disability

6. Self-Care. This category includes activities, which involve personal maintenance and independent daily living (i.e., taking a shower, driving, getting dressed, etc.).

0	1	2	3	4	5	6	7	8	9	10

No
disability

Total
disability

7. Life-Support Activity. This category refers to basic life supporting behaviors such as eating, sleeping, and breathing.

0	1	2	3	4	5	6	7	8	9	10

No
disability

Total
disability

FIGURE 3-8 The Pain Disability Index. (Adapted from Tait RC, Pollard CA, Margolis RB, Duckro PN, Krause SJ (1987) The pain disability index: Psychometric and validity data. Arch Phys Med Rehab, 68: 438–441. With permission).

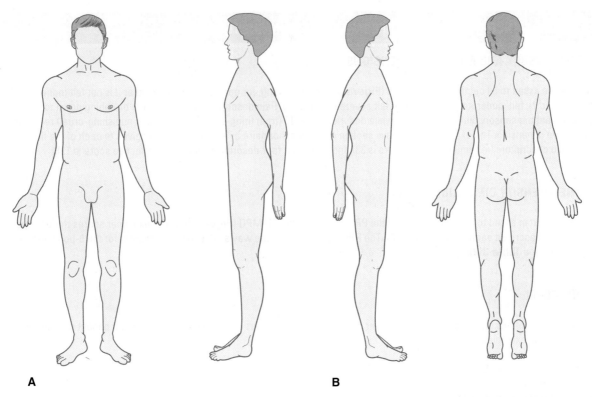

FIGURE 3-9 Assessment of pain location on the body. **(A)** Front and left-side view; **(B)** back and right-side view.

TABLE 3-2	SCORING THE VISUAL ANALOG SCALE, THE 101-POINT NUMERICAL RATING SCALE, AND THE 5-POINT VERBAL RATING SCALE

VISUAL ANALOG SCALE—SCORE: X/10

The examiner scores this tool (**Figure 3-6**) by measuring the distance, using a ruler, in millimeters from the no-pain anchor to the patient's mark. The total length of the scale is 10 cm. For example, a mark placed at 6.2 cm is equivalent to a pain score of 6.2.

101-POINT NUMERICAL RATING SCALE—SCORE: X/100 or %

The examiner scores this tool (**Figure 3-6**) by reporting the number, expressed out of 100, identified by the patient. For example, if the patient answers or writes "40," the score is then 40 or 40%.

5-POINT VERBAL RATING SCALE—SCORE: X/4

The examiner scores this tool (**Figure 3-6**) by assessing the right number (0–4) to the pain adjective identified by the patient. For example, if the patient describes his or her pain as distressing, a score of 2 is given by the examiner.

temperature, blood pressure, heart rate, respiration rate). In other words, when pain is present, clinicians are obliged to respond accordingly and provide adequate management. The broad and complex topic of pain therapy is beyond the scope of this textbook. Consequently, only an overview of the subject is presented in the following paragraphs.

B. GOALS OF PAIN MANAGEMENT

The ultimate goal of any therapeutic intervention is to maximize the patient's quality of life by minimizing his or her suffering while maximizing his or her function. Decreasing pain and maintaining function are thus central to any pain management approach. Although total abolishment of pain

TABLE 3-3	SCORING THE SHORT-FORM MCGILL PAIN QUESTIONNAIRE

FOR THE SENSORY AND AFFECTIVE DIMENSIONS OF PAIN

The patient is asked to fill out the questionnaire (**Figure 3-7**) by indicating, for each descriptor, whether it is not felt (none, 0), felt mildly (circled 1), felt moderately (circled 2), or felt severely (circled 3). Pain descriptors 1–11 (i.e., from throbbing down to splitting) represent the sensory dimension of pain while descriptors 12–15 (from tiring-exhausting down to punishing-cruel) represent the affective dimension. The examiner scores this section of the questionnaire by adding the scores given to each of the first eleven pain descriptors (maximum sensory score is 33) and to the last four descriptors (maximum affective score is 12).

FOR THE INTENSITY DIMENSION OF PAIN

The patient is then asked to fill out the VAS and the PPI sections of the SF-MPQ (**Figure 3-7**). The examiner scores the VAS the same way as described earlier (see **Table 3-2**). The PPI is scored the same way as described previously for the 5-point Verbal Rating Scale (see **Table 3-2**).

SF-MPQ SCORE

After completion of this questionnaire, the examiner may calculate and report one or many of the following patient pain scores. Below are some examples.

Sensory score: 15/33 or 45%
Affective score: 4/12 or 33%
Total SF-MPQ score: 19/45 or 43%
Pain intensity score (VAS): 4.2
Present Pain Intensity score (PPI): 2
The combination of these scores yields the patient's overall pain profile.

TABLE 3-4	SCORING THE PAIN DISABILITY INDEX

The patient is asked to fill out the questionnaire (**Figure 3-8**) by indicating, for each category of disability, the level of disability, on a scale of 0 (no disability) to 10 (maximum disability), caused by his or her current level of pain. Disability descriptors 1–5 relate to physical activities. Descriptors 6 and 7 refer to self-care and life supportability, respectively. The examiner scores this tool by adding up the numbers circled by the patient in relation to each of the seven dimensions of pain disability. The maximum score is 70.

PDI SCORE

After the PDI questionnaire is completed, the examiner may calculate and report on one or many of the following pain disability scores. Below are some examples.

Pain disability: physical activities—score: 24/50 or 48%
Pain disability: self-care—score: 5/10 or 50%
Pain disability: life-supportability—score: 1/10 or 10%
Total PDI score: 30/70 or 43%

is a legitimate therapeutic goal, it is often an *unrealistic one*, especially when caregivers deal with chronic pain.

C. PHARMACOTHERAPY

No one will dispute the fact that the most common therapeutic strategy to manage pain is pharmacotherapy or the use of drugs (Unruh, 2002; Wright et al., 2002; Katz et al., 2005; ACPA, 2005). Like all other pain treatments, pharmacotherapy has its own set of risks and benefits. The major risk associated with most drugs is their side effects on major organs such as the stomach, kidneys, and liver. Another risk, specifically associated with the use of opioid drugs, is addiction. The longer the drug is used, the greater the occurrence of these risks for patients.

D. TOLERANCE, PHYSICAL DEPENDENCE, AND ADDICTION

Physicians must pay particular attention to the phenomena of tolerance, physical dependence, and addiction when considering prolonged management of pain using pharmacotherapy (ACPA, 2005).

1. Tolerance

Tolerance is the condition in which one or more effects of a drug weaken with repeated use of the same dose (ACPA, 2005). This often leads to the prescription of stronger pills.

2. Physical Dependence

Physical dependence occurs when a patient who takes sufficient doses of certain drugs for a significant length of time suffers withdrawal symptoms if the drug is suddenly stopped (ACPA, 2005). Withdrawal symptoms, which should be monitored, may include sweating, runny nose, abdominal cramps, diarrhea, and nervousness.

3. Addiction

Addiction is the irresistible craving for a drug, or loss of control over its use, despite the harm this drug may cause (ACPA, 2005). There are four core elements in true addiction (the 4 Cs): *compulsive* use and preoccupation with the drug and its supply; inability to consistently *control* the quantities used; *craving* the psychic effects of the drug; and *continued* use despite adverse effects from the drug (ACPA, 2005). Physical dependence, therefore, is not addiction.

E. APPROACHES TO PAIN MANAGEMENT

The management of pain rests on two basic approaches: pharmacological and nonpharmacological. The pharmacological approach involves the use of nonopioid, opioid, and adjuvant drugs available over the counter or through a medical prescription. The nonpharmacological approach, on the other hand, refers to the use of surgery, EPAs, and psychotherapy. Presented in **Box 3-4** is an overview of the different drugs and interventions associated with each of these two therapeutic approaches (Unruh, 2002; Wright et al., 2002; American Geriatric Society Panel, 2002; Katz et al., 2005; ACPA, 2005).

1. Pharmacological Approach

Most pain conditions are managed, in the field of medicine, using three families of drugs: nonopioid, opioid, and adjuvant drugs. The term *adjuvant* implies that a drug is given in addition to, or in conjunction with, an oipiod drug to potentiate its analgesic effect.

a. Nonopioid Drugs

Nonopioid drugs include analgesics and nonsteroidal anti-inflammatory drugs (NSAIDs). These drugs are routinely used by patients themselves (e.g., over-the-counter drugs such as Tylenol and Advil) and by treating physicians (e.g., prescription drugs such as Celebrex or Voltaren) to manage mild-to-moderate, acute or chronic, nociceptive, and neuropathic pain. If used for a relatively prolonged period of time, these drugs can cause side effects such as gastric irritation and ulceration. What constitutes a prolonged period of time varies between patients and ranges usually from a few weeks to a few months, depending on the medication.

b. Opioid Drugs

The use of opioid drugs is strictly under a physician's control. Opioid drugs have a much greater pain-suppressing potency than nonopioid drugs and may give rise to physical dependence and addiction. Opioid drugs, or therapeutic narcotics, are used when analgesics and NSAIDs fail to provide adequate pain relief. Opioid drugs, if taken for a relatively long period of time, can cause more serious side effects such as nausea, dizziness, sleepiness, and, in some cases, physical dependence and addiction. As with nonopioid drugs, this period of time varies between patients and depends on the prescription.

c. Adjuvant Drugs

The use of adjuvant drugs is also under the total control of a physician. These drugs are used in conjunction with opioid drugs when adequate pain relief cannot be achieved by narcotics alone. Adjuvant drugs are designed primarily to treat disorders or symptoms often associated with pain, such as depression (antidepressant), epilepsy (anticonvulsant), anxiety (antianxiolytic), and muscle spasm and spasticity (muscle relaxant). Studies have shown that the use of these adjuvant drugs, in combination with opioid drugs, can lead to significantly greater pain relief, especially in severe cases of somatic and neuropathic pain (ACPA, 2005; Curatolo et al., 2002; Unruh, 2002; Wright et al., 2002).

2. Nonpharmacological Approaches

The pharmacological treatment of pain is not a panacea, and when it fails to provide adequate relief other pain management approaches are available. These nonpharmacological approaches comprise three types of therapy: surgery, EPAs, and psychotherapy (see **Box 3-4**).

a. Surgery

Because of its highly invasive and potentially life-threatening nature, surgery is usually restricted to cases in which the use of drugs and EPAs has failed to cure the organic pathology or failed to provide adequate pain relief. The aim of surgery is to repair pathological tissues and organs and often involves partial or total ablation of such tissues. For obvious reasons, pharmacotherapy is always used postsurgically to alleviate surgical pain.

Box 3-4	Common Approaches to Pain Management and Overview of Therapeutic Interventions

PHARMACOLOGICAL

NONOPIOID	OPIOID	ADJUVANT
Analgesic ■ Tylenol *NSAIDs* ■ Aspirin ■ Aleve ■ Advil ■ Motrin ■ Celebrex ■ Vioxx ■ Bextra ■ Naprosen ■ Voltaren	*Narcotic* ■ Dilaudid ■ Demerol ■ MS-Contin ■ Oxy-Contin ■ Talwin	*Antidepressant* ■ Elavil ■ Zoloft ■ Effexor *Anticonvulsant* ■ Neurontin ■ Tegretol ■ Dilantin *Antianxiolytic* ■ Valium ■ Ativan *Muscle relaxant* ■ Flexeril ■ Robaxin ■ Lioresal

NONPHARMACOLOGICAL

SURGERY	ELECTROPHYSICAL AGENTS	PSYCHOTHERAPY
Corrective/ablative	TENS	Cognitive therapy
Arthroplasty	Cryotherapy	Behavioral therapy
Prosthetic implants	Thermotherapy	
Thalamotomy	Laser therapy	
Tractotomy		
Hypothalamotomy		
Peripheral neurectomy		
Sympathectomy		
Rhizotomy		

b. Electrophysical Agents

The use of EPAs covered in this textbook presents a major advantage over the pharmacological and surgical approaches, in that they have no known side effects. However, EPAs also have a major disadvantage, in that their pain-suppressing potency is often weaker and shorter-lasting than that associated with opioid drugs and surgery. Because the pain-suppressing potency of some EPAs, like the use of TENS, may be comparable with that of nonopioid drugs, EPAs appear to be an adequate alternative to nonopioid drugs for the management of mild-to-moderate postsurgical, somatic, and neuropathic pain (Barlas et al., 2006). This is especially true for those patients whose health status (specifically, their stomach, liver, and kidney function) is already compromised and can be further aggravated by taking nonopioid drugs. EPAs are also appealing to those health-conscious patients whose preference is to use pain therapeutics with minimal side effects first, leaving the door open to take drugs later if necessary.

c. Psychotherapy

Finally, the use of psychotherapy, which also has no known side effects, can be of significant help to those patients whose chronic pain has led them to present significant psychological and emotional distress, leaving them unable to experience adequate pain relief or to adequately cope with their pain. Psychotherapy may be the first choice of treatment for those patients who have refused surgery and who just cannot get adequate pain relief using drugs. It may also be the treatment of choice for those patients suffering from chronic pain who have had enough of all the side effects caused by their medications. Psychotherapeutic and cognitive interventions are used primarily in cases of severe chronic organic and nonorganic (true psychogenic) pain.

F. PROPOSED MECHANISMS OF ACTION

It is beyond the scope of this chapter to cover in detail all the proposed mechanisms underlying the therapeutic effects of pharmacological and nonpharmacological treatments. Nonetheless, **Box 3-5** provides an overview of the proposed mechanisms put forward in the literature to explain how nonopioid, opioid, and adjuvant drugs, as well as some EPAs, work to modulate pain. It can be seen that both nonopioid drugs and EPAs share a common mechanism, acting essentially on the inflammatory phase of healing, at the wound site, by altering tissue chemistry. EPAs also have other related mechanisms acting on the injured tissue's vascular and metabolic responses. Opioid and adjuvant drugs also share a similar mechanism, acting on both the peripheral and central nervous system, by altering brain chemistry.

G. MIXTURE OF THERAPEUTIC APPROACHES

Both the pharmacological and nonpharmacological approaches can be used by the treating clinician either in isolation or in combination, depending on the pain condition being treated. The common practice in pain management is to begin with nonopioid drugs and EPAs and then move on to the more potent opioid and adjuvant drugs, and, if necessary, to corrective and ablative surgery if adequate pain relief still cannot be achieved. If the pain becomes intractable, then stimulative (implanted TENS) and drug delivery (implanted pumps) systems are usually considered and used. Psychotherapy and cognitive therapy are usually used in severe chronic cases, when the patient's ability to adequately cope with the pain is compromised and the patient needs psychological and emotional support in addition to better coping skills.

H. PLACEBO ANALGESIA

This chapter on pain cannot end without touching on the important and controversial topic of placebo analgesia because, in some circumstances, placebo treatments can be as effective as real treatment to suppress pain (Roche, 2002; Fields et al., 2006). Among all symptoms related to pathologies, pain appears to be the most common symptom known to respond to placebo therapy (Roche, 2002).

Box 3-5   Proposed Mechanisms of Action of Drugs and Electrophysical Agents

Nonopioid
- At the site of injury
- On the inflammatory phase of healing
- Alter injured tissue chemistry

Opioid
- At the level of the central nervous system
- On endogenous opioid receptors
- Alter spinal cord and brain chemistry

Adjuvant

Antidepressant
- Alter brain chemistry
- Sedative effect, improve sleep
- Reduce depression

Anticonvulsant
- Alter brain chemistry
- Stabilize nerve membrane
- Reduce ectopic discharges

Antianxiolytic
- Alter brain chemistry
- Reduce anxiety

Muscle relaxant
- Alter brain chemistry
- Reduce postinjury muscle spasm and spasticity

Electrophysical Agents
- At the site of injury
- On the inflammatory phase of healing
- Alter chemical, nervous, metabolic, and vascular reactions
- Act as counterirritants

1. Origin

Some believe that the word placebo is derived from the Latin verb *placere*, meaning "to please," whereas others believe it comes from the Latin stem *placebit*, meaning "it will please" (Roche, 2002; Fields et al., 2006). Regardless of its source, common to the origin of this word is its pleasing aspect for the patient.

2. Meaning

The meaning of placebo analgesia is the patient's expectation of effectiveness of the therapeutic intervention he or she is receiving (Fields et al., 2006). There is a body of evidence to suggest that the hope for pain relief and the suggestion that such a relief will come are critical parameters in the generation of placebo analgesia (Fields et al., 2006). Placebo analgesia may be seen as a demonstration of the body's natural tendency to reduce pain, a demonstration that is activated by psychological mechanisms such as conditioning and expectancy (Roche, 2002).

3. Induction of Placebo Analgesia

Placebo analgesia is therapeutically desirable. It is a pain-suppressing response that can be triggered by positive verbal expectations and motivational attitudes and the reduction of anxiety and stress. Placebo analgesia is closely associated with the management of pain using psychotherapy.

4. Nocebo Effect

Opposite to a placebo response is the nocebo response. *Nocebo* is the patient's expectation that his or her treatment is ineffective or that it will make the pain worse (Fields et al., 2006).

5. Scientific Evidence for Placebo Analgesia

Two relatively recent meta-analyses conducted by Hrobjartsson et al. (2001, 2004) have shown little evidence to support the claim that placebo therapies have a significant clinical effect. Both analyses have shown, however, that when placebo therapies had a positive therapeutic response it was for the continuous management of pain, thus giving support to the concept of placebo analgesia.

6. Clinical Importance

Research has shown that both placebo and nocebo responses can significantly affect the outcome of pain therapy. Just as the placebo effect works by making the patient believe he or she will get better, the nocebo effect can serve to make him or her worse. If the patient expects pain relief, he or she will present a placebo analgesia response, regardless of whether a real treatment, a placebo treatment, or no treatment is administered. In contrast, if the patient expects that no relief will be obtained or that the pain may get worse, then a nocebo response will manifest itself.

I. MAXIMIZING QUALITY OF LIFE

Finally, clinicians should always remember that the ultimate goal of pain management is not to try to abolish pain at all costs but, rather, to maximize the patient's quality of life and function by minimizing his or her pain.

CRITICAL THINKING QUESTIONS

Clarification: What is meant by pain, categories of pain, and pain modulation?

Assumptions: You assume that pain has three dimensions and that it is possible to assess, measure, and score these dimensions. How do you justify making that assumption?

Reasons and evidence: The perception, or experience, of nociceptive pain implies the fulfillment of five distinctive physiological phases. How did this come to be?

Viewpoints or perspectives: You agree with the consensus that pain can be objectively and quantitatively assessed and scored. What would someone who disagrees with you say?

Implications and consequences: You state that pain modulation occurs peripherally and centrally. What are you implying by that?

About the question: Is it possible to modulate pain without the use of drugs or surgical procedures? Why do you think I ask this question?

References

Articles

Beyer J, Denyes M, Villarruel A (1992) The creation, validation, and continuing development of the Oucher: A measurement of pain intensity in children. J Pediat Nurs, 7: 335–346

Beyer JE, Knott C (1998) Construct validity estimation of the African-American and Hispanic versions of the Oucher scale. J Pediat Nurs, 13: 20–31

Beyer JE, Turner SB, Jones L, Young L, Onikul R, Bohaty B (2005) The alternate forms reliability of the Oucher pain scale. Pain Manag Nurs, 6:10–17

Bieri D, Reeve R, Champion GD, Addicoat L, Ziegler J (1990) The Faces Pain Scale for the self-assessment of the severity of pain experienced by children: Development, initial validation and preliminary investigation for ratio scale properties. Pain, 41:139–150

Chambers CT, Finley GA, McGrath PJ, Walsh TM (2003) The parent's postoperative pain measure: Replication and extension to 2–6 year-old children. Pain, 105: 437–443

Chambers CT, Reid GJ, McGrath PJ, Finley GA (1996) Development and preliminary validation of a postoperative pain measure for parents. Pain, 68: 307–313

Grunau RVE, Craig KD (1987) Pain expression in neonates: Facial action and cry. Pain, 28: 395–410

Grunau RE, Oberlander T, Holsti L, Whitfield MF (1998) Bedside application of the Neonatal Facial Coding System in pain assessment of premature neonates. Pain, 76: 277–286

Hicks CL, von Baeyer CL, Spafford P, van Korlaar I, Goodenough, B (2001) The Faces Pain Scale-Revised: Toward a common metric in pediatric pain measurement. Pain, 93: 173-–183

Jensen MP, Karoly P, Braver S (1986) The measurement of clinical pain intensity: A comparison of six methods. Pain, 27: 117–126

Jerome A, Gross RT (1991) Pain disability index: Construct and discriminant validity. Arch Phys Med Rehabil, 72: 920–922

Katz J, Melzack R (1999) Measurement of pain. Surg Clin North Am, 79: 231–252

Katz WA, Rothenberg R (2005) Treating the patient in pain. J Clin Rheumatol, 11: S16–S28

Melzack R. (1987) The short-form McGill Pain Questionnaire. Pain, 30: 191–197

Melzack (1975) The McGill pain questionnaire: Major properties and scoring methods. Pain, 1: 277–299

Melzack R, Wall PD (1965) Pain mechanism: A new theory. Science, 150: 971–979

Mense S (2003) The pathogenesis of muscle pain. Cur Pain Headache Rep, 7: 419–425

Tait RC, Pollard CA, Margolis RB, Duckro PN, Krause SJ (1987) The pain disability index: psychometric and validity data. Arch Phys Med Rehabil, 68: 438–441

Review Articles

American Geriatric Society Panel (2002) The management of persistent pain in older persons. J Amer Ger Soc, 50: S205–S224

Bird J (2005) Assessing pain in older people. Nurs Stand, 19: 45–52

Curatolo M, Sveticic G. (2002). Drug combinations in pain treatment: A review of the published evidence and a method for finding the optimal combination. Best Pract Res Clin Anaesthesiol, 16: 507–519

Duhn LJ, Medves JM (2004) A systematic integrative review of infant pain assessment tools. Adv Neonatal Care, 4: 126–140

Hrobjartsson A, Gotzsche PC (2001) Is the placebo powerless? An analysis of clinical trials comparing placebo with no treatment. New Engl J Med, 344: 1594–1602

Hrobjartsson A, Gotzsche PC (2004) Is the placebo powerless? Update of a systematic review with 52 new randomized trials comparing placebo with no treatment. J Intern Med, 256: 91–100

Chapters of Textbooks

Barlas P, Lundeberg T (2006) Transcutaneous electrical nerve stimulation and acupuncture. In: Wall and Melzack's Textbook of Pain, 5th ed. McMahon S, Koltzenburg M (Eds). Churchill Livingstone, Edinburg, pp 583–590

Bielefeld K, Gebhart G (2006) Visceral pain: Basic mechanism. In: Wall and Melzack's Textbook of Pain, 5th ed. McMahon S, Koltzenburg M (Eds). Churchill Livingstone, Edinburg, pp 721–736

Boivie J (2006) Central pain. In: Wall and Melzack's Textbook of Pain, 5th ed. McMahon S, Koltzenburg M (Eds). Churchill Livingstone, Edinburg, pp 1057–1074

Bushnell MC, Apkarian AV (2006) Representation of pain in the brain. In: Wall and Melzack's Textbook of Pain, 5th ed. McMahon S, Koltzenburg M (Eds). Churchill Livingstone, Edinburg, pp 107–124

Craig KD (2006) Emotions and psychobiology. In: Wall and Melzack's Textbook of Pain, 5th ed. McMahon S, Koltzenburg M (Eds). Churchill Livingstone, Edinburg, pp 231–239

Dahl JB, Kehlet (2006) Post-operative pain and its management. In: Wall and Melzack's Textbook of Pain, 5th ed. McMahon S, Koltzenburg M (Eds). Churchill Livingstone, Edinburg, pp 635–651

Devor M (2006) Response of nerves to injury in relation to neuropathic pain. In: Wall and Melzack's Textbook of Pain, 5th ed. McMahon S, Koltzenburg M (Eds). Churchill Livingstone, Edinburg, pp 909–927

Derasari MD (2003) Taxonomy of pain syndromes. In: Pain Medicine: A Comprehensive Review, 2nd ed. Prithvi Raj P (Ed). Mosby, St-Louis, pp 17–22

Dostrovsky JO, Craig AD (2006) Ascending projection systems. In: Wall and Melzack's Textbook of Pain, 5th ed. McMahon S, Koltzenburg M (Eds). Churchill Livingstone, Edinburg, pp 187–203

Flor H, Turk DC (2006) Cognitive and learning aspects. In: Wall and Melzack's Textbook of Pain, 5th ed. McMahon S, Koltzenburg M (Eds). Churchill Livingstone, Edinburg, pp 241–258

Fields Hl, Basbaum AI, Heinricher MM (2006a) Central nervous system mechanisms of pain modulation. In: Wall and Melzack's Textbook of Pain, 5th ed. McMahon S, Koltzenburg M (Eds). Churchill Livingstone, Edinburg, pp 125–142

Fields HL, Price DD (2006b) Placebo analgesia. In: Wall and Melzack's Textbook of Pain, 5th ed. McMahon S, Koltzenburg M (Eds). Churchill Livingstone, Edinburg, pp 361–367

Gagliese L, Melzack R (2006) Pain in the elderly. In: Wall and Melzack's Textbook of Pain, 5th ed. McMahon S, Koltzenburg M (Eds). Churchill Livingstone, Edinburg, pp 1169–1180

Galea MP (2002) Neuroanatomy of the nociceptive system. In: Pain: A Textbook for Therapists. Strong J, Unruh AM, Wright A, Baxter GD (Eds). Churchill Livingstone, Edinburg, pp 13–41

Mantyh PW (2006) Cancer pain: Causes, Consequences and Therapeutic Opportunities. In: Wall and Melzack's Textbook of Pain, 5th ed. McMahon S, Koltzenburg M (Eds). Churchill Livingstone, Edinburg, pp 1087–1097

McGrath PJ, Unruh AM (2006) Measurement and assessment of paediatric pain. In: Wall and Melzack's Textbook of Pain, 5th ed. McMahon S, Koltzenburg M (Eds). Churchill Livingstone, Edinburg, pp 305–315

Melzack R, Katz J (2006) Pain assessment in adult patients. In: Wall and Melzack's Textbook of Pain, 5th ed. McMahon S, Koltzenburg M (Eds). Churchill Livingstone, Edinburg, pp 291–304

Meyer RA, Ringkamp M, Campbell JN, Raja SN (2006) Peripheral mechanisms of cutaneous nociception. In: Wall and Melzack's Textbook of Pain, 5th ed. McMahon S, Koltzenburg M (Eds). Churchill Livingstone, Edinburg, pp 3–34

Parris WC (2003) The history of pain medicine. In: Pain Medicine: A Comprehensive Review, 2nd ed. Prithvi Raj P (Ed). Mosby, St-Louis, pp 3–6

Roche PA (2002) Placebo analgesia—friend not foe. In: Pain: A Textbook for Therapists. Strong J, Unruh AM, Wright A, Baxter GD (Eds). Churchill Livingstone, Edinburg, pp 81–97

Rubertone JA, Barbe M (2005) Wound healing and pain. In: Modalities for Therapeutic Interventions. Michlovitz SL, Nolan TP (Eds). FA Davis Co., pp 15–40

Sikes RW (2004) The physiology and psychology of pain. In: Therapeutic Modalities, 3rd ed. Starkey C (Ed). FA Davis Co, Philadelphia, pp 29–54

Schug SA, Gandham N (2006) Opioids: Clinical use. In: Wall and Melzack's Textbook of Pain, 5th ed. McMahon S, Koltzenburg M (Eds). Churchill Livingstone, Edinburg, pp 443–457

Unruh (2002) Generic principles of practice. In: Pain: A Textbook for Therapists. Strong J, Unruh AM, Wright A, Baxter GD (Eds). Churchill Livingstone, Edinburg, pp 151–167

Weisberg J, Deturk W (2006) Pain. In: Integrated Physical Agents in Rehabilitation, 2nd ed. Hecox B, Andemicael Mehreteab T, Weisberg J, Sanko J (Eds). Prentice Hall, Upper Saddle River, pp 57–71

Wright A (2002) Neurophysiology of pain and pain modulation. In: A Textbook for Therapists. Strong J, Unruh AM, Wright A, Baxter GD (Eds). Churchill Livingstone, Edinburg, pp 43–64

Wright A, Benson HAE, O.Callaghan J (2002) Pharmacology of pain management. In: A Textbook for Therapists. Strong J, Unruh AM, Wright A, Baxter GD (Eds). Churchill Livingstone, Edinburg, pp 307–324

Textbooks

Melzack R, Wall PD (1982) The Challenge of Pain. Penguin Books Ltd, New York

Mense S, Simons DG (2001) Muscle Pain. Understanding its Nature, Diagnosis and Treatment. Lippincott Williams & Wilkins, Philadelphia

Merskey H, Bogduk N (1994) Classification of Chronic Pain. Description of Chronic Pain Syndromes and Definition of Pain Terms, 2nd ed. Elsevier, New York

McMahon S, Koltzenburg M (2006) Wall and Melzack's Textbook of Pain, 5th ed. Churchill Livingstone, Edinburg

Strong J, Unruh AM, Wright A, Baxter GD (2002) Pain: A Textbook for Therapists. Churchill Livingstone, Edinburg

Turk DC, Melzack R (2001) Handbook of Pain Assessment, 2nd ed. The Gilford Press, New York

Other Resources

American Chronic Pain Association (ACPA) (2005) Medication and Chronic Pain—Supplement 2005. American Chronic Pain Association, Rocklin

Electronic Resources

www.iasp-pain.org: Internal Society for the Study of Pain
www.theacpa.org: American Chronic Pain Association
www.ampainsoc.org: American Pain Society
www.painmed.org: American Academy of Pain Medicine

CHAPTER 4

Therapeutic Spectrum of Electrophysical Agents

Learning Objectives

Knowledge: List the cardinal signs and symptoms, and their respective causes, associated with an acute soft-tissue pathology.

Comprehension: Compare the choice of electrophysical agents (EPAs) and related therapeutic interventions used during the first, second, and third stages of tissue healing.

Application: Show how the application of EPAs benefits the healing process of soft tissues.

Analysis: Explain the differences among the therapeutic goals for each stage of healing.

Synthesis: Explain how the judicious and timely use of EPAs may benefit soft-tissue healing.

Evaluation: Discuss the spectrum of EPAs in relation to the future approaches to soft-tissue pathology.

I. THERAPEUTIC SPECTRUM AND PURPOSES

A. SPECTRUM OF ELECTROPHYSICAL AGENTS

The electrophysical agents (EPAs) covered in this textbook have a broad therapeutic spectrum that acts directly on impairment caused by tissue pathologies and indirectly on functional limitations and disabilities that can result from such pathologies (see Chapter 1). They make up, with the use of medication, surgery, therapeutic exercises, mobilizations, and manipulations, the overall spectrum of physical therapeutics for the management of soft-tissue pathology.

B. PURPOSE OF ELECTROPHYSICAL AGENTS

The primary purpose of EPAs is to enhance the natural soft-tissue healing process triggered by pathology (see Chapter 2) while alleviating the pain associated with such pathologies (see Chapter 3). Their secondary purpose is to minimize functional limitations and disabilities resulting from impairments, for example, to accelerate the patient's recovery and return to physical and social activities (see Denegar, 2000; Prentice, 2000; Delforge, 2002a,b; Cameron, 2003; Starkey, 2004; Fedorcyk et al., 2005; Houghton, 2005; Johnson, 2005; Knight et al., 2008a,b).

C. JUDICIOUS AND TIMELY SELECTION

As discussed in Chapter 2, the soft-tissue healing process usually consists of four consecutive and overlapping phases, beginning with the hemostatic phase and followed, in that order, by the inflammatory, proliferative, and remodeling/maturation phases. As is the case with most therapeutic interventions, effective enhancement of this natural tissue healing process through the use of EPAs requires, from the practitioner, a judicious selection and a timely application of these agents (see Section II, Selection Based on Timing).

D. COMBINED THERAPIES

Effective management of soft-tissue pathology rests with the use of combined therapeutic interventions. To use a solo EPA for the management of a case is therefore not recommended. The common clinical practice is to use EPAs in conjunction with, or as a *complement* to, medication and surgery, depending on the severity of the case under treatment. EPAs are also regularly used in conjunction with other therapeutic interventions such as therapeutic exercises, manual therapy techniques including mobilizations and manipulations, and physical conditioning programs.

II. SELECTION BASED ON HEALING PHASES

A. SELECTION AND TIMING

As previously mentioned, the selection and timing of application of EPAs are strongly related to the phases of the healing process (see Chapter 2). To use EPAs *judiciously* means to select the EPAs that will best enhance the current healing phase of the pathological tissue and best minimize the potential functional limitations and disabilities resulting from such pathology. To use it in a timely fashion means to apply them during the period of time in which they will yield optimal results. For example, there is a consensus in the field that the application of cryotherapy immediately after an acute soft tissue injury is the best choice practitioners can make to control the signs and symptoms associated with the first (hemostasis) and second (inflammatory) phases of healing (Knight, 1995). Another example is to use ultrasound therapy to enhance the third (proliferative) and fourth (remodeling/maturation) phases of healing, after the inflammatory phase has subsided.

B. ACUITY OF SOFT-TISSUE WOUNDS

Injury and disease are the primary causes of soft tissue pathology. Wounds may present in their acute, subacute, or chronic state (Chapter 1). How can a practitioner differentiate between these three levels of wound acuity? Generally speaking, the more acute the wound, the more pronounced the signs and symptoms related to the hemostatic and inflammation phases of soft tissue healing. Because the judicious and timely usage of EPAs is closely related to the presence and magnitude of these signs and symptoms, it is important here to briefly describe them.

1. Cardinal Signs and Symptoms

All soft tissue wounds are characterized by cellular and vascular damages. **Table 4-1** lists the cardinal signs and symptoms, and their causes, associated with the acute and subacute states of injury. The presence and magnitude of each of them will depend on the acuity of the pathology, its severity (i.e., amount of tissue damage), and the vascularity of the injured tissues. For example, a recent and moderate injury to a well-vascularized tissue such as skeletal muscle will yield more severe signs and symptoms than a similar injury to a chronic and much less vascularized tissue such as a ligament.

2. RCTDSA

The acronym RCTDSA stands for six signs and symptoms commonly observed in acute and subacute types of soft-tissue pathologies (**Table 4-1**). It includes redness (*Rubor*) and heating (*Calor*) of the skin overlying the

TABLE 4-1	CARDINAL SIGNS AND SYMPTOMS OF ACUTE/SUBACUTE SOFT TISSUE PATHOLOGY
SIGN OR SYMPTOM	**CAUSE**
Erythema (rubor, R)	Skin redness resulting from capillary engorgement
Hyperthermia (calor, C)	Skin heating resulting from erythema
Edema (tumor, T)	Segment enlargement, or swelling, resulting from excess fluid in the interstitial spaces
Pain (dolor, D)	Discomfort or suffering resulting from the activation of nociceptors at wound site
Spasm (S)	Reflex muscle contraction resulting from pain
Abnormal function (A)	Partial-to-total dysfunction of tissue due to cellular damage, as well as due to pain and muscle spasm

wound, coupled with edema (*Tumor*) and pain (*Dolor*). Often associated with these four cardinal signs and symptoms are two additional clinical manifestations: muscle spasm (S) triggered by pain (the vicious pain/spasm circle) and abnormal function (A), the latter being the result of tissue damage causing pain, spasm, and edema.

III. STAGES OF THERAPEUTIC INTERVENTION

A. FRAMEWORK FOR EPA SELECTION

This textbook proposes, as shown in **Boxes 4-1** to **4-3,** respectively, a *three-stage intervention framework,* for using EPAs to treat soft-tissue pathology. These three stages are closely related to the four basic phases of tissue healing (see Chapter 2) and to the cardinal signs and symptoms (see **Table 4-1**) often associated with soft-tissue pathology. The first stage of intervention, described in **Box 4-1**, relates to the control of bleeding and inflammation, that is, to the first and second phases of healing. The second stage, presented in **Box 4-2**, is associated with the enhancement of repair tissue formation and proliferation (i.e., the third phase of healing). The third and final stage of intervention, illustrated in **Box 4-3**, refers to the enhancement of repair tissue remodeling, maturation, and function (i.e., the fourth phase of healing).

B. FIRST STAGE: CONTROLLING BLEEDING AND INFLAMMATION

It is well established in the scientific literature that, if the bleeding and inflammatory responses are not properly controlled, satisfactory wound healing may be delayed and in some circumstances is unlikely to occur (see Chapter 2). Thus, the first stage of therapeutic intervention after acute

tissue damage is to control the hemostatic and inflammatory reactions taking place at the wound site. The evidence from the scientific literature presented in this textbook shows that a broad spectrum of EPAs can be used, as shown in **Box 4-1**, to meet the therapeutic goals associated with this first stage of intervention.

1. Minimizing Wound Bleeding

The use of cryotherapy (see Chapter 8) can minimize wound bleeding *only* if applied immediately after the injury, that is, within the seconds and minutes following it (Knight et al., 2008a,b). Remember that blood clotting is a very rapid physiological phenomenon designed to minimize hemorrhaging. Applying cryotherapy hours after injury, therefore, has very limited effect on wound bleeding.

2. Minimizing Secondary Tissue Damage

Cryotherapy, if applied within the first 24 to 48 hours following soft-tissue damage, can significantly minimize secondary tissue damages (for details, see Chapter 8). Research has shown that primary tissue damages (dead cells) may lead to significant secondary tissue damages involving the viable cells located within the immediate vicinity of the wound, through enzymatic and metabolic changes (see Knight et al., 2008a,b for details). To minimize secondary tissue damage, therefore, is to restrict total tissue damages. The lesser the total amount of tissue damages, the smaller the wound size at the site of injury. The smaller the wound, the faster and better the tissue repair process may be. Cryotherapy, when used in conjunction with other therapeutic interventions such as rest (R) and protection (P), for example, the use of canes, splints, or slings, can further minimize secondary tissue damage. The delivery of anti-inflammatory drugs at the wound site, using iontophoresis therapy (for details, see Chapter 13) is another EPA practitioners can use to minimize secondary tissue damage (**Box 4-1**).

Box 4-1   **First Stage: Controlling Bleeding and Inflammation**

Key Physiological Events

Soft-tissue damage causes bleeding, which triggers a cascade of cellular and chemical responses that lead to blood clotting and to a complex inflammatory response necessary for wound healing.

Therapeutic Goals	Spectrum of Electrophysical Agents
Minimize wound bleeding	Cryotherapy—only if applied immediately or within the first few minutes postinjury
Minimize secondary tissue damage	Cryotherapy[a]—only if applied within the first 24 to 48 hours postinjury Iontophoresis (anti-inflammatory drugs)
Minimize edema	Cryotherapy[b] Intermittent pneumatic compression Cryohydrotherapy
Minimize pain and muscle spasm	Cryotherapy TENS Iontophoresis (analgesic drugs) PRICE

[a]Cryotherapy alone or combined with rest (R) and protection (P)
[b]Cryotherapy alone or combined with compression (C) and elevation (E)
PRICE: Application of *P*rotection, *R*est, *I*ce or cryotherapy, *C*ompression, and *E*levation; TENS, transcutaneous electrical nerve stimulation.

Box 4-2   **Second Stage: Enhancing Scar Tissue Formation and Proliferation**

Key Physiological Events

Angiogenesis and fibroplasia lead to the formation and proliferation of immature repair tissue at the wound site.

Therapeutic Goals	Spectrum of Electrophysical Agents
Promote angiogenesis	Hot pack and paraffin bath therapy
Promote fibroplasia	Fluidotherapy
Enhance local blood flow	Shortwave diathermy therapy
Enhance local cellular metabolism	Ultrasound therapy Thermohydrotherapy Low-level laser therapy Microcurrent therapy High-voltage pulsed-current therapy Ultraviolet therapy
Minimize pain	TENS therapy
Optimize wound contraction	Continuous passive motion therapy Spinal traction therapy

Box 4-3	Third Stage: Enhancing Repair Tissue Remodeling, Maturation, and Function

Key Physiological Events

Immature repair tissue is remodeled, gradually matures, and heals, in most cases, as functional repair tissue.

Therapeutic Goals	Spectrum of Electrophysical Agents
Enhance tissue repair	Ultrasound therapy Low-level laser therapy
Enhance tissue strength and elasticity	Continuous passive motion therapy Spinal traction therapy
Enhance muscle force/endurance	Russian current therapy Interferential current therapy

3. Minimizing Edema

Swelling is the enlargement of a tissue or organ resulting from edema, which is the accumulation of fluids in the interstitial spaces. Cryotherapy can reduce edema at the wound site if applied within the first 24 to 48 hours postinjury. It does this by minimizing secondary tissue damage (Knight et al., 2008a,b). Minimizing secondary damage reduces the amount of free proteins in the wound vicinity which, in turn, leads to less edema formation (for details, see Chapter 8). Edema prevention and reduction can be further enhanced if cryotherapy is used with two other therapeutic interventions, such as elevation (E) and compression (C). The use of intermittent pneumatic compression therapy (see Chapter 22) and cryohydrotherapy (see Chapter 9) can also be used to minimize the formation of postinjury edema.

4. Minimizing Pain and Muscle Spasm

Pain is always, and muscle spasm is occasionally, associated with soft tissue pathology. Pain results from the chemical activation, triggered by the inflammatory response, of nociceptors buried within the tissues located in the vicinity of the wound (see Chapter 3). Muscle spasm results from the vicious pain-spasm cycle, the role of which is to minimize pain by restricting joint movement. Cryotherapy (see Chapter 8) can reduce pain by acting as a counterirritant stimulus (cold over pain) or by acting on the pain nerve fibers (reduce/block nerve conduction). It can reduce muscle spasm by decreasing pain (less pain, less muscle spasm). TENS (see Chapter 14) can be used to modulate pain through its action on the endogenous opiate and gate systems. Iontophoresis (see Chapter 13), using analgesic drugs, can also be employed during this first stage of intervention to modulate pain.

5. PRICE

As stated previously, this first stage of therapeutic intervention aims at controlling tissue bleeding and inflammation. The judicious and timely choice of EPAs, in combination with other therapeutic interventions or approaches, such as elevation and compressions, is critical to the success of therapy during this crucial period of healing. The PRICE approach (Protection, Rest, Ice or cryotherapy, Compression, and Elevation) remains the approach of choice in the field of sports medicine and therapy to manage bleeding and inflammation after acute tissue injury (for details see Knight et al., 2008a,b).

B. SECOND STAGE: ENHANCING REPAIR TISSUE PROLIFERATION AND FORMATION

This second stage of the healing process implies new therapeutic goals designed to enhance repair tissue proliferation and formation. **Box 4-2** lists these goals and the related spectrum of EPAs practitioners can use to achieve them.

1. Promote Angiogenesis, Fibroplasia, Blood Flow, and Metabolism

The proliferation and formation of repair tissues rest on a cascade of interrelated physiological events. *Angiogenesis*, the formation of new blood vessels, and *fibroplasia*, the laying down of repair tissues, are key processes which are optimized by increased blood flow and metabolism at the wound site. Numerous EPAs can be used to achieve these responses or therapeutic goals. The judicious choices are agents that are capable of inducing superficial and deep thermal effects in soft tissues, such as hot packs and paraffin wax (see Chapter 6), fluidotherapy (see Chapter 7), hydrotherapy (see Chapter 9), shortwave diathermy therapy (see Chapter 10), and ultrasound therapy (see Chapter 20). Other EPAs that can be use during this healing stage include low-level laser therapy (see Chapter 11) and ultraviolet therapy (see Chapter 12), microcurrent therapy (see Chapter 15), and high-voltage pulsed-current therapy (see Chapter 16), all of which have the capacity to enhance wound healing.

2. Minimizing Pain and Optimizing Wound Contraction

Decreasing pain (if still present) can best be managed with TENS (see Chapter 14) or one or more of the other thermal agents listed previously. Wound contraction may be improved with the application of continuous passive motion therapy (see Chapter 23) in cases of pathology to the upper and lower limbs, and spinal traction therapy (see Chapter 21) in cases of pathology to the spinal column. These two EPAs can induce the necessary mechanical tensile stress on maturing repair tissue.

D. THIRD STAGE: ENHANCING REPAIR TISSUE REMODELING, MATURATION, AND FUNCTION

As the immature repair tissue gives way to mature and, hopefully, functional tissue, another set of therapeutic goals and therapeutic EPAs must be introduced. The goals during this third stage of intervention, shown in **Box 4-3**, are to encourage optimal remodeling and maturation of these newly formed tissues in order to optimize function. Remodeling and maturation may be enhanced with low-level laser therapy (see Chapter 11) and ultrasound therapy (see Chapter 20). The promotion of maturation and function can also be enhanced with spinal traction therapy (see Chapter 21) and continuous passive motion therapy (see Chapter 22). Finally, the enhancement of repair tissue strength and endurance may also be achieved by means of neuromuscular electrical stimulation (NMES) therapy—through the application of Russian current (see Chapter 17) and interferential current (see Chapter 18) therapy. When the repair tissue is mature and strong enough, the use of the above EPAs is replaced by active functional training and conditioning exercise programs, with the aim of returning the patient to leisure, sport, and work activities.

IV. MANAGEMENT OF SOFT-TISSUE PATHOLOGY

A. TODAY'S APPROACH

The current approach to the therapeutic management of soft tissue pathology is to use conservative treatments, such as therapeutic exercises, manual therapy, and EPAs, and more invasive treatments such as medication and surgery.

B. TOMORROW'S APPROACH

With the rapid advancement of science in the field of soft tissue repair, tomorrow's therapeutic approach will differ drastically from that of today. The following are just a few examples of therapeutic interventions or therapies that may well become common in the next decade.

1. Exogenous Growth Factor Therapy

Research has shown that a well-regulated growth factor cascade is important for the orderly progression of steps in the wound-healing process. Injection of growth factors in patients suffering from soft tissue injury may thus be beneficial.

2. Tissue Replacement

Research in tissue engineering opens the door for replacing injured tissue with tissue constructed in vitro for subsequent implantation in vivo that has similar structural, physiological, and mechanical properties.

3. Gene Therapy

The ability to deliver genes to the cells to improve soft tissue healing outcomes is another therapeutic approach that may be beneficial to millions of patients.

4. Stem Cell Therapy

Stem cell therapy is perhaps the most exciting of all potential treatments. Injecting stem cells into damaged tissue may significantly contribute to the repair and regeneration of soft tissue pathology by optimizing the healing process.

CRITICAL THINKING QUESTIONS

Clarification: What is meant by judicious selection and timely application of EPAs based on a three-stage intervention framework?

Assumptions: You assume that acute soft tissue pathology can be identified on the basis of cardinal signs and symptoms. How do you justify that assumption?

Reasons and evidence: The use of cryotherapy, with or without other therapeutic interventions, is a judicious choice during the first stage of soft tissue repair. Why is this so?

Viewpoints or perspectives: You agree with the suggestion that closely monitoring the presence and magnitude of some of the cardinal signs and symptoms may be one of the best methods for determining the healing phase of soft tissue. What would someone who disagrees with you say?

Implications and consequences: The therapeutic effects of EPAs are best maximized when applied in conjunction with other therapeutic interventions. What are you implying by that?

About the question: Is today's therapeutic approach to the management of soft tissue pathology viable for many years to come? Why do you think I ask this question?

References

Chapters of Textbooks

Cameron MH (2003) Integrating physical agents into patients care. In: Physical Agents in Rehabilitation: From Research to Practice, 2nd ed. Saunders, St-Louis, pp 415–439

Delforge G (2002a) Therapeutic implications: Inflammation and pain. In: Musculoskeletal Trauma: Implications for Sports Injury Management. Human Kinetics, Champaign, pp 53–85

Delforge, G (2002b) Therapeutic implications: Scar formation and maturation. In Musculoskeletal Trauma: Implications for Sports Injury Management. Human Kinetics, Champaign, pp 87–114

Denegar CR (2000) Treatment plan for acute musculoskeletal injuries. In: Therapeutic Modalities for Athletic Injuries. Human Kinetics, Champaign, pp 196–207

Fedorcyk JM, Michlovitz SL (2005) Pain and limited motion. In: Modalities for Therapeutic Interventions, 4th ed. Michlovitz SL, Nolan TP (Eds). FA Davis Co, Philadelphia, pp 185–206

Houghton PE (2005) Tissue healing and edema. In: Modalities for Therapeutic Interventions, 4th ed. Michlovitz SL, Nolan TP (Eds). FA Davis Co, Philadelphia, pp 207–246

Johnson TE (2005) Muscle weakness and loss of motor performance. In: Modalities for Therapeutic Interventions, 4th ed. Michlovitz SL, Nolan TP (Eds). FA Davis Co, Philadelphia, pp 247–270

Knight KL, Draper DO (2008a) Tissue response to injury: Inflammation, swelling and edema. In: Therapeutic Modalities: The Art and Science. Knight, DL, Draper DO (eds.) Lippincott Williams & Wilkins, Philadelphia, pp 38–53

Knight KL, Draper DO (2008b) Immediate care of acute orthopedic injuries. In: Therapeutic Modalities: The Art and Science. Knight, DL, Draper DO (eds.) Lippincott Williams & Wilkins, Philadelphia, pp 54–85

Prentice WE (2002). The healing process and guideline for using therapeutic modalities. In: Therapeutic Modalities for Physical Therapists, 2nd ed. McGraw-Hill, New York, pp 14–27

Starkey C (2004) The injury process. In: Therapeutic Modalities, 3rd ed. FA Davis Co, Philadelphia, pp 2–28

Textbook

Knight KL (1995) Cryotherapy in Sports Injury Management. Human Kinetics, Champaign, IL

Illustrated Glossary of Electrophysical Terminology

Chapter Outline

Learning Objectives

Knowledge: List the main electrical, electromagnetic, and thermodynamic terms related to the use of therapeutic electrophysical agents (EPAs).

Comprehension: Compare the main concepts related to the application of electrical, electromagnetic, and thermal EPAs.

Application: Show the difference between ionizing and nonionizing energy.

Analysis: Explain the difference between electrical, electromagnetic, and thermodynamic with regard to the concept of energy behind the use of EPAs.

Synthesis: Explain the relationship between the electromagnetic spectrum of radiation and the concept of cell ionization.

Evaluation: Discuss the importance of using adequate terminology to better understand the biophysical nature of therapeutic EPAs.

I. BACKGROUND AND PURPOSE

A. CONFUSION

The use of outdated, vague, and erroneous terms, like those listed in **Table 5-1**, to describe electrophysical agents (EPAs) and related concepts and parameters can create significant confusion and misunderstanding among educators, students, clinicians, sales representatives, maintenance and repair technicians, and manufacturers. Many of these terms, unfortunately, are still in use in current corporate brochures as well as in academic textbooks and journals. The crusade to adopt a standardized terminology in the field of therapeutic EPAs is, therefore, far from being over.

B. STANDARD TERMINOLOGY

To address this issue, the American Physical Therapy Association (APTA) commissioned its Section on Clinical Electrophysiology in 1986 to devise a monograph of terminology. The main purpose was to describe electrical current types, waveforms, and other key parameters related to the use and application of electrotherapy. The goal was to foster uniformity of communication in clinical and research applications, product development, and publications.

C. APTA MONOGRAPH

A monograph titled *Electrotherapeutic Terminology in Physical Therapy* was first published by the APTA in 1990 and updated in 2001. This monograph has significantly influenced the electrotherapeutic literature in the United States over the last 15 years as more authors of textbooks and peer-reviewed articles adopted the terminology proposed by APTA.

D. PURPOSE OF THIS CHAPTER

The purpose of this chapter is to provide a comprehensive illustrated glossary of electrophysical terminology to help readers adopt appropriate terms, definitions, and concepts related to the use of therapeutic EPAs. More specifically, the present glossary addresses not only the electrical terminology, as was the case with the APTA monograph (APTA, 2001), but also the terminology related to the electromagnetic and thermodynamic components required for EPAs. In other words, this glossary expands the content of the APTA monograph (2001) by adding terms related to two other types of energy underlying several EPAs. The electrical terminology presented in this chapter conforms to that proposed in the APTA monograph (2001).

II. ELECTRICAL TERMINOLOGY

A. RELEVANCE

The terminology described in this section relates to the study and application of the following EPAs, which generate *electrical energy* and deliver it to soft tissues for therapeutic purposes: iontophoresis (Chapter 13), transcutaneous electrical nerve stimulation (Chapter 14),

TABLE 5-1	EXAMPLES OF RECOMMENDED VERSUS OUTDATED, VAGUE, AND ERRONEOUS TERMINOLOGY
RECOMMENDED TERM	**OUTDATED, VAGUE, OR ERRONEOUS TERM**
Direct current	Galvanic current
Pulsed biphasic asymmetric balanced current	Faradic current
High-voltage pulsed current	High-voltage pulsed galvanic current
Balanced waveform	Zero net DC
Pulse duration	Pulse width; pulse length
Current amplitude	Current intensity
Frequency	Rate
Waveform	Impulse
ON:OFF ratio	Mark:space ratio
Ramp	Surge

microcurrent (Chapter 15), high-voltage pulsed current (Chapter 16), Russian current (Chapter 17), interferential current (Chapter 18), and diadynamic current (Chapter 19). Before considering the terms and concepts described below, it is important to distinguish between electrical and biological currents.

1. Electrical Current
It is the flow (current) of electrons (electricity) from an electron source (stimulator) to the wires and electrodes used to deliver such an electrical current to soft tissues.

2. Biological Current
It is the flow (current) of ions (biological) in the targeted tissues resulting from the passage of an electrical current.

3. Interaction
The flow of electrical current is transformed, within the soft tissues, into a flow of biological current. In other words, electrical energy is transformed into bioelectrical energy for therapeutic purposes.

B. CONSTANT CURRENT (CC)

A constant current (CC) stimulator is a device that delivers an electric current that flows at the same amplitude regardless of changes in tissue impedance over time. Most therapeutic electrical stimulators today are CC type stimulators because they provide a consistent level of current amplitude throughout the therapeutic application, making therapy comfortable for the patient and predictable for the clinician.

C. CONSTANT VOLTAGE (CV)

A constant voltage (CV) stimulator is a device that delivers a source of voltage at the same amplitude regardless of changes in tissue impedance over time. Voltage (V) is the electromotive force, measured in volts, responsible for the movement of electrons within the electrical circuit. It is also referred to as the potential difference between two points in a circuit.

D. OHM'S LAW

The CC and CV concepts described above are based on Ohm's law: voltage (V) = resistance (R) × intensity (I). In keeping with the APTA monograph (2001), the term intensity (I) is replaced here by the term amplitude (A), which is the measure of the magnitude of current. Ohm's law may thus be rewritten as follows: V = R × A. To keep A constant (CC) when R is changing, V is automatically adjusted. To keep V constant (CV) when R is changing, A is automatically adjusted.

E. IMPEDANCE

This term, designated by the letter Z and measured in ohms, refers to the opposition of our biological tissues to the flow of an electrical current. Biophysicists see soft tissues as being made of a mix of several resistors (R) in addition to capacitors (C) and inductors (I). Impedance is thus the total opposition offered by these three sources of opposition, namely, resistance, capacitive reactance, and inductive reactance, to electrical current flow.

1. Resistor (R)
A component made of material that opposes the flow of electrical current (Cook, 1997).

2. Capacitor (C)
A device made of two plates separated by air acting as a dielectric that is capable of storing electrical energy (Cook, 1997).

3. Inductor (I)
A device made of a coil capable of opposing the flow of electrical current (Cook, 1997).

4. Resistance
It is the ability of a resistor, measured in ohms, to oppose current flow *with* dissipation of energy in the form of heat (Cook, 1997). For a given voltage, the greater the resistance (R), the smaller the current amplitude (A) flowing in the conductor or tissue will be.

5. Capacitive Reactance (X_C)
It is the ability of a capacitor (C), measured in ohms, to oppose current flow *without* dissipation of energy (Cook, 1997). It is designated by the symbol X_C. Capacitive reactance is *inversely proportional* to frequency (f) and capacitance (C), as exemplified by the following formula: $X_C = 1/2fC$. Therefore, the greater the current frequency is, the lower the X_C. Capacitance is the ability of a capacitor to store electrical charges, and is measured in units of farad.

6. Inductive Reactance (X_L)
It is the ability of an inductor (L), measured in ohms, to oppose current flow *without* dissipation of energy (Cook, 1997). It is designated by the symbol X_L. Inductive reactance is *proportional* to frequency (f) and inductance (L), as exemplified by the following formula: $X_L = 2fL$. Thus, the higher the current frequency, the higher the X_L is. Inductance is the ability of an inductor to oppose any change in current as the magnetic field produced by the change in current causes an induced countercurrent to oppose the original change. Inductance is measured in units of Henry.

7. Calculation
Impedance (Z) is calculated using the following mathematical formula: $Z = \sqrt{R^2 + X^2}$ (Cook, 1997), where R is the resistance and X, the reactance, is equal to the difference (~) between the inductive and capacitive reactance ($X_L^2 \sim X_C^2$).

8. Rewriting Ohm's Law

In the context of using EPAs for the treatment of soft-tissue pathology, Ohm's law can thus be rewritten as follows: $V = Z \times A$, where the letter Z is substituted for the letter R and the letter A for the letter I.

F. DIRECT CURRENT (DC)

The continuous, unidirectional flow of charged particles, for 1 second or longer, the direction of which is determined by the polarity selected (**Fig 5-1**). Polarity refers to two oppositely charged poles, one positive (+) and the other negative (−). Polarity determines the direction in which current flows.

G. ALTERNATING CURRENT (AC)

The continuous, bidirectional flow of charged particles, for 1 second or longer, relative to the isoelectric (zero) baseline (**Fig 5-2**).

H. PULSED DC/AC CURRENTS

The noncontinuous, interrupted, or periodic flow of direct (DC) or alternating (AC) currents (**Fig 5-3**).

I. CURRENT WAVEFORM

The geometrical description of a DC, AC, pulsed DC, or pulsed AC current. Current waveforms are described as

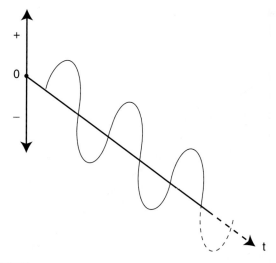

FIGURE 5-2 An alternating sinusoidal current (AC) flowing over time.

either monophasic or biphasic. A biphasic wave is further described as either symmetrical or asymmetrical and as balanced or unbalanced.

1. Monophasic

A pulse or cycle that moves in only one direction (+ or − polarity) from the zero baseline to return to it after a finite time (**Fig 5-4**).

2. Biphasic

A pulse or cycle that moves in one direction and then in the opposite direction from the zero baseline to finally return to that baseline after a finite time (**Fig 5-5**).

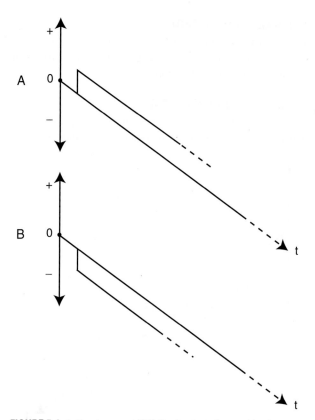

FIGURE 5-1 A direct current (DC) flowing over time and having either a positive **(A)** or a negative **(B)** polarity.

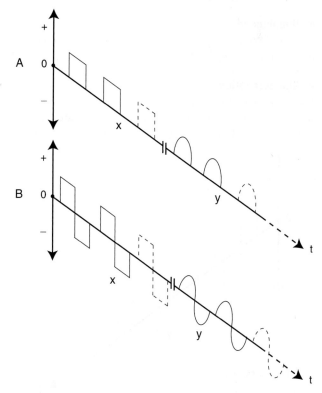

FIGURE 5-3 Pulsed DC (x) and AC (y) monophasic **(A)** and biphasic **(B)** current waveforms.

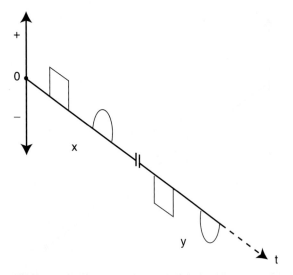

FIGURE 5-4 Monophasic pulses with either positive (x) or negative (y) polarity.

a. Symmetrical
A biphasic pulse or cycle with its positive phase geometrically identical to its negative phase (**Fig 5-6A**).

b. Asymmetrical
A biphasic pulse or cycle with one of its two phases geometrically different from the other (**Fig 5-6B**).

c. Balanced
A biphasic pulse or cycle with equal electrical charges in each phase (**Fig 5-7A**).

d. Unbalanced
A biphasic pulse or cycle with unequal electrical charges in each phase (**Fig 5-7B**).

e. Characteristics
From the above definitions, monophasic waveforms are neither symmetrical nor asymmetrical, but are always unbalanced. Moreover, biphasic waveforms are either

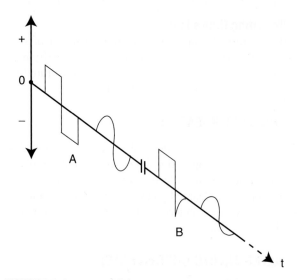

FIGURE 5-6 Symmetrical **(A)** versus asymmetrical **(B)** biphasic pulses.

symmetrical or asymmetrical. Symmetrical waveforms are always balanced, whereas asymmetrical waveforms are either balanced or unbalanced.

J. PHASE

A current flow in one direction for a determined period of time. Current waveforms used in the field of EPAs are either monophasic or biphasic.

1. Phase Duration (PhD)
The determined period of time elapsing from the beginning to the end of one phase (**Fig 5-8**), usually expressed in microseconds or milliseconds.

2. Interphase Duration (IPhD)
The time elapsed between two successive phases (**Fig 5-8**), usually expressed in microseconds or milliseconds.

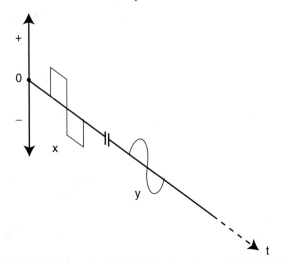

FIGURE 5-5 Biphasic DC (x) and AC (y) pulses.

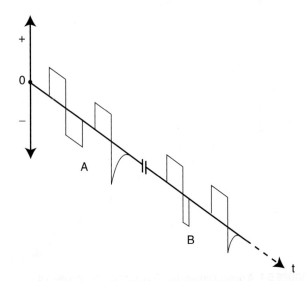

FIGURE 5-7 Balanced **(A)** versus unbalanced **(B)** biphasic pulses.

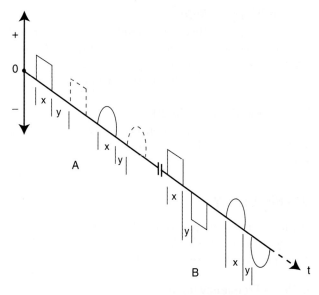

FIGURE 5-8 Phase duration (x = PhD) and interphase duration (y = IPhD) in monophasic **(A)** and biphasic **(B)** pulses.

The term interphase duration is equivalent to interphase interval.

3. Phase Rise Time (PhRT)

The time it takes for the leading edge of a phase to rise from the zero baseline to its maximum amplitude (**Fig 5-9**). This rise time can be as short as a few nanoseconds or as long as a few milliseconds. Phase rise time is related to the property of *nerve accommodation*, a phenomenon in which the threshold of nerve and muscle membrane excitability automatically rises when the membrane is stimulated by a pulse with a slowly increasing phase rise time. Thus, the shorter (or more abrupt) the phase rise time, the lesser the nerve membrane capacity to accommodate the repetition of this phase (or pulse) over time, and the more efficient the stimulating pulse will be.

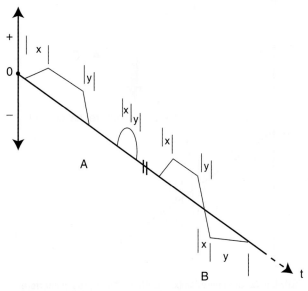

FIGURE 5-9 Phase rise time (x = PhRT) and decay time (y = PhDT) in monophasic **(A)** and biphasic **(B)** pulses.

4. Phase Decay Time (PhDT)

The time it takes for the trailing edge of a phase to decay from maximum amplitude to the zero baseline (**Fig 5-9**), usually expressed in nanoseconds, microseconds, or milliseconds. This decay time can be as short as a few nanoseconds or as long as a few milliseconds.

K. PULSE/CYCLE

A pulse/cycle refers to a current flow in each direction of the phases for a determined period of time. A *pulse* may have one phase (monophasic) or two phases (biphasic). A *cycle* is always made of two phases (biphasic) with a sinusoidal shape. The term cycle is always associated with sinusoidal AC current.

1. Pulse/Cycle Duration

The time elapsed from the beginning to the end of the two phases within a pulse or cycle, including the interphase duration, if present (**Fig 5-10**). Pulse duration (PD) and

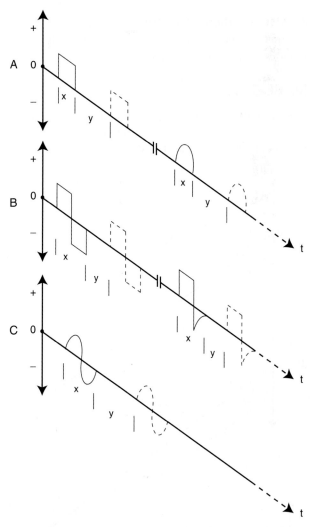

FIGURE 5-10 Pulse/cycle duration (x = PD/CD) and interpulse/intercycle duration (y = IPD/ICD) for monophasic **(A)**, biphasic DC **(B)**, and AC **(C)** current waveforms. Note that for monophasic pulses/cycles, the phase duration and interphase duration are equal to the pulse duration and interpulse duration.

cycle duration (CD) are usually expressed in microseconds or milliseconds.

2. Interpulse/Intercycle Duration

The time elapsed between two successive pulses or cycles (**Fig 5-10**). Interpulse duration (IPD) and intercycle duration (ICD) are usually expressed in microseconds or milliseconds.

L. BURST (Bu)

The successive delivery of pulses or cycles at a preset amplitude, frequency, or duration during a determined period of time. A burst is commonly defined as an interrupted train (see Section P, Train).

1. Burst Duration (BuD)

The time elapsed between the beginning of the first and the end of the last pulse or cycle within the burst (**Fig 5-11**), usually expressed in milliseconds.

2. Interburst Duration (IBuD)

The time elapsed between two successive bursts (**Fig 5-11**), usually expressed in milliseconds.

M. BEAT (Be)

The summation of two or more sinusoidal alternating currents (cycles) delivered at different frequencies and intersecting during a determined period of time.

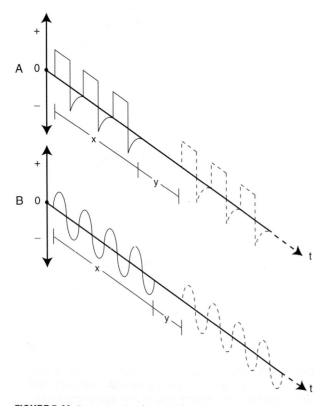

FIGURE 5-11 Burst duration (x = BuD) and interburst duration (y = IBuD) for biphasic DC (**A**) and AC (**B**) current waveforms.

1. Beat Duration (BeD)

The time elapsed between the beginning of the first and the end of the last cycle within the beat (**Fig 5-12**), usually expressed in milliseconds. Beats of current are characteristic of interferential current (see Chapter 18).

2. Interbeat Duration (IbeD)

There is no interbeat duration because each beat ends with the beginning of the next beat, as shown in **Figure 5-12**.

N. FREQUENCY

The number of times per second that a pulse, cycle, burst, or beat will repeat itself. Frequency (f) is inversely related to the period (P) as expressed in $f = 1/P$.

1. Pulse Frequency (pps)

The number of pulses per second (pps). The period (P) is equal to pulse duration (PD) plus interpulse duration (IPD) (**Fig 5-13**).

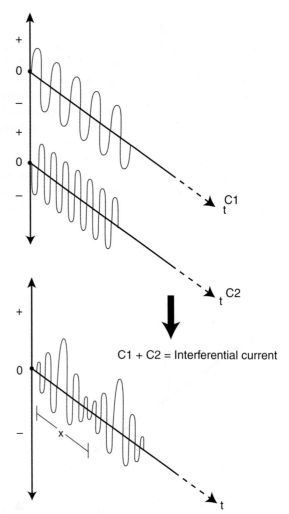

FIGURE 5-12 Beat duration (x = BeD), characteristic of interferential current, resulting from the interference of two sinusoidal currents (C1 and C2) with different cycle frequencies.

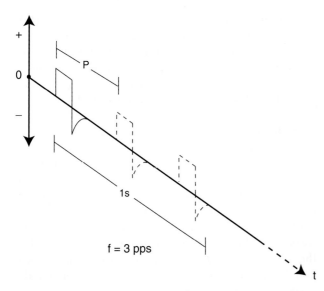

FIGURE 5-13 Pulse frequency (f), in which the period (P) is equal to the pulse duration (PD) plus the interpulse duration (IPD); illustrated is a pulse frequency of 3 pps.

2. Cycle Frequency (cps)

The number of cycles per second (cps). Cycle frequency is commonly expressed in hertz (Hz). The period (P) is equal to cycle duration (CD) plus intercycle duration (ICD) (**Fig 5-14**).

3. Burst Frequency (bups)

The number of bursts per second (bups). The period (P) is equal to the burst duration (BuD) plus interburst duration (IBuD) (**Fig 5-15**).

4. Beat Frequency (beps)

The number of beats per second (beps) determined by the difference between the frequency of both C1 and C2 sinusoidal AC currents (**Fig 5-16**).

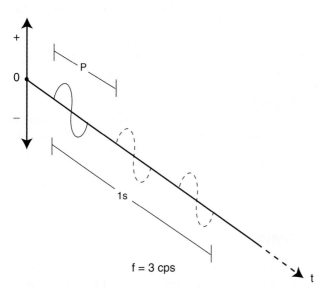

FIGURE 5-14 Cycle frequency (f), in which the period (P) is equal to the cycle duration (CD) plus the intercycle duration (ICD); illustrated is a cycle frequency of 3 cps.

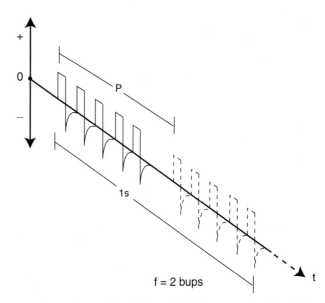

FIGURE 5-15 Burst frequency (f), in which the period (P) is equal to the burst duration (BuD) plus the interburst duration (IBuD); illustrated is a burst frequency of 2 bups.

O. CURRENT AMPLITUDE

The magnitude of current relative to the isoelectric (zero) baseline, expressed in amperes (A). The current amplitude of therapeutic electrical stimulators ranges in micro (μA) to milliamperes (mA).

1. Peak Amplitude (A_{pk})

The maximum or peak current amplitude of one or more phases relative to the zero baseline (**Fig 5-17**), usually expressed in microamperes or milliamperes. A_{pk} is the preferred measurement for charting current amplitude in clinical practice. Because A_{pk} may differ between the positively charged phase and the negatively charged phase,

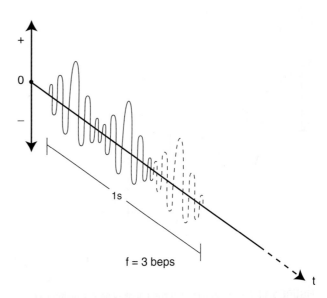

FIGURE 5-16 Beat frequency (f) from an interferential current; illustrated is a beat frequency of 3 beps.

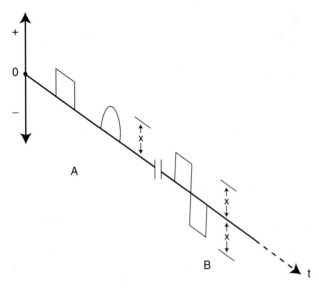

FIGURE 5-17 Measurement of current peak amplitude ($x = A_{pk}$) on monophasic (**A**) and biphasic waveforms (**B**).

practitioners should make a note, in the patient's file, of the polarity of the peak current amplitude used (A_{pk+}; A_{pk-}).

2. Peak-to-Peak Amplitude (A_{pk-pk})
The maximum or peak current amplitude between positively and negatively charged phases (**Fig 5-18**).

3. Average Amplitude (A_{avg})
The average, or mean, current amplitude applied to the tissues over the waveform period (**Fig 5-19**). Measurement of A_{avg} is restricted to pulsed monophasic waveforms because averaging positive and negative charge quantities, as with biphasic symmetrical waveforms, will yield an average current equal to zero. To account for this particular situation, in which A_{avg} equals zero, biophysicists recommend, instead, that current root-mean-square amplitude (A_{rms})

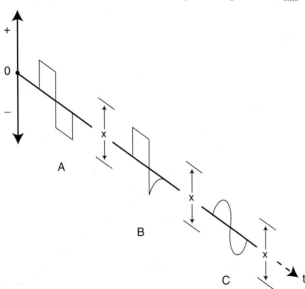

FIGURE 5-18 Measurement of current peak to peak amplitude ($x = A_{pk-pk}$) on biphasic symmetrical (**A**), asymmetrical (**B**), and sinusoidal (**C**) current waveforms.

be measured for all biphasic waveforms. In **Figure 5-19A**, A_{avg} of a monophasic pulsed DC current is calculated as follows: $A_{avg} = A_{pk} \times PD/P$. In this example, the A_{avg} equals 0.3 mA. In **Figure 5-19B**, the A_{avg} of a monophasic pulsed AC current is calculated as follows: $A_{avg} = (A_{pk} \times 0.637) \times CD/P$. In this example, the A_{avg} equals 0.19 mA.

4. Root-Mean-Square Amplitude (A_{rms})
The absolute sum of all phase changes over the waveform period (**Fig 5-20**). A_{rms} is commonly known as the *effective current* acting on the tissues, because it refers to the power-delivery capability of the waveform (power = voltage × current) and, concomitantly, to the amount of electrical energy (energy = power × time) delivered to the tissues. In other words, the electrical power generated by the stimulator remains the same during the entire application, but the amount of electrical energy delivered to the tissues increases over time.

a. A_{rms} Calculation
The A_{rms} value of a biphasic waveform is calculated by squaring the magnitude of each phase, then taking the mean value of the sum of squared magnitudes, then computing the square root value of this previously calculated mean value (**Fig 5-20A**). The period A_{rms} of a biphasic pulsed DC current is calculated as follows: $A_{rms} = (Pulse\ A_{rms} \times PD) / P$. In this example, the period A_{rms} equals 0.3 mA. In **Figure 5-20B**, the period A_{rms} of a biphasic pulsed AC current is calculated as follows: $A_{rms} = (Cycle\ A_{rms} \times CD) / P$. In this example, the period A_{rms} equals 0.21 mA.

b. Thermal Heat
When electrical energy is delivered to tissues, it is converted in part to thermal heat energy at the skin/electrode interface. Therefore, it is clinically important to know the value of A_{rms} delivered by the stimulator, especially if the total duration of the therapeutic application is prolonged over time. This explains why manufacturers limit the maximum A_{rms} generated by their stimulators: to prevent possible heat skin damage under the electrodes.

c. A_{Avg} Versus A_{rms}
Computing the A_{rms} of biphasic currents is comparable to computing the average amplitude (A_{avg}) of monophasic currents, because both measurements reflect the absolute amount of current delivered over time and the amount of heat produced in the tissues during the entire therapeutic application.

P. TRAIN

This term refers to the continuous series (thus the word train) of pulses, cycles, bursts, or beats delivered over time, usually lasting seconds. For example, a train of impulses may be the result of successive bursts delivered at 50 bups for a duration of 5 seconds.

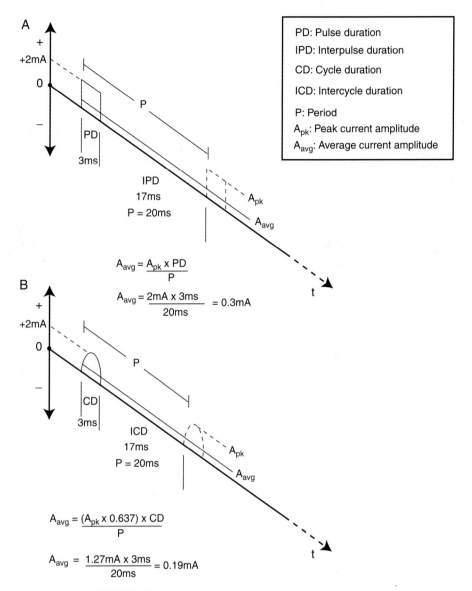

PD: Pulse duration

IPD: Interpulse duration

CD: Cycle duration

ICD: Intercycle duration

P: Period

A_{pk}: Peak current amplitude

A_{avg}: Average current amplitude

$$A_{avg} = \frac{A_{pk} \times PD}{P}$$

$$A_{avg} = \frac{2mA \times 3ms}{20ms} = 0.3mA$$

$$A_{avg} = \frac{(A_{pk} \times 0.637) \times CD}{P}$$

$$A_{avg} = \frac{1.27mA \times 3ms}{20ms} = 0.19mA$$

FIGURE 5-19 Measurement of current average amplitude (A_{avg}) on monophasic rectangular **(A)** and sinusoidal **(B)** waveforms. The 0.637 value corresponds to the surface under the sinewave, or to its integral.

1. ON-Time

The amount of time, measured in seconds, during which a stimulator delivers a train of individual pulses, cycles, bursts, or beats of prescribed amplitude, duration, and frequency during a therapeutic application (**Fig 5-21**). In other words, the ON-time is the period of time during which the stimulator delivers current into the tissue.

2. OFF-Time

The amount of time between two successive trains. In other words, the OFF-time is the period of time during which the stimulator delivers no current to the tissues (**Fig 5-21**).

3. ON:OFF Time Ratio

The ratio of ON-time to OFF-time (**Fig 5-21**), where time is expressed in seconds; for example 10s:50s.

4. Duty Cycle

It is the ratio of ON-time to the summation of ON-time plus OFF-time, expressed as a percentage [(duty cycle = (ON)/(ON + OFF)] × 100 (**Fig 5-21**). For example, a duty cycle of 20% is calculated when the ON- and OFF-times equal 10 and 40 seconds, respectively [(20% = (10s/50s) × 100)].

a. Electrical Versus Electrotherapeutic Duty Cycle

Readers should not confuse the above definition of duty cycle used in the field of EPA with that found in the electrical engineering literature (Cook, 1997). In electrical engineering, the duty cycle is defined as the ratio of pulse duration (PD) to the period duration (P) of the waveform, and is also expressed as a percentage. **Figure 5-22** illustrates the basic differences between an electric and electrotherapeutic duty cycle.

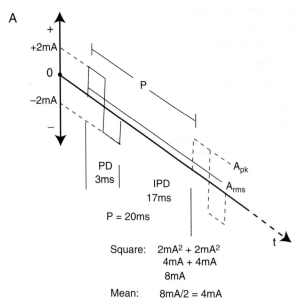

PD: Pulse duration

IPD: Interpulse duration

CD: Cycle duration

ICD: Intercycle duration

P: Period

A_{pk}: Peak current amplitude

A_{rms}: Root-mean-square current amplitude

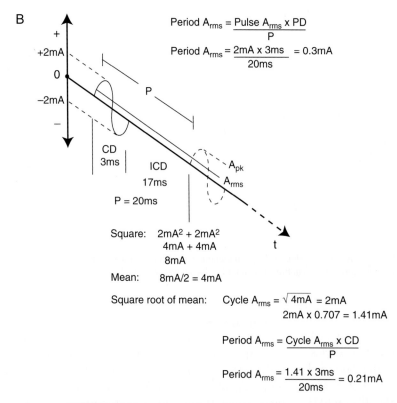

FIGURE 5-20 Measurement of current root-mean-square amplitude (A_{rms}) on biphasic symmetrical rectangular **(A)** and sinusoidal **(B)** waveforms. The 0.707 value corresponds to the sinus value at 90°.

5. Train Ramp-Up and Ramp-Down Time

Ramp-up time is the time elapsed from the onset (or baseline) to plateau current amplitude (or maximum) of the train, whereas ramp-down time is the time elapsed from the plateau current amplitude to zero baseline (**Fig 5-23**). Readers should not confuse these two terms with the terms phase rise-time and decay-time discussed previously.

a. Train ON-time

Current amplitude, when trains of pulses are used, is usually ramped up and down in a linear fashion as shown in **Figure 5-23**). Ramp-up and ramp-down times are adjustable and they usually last approximately 1–3 seconds. Contrary to statements in corporate brochures and textbooks, the train ON-time of a ramped train of pulses, therefore,

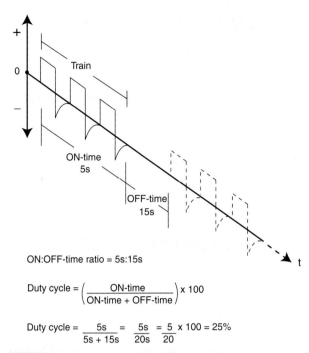

FIGURE 5-21 Measurement of ON:OFF ratio and duty cycle on an unramped train of biphasic asymmetrical pulses.

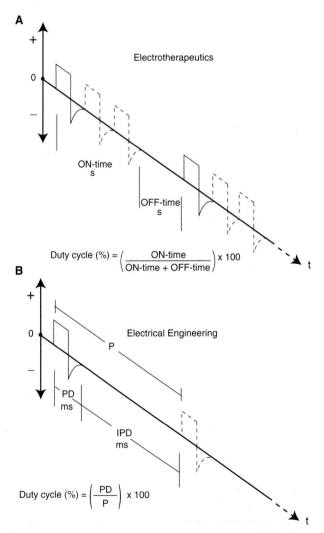

FIGURE 5-22 Comparison between the duty cycle as defined in the field of electrotherapeutics (**A**) versus the field of electrical engineering (**B**).

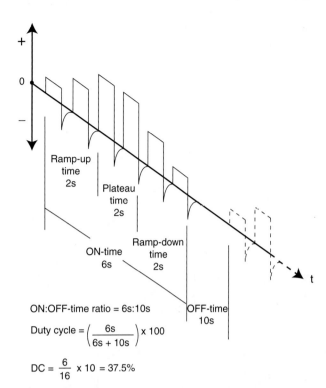

FIGURE 5-23 Measurement of ON:OFF-time ratio and duty cycle on a ramped-up and ramped-down train of biphasic asymmetrical pulses. Note that both the ramp-up and ramp-down times are with the plateau time, part of the train total ON-time.

is equal to the summation of ramp-up time, plateau time, and ramp-down time, because during these three periods of time electrical current is delivered to the tissues. In the example, the train ON-time is 6 seconds and the train OFF-time is 10 seconds.

b. Physiological Mimic

The purpose of *ramping up* the current amplitude of a train of pulses is to mimic the gradual and smooth motor unit recruitment process seen during the early phase of a voluntary contraction. The goal is to maximize patient comfort during the early phase of muscle tetanic contraction by preventing sudden activation of motor units. The rationale behind *ramping down* the current amplitude, on the other hand, is to mimic the end phase of a voluntary contraction, during which motor unit recruitment gradually decreases. This ramping effect increases the effectiveness and safety of treatments by allowing the limb to return to its resting position in a controlled rather than an abrupt motion.

Q. WAVEFORM MODULATION

The random and successive variations of waveform parameters such as current amplitude, pulse duration, and pulse frequency over time (**Fig 5-24**). These parameters can be modulated individually, in pairs, or all together simply by turning a knob. Modulation is a feature on some electrical stimulators, such as TENS units, and is used essentially to optimize comfort while reducing sensory habituation and nerve accommodation to the pattern of stimulation delivered over time.

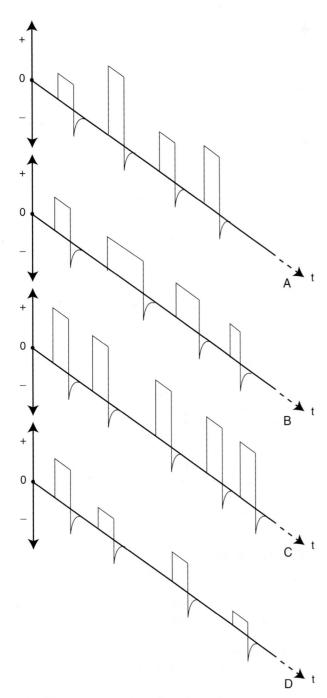

FIGURE 5-24 Examples of current amplitude modulation (**A**), pulse duration modulation (**B**), pulse frequency modulation (**C**), and pulse amplitude combined with pulse frequency modulation (**D**).

III. ELECTROMAGNETIC TERMINOLOGY

A. RELEVANCE

The terminology described in this section relates to the following EPAs, which generate and deliver electromagnetic energy to soft tissues for therapeutic purposes: shortwave diathermy (Chapter 10), low-level laser (Chapter 11), and ultraviolet (Chapter 12) therapy.

B. ELECTROMAGNETIC SPECTRUM

A schematic representation of the spectrum of electromagnetic waves of energies, or radiations, categorized by the magnitude of their frequency, wavelength, and energy (**Table 5-2**). As expected, shortwave diathermy and ultraviolet therapy fall within the shortwave and ultraviolet energy bands of the spectrum, respectively. Low-level laser therapy, on the other hand, falls within the visible and infrared energy bands of the spectrum. The energy per photon (eV) carried by ultraviolet radiation is larger than that carried by visible, infrared, and shortwave radiations because UV photons are delivered at a higher frequency.

C. ELECTROMAGNETIC RADIATION

A stream of photons traveling in a wave-like fashion in space (**Fig 5-25**).

1. Electromagnetic (EM) Waves

Waves form when an electric field couples with a magnetic field perpendicular to it and to the direction of the wave (**Fig 5-25**). The variations of amplitude in both fields are sinusoidal and transverse to the direction of wave travel.

2. Photon

This is the quantum of electromagnetic radiation. According to the wave-particle duality found in quantum physics, a photon may act as either a particle or a wave, as shown in **Figure 5-25**.

D. ELECTROMAGNETIC ENERGY

The energy carried by a single photon, measured in units of electron-volt (eV). One eV is equal to the amount of kinetic energy acquired by an electron accelerated by passing through a potential difference of 1 V. The energy of 1 eV is equal to 1.6×10^{-19} joules. The main difference between the various types of electromagnetic radiation is the amount of energy (eV value) found in their photons, as illustrated in **Table 5-2**. For example, the energy per photon contained in x-rays is much greater than that found in ultraviolet and shortwave rays, respectively.

E. FREQUENCY, WAVELENGTH, AND ENERGY

Photons (particles or waves) travel in space at the speed of light (c), which is equal to 300 million meters per second ($c = 300 \times 10^6$ m/s). The wavelength (λ) of a photon is inversely related to its frequency (f) on the basis of this formula: $\lambda = c/f$ (**Table 5-2**). The energy (E) carried by a photon, on the other hand, is proportional to its frequency (or inversely proportional to its wavelength) on the basis of the following formula: $E = h \times f$, where h is Planck's constant expressed in electron-volt per second (evs). Thus, the higher the frequency, the shorter the wavelength and the higher the energy carried by any given photon (**Table 5-2**).

TABLE 5-2	THE ELECTROMAGNETIC SPECTRUM		
ENERGY TYPE	**FREQUENCY (f)**	**WAVELENGTH (λ)**	**ENERGY PER PHOTON (eV)**
	HIGH	**SHORT**	**HIGH**
	↑	↑	↑
Gamma rays	$>3 \times 10^{19}$ Hz	<1 pm	>1.24 MeV
X-rays	3×10^{16} to 3×10^{19} Hz	10 nm–1 pm	124 eV–1.24 MeV
Ultraviolet	7.5×10^{14} to 3×10^{16} Hz	400 nm–10 nm	3.1 eV–124 eV
Visible	4.0×10^{14} to 7.5×10^{14} Hz	750 nm–400 nm	1.65 eV–3.1 eV
Infrared	3×10^{11} to 4×10^{14} Hz	1 mm–750 nm	0.0012 eV–1.65 eV
Microwave	3×10^{7} to 3×10^{11} Hz	10 m–1 mm	<0.0012 eV
Shortwave	3×10^{6} to 3×10^{7} Hz	100 m–10 m	Negligible
Radio	3×10^{2} to 3×10^{6} Hz	100 km–100 m	Negligible
Electric	1 to 3×10^{2}	>100 km	Negligible
	↓	↓	↓
	LOW	**LONG**	**LOW**
Formula[a]	f = c/λ	λ = c/f	E = h × f

eV = electron-volt; c = speed of light = 300×10^{6} m/s; h = Planck's constant = 4.14×10^{-15} eVs; hc = 1241nm eV.

F. IONIZING VERSUS NONIONIZING RADIATION

The types of radiation found in the electromagnetic spectrum are classified as either ionizing or nonionizing based on the amount of energy their photons carry (**Fig 5-26**). *Ionization* is the process of removing an electron from its orbit. This process is hazardous for living tissues because it alters cell mitosis, potentially leading to cancerous lesions and cell death.

1. Ionizing Radiation

Electromagnetic radiation in which the energy per photon is greater than 30 eV (ter Haar, 2002). This threshold quantum energy, above which cellular ionization will occur, corresponds to all types of radiation with wavelengths of 41 nm and shorter. Ultraviolet rays (extreme), x-rays, and gamma rays are forms of ionizing radiation (**Fig 5-26**). For example, the machines that take x-ray pictures (radiology) produce x-rays with quantum energy of about 120,000 eV or 120 KeV per photon. Other radiation machines that are used to treat cancer by destroying tumor tissue (radiotherapy) are much more powerful, with energies ranging from 2 to 20 million eV (2 to 20 MeV) per photon (**Table 5-2**).

2. Nonionizing Radiation

Radiation associated with levels of energy per photon lower than 30 eV, thus theoretically incapable of causing cellular ionization (**Fig 5-26**). **The types of radiation generated by all the EPAs covered in this textbook are nonionizing in nature**. The EPA closest to the ionizing threshold (30 eV) is ultraviolet C (λ = 180 nm), with a value of 6.8 eV.

G. INTERACTIONS BETWEEN ELECTRO-MAGNETIC RADIATION AND BIOLOGICAL TISSUES

When a beam of radiation or rays or photons comes in contact with biological tissue, as is the case with some EPAs, several interactions can disperse the beam. These interactions are transmission, refraction, absorption, reflection, and scattering.

1. Transmission, Refraction, and Absorption

Illustrated in **Figure 5-27** is a beam of rays with an incident angle of 0° relative to the normal (defined as an imaginary line perpendicular to the surface of the tissue). The beam is transmitted, refracted, and absorbed by the target tissue.

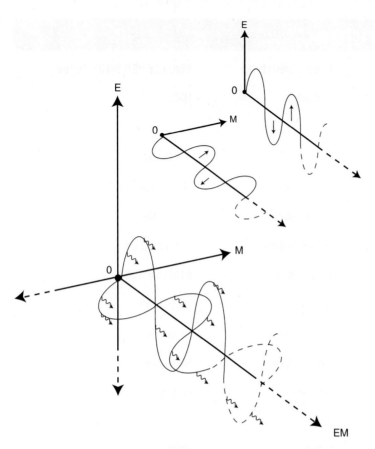

FIGURE 5-25 Electromagnetic wave (EM), resulting from the combination of electric (E) and magnetic (M) currents, showing the wave-photon duality.

Radiation	Energy sources	Usage
	Gamma rays	Radiotherapy
Ionizing		
	X-rays	Radiology
Threshold	Ultraviolet rays – extreme: 30 eV – 41 nm	
	Ultraviolet rays C B A	
Nonionizing	Visible Infrared Microwave Shortwave Radio-wave Electricity	Electrophysical agent

FIGURE 5-26 Electromagnetic ionizing and nonionizing spectrums of therapy. The threshold separating both spectrums is established at 30 eV, which corresponds to extreme UV rays, with a wavelength of 41 nm.

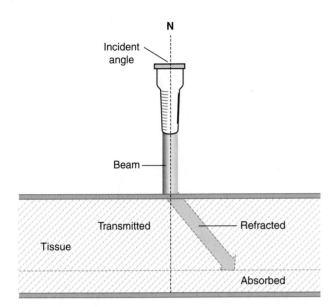

FIGURE 5-27 Geometric interactions between electromagnetic radiation, projected with an incident angle of 0° relative to normal, and soft tissues.

a. Transmission

The process by which a beam of photons passes unaffected through the tissues.

b. Refraction

The change in direction of a propagating beam of photons when passing through the tissues.

c. Absorption

The process by which the photonic energy contained in the refracted beam is retained (absorbed) in the radiated tissues.

2. Transmission, Refraction, Absorption, Reflection, and Scattering

Figure 5-28 shows a beam of rays, delivered at a given incident angle relative to the normal. A large proportion of its photons are transmitted, absorbed, and refracted within the tissue while the remaining portion are reflected off the tissue surface.

a. Reflection

The deflection of a beam of radiation from the surface of the radiated tissue. Reflection occurs only when the incident angle is greater than 0° (**Fig 5-28**).

b. Scattering

The overall dispersal of a beam of radiation in a range of directions, as a result of the above physical interactions, due to the collision of photons with the atoms of radiated tissues. Scattering results from the interaction between reflection and refraction.

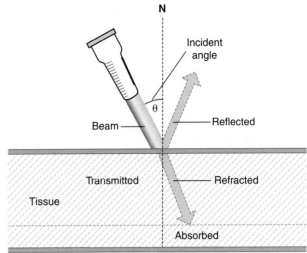

FIGURE 5-28 Geometric interactions between electromagnetic radiation, projected with an incident angle greater than 0° with regard to normal and soft tissues.

H. LAWS GOVERNING THE EFFECTS OF ELECTROMAGNETIC RADIATION

The therapeutic purpose of the various forms of radiant energies emitted by EPAs is to interact with human tissues to cause beneficial physiological and therapeutic effects. The following biophysical laws govern this interaction between the radiating sources and the radiated soft tissues.

1. Grotthus-Draper Law

This law, illustrated in **Figure 5-29**, stipulates that for a radiating energy to have any physiological or therapeutic effect (or response), it must be absorbed by the tissues. Shown in **Figure 5-29A** is a beam of rays not absorbed by the soft tissues, thus inducing no effect. It further states that absorption is inversely related to penetration (or transmission). The greater the absorption of energy by superficial tissues, as illustrated in **Figure 5-29B**, the

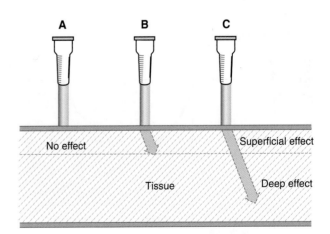

FIGURE 5-29 Grotthus-Draper law.

lesser the penetration (or transmission) of energy in the deeper tissues. Conversely, the lower the absorption in superficial tissues, as shown in **Figure 5-29C**, the greater the penetration of energy in the deeper tissues. This law dictates the relationship between radiating energy absorption and effect (or response), and that between energy absorption and penetration (or transmission).

2. Arndt-Schultz Law

This law, illustrated in **Figure 5-30**, states that no physiological or therapeutic effect (or response) will occur in the target tissues if the amount of radiating energy absorbed (dose) is insufficient to cause such effect (response). It further states that small-to-moderate levels of energy absorption stimulate the effects, whereas stronger doses may be toxic and even lethal for the exposed tissues. This law dictates the relationship between dose and response.

3. Inverse Square Law

This law, illustrated in **Figure 5-31**, stipulates that the intensity (I) of radiation observed from a divergent, or noncollimated, radiating source decreases with the square of its distance (D) from the target tissue, as shown in this formula: $I = 1/D^2$. For example, this means that doubling (D2) the original distance between the source and the target tissue (i.e., from D1 to D2) reduces the intensity of energy to one-quarter (or 25%) of its original value per surface area radiated ($I = 1/1 = 100\%$; $I = 1/2^2 = 1/4 = 25\%$). In other words, the energy twice as far from the source is spread over four times the original area (A), resulting in one-fourth, or 25%, of the intensity per area. Tripling the distance (D3) from the source will further reduce the intensity per area to only one-ninth of the

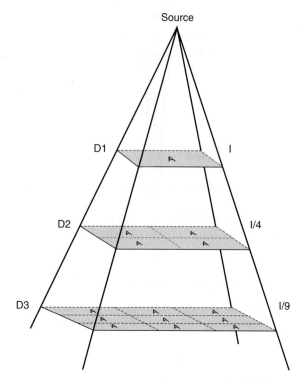

FIGURE 5-31 Inverse square law.

original intensity per area. This law dictates the inverse relationship between distance of exposure and energy exposure per surface area in cases of noncollimated radiating sources. A collimated radiating source, such as a laser, does not obey this law (Chapter 12).

4. Lambert's Cosine Law

This law, illustrated in **Figure 5-32**, states that the amount of radiating energy that can be transmitted and

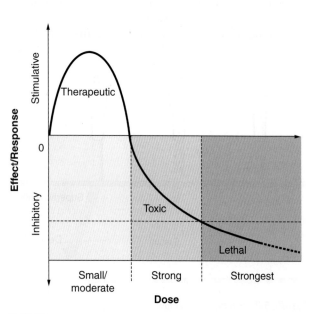

FIGURE 5-30 Arndt-Schultz law.

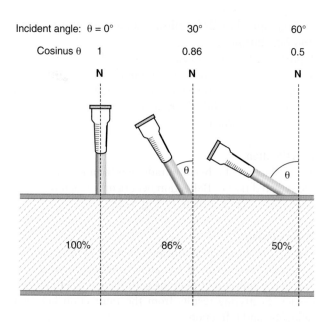

FIGURE 5-32 Lambert's cosine law.

absorbed in the tissue is related to the cosine value the incident angle makes with the normal (N). In other words, the greater the incident angle relative to N, the lesser the amount of radiating energy available to the tissues because of wave reflection. This law is stated as follows: energy available to the tissues = energy from the source $\times$ the cosine of incident angle, and is expressed as a percentage. The examples in **Figure 5-32** show that incident angles of 30° and 60° reduce the amount of energy available to tissues by 14% and 50%, respectively.

IV. THERMODYNAMIC TERMINOLOGY

A. RELEVANCE

The terminology described below relates to the following EPAs, which generate and deliver infrared energy to the exposed soft tissues for therapeutic purposes: hot pack and paraffin bath therapy (Chapter 6), fluidotherapy (Chapter 7), cryotherapy (Chapter 8), and hydrotherapy (Chapter 9).

B. LAWS OF THERMODYNAMICS

Thermodynamics is the branch of physics concerned with the relationship between heat and other forms of energy. Two laws govern the movement of heat between substances.

1. First Law of Thermodynamics

This law states that energy is never lost or gained; it only changes form in any closed system. It is the law of conservation of energy. Hot pack therapy is a good example for illustrating this law. The infrared energy produced by a hot pack is converted into thermal energy in the tissues. The law of conservation of energy stipulates that the energy of the hot pack (i.e., the system energy) is released to the tissues and to the air or atmosphere surrounding the agent (i.e., the surrounding system). The total energy of the system will decrease while that of the surrounding tissues will increase by the same amount. The total energy was never lost or gained, it only changed form.

2. Second Law of Thermodynamics

Heat energy always travels spontaneously from a warmer to a colder substance. For example, the heat of paraffin wax, which is warmer than that of the target tissue, is transmitted to the tissue, which is colder than the paraffin wax. In cryotherapy, the heat of the target tissue is transmitted to the cold pack. In such a case, the heat contained in the target tissues travels to the cryoagent so as to warm it up over time. When the body can no longer replace the heat that is being lost to the cryoagent, the tissues begin to cool.

C. HEAT VERSUS TEMPERATURE

The concept of heat and temperature are often confused. Although related to each other, they are different. It is critical to remember that heat is energy and temperature is a measure of it.

1. Heat

It is the total kinetic energy, or molecular motion, of a substance. The greater the molecular motion of a substance, the more heat it contains. The heat energy of a substance depends on three elements: the speed of its particles (its kinetic energy), the number of particles (its mass), and the capacity of its particles to store heat (its specific heat capacity).

2. Temperature

It is the measurement of the average kinetic energy of a substance. The greater the amount of heat in a substance, the higher its temperature. Temperature depends on one element: the speed of particles (kinetic energy). Thus the greater the kinetic energy of a substance, the higher its temperature will be.

3. Cold Versus Coldness

Cold is the absence of heat. Coldness is the sensation produced by a substance that has less heat or is at lower temperature.

D. HEAT TRANSFER

Thermal energy is measured as heat during heat transfer. The amount of heat transferred (or required) is calculated using the following formula: $q = m \times t° \times c$, where q is the amount of heat transferred (or required), m is the mass of the substance, t° is the change in temperature, and c is the specific heat capacity of the substance.

E. SPECIFIC HEAT CAPACITY (c)

It is the capacity of a substance to store heat (Sekins et al., 1990). Specific heat capacity, designated by the letter c, corresponds to the heat input (cal), in calories, required to increase the temperature of 1 g of a substance by 1°C. Specific heat (c) equals heat input (cal)/(mass (g) $\times$ temperature (°C); its unit is commonly expressed as cal/g°C. The specific heat (c) value of water is 1, because a heat input of 1 calorie is needed to increase 1 gram of pure water by 1°C at 15°C ($1 c = 1$ cal/(1 g $\times$ 1°C)). The higher the specific heat of a substance, the higher its capacity to store heat.

F. THERMAL CONDUCTIVITY (k)

Thermal conductivity is the capacity of a substance to conduct heat (Sekins et al., 1990). It is the quantity of heat (cal) that passes in a unit of time (sec) through a unit area (cm) of a substance whose thickness is unity, when its opposite faces differ in temperature by 1° celcius: its unit is commonly expressed in cal/sec cm°C. The higher the thermal conductivity of a substance, designated by the letter k, the better its ability to conduct heat.

G. THERMOPHYSICAL PROPERTIES

Table 5-3 shows the specific heat capacity (c) and thermal conductivity (k) values of some materials and biological tissues, including water.

1. Comparison Between Materials

The values given in **Table 5-3** show that water at any given temperature (i.e., specific heat) holds approximately 2 times more heat than paraffin oil (1.00 versus 0.45) and conducts heat (i.e., thermal conductivity) approximately 2.5 times more rapidly than paraffin oil (1.42 versus 0.59). The table also shows that air, when compared with water, holds approximately 4 times less heat (0.24 versus 1.00) and conducts heat approximately 70 times more slowly (1.42 versus 0.02).

2. Comparison Between Biological Tissues

Table 5-3 shows that subcutaneous fat, at any given temperature and when compared with the other tissues listed, is the one tissue that holds and conducts heat the least. Fat tissue, because of its poor capacity to conduct heat, acts as a thermal insulator, or barrier, between the skin and the deeper tissues.

3. Clinical Significance

The concepts of specific heat and thermal conductivity explain why humans can more easily tolerate the higher therapeutic temperature range of therapeutic air Fluidotherapy (approximately 48°C or 118°F) and paraffin bath therapy (approximately 55°C or 131°F) than the lower range in hydrotherapy (approximately 40°C or 104°F).

H. MODE OF HEAT TRANSFER

Heat transfer between two substances occurs through four different modes: conduction, convection, radiation, and evaporation (**Fig 5-33**).

TABLE 5-3	THERMOPHYSICAL PROPERTIES OF BIOLOGICAL TISSUES AND PHYSICAL MATERIALS AT 25°C	
	SPECIFIC HEAT (c)[a] (cal/g°C)	**THERMAL CONDUCTIVITY (k)**[b] (cal/sec-cm°C) $\times 10^3$)
Aluminum	0.22	487.00
Rubber	0.48	0.37
Air	0.24	0.02
Paraffin oil	0.45	0.59
Ice	0.46	5.28
Water	**1.00**	**1.42**
Muscle	0.90	1.53
Skin	0.90	0.90
Subcutaneous fat	0.55	0.45
Blood	0.87	1.31
Bone	0.38	2.78

[a]c = The intrinsic capacity of a substance to hold, or store, heat at a given temperature. It is the capacity of a substance to store heat per unit of mass per degree Celsius.
[b]k = The intrinsic capacity of a substance to transmit, or conduct, heat. It is the quantity of heat transmitted in a unit of time through a unit area of a substance whose thickness is unity, when its opposite surfaces differ in temperature by 1°C.
Source: Adapted with permission from Sekins KM, Emery AF (1990) Thermal science for physical medicine. In Therapeutic Heat and Cold, 4th ed. Lehmann JF (Ed). Wilkins & Williams, Philadelphia, pp 62–112.

1. Conduction

Conduction occurs through the physical contact between two solid substances of different temperatures (**Fig 5-33A**). Thermal agents, such as hot packs and paraffin wax, and cryoagents, such as gel packs, use conduction as their mode of heat transfer. Conduction always occurs from the hotter to the colder substance.

a. Thermotherapy

In thermotherapy, using hot packs or paraffin baths, the higher kinetic energy of the warmer substance (the agent) increases, by conduction, the lower kinetic energy of the colder substance (tissue) through microscopic molecular

A. Conduction

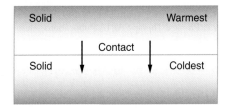

B. Convection

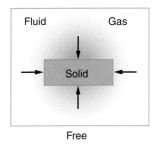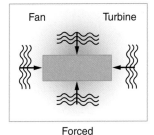

C. Radiation

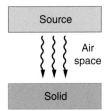

D. Evaporation

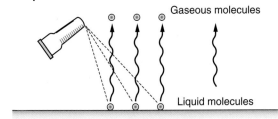

FIGURE 5-33 Modes of heat transfer: conduction (**A**), convection (**B**), radiation (**C**), and evaporation (**D**).

collisions. The resulting heat added to the tissue increases its temperature.

b. Cryotherapy

In cryotherapy, the higher kinetic energy of the warmer substance (tissue) increases, by conduction, the lower kinetic energy of the colder substance (the agent) through microscopic molecular collisions. The tissue thus loses heat, while the cryoagent gains heat.

2. Convection

The second mode, convection, occurs through physical contact between a gaseous or fluid medium (such as air and water) and a solid substance, both at different temperatures (**Fig 5-33B**). Convection can be free (no gaseous or fluid motion) or forced (gaseous or fluid motion). Fluidotherapeutic devices (Chapter 7) and hydrotherapeutic agents (Chapter 9) use convection to transfer their energy to tissues.

a. Free Convection

It is the heating of the solid substance induced solely by the temperature difference between the two substances.

b. Forced Convection

The heating caused when the motion of the fluid or gas is imposed externally by means of a fan (Chapter 7) or a turbine (Chapter 9).

c. Adding or Removing Heat

As in conduction, heat can be added (the agent is warmer than the tissue) or removed (the agent is colder than the tissue) from the tissue by convection.

3. Radiation

The third mode of heat transfer, radiation, occurs in the space between the emitting source at one temperature and the absorbing medium at a different temperature (**Fig 5-33C**). In this nonphysical contact, heat radiates from the hotter to the cooler substance. EPAs such as shortwave diathermy (Chapter 10), low-level laser (Chapter 11), and ultraviolet (Chapter 12) use this mode of heat transfer.

4. Evaporation

The fourth and final mode of heat transfer, evaporation, refers to the transformation, as illustrated in **Figure 5-33D**, from a liquid to a gaseous state (Sekins et al., 1990). For example, when a vapocoolant is sprayed on the skin, as is the case with cryotherapy, the liquid molecules vaporize from the skin surface. The heat to produce this transition is extracted from the skin tissue, which is thus cooled. In other words, if part of a liquid evaporates, it cools the liquid remaining behind because it must extract heat of vaporization from that liquid in order to make the change from liquid to gaseous state.

CRITICAL THINKING QUESTIONS

Clarification: What is meant by the term electromagnetic spectrum when applied in the context of using therapeutic electrophysical agents (EPAs)?

Assumptions: You have assumed that the mode of heat transfer of some agents differs from the modes of other agents. How do you justify that assumption?

Reasons and evidence: The types of radiation within the electromagnetic spectrum are classified according to three basic parameters: frequency, wavelength, and energy per photon. How did this happen?

Viewpoints or perspectives: You agree that the laws governing the effects of electromagnetic radiation on soft tissues are fundamental to the practice of many electrophysical agents. What would someone who disagrees with you say?

Implications and consequences: You state that the concepts of heat and temperature are different although interrelated. What are you implying by that?

About the question: How can the present illustrated glossary of electrophysical terminology further enhance communication between educators, researchers, students, clinicians, distributors, and manufacturers? Why do you think I ask this question?

References

Chapters of Textbooks
Sekins KM, Emery AF (1990) Thermal science for physical medicine. In: Therapeutic Heat and Cold, 4th ed. Lehmann JF, (Ed). Wilkins & Williams, Philadelphia, pp 62–112

ter Harr G (2002) Electrophysical and thermal principles. In: Evidence-Based Practice, 11th ed. Kitchen S (Ed.). Churchill Livingstone, London, pp. 62–112.

Monograph
American Physical Therapy Association (APTA) (2001) Electrotherapeutic Terminology in Physical Therapy. APTA Publications, Alexandria

Textbook
Cook NP (1997) Practical Electricity. Prentice Hall, Upper Saddle River

PART II

Electrophysical Agents

Hot Pack and Paraffin Bath Therapy

Learning Objectives

Knowledge: List the basic considerations associated with the application of hot pack and paraffin bath therapy.

Comprehension: Summarize the physiological and therapeutic effects of hot pack and paraffin bath therapy.

Application: Demonstrate paraffin bath therapy application methods.

Analysis: Explain how to establish objective or quantitative dosimetry with regard to the application of hot pack and paraffin therapy.

Synthesis: Explain the difference between heat and temperature.

Evaluation: Discuss the concepts of specific heat capacity and thermal conductivity and their relevance to the use of hot pack and paraffin bath therapy.

I. RATIONALE FOR USE

A. DEFINITION AND DESCRIPTION

This chapter discusses the use of two therapeutic agents, namely, *hot packs* and *paraffin baths*. These agents fall under the field of *thermotherapy*, which is defined as the application of heat sources, called thermal agents, over skin surface areas for the purpose of heating soft tissues. Hot packs and paraffin baths deliver *moist* heat, as opposed to the dry heat delivered by other thermal electrophysical agents (EPAs) such as fluidotherapy (Chapter 7), shortwave diathermy (Chapter 10), and ultrasound therapy (Chapter 20). The rationale for integrating the discussion of these two agents into a single chapter, therefore, is based on the fact that both deliver moist heat to soft tissues.

1. Superficial Versus Deep Thermotherapy

Historically, thermotherapy has been classified as either superficial or deep in nature. There is a consensus in the EPA literature to define superficial thermotherapy as the heating of soft tissues located within 1 cm from the skin surface (Bell et al., 2002; Knight et al., 2008a,b). Therefore, deep thermotherapy can be logically defined as the heating of soft tissues deeper than 1 cm from the skin surface. Current EPA textbooks classify hot packs and paraffin baths as superficial thermal agents.

2. Superficial Versus Deep Soft Tissues

Research has shown that the application of paraffin baths and fluidotherapy (Chapter 7), which are classified as superficial thermal agents, to the hands and feet of human subjects can induce significant temperature increases not only in the most superficially located tissues (i.e., skin), but also in the deeply located soft tissues (muscles and joint capsules).

3. Potential Confusion

It follows from the above evidence that the use of superficial thermal agents, such as hot packs and paraffin baths, can lead, in some cases, to the therapeutic heating of deeply located soft tissues. When applied over the upper and lower extremities, particularly over the hands, feet, and joint areas (wrist, elbow, ankle, knee) where the fat tissue layer is thinner, it is quite likely that these superficial thermal agents can increase the temperature of the deeper soft tissues. Readers should keep in mind, therefore, that hot pack and paraffin bath therapies can induce superficial as well as deep soft tissue heating.

B. HOT PACKS AND PARAFFIN BATHS

Figure 6-1A shows a typical commercial hot pack; (**B**) shows a paraffin bath filled with a paraffin mixture. Hot packs are manufactured in different sizes and shapes to accommodate different parts of the human body. Paraffin baths are also manufactured in different sizes and are used to treat the distal parts of the upper and lower extremities.

1. Extent of Hot Pack Use

Lindsay et al. (1995) surveyed Canadian private physiotherapy clinics and found hot packs were available in all facilities (100%), with an overall frequency of use of 95.1%. Three years later, Robertson et al. (1998) surveyed more than 200 clinical physiotherapy facilities in Australia and found that hot packs were available in 88% of facilities and were used daily by 73% of all respondents. In 2007, Nussbaum et al. (2007) surveyed 125 Canadian physiotherapists and showed that superficial thermal agents were available to 96% and used by 54% of the respondents. No published survey could be found on the use of hot packs in the United States.

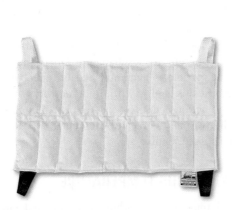

A

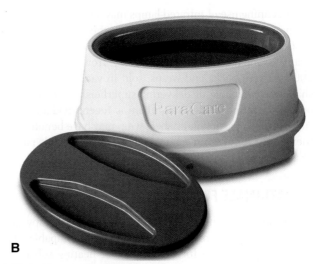

B

FIGURE 6-1 Typical hot pack with hydrocollator unit **(A)** and paraffin bath filled with a paraffin mixture **(B)**. (Courtesy of Chattanooga Group.)

2. Extent of Paraffin Bath Use

The Australian survey by Robertson et al. (1998) revealed that paraffin baths were available in 64% of facilities and were used daily by 28% of the respondents. The Canadian survey by Lindsay et al. (1995) showed this agent to be present in 57.4% of private clinics, with a frequency of use of 11.1%. No literature on the use of hot packs in the United States could be found.

3. Current Use

No literature is available to indicate whether the use of these two thermal agents has increased, decreased, or remained steady. Judging from the fact that these two agents are still covered today in several EPA textbooks (see References) and listed in several brochures published by EPA manufacturers, it is fair to say that their clinical use is still common and widespread. This view is further substantiated by the fact that today, the teaching of hot pack and paraffin bath therapy is still mandatory in the physical therapy academic EPA curricula of many countries, such as Canada (NPAG, 2001), Australia and New Zealand (Chipchase et al., 2005), and the United States (APTA, 2001).

C. INFRARED LAMPS

The popular and routine use of hot packs and paraffin baths stands in clear contrast to the significantly declining use of another classic superficial thermal agent, infrared lamps. In Australia (Robertson et al., 1995), infrared lamps, which generate dry heat, were found in only 39% of the facilities surveyed and were used only 35% of the time. In Canada, Lindsay et al. (1995) found infrared lamps in only 2.2% of the clinics surveyed, with a 0% frequency of use. These results are in keeping with those of Pope et al. (1995) in England, who reported a very low rate of use. Therefore, infrared lamps are not covered in this chapter.

D. MICROWAVEABLE PACKS AND HEAT WRAPS

The declining use of infrared lamps may also be explained by the recent emergence of safe, over-the-counter, easy-to-use, reusable microwaveable packs and disposable heat wraps (Nadler et al., 2002; 2003a,b; Trowbridge et al., 2004). These packs and wraps, sold in various sizes and shapes, are capable of delivering superficial dry or moist heat to localized body areas. There is recent evidence to suggest that a particular dry heat wrap may have beneficial therapeutic effects on acute nonspecific low-back pain (Nadler et al., 2002; 2003a,b).

E. RATIONALE FOR USE

The rationale for hot pack and paraffin bath therapy is to provide practitioners with thermal agents capable of generating *moist heat* for the purpose of heating soft tissues, aside from using hydrotherapy (Chapter 9), and other dry-heat EPAs such as fluidotherapy (Chapter 7), shortwave diathermy (Chapter 10), and ultrasound ther-apy (Chapter 20). It is also to provide practitioners with thermal agents capable of heating large body surface areas (hot packs) and difficult-to-reach body areas such as fingers and toes (paraffin bath).

II. HISTORICAL PERSPECTIVE

A. HOT PACKS

The literature suggests that the therapeutic use of hot packs was introduced during the mid-1950s by Hollander et al. (1949), Horvath et al. (1949), and Erdman et al. (1956).

B. PARAFFIN BATHS

The literature also indicates that paraffin bath therapy was first introduced in the early part of the 20th century by De Sanfort (1915), Humphris (1920), Portmann, (1926), and Zeiter (1939).

C. BODY OF LITERATURE

Despite their routine clinical use over the past 70 or 80 years, the topic of hot pack and paraffin bath therapy has been the subject of a limited number of *articles* (see References), *review articles* (Hardy et al., 1998; Ayling et al., 2000; Brosseau et al., 2006; Robinson et al., 2006), and several *chapters of textbooks* (Jackins et al., 1990; Lehmann et al., 1990; Sekins et al., 1990; Basford, 1998; Hayes, 2000; Bell et al., 2002; Cameron, 2003; Starkey, 2004; Michlovitz et al., 2005; Hecox et al., 2006; Michlovitz et al., 2006; Knight et al., 2008a,b).

III. BIOPHYSICAL CHARACTERISTICS

A. HEAT TRANSFER VIA CONDUCTION

The use of hot pack and paraffin bath therapy is based on the biophysical principle of thermal energy transfer, via conduction, between the agents and the exposed soft tissues. Conduction is defined as the process of internal thermal energy exchange between areas of different temperatures, whereby the exchange of kinetic energy from particle to particle is accomplished by direct molecular collisions (Sekins et al., 1990). In other words, heat transfer by conduction occurs when there is direct contact between the warmer agent and the cooler exposed tissues (for details, see Chapter 5).

B. HEAT VERSUS TEMPERATURE

Heat and temperature, although interrelated, are separate concepts (as discussed in the Illustrated Glossary of Electrophysical Terminology presented in Chapter 5). It is correct to state that the greater the amount of heat

c. Grade III

Evidence based on human *case* studies regardless of their level of randomization and blindness.

3. Strength of Evidence Behind the Agent

The strength of evidence behind the agent, as presented in the research-based indication box, is arbitrarily assessed in this textbook as being *weak, moderate,* or *strong.* For example, the larger the number of studies graded I, regardless of therapeutic benefit, the stronger the scientific evidence behind the agent.

4. Strength of Justification for Usage Behind the Agent

The strength of evidence behind the justification of usage of an agent for individual or groups of pathologies, as listed in the research-based indication box, is arbitrarily assessed in this textbook as being *poor, fair, good,* or *conflicting.* For example, for any given pathology, the larger the number of studies showing therapeutic benefit (Yes) and graded I, "*good*" is the justification of usage of this agent. *Conflicting* justification is reported when similar numbers of studies, with similar grades, repeat therapeutic benefit (Yes) and no benefit (No).

C. STRENGTH OF EVIDENCE AND JUSTIFICATION FOR USAGE OF HOT PACK THERAPY

The results presented in **Box 6-3** show *moderate strength* of evidence for the use of hot pack therapy with all studies graded as II. They also show *poor* to *fair justification* for the use of this thermal agent in a few clinical studies that are beneficial for different pathological conditions.

D. STRENGTH OF EVIDENCE AND JUSTIFICATION FOR USAGE OF PARAFFIN BATH THERAPY

Results from **Box 6-3** further show *moderate strength* of evidence for paraffin bath therapy, with a mix of grade I and II studies. They also show *poor* to *fair justification* for the use of this agent with only half of the studies showing therapeutic benefits.

E. CONTRASTING FACTS

The limited research-based evidence behind these two thermal agents (**Box 6-3**) is in striking contrast to the fact that both have been used clinically for more than eight decades and that their precentage of avai-liability and daily usage still remain high in several countries (see Section IB). Clearly, the justification for the use of these two thermal agents over the past decades has rested as much on the evidence gathered on healthy subjects (**Box 6-1**) as on patients (**Box 6-3**). Until more evidence from research is provided, the routine use of these two thermal agents *cannot be recommended.*

VII. CONTRAINDICATIONS

The contraindications associated with the practice of therapeutic hot pack and paraffin bath therapy are listed in **Table 6-1**. The majority of these contraindications are derived more from clinical common sense than from research studies.

TABLE 6-1	CONTRAINDICATIONS TO HOT PACK (hp) AND PARAFFIN BATH (pb) THERAPY
CONTRAINDICATIONS	**RATIONALE**
Over skin area where sensation to heat is severely impaired (hp, pb)	Risk of cutaneous burn.
Over a cancerous area (hp, pb)	Risk of enhancing tumor growth and metastasis.
Over thrombophlebitic area (hp, pb)	Risk of dislodging blood clot, which may then circulate into the vessels of vital organs, causing serious circulatory problems and, possibly, death (Cameron, 2003).
Over a hemorrhagic area (hp, pb)	Risk of additional bleeding caused by increased blood flow.
Over the abdominal, pelvic, and low-back areas of pregnant women (hb)	Risk of teratogenic effects on fetal development and growth caused by increased local or systemic maternal body temperature.
Over acute and severe inflammatory pathology (hp, pb)	Risk of worsening the condition by aggravating the inflammatory response through increased blood flow resulting from heat application.
Confused and unreliable patients (hp, pb)	Risk of complications during therapy, reducing treatment effectiveness.

VIII. RISKS, PRECAUTIONS, AND RECOMMENDATIONS

The practice of these two thermal agents is not without risk for the patient. The main risks associated with each of them, including some precautions and recommendations designed to improve safety and effectiveness, are listed in **Table 6-2**.

IX. CONSIDERATIONS FOR APPLICATION AND DOCUMENTATION

A. BASIC CONSIDERATIONS

Listed in **Table 6-3** are basic considerations for the practice of hot pack and paraffin bath therapy, which include components of temperature range, coupling media, body application, and application duration.

TABLE 6-2	RISKS, PRECAUTIONS, AND RECOMMENDATIONS FOR HOT PACK (hp) AND PARAFFIN BATH (pb) THERAPY
RISKS	**RATIONALE**
Over an area of impaired blood circulation (hp, pb)	Risk of tissue overheating because the treated area will not be able to cope with the demand for additional and cooler blood flow during treatment.
Over superficial closed and open wounds, including grafted or burn wounds (pb)	Risk of breaking down the immature burn scars and grafts (Head et al., 1977; Helm et al., 1982). To minimize this risk, Burns et al. (1987) proposed the following brushing with wrapping method: (1) keep the paraffin mixture at a constant 47°C (117°F), (2) cover the open wound with a nonadherent, sterile gauze before applying the paraffin, (3) begin to wax the wound and surrounding area using the brushing with wrapping method, and (4) wrap the waxed area in paper or cloth and wait 15–20 mins.
Over superficial closed and open wounds, including grafted or burn wounds (hp)	Risk of breaking down the immature repair tissue. To minimize the risk, first, cover the wound surface with nonadherent, sterile gauze, and then add the necessary insulation through additional layers of toweling before applying the hot pack.
PRECAUTIONS	**RATIONALE**
Hand motor skills and reaction time (hp, pb)	May delay reaction time and decrease tapping speed in healthy subjects (Kaurenen et al., 1997). Inform patients that their hand motor skills may be impaired for a few hours following therapy.
Patients with severe cardiac insufficiency (hp, pb)	May not be able to cope with the increased cardiac demand triggered by the heat-induced increase in blood circulation. Periodic monitoring of vital signs is advised during and after therapy.
Over body areas with superficially located metal implants (hp, pb)	May cause internal soft tissue burns because metals absorb and conduct heat well. Use caution when applying hot pack and paraffin over such body areas.
Preventing fainting (hp, pb)	Some patients may faint during or immediately after a thermotherapy treatment, especially if systemic vasodilation is triggered because of a transient decrease in cerebral blood flow (Cameron, 2003). In such cases, lowering the patient's head while raising the feet will help recovery by increasing cerebral blood flow (Cameron, 2003). Patients suffering from orthostatic hypotension, if treated in the decubitus position, are also likely to experience fainting after treatment. Keep the patient's head elevated with a pillow during therapy, and wait a few minutes after the treatment has ended before allowing the patient to resume the sitting position (Cameron, 2003). Treatment delivered in the sitting position should cause no problem to these patients.
Body part resting on the hot pack as opposed to supporting it	May induce overheating and cutaneous burn if the application is such that the body part rests on top of the hot pack, thus creating higher-pressure contact between the pack and the skin while reducing the towel insulating capacity. Closer monitoring is advised because the skin's ability to dissipate heat is diminished.

(Continued)

TABLE 6-2	CONTINUED
RECOMMENDATIONS	**RATIONALE**
Disrobe the treated body areas and remove all objects, such as jewelry (hp, pb)	Maximize heat transfer and avoid cutaneous burn caused by heating of metal objects.
Inspect the exposed skin area before each treatment (hp, pb)	Assure close monitoring of potential side effects, such as skin irritation and burn caused by the agent.
Conduct skin thermal sensory discrimination testing—**mandatory** (hp, pb)	Minimize risk of cutaneous burn and maximizing dosimetry (see Chapter 25 for details).
Measure temperature differential between the agent and the skin (T°_{ag-s}) before treatment—**mandatory** (hp, pb)	The taking of this measurement is a must in the context of evidence-based practice because it provides quantitative assessment of the thermal dose delivered to the soft tissues (see Chapter 26 for details).
Measure skin temperature differential before and after treatment (T°_{b-a})—**mandatory** (hp, pb)	The taking of this measurement is a must in the context of evidence-based practice because it reveals the extent of soft-tissue heating caused by the thermal agent at the end of treatment (see Chapter 26 for details).
Wash and dry treated body areas before therapy (pb)	Minimize the risk of contaminating the paraffin mixture and optimize heat transfer.
Check on patient regularly during therapy (hp, pb)	Avoid overheating and assure optimal thermal comfort (Fyfe, 1982). Set a timer to warn both the patient and the clinician that the time of therapeutic exposure is over.
Discard used paraffin mixture	Eliminate the risk of contaminating the remaining mixture.
Use separate bath for hand and foot therapy (pb)	Maximize hygiene.
Instruct the patient to keep fingers apart and refrain from moving finger joints during therapy (pb)	Allow complete coating of each finger with wax and avoid the risk of breaking or cracking the hardened paraffin coatings.
Instruct the patient to stay awake during during therapy (hp, pb)	Falling asleep during thermotherapy may occur. Instructing the patient to stay alert will prevent potential skin damage.
Do not repeat application of hot pack	Repeating the application of hot packs every 10 minutes does not lead to further increase of cutaneous temperature. It only causes a slight increase in the subcutaneous and muscular tissue temperature in healthy subjects (Lehmann et al., 1966).
Plug line-powered devices into a GFCI receptacle	Prevent the occurrence of macroshocks (see Chapter 27 for details).
Conduct regular maintenance and calibration procedures (hp, pb)	Ensure optimal therapeutic efficacy and effectiveness. Follow the recommended maintenance schedules outlined by manufacturers.

1. Hot Pack and Cover

Commercial packs, made of hydrophilic silicate gel, absorb and retain the hot water contained in the hydrocollator unit. Water in the hydrocollator unit is maintained at temperatures ranging from 70°C to 76°C (158–168°F). Hot pack therapy always requires a coupling medium, such as a commercial terrycloth cover, that fully covers the pack before it is applied over the treated area, as shown in **Figure 6-3**. These covers are washable and reusable. Dry thick terrycloth towels can be used instead of commercial covers. Application duration is approximately 20 minutes. Hot packs are used primarily over flat and large body areas.

TABLE 6-3	BASIC CONSIDERATIONS FOR THE PRACTICE OF HOT PACK AND PARAFFIN BATH THERAPY	
	HOT PACK	**PARAFFIN BATH**
Basic component	Hydrophilic silicate gel enclosed within canvas.	Mixture of six parts paraffin to one part mineral oil, contained in a thermostatically heated bath.
Temperature range	70°C–76°C (158°F–168°F)	51°C–54°C (124°F–130°F)
Coupling medium	Commercial terrycloth cover or layers of terrycloth towels.	Intact skin: none needed. If minor or superficial wound present: sterile gauze.
Body application	Primarily over flat and large body areas.	Primarily over irregular body areas such as the extremities (wrist/hand; ankle/foot).
Application duration	≈20 min	≈30 min

2. Paraffin Bath

Paraffin is mixed with mineral oil to lower the melting point and the specific heat capacity of the mixture. The bath temperature is maintained at 51°C to 54°C (124°F to130°F). Paraffin bath therapy can be delivered using four different methods (see **Box 6-2** for details). **Figure 6-4** shows the typical paraffin cover observed over a hand that was just immersed in the paraffin bath. Coupling media is necessary only for the treatment of open wounds. Paraffin bath is used primarily for the treatment of extremities and over irregular body areas.

B. PROCEDURES

Safe, effective, and optimal application of these two thermal agents requires that clinicians go through a systematic set of procedures for each and every application. The following is a list of key procedures.

1. Checklists

Before proceeding with treatment, always go through the list of contraindications (**Table 6-1**) and the list of risks, precautions, and recommendations (**Table 6-2**).

2. Thermal Sensory Discrimination Testing

Because skin burn is always a possibility, thermal agents require thermal sensory discrimination testing prior to usage. The steps of this mandatory test are described in Chapter 25. Document the result of this test in the patient's file.

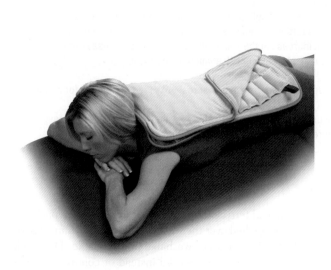

FIGURE 6-3 Commercial hot pack cover. (Courtesy of Chattanooga Group.)

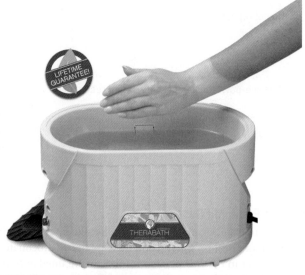

FIGURE 6-4 Typical paraffin cover over the hand following immersion. (Courtesy of WR Medical Electronics.)

3. Skin Inspection and Preparation

Expose the area to be treated and remove any jewelry. Inspect, wash, and dry the skin. Inspect the skin area over which the hot pack will be applied or that will be immersed in the paraffin bath. Any open wound must be covered with sterile gauze.

4. Pack and Bath Preparation

Select a hot pack size and terrycloth cover that best fits the size of the area to be treated. If towels are used, ensure proper layers of toweling (5–10) between the agent and the skin. Select a paraffin bath that best fits the size of the area to be treated. ALWAYS plug the line-powered bath into a ground-fault circuit interrupter (GFCI) receptacle to prevent any risk of macroshock or electrocution (see Chapter 27). Use commercial plastic liners and wraps to cover the immersed extremities to minimize paraffin heat loss.

5. During Treatment

Ensure that the patient is comfortably installed. Check the patient after 5 minutes of application to ensure thermal comfort. Instruct the patient that he or she should feel a warm, as opposed to a hot, sensation during therapy. If necessary, adjust the thickness of coupling to the desired level of heat sensation by adding or removing layers of toweling.

6. Dosimetry

Set the therapeutic dose by measuring the temperature differential between the agent and the skin (T°_{ag-s}) before application. This measurement will reveal how hot the pack or paraffin mixture is. Select dosage levels (T°_{ag-s}) that are capable of inducing heating changes (T°_{b-a}) that will best meet the therapeutic goals. Note that the size of the pack (the larger the size, the more heat it contains for a given temperature), the patient's layer of fat underneath the exposed treatment area, and the application duration influence dosage. Recall that the recommended application duration of hot pack is of 20 minutes and that of paraffin bath may vary greatly depending on the application method used (see **Box 6-2**).

7. End of Treatment

Inspect the exposed skin surfaces for signs of irritation or burn. Question the patient on the level of heat he or she has perceived during treatment in order to qualitatively assess the dose delivered. Any unusual sensation felt by the patient during treatment should be documented in the patient's file. Immerse the used hot pack in the hydrocollator unit. Allow approximately 30 minutes of immersion before using this hot pack again. Peel off the used paraffin and discard into waste bag.

8. Maintenance and Calibration

Optimal functioning of hot packs, hydrocollator units, and paraffin baths can be obtained only through adequate maintenance and calibration. Lack of maintenance can lead to safety issues (see Chapter 27 for details). Lack of periodic calibration can lead to inadequate dosimetry. Follow the manufacturer's recommendations with regard to all issues related to maintenance and calibration.

C. DOCUMENTATION

Adequate record taking in patients' files is expected from all health practitioners. **Table 6-4** shows key parameters to document in the patient's file following hot pack and paraffin bath therapy.

TABLE 6-4	KEY TREATMENT PARAMETERS TO BE DOCUMENTED IN PATIENT'S FILE AFTER HOT PACK OR PARAFFIN BATH THERAPY

Hot Pack Therapy
- Patient skin thermal sensory discrimination testing: record the result (see Chapter 25)
- Application duration: min
- Coupling medium: commercial cover or layers (number) of toweling
- (T°_{ag-s}): °C–°F
- (T°_{b-a}): °C–°F

Paraffin Bath Therapy
- Patient's skin thermal sensory discrimination testing: record the result (see Chapter 25)
- Application method used: description
- Application duration: min; record duration of wrapping and retention, when applicable
- Liner and wrap used: description
- (T°_{ag-s}): °C–°F
- (T°_{b-a}): °C–°F

Case Study 6-1   Subacute Low-Back Pain: Hot Pack Therapy

A 48-year-old male accountant, suffering from subacute low-back pain, consults for treatment. He recalls that his back pain first appeared 2 weeks earlier while lifting a heavy box of documents from the floor of his office. He went to see his physician on the following day. He left the physician's office with a prescription of analgesics, as well as anti-inflammatory and muscle-relaxant drugs. Battling chronic gastric problems for years, this patient wants to stop his drug treatment and replace it with a conservative treatment. There is no past history of back pain. The patient is wearing a pacemaker. The physical exam reveals a man who is underweight (70 kg; 158 pounds) for his height (1.82 m; 72 inches). It further reveals moderate pain over the entire bilateral low-back area as well as a light paravertebral muscle spasm causing difficulty with prolonged sitting at work. There is no neurological sign. Spinal ROM is within the normal range. The patient has reduced his work schedule from 5 to 4 days a week. His goals are to resume prolonged sitting and full-time work without having to take medication.

Evidence-Based Steps Toward the Resolution of This Case

1. **List medical diagnosis.**
   Subacute mechanical low-back pain

2. **List key impairment(s).**
   - Lumbar pain
   - Lumbar paravertebral spasm

3. **List key functional limitation(s).**
   - Difficulty with prolonged sitting

4. **List key disability(ies).**
   - Difficulty with work

5. **Justification for hot pack therapy.**
   Is there justification to use hot pack therapy in this case? This chapter has established that there is moderate strength of evidence behind, and poor to fair justification for, the use of hot pack therapy for soft-tissue pathology (see Section VI). This finding is in clear contradiction with the results of many surveys showing that hot pack therapy is available in the very large majority of clinical facilities and used routinely by a large majority of practitioners. The bottom line therefore is that if hot pack therapy is used for the treatment of soft-tissue pathology, its justification must rest as much on the evidence gathered in healthy subjects (**Box 6-1**) as on patient populations (**Box 6-3**). So where

is the justification for the selection of hot pack as the preferred thermal agent for this case? This textbook recommends the use of this agent for the following reasons. First, the use of shortwave diathermy therapy (Chapter 10) is contraindicated because the patient wears a pacemaker. Ultrasound therapy (Chapter 20) is also ruled out considering the disproportion between the small soundhead size and the much larger symptomatic treatment area. Fluidotherapy (Chapter 7) and paraffin bath therapy are also ruled out considering that the treatment area is large and involves the back area. Hot pack therapy appears as the preferred agent because there is evidence behind its heating effect on soft tissue and that heating can reduce pain, which in turn may reduce muscle spasm. The low-back area is ideal for the application of a hot pack, which can cover large symptomatic area. Considering the fact that this patient is lean (thin fat layer), heat transfer between the hot pack and the paravertebral musculature is maximized. Because EPAs should never be used in isolation or as a sole intervention, hot pack therapy is used here concomitantly with a regimen of manual spinal mobilization coupled with instructions on proper lifting techniques.

6. **Search for contraindications.**
   None is found. Note that in this case, the use of shortwave diathermy therapy (Chapter 10) is contraindicated because the patient is wearing a pacemaker.

7. **Search for risks and precautions.**
   None is found.

8. **Outline the therapeutic goal(s) you and your patient wish to achieve.**
   - Decrease pain
   - Decrease muscle spasm
   - Eliminate drug intake
   - Improve sitting time
   - Improve performance at work

9. **List the outcome measurement(s) used to assess treatment effectiveness.**
   - Muscle spasm: manual palpation
   - Drug intake: pill count in personal diary
   - Pain/sitting and work performance: Modified Oswestry Low-Back Pain Questionnaire

10. **Instruct the patient about what he/she should experience, do, and not do during the hot pack application.**
    - Feel warm sensation over low-back area

- Do not touch or remove the pack
- If a hot or burning sensation is felt, call for help immediately

11. Outline the therapeutic prescription of hot pack based on the evidence available.

There is no evidence from research on which to rely for establishing the prescription in this case. The following prescription, therefore, rests on the other two elements of evidence-based practice, that is, the practitioner's own clinical experience with this agent and pathology and the patient's preference and belief about therapy (see Section VI).

- *Thermal agent:* commercial hydrocollator pack
- *Hot pack size:* 38 × 61 cm (15 × 24 in)—to cover the entire painful area
- *Hot pack temperature:* 70°C (158°F)
- *Treated body area:* over the entire lower back area
- *Patient's positioning:* lying in prone position
- *Coupling media:* commercial cover wrapped in two layers of terrycloth toweling
- *Application duration:* 20 minutes
- *Total number of treatments:* 10 treatments, delivered daily, over a 2-week period separated by a weekend

12. Analyze outcome measurements.

Pre- and posttreatment comparison

- Muscle spasm: absent

- Drug intake: none
- Pain/sitting and work performance: Oswestry score improved by 80%

13. Assess therapeutic effectiveness based on outcome measures.

The results show that the application of 10 hot pack treatments, combined with a therapeutic regimen of spinal mobilization and lifting instructions, delivered over a 2-week period, led to a full recovery. The fact that this patient remained active at work rather than staying at home during his therapy, benefited the therapeutic regimen. The patient is now free of muscle spasm, takes no drugs, and is working full time. Overall, this conservative treatment had a beneficial impact on the patient's disablement status created by the pathology, as illustrated in the **figure below.**

14. State the prognosis.

Excellent if the patient continues to use the proper lifting techniques he learned, both at work and at home. With adequate compliance with these instructions, similar episodes of low-back pain are not likely to recur. If a similar back pain episode was to recur, this patient should consider using an over-the-counter heat wrap, wearable for several hours during daily activities, before relying on medication (see Nadler et al., 2002; 2003 a,b; Trowbridge et al., 2004) or any other conservative intervention.

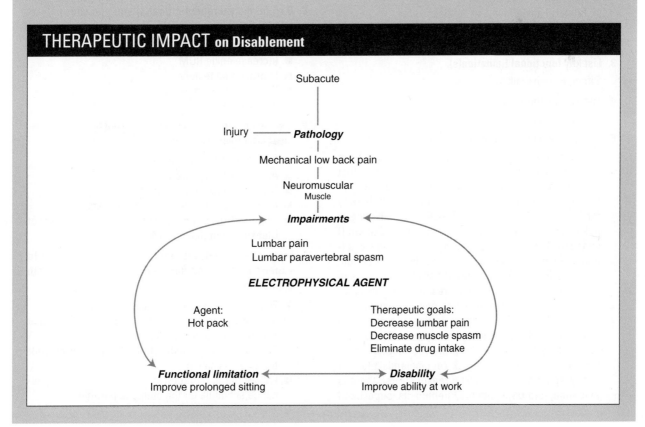

THERAPEUTIC IMPACT on Disablement

A 65-year-old woman, with a long history of moderate rheumatoid arthritis, consults for treatment. Physical exam reveals painful walking, bilateral ankle joint and toe stiffness, light toe deformity, and chapped and dry skin on the feet and ankles. Examination of the upper limbs reveals adequate wrist and hand function. She is under the regular care of her rheumatologist, who has prescribed analgesic and anti-inflammatory drugs for her condition. She wears regular shoes and rubs an over-the-counter cream on her feet and ankles daily to soften her skin. She is concerned about her reduced and declining ability to walk and to perform activities of daily living (ADLs). She is also concerned about the increasing side effects of her medication. Her goals are to reduce drug intake while keeping her mobility. Her favorite social activity is to visit and chat with her friends who live at a walking distance from her home. Her preference is definitively for a home treatment, considering her reduced walking ability and the fact that she has no personal and easy access to public transportation to facilitate any hospital or clinic displacements. She heard from a good friend about the possibility of using home paraffin bath therapy for her arthritic condition. She is convinced that this conservative therapy may help her condition.

Evidence-Based Steps Toward the Resolution of This Case

1. List medical diagnosis.

Rheumatoid arthritis

2. List key impairment(s).

- Painful ankles and feet
- Bilateral ankle/foot joint stiffness
- Reduced bilateral ankle ROM
- Chapped and dry skin overlying ankles and feet

3. List key functional limitation(s).

Difficulty with walking

4. List key disability(ies).

Difficulty with social visits

5. Justification for paraffin bath therapy.

Is paraffin bath therapy the preferred therapeutic option in this case? This chapter has established that there is moderate strength of evidence behind, and poor justification for, the use of paraffin bath therapy for rheumatoid arthritis (see **Box 6-3**). This finding is in keeping with the results of surveys (see Section I) showing that the use of this agent, although available in many facilities, is on the decline. The bottom line therefore is that if paraffin bath therapy is used as treatment, justification must rest on elements other than the evidence from research one can gather from the English-language, peer-reviewed literature (see **Box 6-3**). So where is the justification behind the selection of paraffin bath as the preferred thermal agent for this case? This textbook recommends the use of this agent for the following reasons: First, there is evidence, although limited, behind its superficial

heating effect on soft tissue in healthy subjects (Abramson et al., 1964; Borrell et al., 1980), which suggests that heating can reduce pain and joint stiffness, which in turn may improve function, reduce drug intake, and soften chapped and dry skin (Pils et al., 1991; Sandqvist et al., 2004). In other words, this thermal agent is expected to significantly heat the muscles and periarticular joint structures of the ankle, foot, and toe joints, and to hydrate and soften the skin overlying these joints. Deep heating of these periarticular structures is expected to reduce joint stiffness by decreasing joint viscosity, thus improving walking ability. Second, the irregular surfaces associated with the ankles, feet, and toes are ideal body areas for the application of paraffin mixture, transmitting heat to entire cutaneous surfaces. Third, the fact that this elderly patient prefers a home therapy approach and strongly believes that paraffin bath therapy can improve her condition are other reasons behind the selection of this agent over any other thermal agents. Finally this patient is alert, able to follow instructions, and has adequate upper limb mobility and function to operate a paraffin bath at home. Because EPAs should never be used in isolation or as a sole intervention, paraffin bath is used here concomitantly with a home regimen of passive and active joint (ankle and toes) mobilizations.

6. Search for contraindications.

None is found.

7. Search for risks and precautions.

None is found.

8. Outline the therapeutic goal(s) you and your patient wish to achieve.

- Decrease pain
- Increase ankle ROM
- Improve skin texture
- Decrease drug intake
- Improve walking and ADLs

9. List the outcome measurement(s) used to assess treatment effectiveness.

- Pain: Visual Analog Scale (VAS)
- Ankle ROM: goniometry
- Skin texture: visual assessment
- Drug intake: pill count in personal diary
- Walking/ADLs performance: Arthritic Impact Measurement Scale (AIMS)

10. Instruct the patient about what he/she should experience, do, and not do during the paraffin bath application.

- Feel warm sensation over lower extremities
- If a hot or burning sensation is felt, stop treatment and call the treatment clinician
- Follow the home instruction sheet given by your treatment clinician
- Follow the manufacturer's operation and maintenance schedule for the bath and paraffin

11. **Outline the therapeutic prescription based on the evidence available.**

There is poor evidence from research (**Table 6-3**) on which to rely for establishing the prescription in this case (Hawkes et al., 1985). The following prescription, therefore, rests also on the other two elements of evidence-based practice, that is the practitioner's own clinical experience with this agent and pathology and the patient's preference and belief about therapy (see Section VI). Considering the reduced mobility and age of this patient, a home treatment approach was used. The recommendation is for the patient to rent a paraffin bath for a month. The first four treatments were delivered by the practitioner at home. During these visits, the patient was instructed on how to use the unit, how to do proper maintenance, and how to maximize safety during application. She was also instructed on how to mobilize her ankle and toes after therapy.

- ■ *Thermal agent:* commercial paraffin bath filled with paraffin mixture
- ■ *Paraffin mixture temperature:* 51°C (124°F)
- ■ *Immersed body segments:* ankle and foot
- ■ *Application method:* dip immersion with wrapping
- ■ *Application duration:* 30 minutes
- ■ *Total number of treatments:* 21 treatments, delivered daily, over a 3-week period

12. **Analyze outcome measurements.**

Pre- and posttreatment comparison:

- ■ Pain: decrease VAS score from 6 to 2
- ■ Ankle ROM: Right: increase by 15 degrees; Left: increase by 10 degrees
- ■ Skin texture: softer
- ■ Drug intake: decrease by 25%
- ■ Walking/ADLs performance: AIMS score improved by 60%

13. **Assess therapeutic effectiveness based on outcome measures.**

The results show that 21 consecutive home paraffin bath treatments, combined with a daily self-regimen of ankle and foot mobilization, led to a significant functional gain of ankle ROM, which translated to a much better ability to walk and improved her ability to manage her ADLs and visit her friends. The patient's pain was reduced, her chapped skin resolved, and she reduced her use of drugs. The patient is very satisfied with the results and is looking forward to continuing her paraffin bath therapy at home. Overall, this treatment approach had a beneficial impact on the patient's disablement status created by the pathology, as illustrated in the **figure below**.

14. **State the prognosis.**

There is, unfortunately, no cure for rheumatoid arthritis. Consequently, this elderly patient is looking to a prolonged treatment, lasting months and years, with periodic control of her condition. She is thus advised to purchase, as opposed to renting, the paraffin bath and related accessories. She is again firmly instructed to always plug her paraffin bath into a GFCI receptacle at home so as to ensure full protection against electrical shock. She is also instructed to continue her therapeutic regimen every second day for another month and then to reduce the treatment frequency according to her symptoms and functional ability. The prognosis is good for many years to come if her rheumatoid flares are adequately controlled by her medication.

THERAPEUTIC IMPACT on Disablement

Chronic

Pathology —— Disease

Rheumatoid arthritis

Arthroskeletal
Articular cartilage
Ligaments/tendons

Neuromuscular
Muscle

Impairments

Bilateral ankle-foot pain
Bilateral ankle-foot stiffness
Chapped and dry skin

ELECTROPHYSICAL AGENT

Agent:
Paraffin bath

Therapeutic goals:
Decrease pain
Improve ankle range of motion
Improve skin texture
Decrease drug intake
Improve walking

Functional limitation
Improve walking

Disability
Improve ability to do ADLs

CRITICAL THINKING QUESTIONS

Clarification: What is meant by hot pack and paraffin bath therapy?

Assumptions: Because they are classified as superficial thermal agents, many of your colleagues assume that hot pack and paraffin baths can only induce heating effect in superficial soft tissues. How can you verify or disprove this assumption?

Reasons and evidence: What led you to believe that the subcutaneous fat layer, compared with other soft tissues, is the greatest thermal barrier?

Viewpoints or perspectives: How would you respond to a colleague who says that there is no difference between the concepts of heat and temperature, and thus whatever material or agent has the highest temperature is always the hottest?

Implications and consequences: What generalizations can you make about the use of hot pack and paraffin bath therapy based on the scientific evidence available?

About the question: Why is it important to measure the temperature differential between the agent and the skin (T°_{ag-s}) overlying the treatment area before treatment, and the temperature differential of the skin overlying the treatment area, before and immediately after treatment (T°_{b-a})? Why do you think I ask this question?

References

Articles

Abramson DI, Tuck S, Chu LS, Agustin C (1964) Effects of paraffin bath and hot fomentation on local tissue temperatures. Arch Phys Med Rehab, 45: 87–94

American Physical Therapy Association (APTA) (2001) Guide to physical therapy practice. Phys Ther, 81: 27–34; 105–138

Borrell RM, Parker R, Henley EJ, Masley D, Repinecz M (1980) Comparison of in vivo temperatures produced by hydrotherapy, paraffin wax treatment and fluidotherapy. Phys Ther, 60: 1273–1276

Bromley J, Unsworth A, Haslock I (1994) Changes in stiffness following short- and long-term application of standard physiotherapeutic techniques. Br J Rheumatol, 33: 555–561

Burns SP, Conin TA (1987) The use of paraffin wax in the treatment of burns. Physiother Can, 39: 258–260

Chipchase LS, Williams MT, Robertson VJ (2005) A survey of electrophysical agents's curricula in entry level physiotherapy programs in Australia and New Zealand. NZ J Physioth, 33: 34-47

Cordray YM, Krusen EM (1959) Use of hydrocollator packs in the treatment of neck and shoulder pains. Arch Phys Med Rehab, 39: 105–108

Cosgray NA, Lawrance SE, Mestrich JD, Martin SE, Whalen RL (2004) Effect of heat modalities on hamstring length: A comparison of Pneumatherm, moist hot pack, and a control. J Orthop Sports Phys Ther, 34: 377–384

Dellhag B, Wollersjö I, Bjelle A (1992) Effect of hand exercise and wax bath treatment in rheumatoid arthritis patients. Arthritis Care Res, 5: 87–92

De Sanfort B (1915) Keritherapy: New method of thermal treatment by means of paraffin. M Press, 100: 556, 580

Draper DO, Harris ST, Shulties S, Durrant E, Knight KL, Ricard M (1998) Hot-packs and 1-MHz ultrasound treatments have an additive effect on muscle temperature increase. J Athl Train, 33: 21–24

Erdman WJ, Stoner EK (1956) Comparative heating effects of moistaire and hydrocollator hot packs. Arch Phys Med Rehab, 37: 71–74

Fountain FP, Gersten JW, Sengir O (1960) Decrease in muscle spasm produced by ultrasound, hot packs, and infrared radiation. Arch Phys Med Rehab, 41: 293–297

Fyfe M (1982) Skin temperature, color, and warmth felt, in hydrocollator pack applications to the lumbar region. Aust J Physiother, 28: 12–16

Harris R, Millard JB (1955) Paraffin-wax baths in treatment of rheumatoid arthritis. Ann Rheum Dis, 14: 278–282

Hawkes J, Care G, Dixon JS, Bird HA, Wright V (1985) Comparison of three physiotherapy regimens for hands with rheumatoid arthritis. Br Med J, 291: 1016

Head MD, Helms PA (1977) Paraffin and sustained stretching in the treatment of burns contracture. Burns, 4: 136–139

Helm PA, Kevorkian CG, Lushbaugh M (1982) Burn injury: Rehabilitation management in 1982. Arch Phys Med Rehab, 63: 6–16

Henrickson AS, Fredriksson K, Persson I, Pereira R, Rostedt Y, Westlin N (1984) The effect of heat and stretching on the range of hip motion. J Orthop Sports Phys Ther, 13: 110–115

Hollander JL, Horvath SM (1949) Influence of physical therapy procedures on intra-articular temperature of normal and arthritic subjects. Am J Med Sci, 218: 543–548

Horvath SM, Hollander JL (1949) Intra-articular temperature as measure of joint reaction. J Clin Invest, 28: 469–473

Hoyrup G, Kjorvel L (1986) Comparison of whirlpool and wax treatments for hand therapy. Physiother Can, 38: 79–82

Humphris FH (1920) Melted paraffin wax bath. Br Med J, 2: 397–399

Kaurenen K, Vanharanta H (1997) Effects of hot and cold packs on motor performance on normal hands. Physiotherapy, 83: 340–344

Knight CA, Rutledge CR, Cox ME, Acosta M, Hall SJ (2001) Effect of superficial heat, deep heat, and active exercises warm-up on the extensibility of the plantar flexors. Phys Ther, 81: 1206-1214

Landen BR (1967) Heat or cold for the relief of low back pain? Phys Ther, 47: 1126–1128

Lehmann JF, Silverman DR, Baum BA, Kirk NL, Johnson VC (1966) Temperature distribution in the human thigh produced by infrared, hot pack and microwave applications. Arch Phys Med Rehab, 47: 291–299

Lentell G, Hetherington T, Eagan J, Morgan M (1992) The use of thermal agents to influence the effectiveness of a low-load prolonged stretch. J Orthop Sports Phys Ther, 16: 200–207

Lindsay DM, Dearnes J, McGinley CC (1995) Electrotherapy usage trends in private physiotherapy practice in Alberta. Physiother Can, 47: 30–43

McCray RE, Patton NJ (1984) Pain relief at trigger points: A comparison of moist heat and shortwave diathermy. J Orthop Sports Phys Ther, 5: 175–178

Miller M, Wirth M, Rockwood C (1996) Thawing the frozen shoulder: The "patient" patient. Orthopedics, 19: 849–853

Nadler SF, Steiner DJ, Erasala GN, Hengehold DA, Hinkle RT, Beth Goodale M, Abeln S, Weingand KW (2002) Continuous low-level heatwrap therapy provides more efficacy than ibuprofen and acetaminophen for acute low back pain. Spine, 27: 1012–1027

Nadler SF, Steiner DJ, Petty SR, Erasala GN, Hengehold DA, Weingand KW (2003a) Overnight use of continuous low-level heatwrap therapy for relief of low back pain. Arch Phys Med Rehab, 84: 335–342

Nadler SF, Steiner DJ, Erasala GN, Hengehold DA, Abeln SB, Weingand KW (2003b) Continuous low-level heatwrap therapy for treating acute nonspecific low back pain. Arch Phys Med Rehab, 84: 329–334

Nussbaum EL, Burke S, Johnstone L, Lahiffe G, Robitaille E, Yoshida K (2007) Use of electrophysical agents: Findings and implications of a survey of practice in metro Toronto. Physioth Can, 59: 118–131

Pils K, Graninger W, Sadil F (1991) Paraffin hand bath for scleroderma. Phys Med Rehab, 1: 19–21

Pope GD, Mockett SP, Wright JP (1995) A survey of electrotherapeutic modalities: Ownership and use in the NHS in England. Physiotherapy, 82: 82–91

Portmann U (1926) Electrically heated paraffin bath. Phys Ther, 44: 333–336

Robertson VJ, Spurritt D (1998) Electrophysical agents: Implications of their availability and use in undergraduate clinical placements. Physiotherapy, 84: 335–344

Robertson VJ, Ward AR, Jung P (2005) The effect of heat on tissue extensibility: A comparison of deep and superficial heating. Arch Phys Med Rehab, 86: 519–825

Sandqvist G, Akesson A, Eklund M (2004) Evaluation of paraffin bath treatment in patients with systemic sclerosis. Dis Rehab, 26: 981–987

Stimson CW, Rose GB, Nelson PA (1958) Paraffin bath as thermotherapy: An evaluation. Arch Phys Med Rehab, 39: 219–227

Taylor BF, Waring OA, Brashear TA (1995) The effects of therapeutic application of heat or cold followed by static stretch on hamstring muscle length. J Orthop Sports Phys Ther, 21: 283–286

Trowbridge CA, Draper DO, Feland JB, Hutte LS, Eggett DL (2004) Paraspinal musculature and skin temperature changes: Comparing the ThermaCare heatwrap, the Johnson & Johnson back plaster, and the ABC Warme-Pflaster. J Orthop Sports Phys Ther, 34: 549–558

Williams J, Harvey J, Tannenbaum H (1986) Use of superficial heat versus ice for the rheumatoid arthritic shoulder: A pilot study. Physiother Can, 38: 8–13

Yung P, Unsworth A, Haslock I (1986) Measurement of stiffness in the metacarpophalangeal joint: The effects of physiotherapy. Clin Phys Physiol Meas, 7: 147–156

Zeiter WJ (1939) Clinical application of the paraffin bath. Arch Phys Ther, 20: 469–472

Review Articles

Ayling J, Marks R (2000) Efficacy of paraffin wax baths for rheumatoid arthritic hands. Physiotherapy, 86: 190–201

Brosseau L, Younge KA, Robinson V, Marchand S, Judd M, Wells G, Tugwell P (2006) Thermotherapy for the treatment of osteoarthritis. The Cochrane Library, 3: 1–18

Hardy M, Woodall W (1998) Therapeutic effects of heat, cold, and stretch on connective tissue. J Hand Ther, 11: 148–156

Robertson VA, Brosseau L, Casimiro L, Judd MG, Shea BJ, Tugwell P, Wells G (2006) Thermotherapy for treating rheumatoid arthritis. The Cochrane Library, 3: 1–53

Chapters of Textbooks

Basford JR (1998) Physical agents. In: Rehabilitation Medicine: Principles and Practice. DeLisa JA, Gans BM (Eds). Lippincott-Raven Publishers, Philadelphia, pp 483–503

Bell GW, Prentice WE (2002) Infrared modalities. In: Therapeutic Modalities for Physical Therapists, 2nd ed. Prentice WE (Ed). McGraw-Hill Health Profession Division, New York, pp 201–269

Cameron MH (2003) Thermal agents: Cold and heat. In: Physical Agents in Rehabilitation. From Research to Practice, 2nd ed. WB Saunders, Philadelphia, pp 161–173

Hayes KW (2000) Superficial heat. In: Manual for Physical Agents, 5th ed. Hayes KW (ed.) Prentice Hall Health, Upper Saddle River, pp 3–20

Hecox B, Sanko JP (2006) Superficial thermotherapy. In: Integrating Physical Therapy in Rehabilitation, 2nd ed. Hecox B, Mehreteab TA, Weisberg J, Sanko J (Eds). Pearson Prentice Hall, Upper Saddle River, pp 153–160

Jackins S, Jamieson A (1990) Use of heat and cold in physical therapy. In: Therapeutic Heat and Cold, 4th ed. Lehmann JF (Ed). Williams & Wilkins, Baltimore, pp 645–651

Knight KL, Draper DO (2008a) Principles of heat for thermotherapy. In: Therapeutic Modalities: The Art and Science. Lippincott Williams & Wilkins, Philadelphia, pp 188–199

Knight KL, Draper DO (2008b) Application procedures: Superficial thermotherapy. In: Therapeutic Modalities: The Art and Science. Lippincott Williams & Wilkins, Philadelphia, pp 200–214

Lehmann JF, DeLateur BJ (1990) Therapeutic heat. In: Therapeutic Heat and Cold, 4th ed. Lehmann JF (Ed). Williams & Wilkins, Baltimore

Michlovitz SL, Rennie S (2005) Heat therapy modalities: Beyond fake and bake. In: Modalities for Therapeutic Interventions, 4th ed. Michlovitz SL, Nolan TP (Eds). FA Davis, Philadelphia, pp 61–78

Michlovitz SL, Von Nieda K (2006) Therapeutic heat and cold. In: Physical Agents: Theory and Practice, 2nd ed. Behrens BJ, Michlovitz SL (Eds). FA Davis Co, Philadelphia, pp 36–55

Sekins KM, Emery AF (1990) Thermal science for physical medicine. In: Therapeutic Heat and Cold, 4th ed. Lehmann JF (Ed). Williams & Wilkins, Baltimore, pp 62–112

Starkey C (2004) Clinical application of thermal modalities. In: Therapeutic Modalities, 3rd ed. FA Davis, Philadelphia, pp 124–154

Monographs

National Physiotherapy Advisory Group (NPAG) (2001) Physiotherapy Entry-Level Education in Canada. Defining a Vision. Canadian Physiotherapy Association, Toronto

Fluidotherapy

Chapter Outline

Learning Objectives

Knowledge: List the key parameters of Fluidotherapy that should be documented in the patient's file after each treatment.

Comprehension: Compare the heat transfer properties and thermal responses of Fluidotherapy to those of hot pack and paraffin bath therapy.

Application: Demonstrate the procedures required to ensure safe and effective application of Fluidotherapy.

Analysis: Explain the concept of fluidization.

Synthesis: Explain the proposed mechanisms behind the physiological and therapeutic effects attributed to Fluidotherapy.

Evaluation: Discuss the strength of scientific evidence behind the therapeutic justification of Fluidotherapy for the treatment of soft tissues.

I. RATIONALE FOR USE

A. DEFINITION AND DESCRIPTION

Fluidotherapy is a trademarked name coined in 1973 by an American chemical engineer named Ernest Henley. Fluidotherapy is defined as the use of a fluidized bed of organic particles, thus the term *fluido*, for the delivery of heat for therapeutic purposes. It is described as a dry-heating agent that transfers heat to the treated parts by convection. The device allows finely divided particles to circulate around the treated area by a warm air current, creating a fluidlike medium.

B. FLUIDOTHERAPY DEVICE

Figure 7-1 shows three different models of Fluidotherapy devices with a container, filled with finely divided particles of cellulose, called *Cellex,* to be emptied into the device's chamber. These line-powered devices are designed to treat the upper and lower limbs.

C. RATIONALE FOR USE

The rationale behind the development and application of Fluidotherapy was the desire to provide clinicians with an effective alternative to the traditional therapeutic application of moist heat agents, such as hot pack and paraffin bath therapy (see Chapter 6), and hydrotherapy (see Chapter 9). The goal was also to develop a *dry*-heating agent capable of inducing significant heat transfer in soft tissues using means other than electromagnetic energy, such as short-wave diathermy therapy (see Chapter 10), and mechanical energy, such as ultrasound therapy (see Chapter 20).

II. HISTORICAL PERSPECTIVE

A. DISCOVERY

Fluidotherapy was first conceived in 1972 by an American chemical engineer named Ernest Henley. He was unimpressed by the capacity of existing moist thermal therapeutic agents, such as hot-pack and paraffin bath therapy (see Chapter 6), to deliver heat to soft tissues. Henley sought to develop a new dry thermal agent that would transfer a greater quantity of heat to superficial as well as deep soft tissues (Henley, 1991).

B. CONCEPT OF FLUIDIZATION

Drawing on his engineering knowledge of the good thermal conductivity of fluidized beds for heat transfer in industry, Henley adapted the industrial concept of fluidization to the field of therapeutics, coining the trademarked name Fluidotherapy. The first Fluidotherapy device is reported to have been built in 1974 and to have been first tested clinically at the Saint Anthony Center Hospital in Houston, Texas.

C. FIRST HUMAN STUDY

In 1977, Borrell and colleagues published the results of what appears to be the first study of Fluidotherapy conducted on human subjects (Borrell et al., 1977). This group of authors, which included Ernest Henley, reported on the heat transfer capabilities of this agent compared with those of traditional paraffin baths (see Chapter 6) and warm whirlpool tubs (see Chapter 9).

D. BODY OF LITERATURE

An exhaustive search of the English-language, peer-reviewed scientific literature reveals that the topic of Fluidotherapy has been the subject of few *articles* (Borrell et al., 1977, 1980; Valenza et al., 1979; Alcorn et al., 1984; Kelly et al., 2005), *review articles* (Henley, 1991; Herrick et al., 1992), and *short chapters of textbooks* (Rennie et al., 1996; Bell et al., 2002 Hecox et al., 2006).

III. BIOPHYSICAL CHARACTERISTICS

A. FLUIDIZATION

The biophysical principle behind the clinical use of Fluidotherapy is fluidization (Henley, 1991). To fluidize

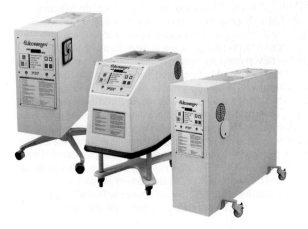

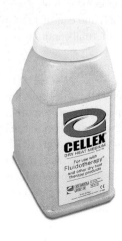

FIGURE 7-1 Typical Fluidotherapy devices, shown with a container of fine organic particles called Cellex. (Courtesy of Chattanooga Group.)

something means that finely divided particles, activated by a flow of warm air, are caused to acquire the characteristics of a fluid.

B. DEVICE COMPONENTS

Figure 7-2 shows the basic components of a typical Fluidotherapy device. Such a device brings a bed of fine cellulose particles to a fluidized state that induces the desired physiological and therapeutic effects on soft tissues.

C. FORCED CONVECTION

Fluidotherapy is the use of a dry thermal agent which transfers its energy, in the form of heat, to soft tissues by the process of forced convection. That is, the heat transfer takes place through forced movements, or agitation, of heated air and cellulose particles in the unit chamber, which together are circulated, as shown in **Figure 7-2B**, around the body part during treatment.

D. HEAT TRANSFER

A limb immersed in a fluidized bed of a different temperature than itself will experience a heat transfer rate many times greater than it would if immersed in a warm airbed alone (Henley, 1991; Borrell et al., 1977, 1980). This is because the particles make physical contact with the immersed limb, thus enhancing the heat transfer.

E. SPECIFIC HEAT CAPACITY AND THERMAL CONDUCTIVITY

These two biophysical concepts, defined and described in Chapter 5, are important concepts related to the practice of Fluidotherapy. Briefly, specific heat capacity (c) is the ability of a substance to hold, or store, heat at a given temperature. Thermal conductivity (k), on the other hand, is the ability of a substance to transmit, or conduct, heat.

1. Air Versus Paraffin

Why is it that, if you immerse one of your hands in a Fluidotherapy chamber of a given temperature and the other in a paraffin bath (see Chapter 6) of the same temperature, the paraffin bath feels hotter than the air chamber? Because paraffin holds approximately 2 times more heat (higher specific heat capacity; c = 0.45 versus 0.24) and conducts heat approximately 30 times faster (higher thermal conductivity; k = 0.59 versus 0.02) than air.

2. Air Versus Water

Why is it that, if you immerse one of your hands in a Fluidotherapy chamber of a given temperature and the other in a water tub (see Chapter 9) of the same temperature, the water tub feels much hotter than the air chamber? Because water holds approximately 4 times more heat (higher specific heat capacity; c = 1.00 versus 0.24) and conducts heat approximately 70 times faster (higher thermal conductivity; k = 1.42 versus 0.02) than air.

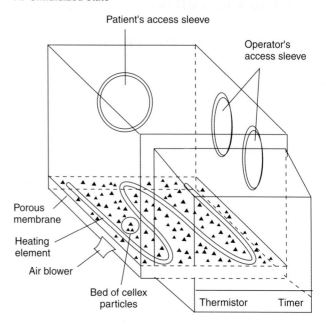

A. Unfluidized state

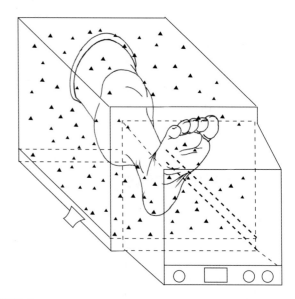

B. Fluidized state

FIGURE 7–2 A typical Fluidotherapy unit is made of the following components: (1) a chamber made of steel, plastic, or glass containing the fluidized medium, represented by a bed of cellulose particles, which rests on a porous membrane at the bottom of the chamber; (2) an air blower unit; (3) a heating element; (4) access sleeves for the patient and clinician; (5) a thermistor; and (6) a timer. **A:** *Unfluidized state.* The device is turned off, and as a result the Cellex particles lie resting against the porous membrane. **B:** *Fluidized state.* The heating element and the air blower are turned on. The bed of particles is now agitated, and the particles are suspended in the heated air chamber, free to move around the treated body segment. The amount of heat, the blower speed, and the timer are under the control of the operator. Cellulose particles, commercially known as Cellex particles, are derived from corncobs, which are made of natural and organic cellulose (Herrick et al., 1992). Manufacturers of Fluidotherapy units describe these particles as environmentally safe and recyclable.

IV. PHYSIOLOGICAL AND THERAPEUTIC EFFECTS

A. THERMOMECHANICAL EFFECTS

The proposed physiological and therapeutic effects associated with the use of Fluidotherapy (Henley, 1991; Kelly et al., 2005) are summarized in **Figure 7-3**. These effects are described as thermal and mechanical in nature.

1. Thermal Effect

The main physiological effect attributed to this EPA is thermal, through the heating of soft tissues. **Table 7-1** summarizes the results gathered by Borrell et al. (1980) on four healthy subjects, which provide scientific evidence for the heating effect of Fluidotherapy. These results show Fluidotherapy to be more effective than paraffin baths and warm whirlpool tubs at inducing absolute temperature increases in peripheral joint capsules and muscles. Borrell et al. (1977) reported the average heat absorption induced by Fluidotherapy to be approximately threefold greater than that of paraffin baths and warm water (17.2, 5.6, and 4.8 BTUs, respectively) after 15 minutes of continuous application of each of these three agents to a hand. The results of a recent study (Kelly et al., 2005) conducted on a cohort of 7 healthy subjects also provide evidence that Fluidotherapy, when delivered at a temperature of approximately 47°C for 20 minutes, can increase skin temperature by 5°C when compared with a similar-size control group.

2. Mechanical Effect

A second physiological effect attributed to Fluidotherapy is mechanical, through the gentle rubbing effect the fine particles have on the surface of the skin (Henley, 1991; Kelly et al., 2005).

B. COMBINED EFFECTS

The thermal effect of Fluidotherapy is proposed to enhance tissue healing and decrease pain (Henley, 1991; Kelly et al., 2005). Its mechanical effect is proposed to decrease hypersensitive skin areas (Henley, 1991).

V. DOSIMETRY

A. DOSAGE

The thermomechanical dose delivered during treatment is determined by setting the following parameters on the device's console. The combined effects of air temperature and agitation of particles in the chamber cause the phenomenon of fluidization on the immersed limb.

1. Operating Temperature

Set the desired temperature, which normally ranges between 43°C and 52°C (110°F and 126°F).

2. Air Agitation Speed

Set the desired speed, which ranges from 0% to 100% (5% increments).

3. Operating Mode

Select between continuous or pulsed mode.

4. Dose

This value, or dose, is the temperature differential between the agent (ag) operating temperature and the exposed skin (s) surface; it corresponds to $T°_{ag-s}$. This setting is done easily and quickly using a noncontact, portable, infrared thermometer, as described in Chapter 26.

5. Application Duration

Recommended duration is approximately 20 minutes.

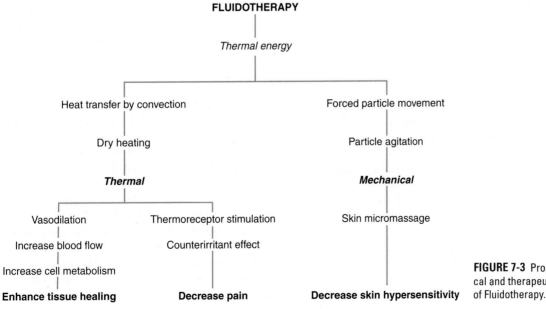

FIGURE 7-3 Proposed physiological and therapeutic effects of Fluidotherapy.

TABLE 7-1	SUMMARY OF RESULTS OBTAINED BY BORRELL AND COLLEAGUES		
	FLUIDOTHERAPY	**PARAFFIN BATH**	**HYDROTHERAPY**
Type of heat	Dry	Moist	Moist
Energy transfer mode	Forced convection	Passive conduction	Passive conduction
Agent temperature	47.8°C (118°F)	55.0°C (131°F)	38.8°C–40°C (102°F–104°F)
Application duration	20 min	20 min	20 min
Number of subjects	4	4	4
Body areas investigated	Hand/foot	Hand/foot	Hand/foot
Maximum temperature rise (depth, 0.5 cm), joint capsule[a]	9.0°C (16.2°F)	7.5°C (13.5°F)	6.0°C (10.8°F)
Maximum temperature rise (depth, 1.2 cm), muscle[b]	5.2°C (9.5°F)	4.5°C (8.1°F)	4.3°C (7.7°F)

Borrell et al. (1980) state that each curve in their figures 2–5 represents single subject measurement. No descriptive data and statistics are provided to explain the intersubject variability of these measurements.
[a]Metacarpophalangeal and metatarsophalangeal joints; probe tip located 0.5 cm beneath the skin surface.
[b]Flexor hallucis brevis muscle; probe tip located 1.2 cm beneath the skin surface.

B. QUANTITATIVE DOSIMETRY

The evidence-based practice of Fluidotherapy requires that the therapeutic dose administered to a patient during therapy be *quantitatively* assessed. To qualitatively assess dosage level by simply asking the patient about his or her perception of heat during treatment, currently a routine practice, is not enough. A simple, practical, and rapid way to quantitatively assess thermal dosage is to measure two temperature differentials, namely, the temperature difference between the agent (ag) and the exposed skin (s) surface (T°_{ag-s}) and the temperature differential between the exposed skin surface before (b) and after (a) treatment (T°_{b-a}). Chapter 26 shows how these two measurements are taken using a portable infrared surface thermometer.

1. Case Example

The Fluidotherapy unit's operating temperature is set at 48°C (118°F) and the exposed skin surface measured at 30°C (86°F). The thermal dose delivered is the temperature difference between the agent and the skin (T°_{ag-s}), 18°C (22°F), which represents its *potential* heating effect. Immediately after treatment, the exposed skin temperature is measured at 36°C (97°F); the *actual* skin heating effect (T°_{b-a}) of this dosage was +6°C (+11°F).

2. To Sum Up

In the context of evidence-based practice, it is useful to ask the patient how warm the thermal agent felt during and after treatment. But it is even better to supplement this qualitative information with actual temperature measurements. This textbook strongly encourages practitioners to supplement their qualitative approach with the suggested quantitative approach. It is easy and practical, and not time-consuming, to take these temperature measurements using an infrared portable thermometer.

VI. EVIDENCE FOR INDICATIONS

A. GUIDED BY EVIDENCE

Dictionaries generally define *evidence* as anything that establishes a fact or gives reason to believe something. The aim of this textbook is to present scientific evidence behind therapeutic EPAs. To be guided by evidence is the process of integrating evidence from research, however imperfect or scarce this evidence may be, with clinical experience and patients' values. In other words, the *evidence-based practice* of EPA requires practitioners to consider the evidence from research, in addition to their own clinical experience and the patient's own preference and beliefs about a given EPA, when the time comes to justify, prescribe, and apply the therapeutic agent. To be guided by evidence is a process, not a search for the absolute truth. Finally, a lack of evidence from research behind any given EPA does not mean that this EPA should never be used. What it means is that no statement can be made on its therapeutic effectiveness and that until more evidence from research is presented, its routine use cannot be recommended.

B. EVIDENCE FROM HUMAN RESEARCH

Box 7-1 provides evidence for Fluidotherapy based on an exhaustive search of published English-language, peer-reviewed literature on human research. The term *indication* refers to a list of pathologies for which Fluidotherapy is used. Ratings of therapeutic benefit (Yes or No) and grading of the strength of scientific evidence (I, II, or III), including the reference, are included for each pathological condition.

1. Rating Therapeutic Benefit

The rating, expressed as Yes or No, is based on the overall conclusion(s) reached on the issue of therapeutic effectiveness by the author(s) who conducted the peer-reviewed study.

2. Grading Strength of Evidence

The grading, numerically classified as I, II, and III, is based on the type of research methodology or experimental design used by the author(s). All the studies listed are human studies published in English-language, peer-reviewed journals. It follows that the strength of evidence in studies graded I is stronger than in those graded II, which itself is stronger than in those graded III.

a. Grade I

Evidence based on human *controlled* studies, regardless of their level of randomization and blindness.

b. Grade II

Evidence based on human *noncontrolled* studies, regardless of their level of randomization and blindness.

c. Grade III

Evidence based on human *case* studies, regardless of their level of randomization and blindness.

3. Strength of Evidence Behind the Agent

The strength of evidence in favor of the agent, as presented in the research-based indication box, is arbitrarily assessed in this textbook as being *weak, moderate,* or *strong.* For example, the larger the number of studies graded I, regardless of therapeutic benefit, the stronger the scientific evidence in favor of the agent.

4. Evidence Justifying Usage of the Agent

The strength of evidence justifying usage of the agent for individual pathologies or groups of pathologies, as listed in the research-based indication box, is arbitrarily assessed in this textbook as being *poor, fair, good,* or *conflicting.* For example, when a large number of studies on an agent show therapeutic benefit (Yes) and are graded I, for any given pathology, the justification for usage of this agent for this pathology is assessed as *good. Conflicting* justification is reported when similar numbers of studies, with similar grades, show therapeutic benefit (Yes) and no benefit (No).

C. STRENGTH OF EVIDENCE AND JUSTIFICATION FOR USAGE OF FLUIDOTHERAPY

The results gathered in **Box 7-1** show *weak* strength of evidence behind Fluidotherapy, with only two clinical studies graded as II and III, respectively. They also show *poor* justification for the use of this thermal agent with, again, only two clinical studies, both beneficial for different pathologies. To sum up, the body of evidence presented strongly suggests that until more evidence from research is provided, the routine usage of Fluidotherapy *cannot be recommended.*

VII. CONTRAINDICATIONS

The contraindications associated with the practice of Fluidotherapy are listed in **Table 7-2**. These contraindications are based more on clinical common sense than on evidence from research.

VIII. RISKS, PRECAUTIONS, AND RECOMMENDATIONS

The practice of Fluidotherapy is not without risks for patients. The main risks associated with this EPA, as well as some precautions and recommendations designed to improve safety and effectiveness, are listed in **Table 7-3**.

Box 7-1	Research-Based Indications for the Use of Fluidotherapy			
PATHOLOGY		**BENEFIT**	**GRADE**	**REFERENCE**
Sickle cell anemia in children: decrease pain and improve mobility		Yes	II	Alcorn et al., 1984
Podiatric conditions: increase blood circulation		Yes	III	Valenza et al., 1979

TABLE 7-2	CONTRAINDICATIONS TO FLUIDOTHERAPY
CONTRAINDICATIONS	**RATIONALE**
Over skin area where sensation to heat is severely impaired	Risk of cutaneous burn.
Over a cancerous area	Risk of enhancing tumor growth and metastasis.
Over thrombophlebitic area	Risk of dislodging blood clot, which may then circulate into the vessels of vital organs, causing serious circulatory problems and, possibly, death.
Over hemorrhagic area	Risk of additional bleeding caused by increased blood flow in area.
Over acute and severe inflammatory pathology	Risk of worsening the condition by aggravating the inflammatory response through increased blood flow resulting from heat application.
With confused and unreliable patients	Risk of complications during therapy, reducing treatment effectiveness.

TABLE 7-3	RISKS, PRECAUTIONS, AND RECOMMENDATIONS FOR FLUIDOTHERAPY
RISKS	**RATIONALE**
Over an area of impaired blood circulation	Risk that the treated area will not be able to cope with the demand for additional and cooler blood flow needed during heat application to prevent tissue overheating.
With cases of systemic infectious diseases	Risk of increased core body temperature, which may increase fever (Henley, 1991; Herrick et al., 1992).
Failure to perform required maintenance	Risk of cellulose particles entering the unit's heat chamber, causing severe injury to the patient and smoke damage to the facility and the device.
Used in the presence of flammable anesthetics	Risk of explosion.
PRECAUTIONS	**RATIONALE**
Over an open wound	Cellulose particles may embed in the wound increasing the risk of cross-contamination. Always cover a wound with a nonpermeable dressing before treatment.
Cases in which the limb is covered with splints, bandages, tapes, and/or contains orthopedic pins, plastic joint replacements, or artificial tendons	May cause uneven heat distribution within the tissues. Additional supervision during treatment is advised.
All entry ports	Cellulose particles may escape the device's chamber if all entry ports are not properly sealed before turning on the device.

(Continued)

TABLE 7-3	CONTINUED

RECOMMENDATIONS	RATIONALE
Disrobe the treated body areas and remove all objects, such as jewelry	Although Fluidotherapy can be administered in the presence of clothing and metallic objects, undressing the exposed body part will maximize heat transfer (Henley, 1991). The removing of externally worn objects is always indicated before therapy.
Inspect the exposed skin area before each treatment (hp, pb)	Assure close monitoring of potential side effects, such as skin irritation and burn caused by the agent.
Conduct skin thermal sensory discrimination testing—**mandatory**	Minimize risk of cutaneous burn and maximizing dosimetry. This test is described in Chapter 25.
Wash and dry treated body areas before paraffin bath therapy	Minimize the risk of contaminating the device's chamber and organic particles and optimizing heat transfer.
Measure temperature differential between the agent and the skin (T°_{ag-s}) before treatment—**mandatory**	The taking of this measurement is a must in the context of evidence-based practice because it provides quantitative assessment of the thermal dose delivered to the soft tissues (see Chapter 26 for details).
Measure skin temperature differential before and after treatment (T°_{b-a}) – **mandatory**	The taking of this measurement is a must in the context of evidence-based practice because it reveals the extent of soft-tissue heating caused by the thermal agent at the end of treatment (see Chapter 26 for details).
Assure that all entry ports are sealed properly and instruct the patient to shake the treated body part prior to removing it from the chamber	Minimize organic particles lost.
Plug line-powered devices into a GFCI receptacle	Prevent the occurrence of macroshocks (see Chapter 27 for details).
Conduct regular maintenance and calibration procedures	Ensure optimal therapeutic efficacy and effectiveness. Follow the recommended maintenance schedules outlined by manufacturers.

IX. CONSIDERATIONS FOR APPLICATION AND DOCUMENTATION

A. KEY CONSIDERATIONS

Listed in **Box 7-2** are the main advantages and disadvantages associated with the application of Fluidotherapy. A key advantage is that thermotherapy can be delivered without the use of plumbing and toweling.

B. CASE EXAMPLES

Contrary to hot pack and paraffin bath therapy (see Chapter 6), which deliver moist heat to small/large flat body surfaces (hot packs) or to the extremities (ankle/feet, wrist/hands), Fluidotherapy devices can deliver dry heat to the entire upper (arm, forearm, wrist, and hand) and lower (thigh, leg, ankle, and foot) limbs. **Figure 7-4** shows case applications to unilateral upper limb (**A**), bilateral upper

limbs (**B**), and unilateral lower limb (**C**). In all cases the patient sits in front of the device and then immerses his or her bare upper or lower limb into the unit chamber.

C. PROCEDURES

Safe, effective, and optimal application of Fluidotherapy requires that clinicians go through a systematic set of procedures for each and every application. The following is a list of such procedures.

1. Checklists

Before proceeding with the treatment, always go through the list of contraindications (**Table 7-2**) and the list of risks, precautions, and recommendations (**Table 7-3**).

2. Thermal Sensory Discrimination Testing

Because skin burn is always a possibility, thermal agents require thermal sensory discrimination testing prior

Box 7-2	Advantages and Disadvantages of Fluidotherapy

Advantages

Unit is convenient and easy to operate.

Limb can be positioned in the horizontal plane, minimizing the effect of gravity.

Higher temperature is used, because dry heat is better tolerated than moist heat.

Heat is distributed over the entire limb surface area.

Unit can be placed anywhere in the service area, department, or clinic.

Free limb movement is possible during the entire treatment session.

Access ports allow clinicians to use their hands to mobilize the limb.

Minimal to no pressure is applied to the treated area.

Treatment over an open wound is possible if the wound is sealed and protected from cellulose particles.

Temperature and particle agitation is controlled by the operator.

Temperature is kept constant throughout the treatment session.

Unit requires no water plumbing or toweling.

Disadvantages

Devices are relatively expensive to purchase.

Treatment is limited to distal upper and lower extremities.

Devices are relatively large, requiring appropriate floor space to accommodate them.

---

to usage. The conduct of this mandatory test is described in Chapter 25. Document the result of this test in the patient's file.

3. Skin Inspection and Preparation

Undress the limb to be treated and remove any jewelry. Inspect, wash, and dry the skin. Open wounds must be covered with sterile gauzes to avoid particles from touching them.

4. Device Preparation

Plug the line-powered device into a ground-fault circuit interrupter (GFCI) receptacle to prevent the risk of

any macroshock or electrocution during treatment (see Chapter 27). Preheat the device. Ask the patient to immerse his or her limb into the device's chamber. Ensure that all entry ports are properly sealed.

5. During Treatment

Ensure that the patient is comfortably installed and instruct him or her not to touch the device. Instruct the patient to exercise or not exercise the limb during therapy. The treated body part may or may not be manipulated, or mobilized, by the treating clinician during the application.

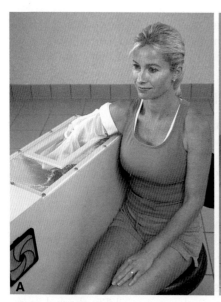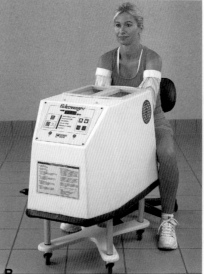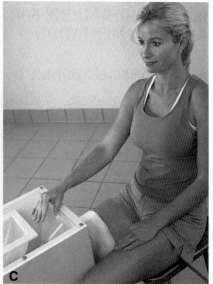

FIGURE 7-4 Applications of Fluidotherapy over one upper limb **(A)**, two upper limbs simultaneously **(B)**, and one lower limb **(C)**. (Courtesy of Chattanooga Group.) Practitioners can use the other unused ports to manipulate the limb in the chamber during treatment.

6. Dosimetry

Set the therapeutic dose by choosing the mode of application (continuous or pulsed), temperature level, air agitation speed, and application duration. Measure the temperature gradient between the agent and the skin ($T°_{ag-s}$) before application and the skin temperature gradient before and after ($T°_{b-a}$) treatment, using an infrared thermometer (see Chapter 26). The device's temperature is obtained from the console built-in thermometer. These temperature differentials will reveal how hot (i.e., heating potential) the EPA was before application and how hot the skin (actual tissue heating) was at the end of treatment, thus providing quantitative dosimetry. Select dosage levels ($T°_{ag-s}$) that are capable to induce tissue-heating changes ($T°_{b-a}$) that will best meet the therapeutic goals.

7. End of Treatment

Ask the patient to lightly shake his or her immersed limb in the chamber, so as to remove Cellex particles from the skin surface, before pulling it out of the chamber. Inspect the exposed skin surface for signs of irritation or burn. Question the patient on the level of heat he or she has perceived during treatment in order to qualitatively assess the dose received. Any unusual sensation felt by the patient during treatment should be documented in the patient's file.

8. Maintenance and Calibration

Optimal functioning of the Fluidotherapy device can only be obtained through adequate maintenance and calibration. Lack of maintenance can lead to safety issues (see Chapter 27). Lack of periodic calibration can lead to inadequate dosimetry. Follow the manufacturer's recommendation with regard to the device's maintenance and calibration.

D. DOCUMENTATION

Adequate record taking in the patient's file is expected from all health practitioners. **Table 7-4** shows key parameters to document in the patient's file following Fluidotherapy.

TABLE 7-4	KEY TREATMENT PARAMETERS TO BE DOCUMENTED IN PATIENT'S FILE AFTER FLUIDOTHERAPY

- Skin thermal sensory testing: record the result (see Chapter 25)
- Operating mode: continuous or pulsed; if pulsed, record ON:OFF ratio
- Temperature setting: °C–°F
- Operating air agitation speed: % of maximum
- Immersed body area: description
- Application duration: min
- Temperature differential between the agent and the skin before application ($T°_{ag-s}$): °C–°F
- Temperature differential between skin surface before and after application ($T°_{b-a}$): °C–°F

Case Study 7-1   Osteoarthritis

A 60-year-old retired woman suffering from osteoarthritis consults for treatment. Her main complaints are increasing pain and general joint stiffness over her right and left elbow, wrist, and hand areas, causing her increasing difficulties with her activities of daily living (ADLs), including personal hygiene. She also complains of her increasing inability to do her shopping and carry bags. Physical examination reveals no warmth and no swelling over her painful joints and a relatively large open skin wound over the lateral side of her left index finger, from a recent cut with a kitchen knife. The wound is covered with a Band-Aid. She reports taking oral analgesics for years, but over the past 6 months they have started to give her gastric irritation. She is aware that the therapeutic application of moist heat, in the form of paraffin bath (see Chapter 6), may help her condition, but she worries that, because her two hands are affected, she will not be able to adequately perform paraffin bath therapy at home, which would have to be done daily on both her hands. Her preference is to receive dry heat over all of her painful body areas. Her goal is to be able to adequately perform personal hygiene and do most of her ADLs, as well as shopping, while reducing her daily use of oral analgesics.

Evidence-Based Steps Toward the Resolution of This Case

1. List medical diagnosis.

- Osteoarthritis

(Continued)

Case Study 7-1   Continued

2. List key impairment(s).

- Bilateral elbow, wrist, and hand pain
- Bilateral elbow, wrist, and finger joint stiffness

3. List key functional limitation(s).

- Difficulty with personal hygiene
- Difficulty with ADLs

4. List key disability/disabilities.

- Difficulty with shopping

5. Justification of Fluidotherapy.

Is there justification for the use of Fluidotherapy in this case? This chapter has established that there is weak strength of evidence behind and poor justification for the use of Fluidotherapy for soft-tissue pathology and that, consequently, its routine application cannot be recommended until more evidence is presented (see Section VI). The bottom line therefore is that if Fluidotherapy is used today for the treatment of this arthritic condition, its justification must rest on elements other than the evidence one can gather from the English-language, peer-reviewed human literature (**Box 7-1**). So where is the justification for the selection of Fluidotherapy as the preferred thermal agent for this case? This textbook recommends the use of this agent for the following reasons: First, the pathology is chronic and there is no evidence of inflammation. Second, the patient's preference is for the use of a dry thermal agent that would heat up all of her painful body areas, that is, from her elbows to her fingertips. Considering the large and bilateral treatment areas to be covered, the use of other dry-heat agents, such as shortwave diathermy (Chapter 10) or ultrasound therapy (Chapter 20), is ruled out. Hot pack therapy (Chapter 6) is not an option because it will require multiple simultaneous applications. Paraffin bath therapy (Chapter 6) is also not an option because immersion of elbow and forearm areas is impossible. Fluidotherapy, therefore, appears to be the preferred agent because there is evidence, although limited (see **Table 7-1**), of its heating effect on healthy human upper-limb tissues (Borrell et al., 1977, 1980; Kelly et al., 2005). Fluidotherapy is expected to induce significant heating of superficial and deep joint structures, such as joint capsules, including muscles and ligaments. Together these effects are expected to decrease pain by reducing joint stiffness, thus leading to more functional upper limb ability. Because EPAs should never be used in isolation or as a sole intervention, Fluidotherapy is used here concomitantly with a regimen of passive elbow, wrist, and finger stretching done by the clinician during treatment and by a regimen of active elbow, wrist, hand, and finger exercises done by the patient at home.

6. Search for contraindications.

None is found.

7. Search for risks and precautions.

This patient has an open wound over the left index finger. This wound must be sealed with a nonpermeable dressing before each treatment until it is completely healed. This will prevent the flowing of Cellex particles from invading the wound during the treatment.

8. Outline the therapeutic goals you and your patient wish to achieve.

- Decrease pain
- Decrease elbow, wrist, and hand joint stiffness
- Decrease use of oral analgesics
- Improve ability to perform personal hygiene and ADLs
- Improve ability to shop

9. For each therapeutic goal, list which outcome measurement(s) you will use to assess treatment effectiveness.

- Pain: Numerical Rating Scale 101 (NRS-101)
- Joint stiffness: goniometry
- Drug intake: pill count in personal diary
- Personal hygiene / ADL / shopping performance: arthritic impact measurement scale (AIMS) and patient-specific function scale (PSFS)

10. Instruct the patient about what he or she should experience, do, and not do during the application of Fluidotherapy.

- Feel warm sensation over immersed upper limbs
- Feel stretching over the wrist and finger joints as the clinician manipulates the joints in the unit's chamber during treatment
- In the absence of clinician, gently mobilize the elbow, wrist, and fingers in the device's chamber during treatment

11. Outline your therapeutic prescription based on the evidence available.

There is no evidence from research (**Box 7-1**) for establishing the prescription of Fluidotherapy in this case. The following prescription, therefore, rests on the evidence provided by Borrell et al. (1977, 1980) and Kelly et al. (2005) in healthy subjects. It is also based on the patient's preference for dry heat as well as on the practitioner's clinical experience with this agent and pathology.

- **Fluidotherapy unit type:** upper extremity unit
- **Operating mode:** continuous
- **Operating temperature:** 48°C (118°F)
- **Air agitation speed:** 75% of maximum
- **Immersed body segments**
  - Right and left elbow, forearms, wrists, and hands
  - Immersion of left followed by right upper limb
  - Gauze applied over wound of left index finger
- **Application duration:** 20 minutes
- **Total number of treatments:** 15 treatments, delivered 5 times per week, over a 3-week period

12. **Analyze outcome measurements.**

Pre- and posttreatment comparison:

- Pain: decreased NRS-101 score from 75 to 20
- Joint stiffness
  - Elbow flexion/extension ROM: Increase of 8° (left) and 12° (right)
  - Wrist flexion/extension ROM: Increase of 3° (left) and 7° (right)
- Drug intake: decrease count by 30%
- Personal hygiene/ADLs/shopping performance: improved AIMS score by 65%; improved PSFS score by 70%.

13. **Assess therapeutic effectiveness based on outcome measures.**

The results show that 15 Fluidotherapy treatments, combined with passive and active joint stretching regimens, delivered over a 3-week period, led to significant therapeutic benefit. In addition to improvement in elbow and wrist mobility, the main benefits were drug intake reduction, decrease in pain, and improved performance in regard to personal hygiene, ADLs, and shopping activities. She is very satisfied with these results. Overall, this treatment approach had a beneficial impact on the patient's disablement status created by the pathology, as illustrated in the **figure below**.

14. **State the prognosis.**

Because there is no cure for such a condition, the prognosis is a continued management of her residual pain and joint stiffness, using drugs and conservative interventions, for the months and years to come. The patient is advised to stay mobile by continuing to do her personal, home, and shopping activities, knowing very well that some level of pain will always persist. She is also advised to apply, when the pain is too strong, microwavable dry-heat pads over the painful joints when resting at home. Finally she is asked to consult again if her arthritic upper limb condition was to deteriorate further.

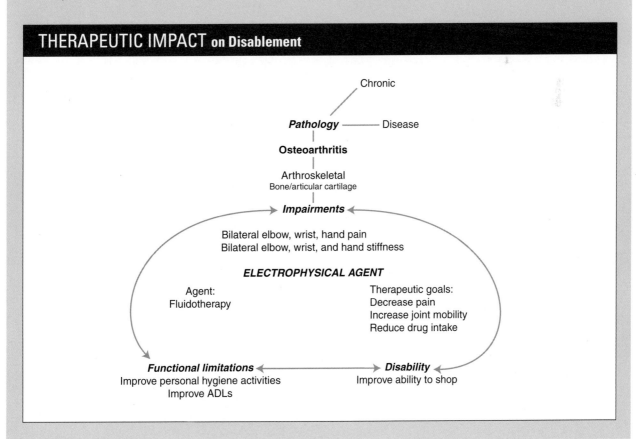

THERAPEUTIC IMPACT on Disablement

CRITICAL THINKING QUESTIONS

Clarification: What is meant by Fluidotherapy?

Assumptions: You have assumed Fluidotherapy may be as effective as other moist therapeutic heating agents, such as hot packs and paraffin baths, in substantially heating superficial and deep soft tissues. How do you justify that assumption?

Reasons and evidence: What led you to believe that the heat transfer mode in Fluidotherapy is forced convection?

Viewpoints or perspectives: How would you respond to a colleague who says that the use of Fluidotherapy devices has more disadvantages than advantages?

Implications and consequences: What are the implications and possible consequences of not adequately covering an open wound in the exposed limb and of not performing regular maintenance on the Fluidotherapy device?

About the question: Is it true that Fluidotherapy is the only EPA capable of delivering dry heat to soft tissues? Why do you think I ask this question?

References

Articles

Alcorn R, Bowser R, Henley EJ, Holloway V (1984) Fluidotherapy and exercise in the management of sickle cell anemia: A clinical report. Phys Ther, 64: 1520–1522

Borrell RM, Henley EJ, Ho P, Hubbell MK (1977) Fluidotherapy: Evaluation of a new heat modality. Arch Phys Med Rehab, 58: 69–71

Borrell RM, Parker R, Henley EJ, Masley D, Repinecz M (1980) Comparison of in vivo temperatures produced by hydrotherapy, paraffin wax treatment, and Fluidotherapy. Phys Ther, 60: 1273–1276

Kelly R, Beehn C, Hansford A, Westphal KA, Halle JS, Greathouse DG (2005) Effect of Fluidotherapy on superficial radial nerve conduction and skin temperature. J Orthop Sports Phys Ther, 35: 16–23

Valenza J, Rossi C, Parker R, Henley EJ (1979) A clinical study of a new heat modality: Fluidotherapy. J Am Podiatr Assoc, 69: 440–442

Review Articles

Henley EJ (1991) Fluidotherapy. Crit Rev Phys Rehab Med, 3: 173–195

Herrick RT, Herrick S (1992) Fluidotherapy: Clinical applications and techniques. Ala Med, 61: 20–25

Chapters of Textbooks

Bell GW, Prentice WE (2002) Infrared modalities. In: Therapeutic Modalities for Physical Therapists. Prentice WE (Ed). McGraw-Hill, New York, pp 233–235

Hecox B, Sanko JP (2006) Superficial thermotherapy. In: Integrating Physical Agents in Rehabilitation, 2nd ed. Hecox B, Mehreteab TA, Weisberg J, Sanko J (Eds). Pearson Prentice Hall, Upper Saddle River, New Jersey, pp 160–162

Rennie GA, Michlovitz SL (1996) Biophysical principles of heating and superficial heating agents. In: Thermal Agents in Rehabilitation, 3rd ed. Michlovitz SL (Ed). FA Davis, Philadelphia, pp 122–124

Cryotherapy

Chapter Outline

Learning Objectives

Knowledge: List and describe the various cryoagents practitioners use to deliver cryotherapy.

Comprehension: Explain the biophysical principles and concepts underlying the use of cryotherapy for managing soft tissue pathologies.

Application: Show the methods practitioners can use to deliver cryotherapy.

Analysis: Explain the proposed physiological and therapeutic effects of cryotherapy.

Synthesis: Explain the rationale behind each of the elements practitioners must consider when calculating the dosimetry of a cryoagent.

Evaluation: Discuss the strength of the English-language-based scientific evidence supporting the use of cryotherapy for managing soft tissue pathologies.

I. RATIONALE FOR USE

A. DEFINITION AND DESCRIPTION

The term *cryotherapy* is derived from the Greek word *cryos*, meaning cold, and refers to lowering the temperature of soft tissue for therapeutic purposes. In this textbook, cryotherapy refers to the *percutaneous,* or *surface,* application of cryoagents resulting in the withdrawal of heat from the body, causing a reduction in the temperature of soft tissue. The use of cryotherapy for surgical purposes (tissue destruction) is beyond the scope of this chapter.

B. CRYOAGENTS

Several cryotherapy agents have been developed and marketed over the past five decades. This chapter focuses on the most commonly used agents: ice packs, icicles, gel packs, instant cold packs, vapocoolant sprays, cryocompression-controlled devices, and cryotemperature-controlled devices. A sample of each is shown in **Figure 8-1**. Readers will notice that the use of water-based cryoagents, in which cold *water* is the thermal medium, as with cold baths and tubs, is covered in the chapter on hydrotherapy (Chapter 9).

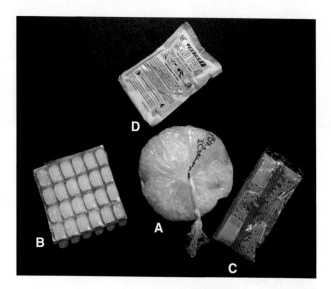

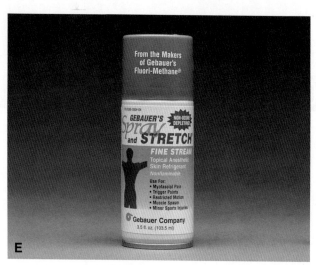

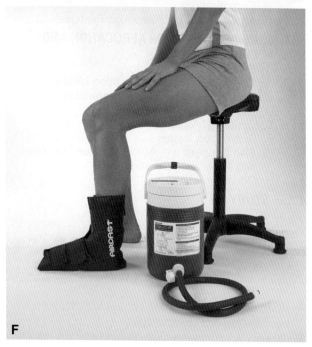

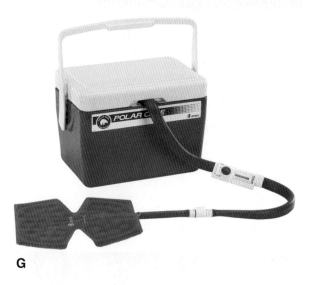

FIGURE 8-1 Common cryoagents: (**A**) ice pack, (**B**) icicles, (**C**) gel pack, (**D**) instant cold pack, (**E**) vapocoolant spray, (**F**) cryocompression-controlled unit, (**G**) cryotemperature-controlled unit. (A to D: Reprinted with permission from Knight, KL and Draper DO. Therapeutic Modalities. Baltimore, Maryland: Lippincott Williams & Wilkins, 2008; E: Courtesy of Gebauer Co.; F: Courtesy of Aircast Global Corp.; G: Courtesy of Breg Inc.)

C. RATIONALE FOR USE

The therapeutic use of cryoagents relates primarily to the treatment of acute and subacute soft-tissue pathology, characterized by the two early phases of tissue repair—hemostatic and inflammatory (see Chapter 2). It is hypothesized that by decreasing soft-tissue temperature, cryotherapy promotes the regulation of these two important phases, thus aiding in the process of tissue repair and recovery. Moreover, cooling other soft tissues, such as peripheral nerves of the nociceptive and gamma systems, provides the rationale for using this electrophysical agent (EPA) to manage pain and spasticity.

II. HISTORICAL PERSPECTIVE

A. FOUNDATIONS

Cryotherapy dates back to the ancient Greeks and Romans, who used snow and natural ice to treat a variety of health problems (Knight, 1995). During the mid-1950s, the clinical use of various cryoagents emerged under the leadership of physical therapists and athletic trainers for the treatment of various acute and subacute soft-tissue pathologies (Knight, 1995).

B. FORMAL RECOGNITION

Acceptance of cryotherapy by the health-care mainstream came during the early 1960s after Grant (1964) and Hayden (1964) showed its benefits for the treatment of various musculoskeletal injuries in military populations. The results of their studies were important to the formal establishment and recognition of cryotherapy as an integral part of physical medicine, physical therapy, athletic therapy, and sports medicine.

C. BODY OF LITERATURE

Over the past three decades, cryotherapy has been the subject of several *articles* (see References), *review articles* (Hocutt, 1981; McMaster, 1982; Teppermann et al., 1983; Kowal, 1983; Meeusen et al., 1986; Kellett, 1986; Airhihenbuwa et al., 1987; McLean, 1989; Halvorson, 1990; Chapman, 1991; Nanneman, 1991; Rivenburg, 1992; Hayes, 1993; Cook et al., 1994; Ernst et al., 1994; McDowell et al., 1994; Swenson et al., 1996; Hardy et al., 1998; Kerr et al., 1999; MacAuley, 2001a,b; Merrick, 2002; Daanen, 2003; Hubbard et al., 2004a,b; Bleakley et al., 2004; Allen, 2006; French et al., 2006), and *chapters of textbooks* (Lehmann et al., 1990; Low et al., 1990; Sekins et al., 1990; Hayes et al., 2000; Bell et al., 2002; Cameron, 2003; Starkey, 2004; Michlovitz, 2005; Michlovitz et al., 2006; Hecox et al., 2006; Knight et al., 2008a,b). Kenneth Knight's textbook (1995), although written in the mid-1990s, still merits special mention because it is the only textbook available that exclusively deals with the theory and practice of cryotherapy.

III. BIOPHYSICAL CHARACTERISTICS

A. HEAT ABSORPTION AND TRANSFER

The biophysical foundation of cryotherapy rests on the concepts of heat absorption and heat transfer. The field of thermodynamics stipulates that heat transfer is always unidirectional, occurring from *high* to *low*. Cryoagents, therefore, do not transfer their coldness to the warmer soft tissues. Instead, soft tissues cool by losing their heat to the cryoagents. In other words, this transfer of tissue heat to the cryoagent causes tissue cooling.

B. SUPERFICIAL VERSUS DEEP TISSUE COOLING

Superficial tissues, such as skin, cool down by losing heat to the cryoagents. Deeper tissues, such as muscle and joint structures, cool in a similar fashion by losing their heat to the more superficial tissues, which have been previously cooled by the cryoagent (Merrick et al., 2003). Located in between the superficial and deep tissues is the subcutaneous fat tissue, which plays an important role in the process of heat transfer.

C. SUBCUTANEOUS FAT TISSUE

As stated above, deep tissue cooling can occur only if some of their heat is absorbed and lost to the cooler superficial tissues. This process is inevitably influenced by the thickness of subcutaneous fat tissue that separates the superficial from the deep soft tissues in the treated area.

1. Fat Thermal Conductivity

The ability of soft tissues to conduct heat is determined by its thermal conductivity (k). Subcutaneous fat (k = 0.45) conducts heat approximately 2 times less than skin (k = 0.90) and 3 times less than muscle (k = 1.53). This means that the thicker the subcutaneous layer, the greater the thermal barrier between superficial (skin) and deeper tissues, such as muscle, ligament, tendon, and joint capsule.

2. Fat and Deep Tissue Cooling

There is strong experimental evidence to show that a significant inverse relationship exists between subcutaneous fat tissue thickness and rate of intramuscular temperature change (Lowden et al., 1975; Johnson et al., 1979; Zemke et al., 1998; Myer et al., 2001). This means that for any given cryoagent, the thinner the subcutaneous fat layer is, the greater the rate and extent of deeper tissue cooling.

3. Fat and Application Duration

Experimental evidence also suggests a direct relationship between adipose thickness and required application duration or cooling time (Otte et al., 2002). This means that to cool deeper tissues covered by a thick subcutaneous fat layer, a longer application period is required so that cooler superficial tissues can extract more heat from the warmer deep tissues. In other words, the greater the superficial tissue cooling is, the greater the deep tissue cooling will be.

D. HEAT TRANSFER MODES

Heat transfer in cryotherapy occurs via two modes: conduction and evaporation.

1. Conduction

Heat transfer by conduction occurs when there is direct contact between the surface of the cryoagent and the skin surface over which it is applied (see Chapter 5). All the cryoagents covered in this chapter, with the exception of vapocoolant spray, work using this form of heat transfer.

2. Evaporation

Heat transfer by evaporation occurs through the conversion of a substance from a liquid to a vapor state (Sekins et al., 1990). For example, when the vapocoolant liquid spray hits the surface of the skin, it is heated by the warm skin, thus changing its physical state from liquid to vapor. During this process of evaporation, the skin loses heat, resulting in its cooling (see Chapter 5).

E. HEAT EXTRACTION

The biophysical process behind cryotherapy involves the extraction of heat from soft tissues to cool them for therapeutic purposes. The greater the amount of heat extracted by the cryoagent, the greater the soft tissue cooling effect will be.

IV. PHYSIOLOGICAL AND THERAPEUTIC EFFECTS

A. GENERAL EFFECTS

The proposed physiological and therapeutic effects of cryotherapy are listed in **Figure 8-2**.

1. Cooling

The initial and primary effect of cryotherapy is the cooling of soft tissues, which occurs usually within the first 20 minutes of application. Tissue cooling is caused by the extraction or withdrawal of heat from the exposed tissue by the cryoagent. This cooling effect induces significant vascular and neural responses that may last as long as a few hours, or until full tissue rewarming occurs (see Knight, 1995; Knight et al. 2008a,b).

2. Cold-Induced Vasodilation

The subsequent and secondary effect is cold-induced vasodilation (CIVD). This effect is a response to tissue cooling, which, under some particular circumstances (intense cooling) and for some specific organs or body areas (such as hand and foot, nail bed, elbow, lips, cheeks, ears, and nose), may prevent cold-induced tissue damage (see Iida, 1949; Daanen et al., 1997; Daanen, 2003).

B. COOLING

Tissue cooling causes several physiological effects, which may induce therapeutic responses that decrease blood flow, cell metabolism, secondary tissue damage, edema, pain, muscle spasm, and spasticity (see the following subsections).The application of a cryoagent over a skin surface area triggers the reflex activation, or depolarization, of several sympathetic adrenergic nerve fibers. The depolarization of these nerve fibers leads to release of their neurotransmitter, norepinephrine, on the adrenergic receptors of smooth muscles surrounding blood vessels, which in turn causes a *powerful reflex vasoconstriction*.

1. Decrease Blood Flow

There is evidence to show that vasoconstriction decreases blood flow to soft tissues by reducing the lumen (or diameter) of blood vessels; the smaller the lumen, the less the amount of blood flowing per unit of time (Knight, 1995; Daanen, 2003).

2. Decrease Cell Metabolism

There is also evidence to show that reducing tissue temperature (cooling it) reduces cell metabolism, which in turn further reduces the tissue's oxygen requirement (Knight et al., 2008a,b).

3. Decrease Secondary Tissue Damage

Primary tissue damage refers to the cellular damages (dead cells) caused by injury or disease, found at the site of the wound. There is a consensus in the field of cryotherapy that the key therapeutic effect caused by this powerful reflex vasoconstriction decreases cell metabolism, as shown in **Figure 8-2**, which in turn will decrease secondary tissue damage (see Knight, 1995; Merrick, 2002; Knight et al., 2008a,b). *Secondary* tissue damages refer to cellular damages caused to nondamaged or healthy cells within, and at the periphery of, the wound. Because soft tissues have a very limited time window during which they can survive ischemia (lack of blood) and hypoxia (lack of oxygen), the time period between the initial injury and the first application of cryotherapy is *critical*. There is a consensus that, *when applied as soon as possible after injury*, that is, within the first *24 to 48 hours*, cryotherapy makes a greater contribution to tissue repair by limiting the extent of secondary tissue damage (Knight, 1995; Knight et al., 2008a,b). When the tissue temperature is lowered, the rate of cellular metabolism is slowed down, and thus the

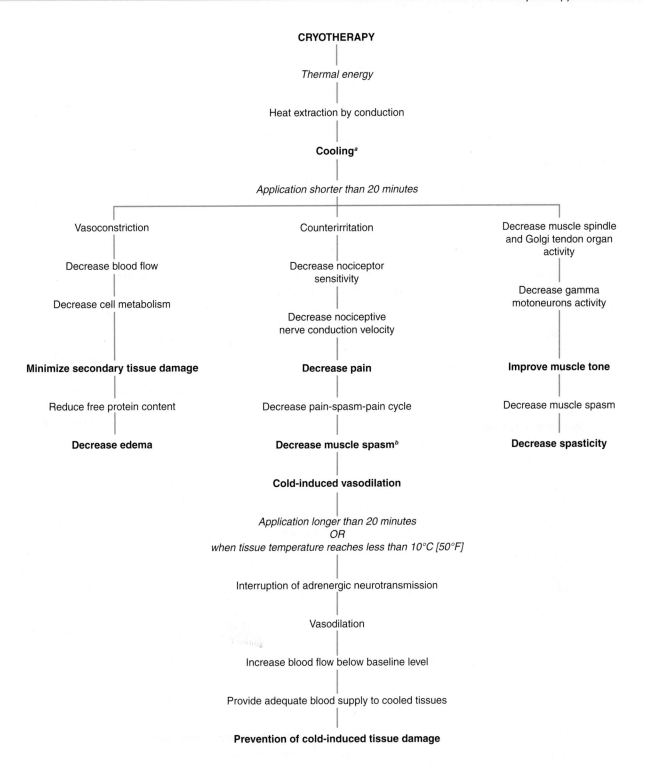

FIGURE 8-2 Proposed physiological and therapeutic effects of cryotherapy.

[a]primary effect: [b]secondary effect

oxygen requirement of local tissues is reduced. Consequently, cellular necrosis in tissues that are unaffected by the original injury may be minimized, which would limit the extent of necessary tissue repair (Knight, 1995; Knight et al., 2008a,b). In other words, when the metabolism of uninjured cells within the wound and of healthy or normal cells surrounding the wound is slowed down, their reliance on oxygen is reduced, which enables them to better face the temporary period of hypoxia caused by the impaired blood flow at the trauma site, or organ, affected.

4. Decrease Edema Formation

Swelling is the enlargement of a tissue or organ resulting from edema, which is the accumulation of fluids in the interstitial spaces. Cryotherapy can decrease edema at the wound site if applied *within the first 24 to 48 hours postinjury*. It does this, as illustrated in **Figure 8-2**, by minimizing secondary tissue damages (Knight et al., 2008a,b). Minimizing secondary damages reduces the amount of free proteins in the wound vicinity, which in turn leads to less edema formation.

5. Decrease Pain

Cryotherapy can decrease pain, as shown in **Figure 8-2**, through the following three physiological processes.

a. Counterirritation

This process involves substituting one form of irritation (pain) with another form of irritation (cold). In other words, during cryotherapy the sensation of pain is counteracted, or replaced, by the sensation of coldness, thus diminishing the patient's perception of pain.

b. Nociceptive Hyposensitivity

The second process, resulting from cooling, reduces the release of pain-sensitizing substances in the injured area, thus decreasing nociceptor sensitivity and pain (Allen, 2006).

c. Nerve Fiber Conduction Velocity

The final process relates to the transient reduction, or blocking, of the conduction velocity of pain nerve fibers.

6. Decrease Muscle Spasm

Cryotherapy can reduce the protective muscle spasm that follows injury by decreasing the pain-spasm-pain cycle.

7. Decrease Spasticity

Cryotherapy is presumed to decrease spasticity, or muscle tone, by decreasing the activity of the gamma motor neuron system, which is regulated by muscle spindle and Golgi tendon organ activity.

C. COLD-INDUCED VASODILATION

The secondary effect of cryotherapy usually observed with prolonged applications leading to soft-tissue temperatures decreasing below 10°C (50°F) is termed *cold-induced vasodilation*. CIVD can be defined as a vasodilation of cold-exposed blood vessels, in particular the arteriovenous anastomoses (AVAs) found in specific body areas, such as the hands and feet, and organs usually exposed without protection to cold, such as our lips, cheeks, ears, and nose (Daanen, 2003). This effect, much discussed in the field of cryotherapy and human exposure to cold, is still the subject of controversy (Daanen, 2003; Knight et al., 2008a) and, as a result, deserves further clarification. The main controversy is over the magnitude of vasodilation and whether this physiological response is strong enough to negate the therapeutic purpose of cryotherapy, which is to cool soft tissues. This controversy stems from an early

study by Clarke et al. (1958), which suggested that cryotherapy leads to a significant increase in blood flow that actually exceeds baseline values over time.

1. Hunting Response

CIVD was first observed by Lewis (1930). Experimentally measuring human finger temperatures during and after immersion in ice-cold water, Lewis observed cycles of increase/decrease in skin temperature, which were interpreted as cycles of vasoconstriction and vasodilation. To describe this cold-induced effect, he coined the term *hunting response*, hypothesizing that this cycling vascular effect was triggered by the release of a so-called H substance, similar in action to histamine at the site of injury.

2. Revisiting the Hunting Response

As pointed out by Knight (1995), many in the field have mistakenly inferred from Lewis' work that the magnitude of this CIVD response was large enough not only to reestablish the initial blood flow at the injury site (i.e., to reestablish the baseline level), but also to actually yield a net increase in blood flow at this site, thus negating the cooling effect of cryotherapy. The clinical implication of this belief is that the application of cryotherapy should be brief to avoid such a late vasodilation. To answer these concerns, Knight and colleagues (1980, 1981) revisited this issue by replicating Lewis' original experiments in healthy humans.

a. Low-Magnitude Response

Knight et al. (1980, 1981) showed that the relatively small and irregular skin temperature changes measured by Lewis when the subject's fingers remained immobile in still (unstirred) ice-cold water were due to the formation of a "blanket" of warm water trapped around the fingers as the body part gave up heat to the water surrounding it. Stirring the ice water during the experiment, thus removing this blanket of warm water, led to smaller average temperature fluctuations, from a mean value of 2.1 ± 2.0°C (mean ± SD) for unstirred water to a mean value of 1.6 ± 2.0°C for stirred water. Similar small and nonstatistically significant mean temperature changes (2°C) were also recorded by Daanen et al. (1997) in a similar study on healthy human subjects.

b. Little Physiological Significance

The fact that measurement errors around the mean values (see above) are as large as the mean values themselves led Knight (1995) to conclude that these skin temperature changes of approximately 2°C after prolonged cold immersion have little physiological and therapeutic significance. In other words, this cold-induced vasodilation, or hunting reaction, leads to only a small blood flow increase in the cooled tissues.

3. Body Core Temperature

Cold-induced vasodilation is a complex response, which may be related to body core temperature. Daanen et al.

(1997, 2003) showed that a cooler body core temperature in comparison to a warmer one before cold immersion is associated with decreased magnitude and frequency of the CIVD response. This finding contradicts the opinion of many who believe that the purpose of CIVD is to prevent excessive tissue cooling in victims suffering from hypothermia.

4. Blood Flow Changes

The effect of cryotherapy on human blood flow has been extensively studied since the release of Lewis' article in 1930, and the results provide evidence for a cold-induced vasodilation effect (see Bancroft et al., 1943; Greenfield et al., 1950; Duff et al., 1953; Clarke et al., 1958; Abramson et al., 1966; Aizawa et al., 1979; Ho et al., 1994). Together, the results of these studies reveal that this cyclic increase in blood flow, caused by late-induced vasodilation, always remains below baseline values, suggesting that the net effect of cryotherapy is one of vasoconstriction leading to soft-tissue cooling. Practitioners, therefore, need not be concerned that this CIVD response will negate the cooling effect of cryotherapy and should not limit cryotherapy application to short application durations.

5. Recap

The scientific evidence presented in this chapter strongly suggests that the purpose of CIVD, a genuine human physiological phenomenon, is to provide more warmed blood to specific body areas, such as the hands and feet, lips, cheeks, ears, and nose, which are often exposed to intense cold without protection (see Daanen, 2003). The net effect is to prevent cold-induced tissue damage, such as a frostnip or frostbite (Iida, 1949; Daanen, 2003). CIVD is presumed to be caused by a sudden decrease in the release of neurotransmitters from the sympathetic nerves to the muscular coat of the AVAs due to local cold (Daanen, 2003). AVAs, found primarily in the skin overlying the hands and feet as well as other organs such as lips, cheeks, ears, and nose, are specific thermoregulatory vascular structures that regulate blood flow in cold and hot conditions (Daanen, 2003). Finally, the present body of scientific evidence suggests that CIVD is more likely to occur when the extremities (hands and feet) are subjected to cryotherapy by means of immersion in cold water (see cryo-hydrotherapy, Chapter 9). Practitioners can feel reassured that the presence of a CIVD response in the extremities (hands and feet), during and following cryotherapy, does not negate the prime cooling effect of this agent.

V. DOSIMETRY

A. DOSAGE

The dose is determined by selecting and setting the following five parameters: cryoagent type, temperature differential between the agent and the treated skin area

(T_{a-s}), application duration, application method, and coupling medium.

1. Cryoagent Types

Listed and described in **Box 8-1** are the most common types of cryoagents used today to deliver cryotherapy. The selection of one cryoagent over another depends on the size and location of the pathology.

a. Ice and Gel Pack

These agents, available in different sizes and shapes, are reusable and relatively inexpensive.

b. Icicle

This agent, disposable and inexpensive, is used primarily for the treatment of localized and small injured body areas.

c. Instant Cold Pack and Vapocoolant Sprays

Relatively more expensive and not reusable, instant cold packs (also known as instant chemical packs) are rarely used. When they are used, it is usually in emergency situations when none of the above cryoagents are available for immediate application. Also relatively expensive and disposable are vapocoolant sprays, used to treat trigger points and myofascial pain (see Travell and Simons (1999a,b) for details).

d. Cryocompression- and Cryotemperature-Controlled Devices

These two reusable and much more expensive agents are used primarily for the treatment of acute and postoperative surgical conditions. Cryocompression-controlled devices deliver cold with controlled compression. Cryotemperature-controlled devices, on the other hand, deliver cold at preset and constant temperatures.

2. Temperature Differential ($T°_{ag-s}$)

The temperature differential between the agent (ag) and the exposed skin surface (s) is the dose delivered to soft tissues. This setting is done easily and quickly using a noncontact, portable infrared thermometer, as described in Chapter 26. The larger the dose, the greater its ability to cool soft tissues by extracting heat from them.

3. Application Duration

Recommended application durations range between 10 and 30 minutes, and vary with the application methods (see below). Practically speaking, the longer the cryoagent is applied, the greater its cooling potential. In other words, the longer the cryoagent is in contact with the skin, the more time it has to extract heat from soft tissues.

4. Application Methods

Listed and described in **Box 8-2** are the most common methods of application used today to deliver cryotherapy, with recommendations on application duration for each method. The method used to apply cryotherapy will influence the cooling potential of the agent used.

Box 8-1 Common Cryoagents

Ice Pack

A mixture of crushed ice and water enclosed in a commercial linen or plastic bag (**Fig 8-1A**) or wrapped in a terry cloth towel (custom pack).

Icicle

Frozen water contained in a commercial plastic wrap (**Fig 8-1B**).

Gel Pack

Commercial mixture of water and antifreeze, forming a gel mixture, enclosed in a flexible vinyl cover (**Fig 8-1C**). Gel packs always remain in a semisolid state despite their being stored at below-freezing temperatures.

Instant Cold Pack

A mixture of two chemical substances, each contained in a separate bag (one smaller bag inside the other) and both enclosed in a flexible plastic cover (see **Fig 8-1D**). When the chemical pack is squeezed, the smaller bag ruptures, allowing its contents to mix with the other chemical substance stored in the larger bag and causing an instant cold reaction. These compresses are marketed under brand names such as Instant Chemical Packs. They can only be used once and are not recommended unless no other choice is available (Knight, 1995). *Caution:* These packs may cause chemical burns if their contents leak from the bag onto the skin during treatment.

Vapocoolant Spray

Coolant liquid, contained in a pressurized canister and activated manually by a valve (see **Fig 8-1E**). These sprays are marketed under brand names such as *ethyl chloride, fluorimethane,* and, more recently, as *Spray and Stretch* spray. *Caution:* Ethyl chloride is a highly flammable and explosive pressurized liquid, possibly toxic for the environment, and if inhaled (Kraus, 1941; Simons et al., 1989). Fluori-methane, in contrast, is nonflammable, nonexplosive, and nontoxic, but because it is made of chlorofluorocarbons, represents a danger to the environment: the destruction of the ozone layer (Vallentyne et al., 1988). To eliminate all the potential risks noted above, the manufacturer has devel-

oped a third-generation vapocoolant spray, as illustrated in **Figure 8-1E**, named *Spray and Stretch.* This spray is non–ozone-depleting and can be used in facilities that restrict the use of flammable components.

Cryocompression-Controlled Device

Continuous and controlled delivery of pressurized cold water, circulating in specially designed sleeves, wrapped around the injured body parts (see **Fig 8-1F**). The device contains three basic components: A *cuff,* wrapped around the injured area, a *reservoir,* holding the ice–water mixture, and a flexible *tube,* used for the exchange of water between the cuff and the canister. Elevating the cooler above the injured part fills and pressurizes the cuff. Compression is controlled by gravity and is proportional to the elevation of the canister. For example, if the canister is positioned 90 cm (30 in.) above the cuff during treatment, the applied compression will be approximately 54 mmHg (2.5 cm or 1 in. = 1.8 mmHg). These cryoagents are marketed under brand names such as *Cryo-Cuff* and *AutoChill. Caution:* As the water in the cuff gradually warms up over time by the heat extracted from the body area, it must be exchanged or flushed out approximately every 2 hours, either manually or automatically, via an electrical pump. The ice in the reservoir must also be refilled approximately every 6 hours to maintain the cold water temperature in the cuff.

Cryotemperature-Controlled Device

Continuous and controlled temperature delivery of cold water, circulating in specially designed pads, applied against injured body areas (see **Fig 8-1G**). This device comprises four basic components: a flexible *pad* that is filled with cold water and applied over the injured area; a *reservoir* that holds the ice and water mixture; a flexible *tube,* which links the reservoir to the pad; and an *electrical submersible pump with an in-line thermometer and flow valve* to control temperature within the range of 1.7°C to 21°C (35°F to 70°F). These devices are marketed under brand names such as *Polar Care Unit* and *Iceman Cold Unit. Caution:* The ice in the reservoir must be replenished approximately every 10 hours to allow the device to maintain the preset cold water temperature in the pad for the entire duration of the treatment.

a. Cryostatic

This classic method, characterized by the static and continuous contact of the agent with the injured body area for the entire treatment duration, is by far the most common.

b. Cryokinetics

This method, described by Knight (1995, Knight et al., 2008b), involves repeated applications of cold interrupted by sessions of active exercises. Its purpose is to accelerate

Box 8-2   Application Methods

Cryostatic

Continuous and static application over the injured area. The recommended application duration ranges between 12 and 30 minutes.

Cryokinetics

Repeated applications, interrupted by sessions of voluntary exercises, within the treatment session. Cryokinetics consists of a systematic combination of three to five cold applications, with each application followed by a session of graded and progressively active exercises involving muscles related to the site of injury. The recommended application durations are approximately 20 minutes for the initial application and 5 minutes for each of the subsequent four applications, with each session of active exercise lasting approximately 3 minutes (Knight, 1995).

Cryomassage

Continuous massaging of the skin surface overlying the injured area. The recommended application duration ranges between 10 and 30 minutes.

Cryostretch

Repeated applications, interrupted by sessions of voluntary/passive stretching exercises, within the treatment session. This method consists of a systematic combination of two to three cold applications, with each application followed by a session of voluntary/passive stretching exercises involving muscles related to the site of injury. The recommended application duration is approximately 20 minutes for the initial application and 5 minutes for each of the next two applications, with each session of active/passive stretching exercise lasting approximately 3 minutes (Knight, 1995).

Compression Controlled

Single or repeated applications of a pressurized cold sleeve wrapped over the injured area. The recommended application duration is approximately 2 hours per application. If the application needs to be repeated, the water in the sleeve, warmed up by the body part, must be flushed out and replaced by fresh ice-cold water from the reservoir.

Temperature Controlled

Single or repeated applications of a cold pad, maintained at a preset temperature, over the injured area. The recommended duration is for several hours, ranging up to 10 hours per application, as long as the operating temperature is set between $7.2°C$ and $12.8°C$ ($45°F$ to $55°F$). The manufacturer cautions that such a device should *never* be applied at water temperatures below $7.28°C$ ($45.8°F$) for longer than 20 minutes, to prevent cold-related injuries.

Intermittent Cold with Stretch

Repeated stroking applications of cold over the injured area, followed immediately by a series of manual passive stretching exercises. It is important to remember that with this application, *stretch is the therapeutic action, whereas cold is the distraction* (Simons et al., 1989, p. 127). Durations of cold application may range between 30 and 90 seconds, whereas passive stretching exercises may range between 1 and 2 minutes. The number of applications will vary according to the acuity and severity of the condition under treatment.

Cryoimmersion

Continuous immersion of the injured body part in cold water (see Chapter 9).

Contrast Immersion

Alternating or contrasting immersions of the injured body part in cold and hot water (see Chapter 9).

---

return to function by introducing voluntary muscle contractions early in the rehabilitation process.

c. Cryomassage
This method involves continuous manual massaging of small body areas using ice cups or icicles.

d. Cryostretch
The method, also described by Knight (1995; Knight et al., 2008b), involves repeated applications of cold interrupted by sessions of active/passive stretching exercises. Its purpose is to accelerate range of motion recovery by means of stretching exercises early in the rehabilitation process.

e. Compression Controlled
The compression-controlled method combines the simultaneous application of cryotherapy and gravity-induced controlled-compression therapy. It differs from the previous methods in that it provides continuous controlled compression over the injured area during cryotherapy.

f. Temperature Controlled

This method combines the continuous and controlled delivery of cold at a preset temperature. It differs from all the above methods in that it delivers cryotherapy at a preset temperature for the entire treatment duration. It is the only cryoagent that is not warmed up by the body heat over time, since the preset cold water temperature is constantly circulating in the cryotemperature-controlled unit's pad.

g. Intermittent Cold With Stretch

Originally known as *intermittent spray and stretch method,* because a vapocoolant spray was used, this method has recently been renamed as *intermittent cold* (because cryoagents other than vapocoolant sprays can be used) *with stretch* method (see Travell et al., 1999a). It is defined as the repeated applications of cold, using any cryoagent for a short period of time, followed immediately by a series of passive stretching maneuvers.

h. Immersion and Contrast Immersion

The cryoimmersion method involves the immersion of a body part, or segment, into cold water. The contrast immersion method, commonly known as the *contrast bath* method, involves the repeated immersion of a body part into cold and warm water; hence the name *contrast.* Because water (hydro) makes direct contact with the skin, both methods are covered in detail in the chapter on hydrotherapy (Chapter 9). Note that these two immersion methods can be used to deliver cryo-hydrotherapy (cold water) and thermo-hydrotherapy (warm water), as described in Chapter 9, on hydrotherapy.

5. Coupling Medium

All the cryoagents described in this chapter, with the exception of one, the gel pack, can and should be applied *without* the use of a coupling medium, that is, directly over the bare skin area to maximize soft-tissue cooling (Knight, 1995; Tsang et al., 1997; Janwantanakul, 2004). Because the temperature of the gel pack may be below the freezing point, there exists a risk of causing cold-induced skin damage, such as frostnip and frostbite, especially if the gel pack is left in place for a long period of time (Nadler et al., 2003; Janwantanakul, 2004).

a. Rule of Thumb for Coupling Media

The use of coupling media should be restricted as much as possible if the purpose is to obtain maximum deep tissue cooling within the shortest application duration. If coupling media are used, practitioners must either increase the cryo-dose or temperature differential between the agent and the skin ($T°_{ag-s}$) before application or increase the total application duration to maximize cooling.

b. Coupling for Gel Pack

Because commercially made gel packs are normally chilled to less than 0°C (32°F) before use, Knight (1995) recommends placing a layer of damp cloth between the pack and the exposed skin surface and limiting the application to 30 minutes.

c. Tolerance to Cold

Tolerance to cold stimuli varies greatly between patients. The level of tolerance to cryotherapy can be increased by the use of layers of damp toweling between the cryoagent and the skin surface, which are then gradually removed. Tolerance can also be improved if the practitioner takes the time to explain to patients the various cold sensations they will experience during therapy. Research has shown that cryotherapy is first felt as a sensation of intense cold, followed by a burning/aching sensation, which is then followed by a sensation of local aching and numbness (Hocott, 1982; Knight, 1995). Finally, it will greatly enhance the patient's tolerance if he or she knows what to expect during cryotherapy.

B. SUBCUTANEOUS FAT TISSUE THICKNESS

Another important dosimetric parameter to consider is the thickness of subcutaneous fat tissue between the surface and deep soft tissues at the site of injury. Research has shown an inverse relationship between fat thickness and the extent of deep tissue cooling and a direct relationship between fat tissue thickness and required application duration (Myrer et al., 2001). In other words, if the purpose is to maximize deep tissue cooling in the presence of a thick subcutaneous fat tissue, a longer application period is required.

C. QUANTITATIVE DOSIMETRY

The evidence-based practice of cryotherapy dictates that the therapeutic dose administered to the patient be *quantitatively* assessed. To *qualitatively* assess the dosage level by simply asking the patient about his or her perception of cold during treatment, as is done by practitioners routinely at present, is not enough. A simple, practical, and rapid way to quantitatively assess thermal dosage is to measure two temperature differentials, namely, the temperature difference between the agent (ag) and the exposed skin (s) surface ($T°_{ag-s}$) and the temperature differential between the exposed skin surface before (b) and after (a) treatment ($T°_{b-a}$). Chapter 26 shows how to take these two measurements using a portable infrared surface thermometer.

1. Case Example

The ice pack is measured at 5°C (41°F) and the exposed skin surface at 30°C (86°F). The thermal dose delivered ($T°_{ag-s}$) equals 25°C (41°F), which represents its *potential* cooling effect. Immediately after treatment, the exposed skin temperature is measured at 12°C (54°F); the *actual* skin heating effect ($T°_{b-a}$) of this dosage was −18°C (−32°F).

2. Recap

In the context of evidence-based practice, it is useful to ask the patient how cold the thermal agent feels against the body parts, during and after treatment, but it is better to supplement this qualitative information with actual temperature measurements This textbook strongly encourages practitioners to supplement their qualitative approach with the suggested quantitative approach. It is easy and practical, and not time-consuming, to take these temperature measurements using an infrared portable thermometer.

VI. EVIDENCE FOR INDICATIONS

A. GUIDED BY EVIDENCE

Dictionaries generally define *evidence* as anything that establishes a fact or gives reason to believe something. The aim of this textbook is to present scientific evidence behind therapeutic EPAs. To be guided by evidence is the process of integrating the evidence from research, however imperfect or scarce this evidence may be, with clinical experience and patients' values. In other words, the *evidence-based practice* of EPA requires practi-

tioners to consider the evidence from research, in addition to their own clinical experience and the patient's own preference and beliefs, when the time comes to justify, prescribe, and apply the therapeutic agent. To be guided by evidence is a process, not a search for the absolute truth. Finally, lack of evidence from research behind any given EPA does not mean that this EPA should never be used. What it means is that no statement can be made on its therapeutic effectiveness and that until more evidence from research is presented, its routine use cannot be recommended.

B. EVIDENCE FROM HUMAN RESEARCH

Box 8-3 provides evidence for cryotherapy based on an exhaustive search of published English-language, peer-reviewed literature on human research. The term *indication* refers to a list of pathologies for which cryotherapy is used. Ratings of therapeutic benefit (Yes or No) and grading of the strength of scientific evidence (I, II, or III), including the reference, are included for each pathological condition.

Box 8-3	Research-Based Indications for the Use of Cryotherapy		
PATHOLOGY	**BENEFIT**	**GRADE**	**REFERENCE**
Postoperative knee arthroplasty	Yes	I	Ohkoshi et al. (1999)
	Yes	I	Martin et al. (2001)
	Yes	I	Barber et al. (1998)
	Yes	I	Cohn et al. (1989)
	Yes	I	Levy et al. (1993)
	Yes	I	Morsi (2002)
	Yes	I	Webb et al. (1998)
	Yes	I	Bert et al. (1991)
	Yes	II	Shelbourne et al. (1994)
	Yes	II	Schroder et al. (1994)
	Yes	II	Hecht et al. (1983)
	Yes	II	Whitelaw et al. (1995)
	Yes	II	Lessard et al. (1997)
	Yes	II	Sanchez-Inchausti et al. (2005)
	No	I	Daniel et al. (1994)
	No	I	Dervin et al. (1998)
	No	I	Edwards et al. (1996)
	No	I	Konrath et al. (1996)
	No	I	Leutz et al. (1995)
	No	I	Scarcella et al. (1995)
	No	I	Zaffagnini et al. (1998)
	No	II	Walker et al. (1991)
	No	II	Healy et al. (1994)

(Continued)

Box 8-3   Continued

PATHOLOGY	BENEFIT	GRADE	REFERENCE
Ankle sprain	Yes	I	Sloan et al., (1989)
	Yes	II	Weston et al., (1994)
	Yes	II	Basur et al., (1976)
	Yes	II	Wilkerson (1991)
	Yes	II	Wilkerson et al., (1993)
	Yes	II	Michlovitz et al., (1988)
	Yes	II	Hocutt et al., (1982)
	Yes	II	Pincivero et al., (1993)
	Yes	II	Cote et al., (1988)
	Yes	II	Bleakley et al., (2006)
	Yes	III	Starkey (1976)
Spasticity	Yes	II	Price et al., (1993)
	Yes	II	Boes (1962)
	Yes	II	Hedenberg (1970)
	Yes	II	Knuttson (1970a,b)
	Yes	II	Miglietta (1973)
	Yes	II	Miglietta (1964)
	Yes	II	DonTigny et al., (1962)
	Yes	II	Kelly (1969)
	Yes	III	Hartvikksen (1962)
	Yes	III	Basset et al., (1958)
Muscle spasm/myofascial pain	Yes	II	Travell (1952)
	Yes	II	Mennell (1976)
	Yes	III	Nielsen (1978, 1981)
Postexercise delayed muscle soreness	Yes	I	Denegar et al., (1992)
	No	I	Yackzan et al., (1984)
	No	I	Isabell et al., (1992)
Mixed cases of joint sprain, tendon strain, and muscle contusion	Yes	II	Hayden (1964)
	Yes	II	Grant (1964)
Postsurgical hip arthroplasty	Yes	I	Saito et al., (2004)
	No	I	Scarcella et al., (1995)
Musculoskeletal pain	Yes	II	Kraus (1941)
	Yes	II	Modell et al., (1952)
Headache/migraine	Yes	II	Robbins (1989)
	Yes	II	Diamond et al., (1986)
Low back pain	Yes	II	Melzack et al., (1980b)
	Yes	II	Landen (1967)

(Continued)

Box 8-3   Continued

PATHOLOGY	BENEFIT	GRADE	REFERENCE
Postoperative shoulder	Yes	I	Singh et al., (2001)
	Yes	I	Speer et al., (1996)
Multiple sclerosis	Yes	II	Kinnman et al., (2000a)
	Yes	II	Kinnman et al., (2000b)
Chronic osteoarthritis	Yes	II	Halliday Pegg et al., (1969)
Postsurgical low back pain	Yes	I	Brandner et al., (1996)
Rheumatoid arthritic shoulder	Yes	II	Williams et al., (1986)
Rheumatoid arthritic knee	Yes	II	Kirk et al., (1968)
Osteoarthritic knee	Yes	II	Clarke et al., (1974)
Postorthopedic surgical cases	Yes	II	Schaubel (1946)
Postsurgical hand disorders	Yes	II	Showman et al., (1963)
Acute stiff neck	Yes	II	Travell (1949)
Pain after tooth extraction	Yes	II	Bastian et al., (1998)
Postoperative cesarean section	No	II	Amin-Hanjani et al., (1992)
Bicipital tendinitis	Yes	III	Lane (1971)
Dental pain	Yes	II	Melzack et al., (1980)
Rheumatoid arthritis	Yes	II	Curkovic et al., (1993)
Postfracture compartment pressure	Yes	II	Moore et al., (1977)
Trigeminal neuralgia	Yes	II	De Coster et al., (1993)
Myofascial masticatory pain	Yes	II	Burgess et al., (1988)
Muscle contusion	Yes	III	Kalenak et al., (1975)
Foot and ankle trauma	Yes	II	Stockle et al., (1997)
Postoperative foot surgery	Yes	II	Scheffler et al., (1992)
Postsurgical rheumatoid hands	No	I	Rembe (1970)
Postlaparotomy pain	No	I	Finan et al., (1993)
Postarthroscopic patellar tendon	Yes	II	Barber (2000)
Post–carpal tunnel release	Yes	II	Hochberg (2001)

1. Rating Therapeutic Benefit

The rating, expressed as Yes or No, is based on the overall conclusion(s) reached on the issue of therapeutic effectiveness by the author(s) who conducted the peer-reviewed study.

2. Grading Strength of Evidence

The grading, numerically classified as I, II, and III, is based on the type of research methodology, or experimental design used by the author(s). All the studies listed are human studies published in English-language, peer-reviewed journals. It follows that the strength of evidence in studies graded I is stronger than in those graded II, which itself is stronger than in those graded III.

a. Grade I

Evidence based on human *controlled* studies, regardless of their level of randomization and blindness.

b. Grade II

Evidence based on human *non-controlled* studies, regardless of their level of randomization and blindness.

c. Grade III

Evidence based on human *case* studies, regardless of their level of randomization and blindness.

Strength of Evidence Behind the Agent

The strength of evidence behind the agent, as presented in the research-based indication box, is arbitrarily assessed in this textbook as being *weak, moderate,* or *strong.* For example, the larger the number of studies graded I, regardless of therapeutic benefit, the stronger the scientific evidence in favor of the agent.

Strength of Justification of Usage Behind the Agent

The strength of evidence justifying usage of the agent for individual pathologies or groups of pathologies, as listed in the research-based indication box, is arbitrarily assessed in this textbook as being *poor, fair, good,* or *conflicting.* For example, when a larger number of studies on an agent shows therapeutic benefit (Yes) and are graded I, for any given pathology, the justification for usage of this agent for this pathology is assessed as *good. Conflicting* justification is reported when similar numbers of studies, with similar grades, report therapeutic benefit (Yes) and no benefit (No).

C. STRENGTH OF EVIDENCE AND JUSTIFICATION FOR USAGE OF CRYOTHERAPY

The results gathered in **Box 8-3** show *moderate* strength of evidence behind the use of cryotherapy, with the majority of studies graded as II. They also show that the body of research on the effectiveness of cryotherapy has concentrated on the management of three conditions: postoperative knee arthroplasty, ankle sprain, and spasticity. The body of evidence presented in **Box 8-3** also shows that justification for the usage of cryotherapy is *conflicting* for cases of postoperative knee arthroplasty and *fair* to *good* for cases of ankle sprain and spasticity. Moreover, the justification for the usage of this therapeutic agent for the remaining pathologies listed in this box is *weak.* Until more evidence from research is provided with regard to those remaining pathologies, or any other pathology, the routine use of cryotherapy for such pathologies *cannot be recommended.*

VII. CONTRAINDICATIONS

The contraindications associated with the practice of cryotherapy are shown in **Table 8-1**. To determine whether a patient is allergic to cryotherapy, it is essential that the practitioner questions the patient about his or her past reactions to cold exposure and, subsequently, conducts the ice-cube test (see below).

TABLE 8-1	CONTRAINDICATIONS TO CRYOTHERAPY
CONTRAINDICATIONS	**RATIONALE**
Over skin areas where sensation of cold is severely impaired	Risk of cutaneous damage or burn (frostnip to frostbite).
Cold-induced urticaria (cold allergy) or cold hypersensitivity	Risk of triggering local skin reactions, such as wheal or patches, or systemic allergic reactions, such as sneezing and dysphasia, in addition to moderate-to-severe itching (Day, 1974; Escher et al., 1992, Knight 1995). A simple diagnostic tool for cold urticaria is the *ice-cube test.*
Raynaud's disease or phenomenon	Risk of further enhancing the vasoconstrictive spasm, which, if prolonged, is likely to aggravate digital cyanosis and eventually lead to ischemic necrosis (Bolster et al., 1995).
Cryoglobulinemia	Risk of aggravating the condition, which is characterized by the aggregation of serum proteins in the small distal vessels after cold applications, resulting in impaired blood circulation, possibly causing ischemia and, in the worst case, gangrene.

(Continued)

TABLE 8-1	CONTINUED

CONTRAINDICATIONS	RATIONALE
Paroxysmal cold hemoglobinuria	Risk of aggravating the condition, which is characterized by the undesirable release of hemoglobin in the urine, resulting from the rapid breakdown, or lysing, of many blood cells after cold applications.
Over open dermal wounds	Risk of further slowing or delaying the repair process because cold induces vigorous dermal vasoconstriction, reducing blood flow and metabolism.
Over peripheral vascular disease areas	Risk of further reducing the vascular supply to the area, caused by cold-induced vasoconstriction, leading to unnecessary pain and possible tissue necrosis.
Confused or unreliable patients	Risk of complications during therapy, reducing treatment effectiveness.

VIII. RISKS, PRECAUTIONS, AND RECOMMENDATIONS

A. RISKS

The practice of cryotherapy is not without risks for the patient. The main risk associated with this agent, as well as some precautions and recommendations designed to improve safety and effectiveness, are listed in **Table 8-2**.

B. COMPLICATIONS

A recent study by Nadler et al. (2003) revealed that of 362 complications documented by athletic trainers after the application of various electrophysical agents (EPAs), 42% were related to cryotherapy. The most common complications were cold-induced allergic reaction (urticaria; n = 86), skin damage (frostnip to frostbite; n = 23), and intolerance to cold-induced pain (n = 16). These findings differ from those documented in the peer-reviewed literature where most complications were related to cold-induced peripheral nerve injuries (see **Table 8-2**). The fact that no case of nerve injury was reported in this survey implies that either the respondents were well aware of this complication (i.e., they were fully prevented) or such nerve injuries were underreported or missed during the course of assessing athletic injuries (Nadler et al., 2003).

C. IMPLICATIONS FOR THERAPEUTIC EXERCISES

Although cryotherapy reduces the sensation of pressure, its use is not contraindicated as an analgesic before submaximal rehabilitative exercise programs (Rubley et al., 2002). Moreover, when supervising therapeutic exercise regimens, clinicians must recognize that cryotherapy may make joints stiffer and lessen the patient's sensitivity to position (Uchio et al., 2003). Finally, motor function may

be enhanced after ankle joint cooling partly because of decreased residual pain, combined with facilitation of the motor neuron pools (soleus) that may have been affected by the joint injury (Hopkins et al., 2002).

IX. CONSIDERATIONS FOR APPLICATION AND DOCUMENTATION

A. SELECTION OF CRYOAGENTS

Practitioners can choose between various inexpensive and more costly commercial cryoagents to deliver cryotherapy (see **Fig 8-1** and **Box 8-1**). Selection of one cryoagent over another, as shown in **Table 8-3**, is influenced by two criteria: the size and surface of the area to be treated and the extent and acuity of the pathology.

B. CRYOAGENTS VERSUS APPLICATION METHODS

The choice of cryoagent is also guided by the application methods used, and vice versa, as shown in **Table 8-4**.

C. REQUIRED TESTS AND MEASUREMENTS

The evidence-based practice of cryotherapy requires some prediagnostic tests to be done and key physiological measurements to be taken before, during, and after therapy.

1. The Ice-Cube Test

A simple and effective prediagnostic test, called the ice-cube test, is available to determine whether the patient suffers from cold urticaria, also called cold hypersensitivity, or cold allergy (Harvey, 1992). This test, conducted before the first application, consists of massaging the skin with an ice cube for approximately 3 minutes. A normal reddish patch, or skin erythema, should occur over the massaged area within 5 minutes of the initiation of ice

TABLE 8-2	RISKS, PRECAUTIONS, AND RECOMMENDATIONS FOR CRYOTHERAPY

RISKS	RATIONALE
Over an area of impaired blood circulation	Risk of causing a frostnip or chilblain lesion, characterized by blanching of the skin, combined with a tingling and burning sensation (Knight, 1995). This skin lesion is temporary and reversible by slow and gentle rewarming of the exposed skin area (Knight, 1995). There is also a risk of causing a frostbite, which is characterized by the freezing of the skin and subcutaneous tissues (superficial), or the freezing of the skin, subcutaneous, muscle, and blood vessels (deep), if a very cold agent is applied directly over the skin for a prolonged and continuous period of time (Knight, 1995; Hoiness et al., 1998). Cases of frostbite due to the inadequate application of cryoagents have been reported (Proulx, 1976; Stevens et al., 1978; Quist et al., 1996; O'Toole et al., 1999; Graham, 2000; Cuthill et al., 2006; McGuire et al., 2006).
Over the thoracic area in patients with coronopathies	Risk of causing a reflex constriction of the coronary arteries. Seek the treating cardiologist's opinion, if necessary, before administering cryotherapy.
With hypertensive patients	Risk of inducing a transient increase of blood pressure when cooling larger areas and/or multiple sites.Continuous monitoring of blood pressure is advised both during and after treatment. Seek the treating cardiologist's opinion, if necessary, before administering cryotherapy.
Over superficial peripheral nerves	Risk of damaging peripheral nerve fibers causing transient neuropathies, such as neurapraxia, axonotmesis, and neurotmesis (Drez et al., 1981; Parker et al., 1983; Collins et al., 1986; Green et al., 1989; Bassett et al., 1992; Malone et al., 1992; Covington et al., 1993; Moeller et al., 1997).
With hemiplegic patients	Risk of producing myocardial ischemia (Lorenze et al., 1960).

PRECAUTION	RATIONALE
With very young and very old patients	May lead to improper dosimetry and skin damage because of immature (young) or impaired (elder) thermal regulation and difficulty to communicate cold sensation (young and elder). Elderly patients have a decreased ability to maintain normal body thermoregulation because of their reduced ability to shiver and, thus, to produce heat (Leblanc et al., 1978) and because of their impaired vasoconstriction to conserve heat (Collins et al., 1977).

RECOMMENDATIONS	RATIONALE
Disrobe the treated body area and remove all objects, such as jewelry	To maximize heat transfer.
Inspect the exposed skin area before and after each treatment	To ensure close monitoring of potential cold-induced tissue damage (frostnip to frostbite).
Conduct skin thermal sensory discrimination testing— **mandatory**	To minimize the risk of cold-induced tissue damage and maximize dosimetry (see Chapter 25 for details).
Conduct the ice-cube test— **mandatory**	To determine if the patient presents cold urticaria or cold allergy.
Conduct the nail bed test (when applicable)	This test should be performed before application of cryotherapy with patients who have a history of moderate-to-severe peripheral vascular disorders, to determine if peripheral blood flow is adequate in the treated area.
Measure skinfold thickness (when applicable)	These measurements should be taken on overweight and obese patients to determine the proper application duration because subcutaneous fat layer interferes with heat loss from deep tissues. The greater the skinfold thickness of the treated body area, the longer the application duration should be (Otte et al., 2002).

(Continued)

TABLE 8-2   CONTINUED

RECOMMENDATIONS	RATIONALE
Take blood pressure measurements (when applicable)	These measurements should be taken on patients suffering from cardiovascular and cardiorespiratory disorders because cryotherapy may increase blood pressure beyond safe levels.
Measure temperature differential between the agent and the skin ($T°_{ag-s}$) before treatment—**mandatory**	The taking of this measurement is a must in the context of evidence-based practice because it provides quantitative assessment of the thermal dose delivered to the soft tissues (see Chapter 26 for details).
Measure skin temperature differential before and after treatment ($T°_{b-a}$)—**mandatory**	The taking of this measurement is a must in the context of evidence-based practice because it reveals the extent of soft-tissue heating caused by the thermal agent at the end of treatment (see Chapter 26 for details).
Do not use compressive measures with gel pack	Do not secure these cryoagents, stored below freezing (0°C–32°F), using compressive bandages, because this combination is likely to cause frostbite (Knight, 1995). Compression of cryoagents against the skin surface produces significantly cooler temperatures at all tissue depths (Merrick et al., 1993).
Do not use a coupling medium with cryoagents—with the exception of gel pack	Usage of cryoagents over dry/wet coupling media significantly reduces soft-tissue cooling because of their insulation effect, thus reducing the overall effectiveness of cryotherapy (Lavelle et al., 1985; Belitsky et al., 1987; Culp et al., 1995; Metzman et al., 1996). If coupling media are used, prolong the total application duration to obtain the desired tissue cooling. Recall that the application of a gel pack always requires a coupling medium because its temperature is below the freezing point; hence, the increased risk of causing a frostnip or frostbite (Knight, 1995).
Beware of inconsistent instructions given to patients with regard to a cryocompression-controlled unit	Inconsistent instructions given to a patient related to the use of this device have led to the development of a compartment syndrome (Khajavi et al., 2004). Practitioners should be familiar with the manufacturer's recommendations and safe use of such cryoagents before use.
Increase application duration of cryotherapy if applied immediately after exercise	Exercise before cooling increases the application duration needed to decrease intramuscular temperature (Long et al., 2005). Applications of 30 min or longer are needed to deeply cool large muscle mass (Knight et al., 2000).
Limit the use of *to-go* ice pack	Wrapping a "*to-go*" ice pack over active leg muscles (walking) does not induce intramuscular temperature change, despite skin cooling, as does the application of cryotherapy while resting (Bender et al., 2005).
Increase application durations with greater adipose tissue (skinfold) thickness	A 25-min application duration may be adequate for skinfolds of 20 mm or less; a 40-min application is required to produce similar results in patients with skinfolds between 21 and 30 mm, and a 60-min application is required for patients with skinfolds of 30–40 mm to produce similar results (Otte et al., 2002).
Do not use compressive elastic bandages to secure cryoagents over superficial peripheral nerves	The evidence from the literature suggests that the compressive effect of the elastic bandage, and not the cooling of the nerve per se, is what causes peripheral nerve damage (Knight, 1995).
Drape patients if multiple cryoagents are used simultaneously	Prevent unnecessary heat loss of body heat and shivering during treatment.
Plug line-powered devices into a GFCI receptacle	Prevent the occurrence of macroshocks (see Chapter 27 for details).
Conduct regular maintenance and calibration procedures.	Ensure optimal therapeutic efficacy and effectiveness. Follow the recommended maintenance schedules outlined by manufacturers.

TABLE 8-3	CRITERIA FOR SELECTING CRYOAGENTS		
AGENT	**CRITERIA**		
	BODY SURFACE AREA		**ACUITY OF CONDITION**
Ice pack/gel pack	Large/regular body areas		Acute/subacute
Icicle	Small/irregular body areas		Acute/subacute
Instant cold pack	Small body areas		Acute
Vapocoolant spray	Small/large body areas		Acute/subacute/chronic
Cryocompression-controlled unit	Peripheral articulations		Acute/subacute/postsurgical
Cryotemperature-controlled unit	Peripheral articulations		Acute/subacute/postsurgical

massage. If this reddish patch is replaced by a wheal (localized skin edema) that covers the tested surface area, the test is *positive* (Harvey, 1992). In this case, it is strongly recommended that the patient be referred to an allergist for confirmation of the diagnosis. Note that the skin redness observed during and after cryotherapy is a normal physiological response to cold and therefore should not be interpreted as a sign of cold urticaria or cold-induced vasodilation. This reddening of the skin is caused by the increase in oxyhemoglobin concentration in the blood, which results from the decrease in oxygen–hemoglobin dissociation that occurs at lower temperatures.

2. Nail Bed Test

The use of cryotherapy over the extremities requires adequate blood flow regulation. Another simple and effective prediagnostic test to assess blood flow at these levels is the nail bed test (Starkey, 2004). This test, conducted before the first application, consists of exerting finger pressure over the nail bed of fingers or toes, which will flush out the blood, making the compressed nail bed area pale and white. Rapidly releasing the test finger pressure allows the blood to flush back into the nail bed, thus restoring its original reddish color. The test is positive if releasing pressure on the finger fails to restore the nail bed's original color within a few seconds, which suggests peripheral circulatory problems. Further comprehensive vascular assessment is thus required to determine if severe occlusive vascular disorder is present, in which case cryotherapy is contraindicated.

3. Blood Pressure Measurement

Cryotherapy may induce in some patients significant cardiovascular responses, including blood pressure changes. The diastolic and systemic blood pressure before, during, and after therapy must be measured and monitored,

TABLE 8-4	CRYOAGENTS AND RELATED APPLICATION METHODS
AGENT	**METHOD(S)**
Ice pack/gel pack	Cryostatic, cryokinetic
Icicle	Cryomassage, intermittent cold and stretch
Instant cold pack	Cryostatic
Vapocoolant spray	Intermittent cold and stretch
Cryocompression-controlled unit	Compression controlled
Cryotemperature-controlled unit	Temperature controlled

especially for patients who have a history of cardiovascular or cardiorespiratory disorders or both.

4. Skinfold Measurement

Because the thickness of subcutaneous fat tissue at the treated area may significantly decrease the cooling of deeper soft tissues (Myrer et al., 2001), the practitioner must measure the skinfold thickness using a hand caliper before the first application of cryotherapy, especially in overweight and obese patients. This objective skinfold measurement will guide the dosimetry for treatment, helping practitioners to select appropriate temperature differentials, as well as proper application methods and application durations.

D. CASTS, BANDAGES, AND DRESSINGS

Cryoagents may be applied over synthetic and plaster casts as well as over common bandages and dressings (Kaempffe, 1989; Metzman et al., 1996; Weresh et al., 1996; Okcu et al., 2006). In such cases, application duration needs to be significantly prolonged (for as long as 60 minutes) to significantly reduce soft-tissue temperature.

E. COUPLING MEDIUM

The common media used in cryotherapy are layers of dry or damp toweling.

1. Icicle, Instant Cold Pack, and Vapocoolant Spray

These cryoagents are applied directly over the treated bare skin area and thus require *no* coupling medium. These agents are used to provide an immediate cooling effect where fast thermal transfer is required.

2. Ice Pack

No coupling is needed as long as the pack is properly applied and the patient is able to tolerate the initial thermal shock that comes with its application.

3. Gel Pack

Because its temperature is below 0°C (32°F), a coupling medium (layers of toweling) is required for the first 5 minutes in order to prevent a frostnip and possibly a frostbite. As the agent warms up, the coupling medium should be removed to optimize soft-tissue cooling.

4. Cryocompression- and Cryotemperature-Controlled Devices

A medium, such as a cotton wrap, may be needed, depending on the clinical situation (see the manufacturer's recommendations).

a. Postoperatively

The surgical wound and the entire skin surface in contact with the sleeve or pad must be covered by a protective coupling medium before application.

b. Nonsurgical Case

No coupling medium is needed as long as the exposed skin is regularly and periodically inspected during treatment.

F. APPLICATION ISSUES

Because cryotherapy can be applied in a variety of ways, several application *issues* have been investigated. Presented below are the results found for some of them.

1. Moderate Walking

Moderate walking after a 20-minute ice-pack application significantly enhanced rewarming of the triceps surae in healthy subjects (Myrer et al., 2000).

2. Ice Massage Versus Cryostatic Method

Both ice massage and the cryostatic method are effective in decreasing intramuscular temperature. Ice massage, however, appears to cool muscle more rapidly (Zemke et al., 1998).

3. Immersion Versus Cryostatic Method

Immersion in cold water at 10°C (50°F) for 20 minutes is superior to application of an ice pack for 20 minutes in maintaining prolonged, significant temperature reduction after treatment (Myrer et al., 1998).

4. Prolonged and Intermittent Application Versus Single Cold Application

Prolonged, intermittent cold application (20 min ON, 10 min OFF, 10 min ON, 10 min OFF, 10 min ON) is superior in producing a sustained reduction in blood flow, because it retards the rebound or increase in blood flow that occurs after a single cold application (Karunakara et al., 1998).

5. Application Duration

The cooling effect is time dependent and can be enhanced three- to fourfold by increasing the application duration by 5 to 25 minutes (Ho et al., 1995).

6. Core Body Temperature

Applications of cryotherapy over large body parts are more likely to alter core body temperature than over the extremities (Palmieri et al., 2006). A 20-minute cryotherapy treatment applied to the ankle did not alter core temperature (Palmieri et al., 2006).

7. Cooling Versus Rewarming Time Ratio

Rewarming time should be at least twice as long as cooling time, to yield an ON:OFF application ratio of 1:2, so that excessive cooling due to repeated applications is avoided (Knight, 1995). Reapplication of cryotherapy, if too frequent, increases the possibility of too much tissue cooling, thus affecting the healing process (Post et al., 1992).

8. Skin Versus Knee Intra-articular Temperature Changes

Skin temperature must be lowered to approximately 20°C (68°F) to obtain demonstrable temperature changes in intra-articular regions of the human knee (Dahlstedt et al., 1996).

9. Motor Performance

Cryotherapy can be used safely before strenuous exercise without altering the sense of proprioception (Ingersoll et al., 1992; Isabell et al., 1992; La Riviere et al., 1994; Knight et al., 1994; Evans et al., 1995; Thieme et al., 1996; Tremblay et al., 2001).

10. Muscle Assessment

Because muscle cooling affects muscle performance (Ruiz et al., 1993), the practitioner must assess muscle force before treatment or 4 hours after treatment, and should not return athletes to competition immediately after cryotherapy.

G. SKIN TEMPERATURE, ADIPOSE TISSUE THICKNESS, AND APPLICATION DURATION

The combination of skin temperature, adipose tissue thickness, and application duration must be considered when prescribing cryotherapy because none of them, taken individually, is a good predictor of deep tissue cooling (Jutte et al., 2001). Consequently, to optimize deep soft-tissue cooling, a combination of high skin temperature, a thin layer of adipose tissue, and long application duration is required.

H. DOCUMENTATION

All health practitioners are expected to record adequate information in patients' files. **Table 8-5** shows the key parameters to be documented in the patient's file following cryotherapy.

TABLE 8-5	KEY TREATMENT PARAMETERS TO BE DOCUMENTED IN PATIENT'S FILE AFTER CRYOTHERAPY

- Skin thermal sensory testing: record the result (see Chapter 25)
- Ice-cube test: result (negative or positive)
- Nail bed test (when applicable): result (negative or positive)
- Skinfold thickness scores (when applicable): mm
- Blood pressure scores (when applicable): mm Hg
- Type of cryoagents: description
- Application method: description
- Application duration: min
- Coupling media (when applicable): layers (number) of toweling
- Cryocompression: level (height [cm] of reservoir from sleeve or mmHg)
- Cryotemperature controlled: preset value (°C–°F).
- ($T°_{ag-s}$); °C–°F
- ($T°_{b-a}$); °C–°F

Case Study 8-1   Ankle Sprain

A 20-year-old college football player who sustained a moderate right-ankle sprain approximately 45 minutes earlier is referred for immediate treatment. The physical examination reveals all the cardinal signs of an acute traumatic soft-tissue lesion. There is no evidence of bone fracture or ligament rupture. The patient complains of pain at rest and particularly during ankle mobilization. He has difficulty bearing weight and walking. He is limping. This athlete is new to the team and to your sports clinic. Questioned about his past experience with cryotherapy, he explains that sometimes a significant reddish patch over his exposed skin has occurred together with some kind of skin edema. He adds that these skin reactions went away a few hours after exposure. You wonder if he may be allergic to cold. His goal is to return to play as soon as possible.

Evidence-based Steps Toward the Resolution of This Case

1. List medical diagnosis.
   Grade II inversion ankle sprain

2. List key impairment(s).

   - Lateral ankle ligament sprain
   - Ankle pain
   - Ankle swelling

3. List key functional limitation(s).

   - Difficulty to bear weight
   - Difficulty to walk and run

4. **List key disabilities.**
   - Unable to play football

5. **Justification for cryotherapy.**

   Is there justification to use cryotherapy in this case? This chapter has established that there is moderate strength of evidence and fair-to-good justification for the use of cryotherapy therapy for soft-tissue pathology, particularly for acute pathology (see Section VI). This textbook recommends the use of this agent for the following reasons. First, the pathology is acute, and cooling effects of soft tissues surrounding the site of injury are needed to minimize secondary tissue damage, which in turn will facilitate healing. Second, there is evidence that cryotherapy can benefit ankle sprain (Basur et al., 1976; Starkey, 1976; Hocutt et al., 1982; Cote et al., 1988; Michlovitz et al., 1988; Sloan et al., 1989; Wilkerson, 1991; Pincivero et al., 1993; Wilkerson et al., 1993; Weston et al., 1994; Bleakley et al., 2006). The cryoagent, because it is applied within 2 hours postinjury, is expected to regulate the inflammatory healing response by reducing tissue metabolism, thus minimizing secondary tissue damage as well as the cardinal signs and symptoms of inflammation. Such effects are expected to promote healing by quickly promoting ankle mobility. Because EPAs should never be used in isolation or as a sole intervention, cryotherapy (I for ice) is used here concomitantly with a regimen of protection (P), rest (R), compression (C), and elevation (E). In other words, the well-known therapeutic approach for acute soft-tissue pathology in sports therapy, described as PRICE, is applied in the present case.

6. **Search for contraindications.**

   The patient reports past episodes of transient skin edema following cryotherapy. The ice-cube test is performed. The result is negative. Further inquiries by the football team's physician reveal no additional element consistent with a diagnosis of cold urticaria. Cryotherapy is thus safe for this patient.

7. **Search for risks and precautions.**
   None is found.

8. **Outline the therapeutic goal(s) you and your patient wish to achieve.**
   - Decrease pain
   - Decrease edema
   - Decrease secondary tissue damage
   - Improve weight bearing
   - Improve walking and running performance
   - Accelerate return to play football

9. **For each therapeutic goal, list the outcome measurement(s) used to assess treatment effectiveness.**
   - Pain: Visual Analog Scale (VAS)
   - Swelling: volumetry
   - Weight bearing/walking/running performance: Patient-Specific Functional Scale (PSFS)

10. **Instruct the patient about what he or she should experience, do, and not do during the application of cryotherapy.**
    - Feel change in sensation from cold, to burning, to aching, and to numbness
    - Do not touch or remove the agent
    - If unbearable cold sensation is felt, call for help immediately

11. **Outline the therapeutic prescription of cryotherapy based on the evidence available.**

    The following prescription is based on the evidence presented in the following articles on the usage of cryotherapy for ankle sprain (Basur et al., 1976; Starkey, 1976; Hocutt et al., 1982; Cote et al., 1988; Michlovitz et al., 1988; Sloan et al., 1989; Wilkerson, 1991; Wilkerson et al., 1993; Pincivero et al., 1993; Weston et al., 1994; Bleakley et al., 2006). It is also based on the practitioner's clinical experience with this agent for similar cases of ankle sprain.

    - *Cryoagent:* ice (I) pack filled with crushed ice and water
    - *Ice-pack size:* 25 × 25 cm (10 × 10 in)
    - *Ice-pack temperature:* 2°C (35°F)
    - *Treated body area:* lateral aspect of traumatized ankle
    - *Patient's positioning:* lying in supine position; right lower limb elevated (E)
    - *Coupling medium:* none in order to induce rapid and intense soft-tissue cooling
    - *Application method:* cryostatic (first day); cryokinetic (following days)
    - *Application duration:* 20 minutes
    - *Application frequency per day:* First day: every 3 hours, except while sleeping;

    Other days: Every 6 hours, except while sleeping

    - *Total number of treatments:* 16 treatments delivered over 4 consecutive days
    - *Between treatments:* At rest (R) the affected lower limb is kept elevated (E) and the ankle joint compressed (C). During ambulation, the ankle joint is protected (P) by the use of a pair of crutches.

12. **Analyze outcome measurements.**
    Pre- and posttreatment comparison:

    - Pain: decreased VAS score from 8 to 2
    - Swelling: decreased volume by 75%
    - Weight bearing/walking/running: improved PSFS by 80%

(Continued)

Case Study 8-1   **Continued**

13. Assess therapeutic effectiveness based on outcome measures.

The results show that the application of 16 cryotherapy (I) treatments, combined with a regimen of ankle protection (P), rest (R), compression (C), and elevation (E) (i.e., PRICE), delivered daily over a 4-day period, led to significant control over the inflammatory response to trauma, preparing soft tissues for the proliferative and maturation phases of healing. Because cryotherapy was applied within hours following trauma, secondary tissue damages were minimized, which led to less ankle swelling, in addition to improving weight bearing, walking, and running abilities. Cryotherapy was first delivered using the cryostatic method (first day) and then using the cryokinetic method (following days). Overall, this conservative treatment had a beneficial impact on the patient's disablement status created by the pathology, as illustrated in the **figure below**.

14. State the prognosis.

The prognosis is excellent if this young athlete complies with his forthcoming rehabilitation program (ankle strengthening to fast walking and running). Full recovery is expected. This patient will gradually resume his regular football training schedule and should be ready to resume full competition over the next 2 weeks.

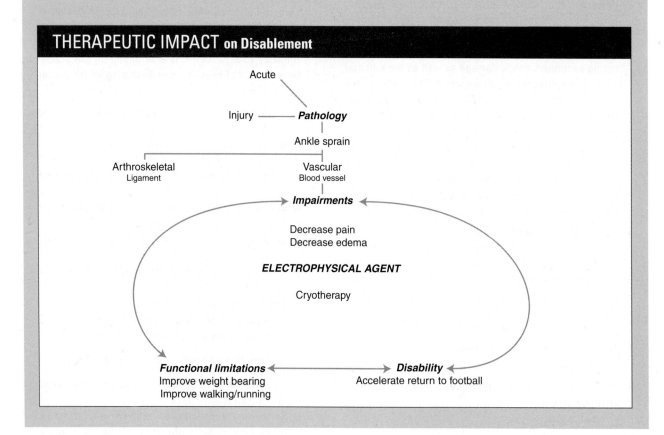

THERAPEUTIC IMPACT on Disablement

Acute

Injury —— *Pathology*

Ankle sprain

Arthroskeletal
Ligament

Vascular
Blood vessel

Impairments

Decrease pain
Decrease edema

ELECTROPHYSICAL AGENT

Cryotherapy

Functional limitations
Improve weight bearing
Improve walking/running

Disability
Accelerate return to football

Case Study 8-2 — Postoperative Anterior Cruciate Ligament Knee Reconstruction

A 32-year-old male amateur soccer player was involved in a collision with another player during a match. The collision caused the rupture of the anterior cruciate ligament (ACL) of his right knee joint. He is referred for immediate postoperative treatment following ACL surgical reconstruction. The physical examination, done hours after surgery, reveals all the signs of a traumatic inflammatory reaction caused by both the pathology (tissue damage) and the surgical procedure. The injured foot and toes feel cooler than normal. Knee swelling is important. According to information in the file, this patient may have a history of a mild, and undiagnosed, occlusive peripheral vascular disorder affecting particularly his lower limbs. The patient is resting fully awake in his hospital bed awaiting your visit. The knee is wrapped with surgical bandages. The surgeon prescribed the usual regimen of medication, which includes analgesics and anti-inflammatory drugs. The patient's immediate goals are to reduce pain, while taking the minimal number of pills, and then resume weight bearing and free walking in his room as soon as possible. He is anxious to be discharged from the hospital and receive treatment in a private sport clinic not far from his home. His later goals are to return, within the next few weeks, to his normal home and work activities as a lawyer. His ultimate goal is to be able, one day, to resume playing soccer.

Evidence-based Steps Toward the Resolution of This Case

1. **List medical diagnosis.**
   Complete right ACL rupture

2. **List key impairment(s).**
   - ACL rupture
   - Surgical wound
   - Knee pain
   - Knee swelling

3. **List key functional limitation(s).**
   - Unable to mobilize the knee
   - Unable to bear weight
   - Unable to walk
   - Unable to resume activities of daily living (ADLs)

4. **List key disabilities.**
   - Unable to work
   - Unable to play soccer

5. **Justification for cryotherapy.**
   Is there justification to use cryotherapy in this case? This chapter has established that as a whole there is mod-

erate strength of evidence and fair-to-good justification for the use of cryotherapy therapy for soft-tissue pathology, particularly for acute pathology (see Section VI). More specifically, scientific evidence reveals conflicting evidence for justifying the use of cryotherapy for postoperative ACL knee reconstruction (**Box 8-3**). Despite conflictual evidence, this textbook, nonetheless, recommends the use of this agent for the following reasons. First, the pathology (ACL rupture) and the surgical wound are acute, and cooling effects of soft tissues surrounding the site of injury and surgical wound are needed to minimize secondary tissue damage, which in turn will facilitate healing. Second, there is substantial evidence from research to show that cryotherapy may be beneficial for this type of pathology (Hecht et al., 1983; Cohn et al., 1989; Bert et al., 1991; Levy et al., 1993; Schroder et al., 1994; Shelbourne et al., 1994; Whitelaw et al., 1995; Lessard et al., 1997; Barber et al., 1998; Webb et al., 1998; Ohkoshi et al., 1999; Martin et al., 2001; Morsi, 2002; Sanchez-Inchausti et al., 2005). Third, the cryoagent, because it is applied within 24 to 48 hours postsurgery, is expected to regulate the inflammatory healing response by reducing tissue metabolism, thus minimizing secondary tissue damage as well as the cardinal signs and symptoms of inflammation, such as pain and edema. Such effects are expected to promote healing by quickly promoting knee mobility. Because EPAs should never be used in isolation or as a sole intervention, cryotherapy (I) is used here concomitantly with a regimen of protection (P), rest (R), compression (C), and elevation (E). In other words, the well-known therapeutic approach for acute soft-tissue pathology in sports therapy, described as PRICE, is applied in the present case. A regimen of bedside passive and active knee mobilization is also used. Because the pathology is acute and swelling is important, the cryotemperature-controlled device, which can deliver continuous cryotherapy (for hours) at a preset temperature, is recommended.

6. **Search for contraindications.**
   None is found.

7. **Search for risks and precautions.**
   The history of this patient reveals that he may be suffering from a mild case of peripheral vascular disorder affecting his lower limbs because his injured lower limb is much cooler than the other noninjured limb (see above). The *nail test* is thus performed on the big toe of both limbs. The results are negative. There is no risk involved in the use of cryotherapy for this patient.

(Continued)

Case Study 8-2   Continued

8. **Outline the therapeutic goal(s) you and your patient wish to achieve.**

   - Decrease pain
   - Decrease secondary tissue damage
   - Decrease swelling
   - Decrease drug intake
   - Improve knee mobility
   - Improve weight bearing and walking
   - Accelerate return to full ADLs, work, and possibly soccer

9. **For each therapeutic goal, list the outcome measurement(s) you will use to assess treatment efficacy based on research literature.**

   - Pain: Visual Rating Scale—5 (VRS-5)
   - Swelling: volumetric tape
   - Drug intake: pill count in personal diary
   - Weight bearing/walking performance: Patient-Specific Functional Scale (PSFS)

10. **Instruct the patient about what he or she should experience, do, and not do during the application of cryotherapy.**

    - Feel sensation from cold, to burning, to aching, and to numbness
    - Do not touch or remove the agent
    - If intense cold (burning sensation) is felt, call for help immediately
    - The agent will be in place for several hours everyday

11. **Outline the therapeutic prescription based on the evidence available.**

    The prescription is based on the following clinical studies conducted on the use of cryotherapy for post-operative ACL knee reconstruction (Hecht et al., 1983; Cohn et al., 1989; Bert et al., 1991; Levy et al., 1993; Schroder et al., 1994; Shelbourne et al., 1994; Whitelaw et al., 1995; Lessard et al., 1997; Barber et al., 1998; Webb et al., 1998; Ohkoshi et al., 1999; Martin et al., 2001; Morsi, 2002; Sanchez-Inchausti et al., 2005). It is also based on the practitioner's clinical experience with cryotherapy for similar cases.

    - *Cryoagent:* cryotemperature-controlled device (see **Fig 8-1D**)
    - *Preset pad temperature:* first 3 hours postoperatively: 8°C (46°F); next 3 hours post-op and thereafter: 9°C (48°F)
    - *Pad type:* commercial adult-size knee pad
    - *Treated body area:* total knee joint area

- *Coupling media*
  - Directly over wound: sterile gauze dressing
  - Around knee joint: compressive crepe bandage
- *Application method:* cryostatic
- *Application frequency and duration:*
  - Post-op–fourth day: continuous application; interruption only for knee mobilization, partial weight bearing, and short walking
  - Fifth–eighth day (or until discharge from hospital):
    - While awake: 1 hour every 2 hours
    - While asleep: continuous application
- *Total treatment duration:* 8 days (discharge from hospital)

12. **Collect outcome measurements.**

    Pre- and posttreatment comparison:

    - Pain: decreased VRS-5 score from 4 to 2
    - Swelling: volume score decreased by 80%
    - Analgesic intake: pill count decreased by 70%
    - Weight bearing/walking performance: improved PSFS score by 50%

13. **Assess therapeutic effectiveness based on outcome measures.**

    The results show that the application of cryotherapy, combined with a regimen of PRICE and periods of knee mobilization and short ambulation, delivered daily for several hours and over 8 consecutive days, led to significant control over the inflammatory response, preparing soft tissues for the proliferative and maturation phases of healing. The continuous application of cryotherapy, at a preset temperature, postsurgery, was beneficial in minimizing secondary tissue damage, thus accelerating healing and return to function. It was also beneficial in decreasing drug intake by 70%. The patient in now able to walk, using crutches, and is ready to return home. Overall, this treatment approach had a beneficial effect on the patient's disablement status created by the pathology, as illustrated in the **figure** on page 145.

14. **State the prognosis.**

    The prognosis is excellent if the patient complies with his forthcoming rehabilitation program until he is fully recovered. Healing of reconstructed ligaments takes months and is often imperfect. This patient will gradually return to his daily home activities, and then resume his office work as a lawyer. Considering the patient's age (32 years) and the fact that soccer is demanding on knee joints, he is advised to give up this sport and take up another sport that would be less demanding on his reconstructed knee joint.

THERAPEUTIC IMPACT on Disablement

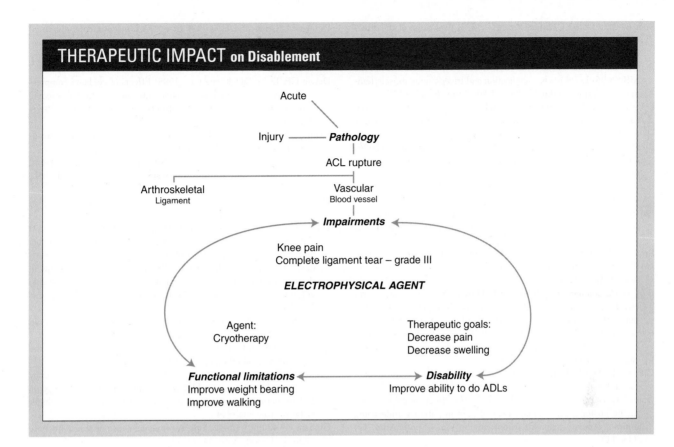

Acute

Injury ———— *Pathology*

ACL rupture

Arthroskeletal
Ligament

Vascular
Blood vessel

Impairments

Knee pain
Complete ligament tear – grade III

ELECTROPHYSICAL AGENT

Agent:
Cryotherapy

Therapeutic goals:
Decrease pain
Decrease swelling

Functional limitations
Improve weight bearing
Improve walking

Disability
Improve ability to do ADLs

CRITICAL THINKING QUESTIONS

Clarification: What is meant by cryotherapy?

Assumptions: You have assumed that cryotherapy is effective in preventing secondary tissue damage following trauma. How do you justify that assumption?

Reasons and evidence: What led you to believe that applying a cryoagent over the skin will cool superficial and deep soft tissues? If this is true, by which mechanism does it occur?

Viewpoints or perspectives: How would you respond to a colleague who says that the late cold-induced vasodilation (CIVD) effect should be avoided at all costs because it significantly diminishes the prime effect of cryotherapy, which is to cool soft tissues?

Implications and consequences: What are the implications of (a) applying a cryoagent using a coupling medium and (b) applying a cryoagent without a coupling medium over a body part that has a thick layer of adipose tissue?

About the question: Should practitioners using cryotherapy not be concerned with the issue of cold urticaria and seriously concerned with frostbite and peripheral nerve injury? Why do you think I ask this question?

References

Articles

Abramson DI, Chu LS, Tuck S, Lee SW, Richardson M (1966) Effect of tissue temperature and blood flow on motor nerve conduction velocity. JAMA, 198: 1082–1088

Aizawa Y, Shibata A, Tajiri M, Hirasawa Y (1979) Reflex vasoconstriction to a cold stimulus for non-invasive evaluation of neurovascular function in man. Jpn Heart, 20: 301–305

Amin-Hanjani S, Corcoran J, Chatwani A (1992) Cold therapy in the management of postoperative cesarean section pain. Am J Obstet Gynecol, 167: 108–109

Bancroft H, Edholm OG (1943) The effect of temperature on blood flow and deep temperature in the human forearm. J Physiol, 102: 5–20

Barber FA (2000) A comparison of crushed ice and continuous flow cold therapy. Am J Knee Surg, 13: 97–101

Barber FA, McGuire DA, Click S (1998) Continuous-flow cold therapy for outpatient anterior cruciate ligament reconstruction. Arthroscopy, 14: 130–135

Basset SW, Lake BM (1958) Use of cold applications in the management of spasticity. Phys Ther Rev, 38: 333–334

Bassett FH, Kirkpatrick JS, Englehartd DL, Malone TR (1992) Cryotherapy-induced nerve injury. Am J Sports Med, 20: 516–518

Bastian H, Soholm B, Marker P, Eckerdal A (1998) Comparative study of pain control by cryotherapy of exposed bone following extraction of wisdom teeth. J Oral Sci, 40: 109–113

Basur RL, Shephard E, Mouzas GL (1976) A cooling method in the treatment of ankle sprains. Practitioner, 216: 708–711

Belitsky RB, Odam SJ, Hubley-Kozey C (1987) Evaluation of the effectiveness of wet ice, dry ice, and cryogen packs in reducing skin temperature. Phys Ther, 67: 1080–1084

Bender AL, Kramer EE, Brucker JB, Demchak TJ, Cordova ML, Stone MB (2005) Local ice-bag application and triceps surea muscle temperature during treadmill walking. J Athl Train, 40: 271–275

Bert JM, Stark JG, Maschka K, Chock C (1991) The effect of cold therapy on morbidity subsequent to arthroscopic lateral retinacular release. Orthop Rev, 20: 755–758

Bleakley CM, McDonough SM, MacAuley DC, Bjordal J (2006) Cryotherapy for acute ankle sprains: A randomized controlled study of two different icing protocols. Br J Sports Med, 40: 700–705

Boes MC (1962) Reduction of spasticity by cold. J Am Phys Ther Assoc, 42: 29–32

Bolster MB, Maricq HR, Leff RL (1995) Office evaluation and treatment of Raynaud's phenomenon. Cleve Clin J Med, 62: 51–61

Brandner B, Munro L, Bromley LM, Hetreed M (1996) Evaluation of the contribution to postoperative analgesia by local cooling of the wound. Anaesthesia, 51: 1021–1025

Burgess JA, Sommers EE, Truelove EL, Dworkin SF (1988) Short-term effect of two therapeutic methods on myofascial pain and dysfunction of the masticatory system. J Prosthet Dent, 60: 606–610

Clarke GR, Willis LA, Stenner L, Nichols PJ (1974) Evaluation of physiotherapy in the treatment of osteoarthrosis of the knee. Rheumatol Rehab, 13: 190–197

Clarke RH, Hellon R, Lind A (1958) Vascular reactions of the human forearm to cold. Clin Sci, 17: 165–179

Cohn BT, Draeger RI, Jackson DW (1989) The effects of cold therapy in the postoperative management of pain in patients undergoing anterior cruciate ligament reconstruction. Am J Sports Med, 17: 344–349

Collins KJ, Dore C, Exton-Smith AN, Fox RH, McDonald IC, Woodward PM (1977) Accidental hypothermia and impaired temperature homeostasis in the elderly. Br Med J, 1(6057): 353–356

Collins K, Storey M, Peterson K (1986) Peroneal nerve palsy after cryotherapy. Physician Sportsmed, 14(5): 105–108

Cote DJ, Prentice WE, Hooker DN, Shields EW (1988) Comparison of three treatment procedures for minimizing ankle sprain swelling. Phys Ther, 68: 1072–1076

Covington DB, Bassett FH (1993) When cryotherapy injures. Physician Sportsmed, 21(3): 78, 82, 84, 93

Culp R, Taras J (1995) The effect of ice application versus controlled cold therapy on skin temperature when used with postoperative bulky hand and wrist dressings: A preliminary study. J Hand Ther, 8: 249–251

Curkovic B, Vitulic V, Babic-Naglic D, Durrigl T (1993) The influence of heat and cold on the pain threshold in rheumatoid arthritis. Z Rheumatol, 52: 289–291

Cuthill JA, Cuthill GS (2006) Partial-thickness burn to the leg following application of cold pack: Case report and results of a questionnaire survey of Scottish physiotherapists in private practice. Physiotherapy, 92: 61–65

Daanen HA, Van de Linde FJ, Romet TT, Ducharme MB (1997) The effect of body temperature on the hunting response of the middle finger skin temperature. Eur J Appl Physiol, 76: 538–543

Dahlstedt L, Samuelson P, Dalen N (1996) Cryotherapy after cruciate knee surgery: Skin, subcutaneous and articular temperatures in 8 patients. Acta Orthop Scand, 67: 255–257

Daniel DM, Stone ML, Arendt DL (1994) The effect of cold therapy on pain, swelling, and range of motion after anterior cruciate ligament reconstructive surgery. Arthroscopy, 10: 530–533

Day MJ (1974) Hypersensitive response to ice massage: Report of a case. Phys Ther, 54: 592–593

De Coster D, Bossuyt M, Fossion E (1993) The value of cryotherapy in the management of trigeminal neuralgia. Acta Stomatol Belg, 90: 87–93

Denegar CR, Perrin DH (1992) Effect of transcutaneous electrical nerve stimulation, cold, and a combination on pain, decreased range of motion, and strength loss associated with delayed muscle soreness. J Athl Train, 27: 200–206

Dervin GF, Taylor DE, Keene GC (1998) Effects of cold and compression dressings on early postoperative outcomes for the arthroscopic anterior cruciate ligament reconstruction patient. J Orthop Sports Phys Ther, 27: 403–406

Diamond S, Freitag FG (1986) Cold as an adjunctive therapy for headache. Postgrad Med, 79: 305–309

DonTigny RL, Shelton KW (1962) Simultaneous use of heat and cold in treatment of muscle spasm. Arch Phys Med Rehab, 43: 148–150

Drez D, Faust DC, Evans JP (1981) Cryotherapy and nerve palsy. Am J Sports Med, 9: 256–257

Duff F, Greenfield AD, Shepherd JT, Thompson ID, Whelan RF (1953) The response of vasodilator substances on blood vessels in fingers immersed in cold water. J Physiol, 121: 46–54

Edwards DJ, Rimmer M, Keene GC (1996) The use of cold therapy in the postoperative management of patients undergoing arthroscopic anterior cruciate ligament reconstruction. Am J Sports Med, 24: 193–195

Escher S, Tucker A (1992) Preventing, diagnosing, and treating cold urticaria. Physician Sportsmed, 20 (12): 73–84

Evans TA, Ingersoll C, Knight K, Worrell T (1995) Agility following the application of cold therapy. J Athl Train, 30: 231–234

Finan MA, Roberts WS, Hoffman MS, Fiorica JV, Cavanagh D, Dudney BJ (1993) The effects of cold therapy on postoperative pain in gynecologic patients: A prospective, randomized study. Am J Obstet Gynecol, 168: 542–544

Graham CA (2000) Frozen chips: An unusual cause of severe frostbite injury. Br J Sports Med, 34: 382–384

Grant AE (1964) Massage with ice (cryokinetics) in the treatment of painful conditions of the musculoskeletal system. Arch Phys Med Rehab, 45: 233–238

Green GA, Zachazewski JE, Jordan SE (1989) Peroneal nerve palsy induced by cryotherapy. Physician Sportsmed, 17: 63–70

Greenfield AD, Shepherd JT (1950) A quantitative study of the response to cold of the circulation through the fingers of normal subjects. Clin Sci, 9: 323–334

Halliday Pegg SM, Littler TR, Littler MD (1969) A trial of ice therapy and exercise in chronic arthritis. Physiotherapy, 55: 51–56

Hartvikksen K (1962) Ice therapy in spasticity. Acta Neurol Scand, 38: 79–84

Harvey CK (1992) An overview of cold injury. J Am Podiatr Med Assoc, 82: 436–438

Hayden CA (1964) Cryokinetics in an early treatment program. J Am Phys Ther Assoc, 44: 940–943

Healy WL, Seidman J, Pfiefer B, Brown DG (1994) Cold compressive dressing after total knee arthroplasty. Clin Orthop, 299: 143–146

Hecht PJ, Bachmann S, Booth RE, Rothman RH (1983) Effects of thermal therapy on rehabilitation after total knee arthroplasty. Clin Orthop, 178: 198–201

Hedenberg L (1970) Functional improvement of the spastic hemiplegic arm after cooling. Scand J Rehab Med, 2: 154–158

Ho SS, Coel MN, Kagawa R, Richardson AB (1994) The effect of ice on blood flow and bone metabolism in knees. Am J Sports Med, 22: 537–540

Ho SS, Illgen R, Meyer R (1995) Comparison of various icing times in decreasing bone metabolism and blood flow in the knee. Am J Sports Med, 23: 74–76

Hochberg J (2001) A randomized prospective study to assess the efficacy of two cold-therapy treatments following carpal tunnel release. J Hand Ther, 3: 208–215

Hocutt JE, Jaffe R, Rylander CR, Beebe JK (1982) Cryotherapy in ankle sprains. Am J Sports Med, 10: 316–319

Hoiness PR, Hvaal K, Engebretsen L (1998) Severe hypothermic injury to the foot and ankle caused by continuous cryocompression therapy. Knee Surg Sports Traumatol Arthrosc, 6: 253–255

Hopkins JT, Stencil R (2002) Ankle cryotherapy facilitates soleus function. J Orthop Sports Phys Ther, 32: 622–627

Iida T (1949) Studies concerning vascular reaction to cold (Part I): Physiological significance of vascular reaction to cold. J Physiol Soc Jpn, 11: 73–78

Ingersoll CD, Knight KL, Merrick MA (1992) Sensory perception of the foot and ankle following therapeutic applications of heat and cold. J Athl Train, 27: 231–234

Isabell WK, Durrant E, Myrer W, Anderson S (1992) The effects of ice massage and exercise on the prevention and treatment of delayed onset muscle soreness. J Athl Train, 27: 208–217

Janwantanakul P (2004) Different rate of cooling time and magnitude of cooling temperature during ice bag treatment with and without damp towel wrap. (Phys Ther Sports, 5: 156–161

Johnson DJ, Moore S, Moore J, Oliver RA (1979) Effect of cold submersion on intramuscular temperature of the gastrocnemius muscle. Phys Ther, 59: 1239–1242

Jutte LS, Merrick MA, Ingersoll CD, Edwards JE (2001). The relationship between intramuscular temperature, skin temperature and adipose thickness during cryotherapy and rewarming. Arch Phys Med Rehab, 82: 845–850

Kaempffe FA (1989) Skin surface temperature reduction after cryotherapy to a casted extremity. J Orthop Sports Phys Ther, 10: 448–450

Khajavi K, Pavelko T, Mishra AK (2004) Compartment syndrome arising from use of an electronic cooling pad. Am J Sports Med, 32: 1538–1541

Kalenak A, Medlar CE, Fleagle SB, Hochberg WJ (1975) Treating thigh contusions with ice. Physician Sportsmed, 3 (3): 65–67

Karunakara RG, Lephart SM, Pincivero DM (1998) Changes in forearm blood flow during single and intermittent cold application. J Orthop Sports Phys Ther, 29: 177–180

Kelly M (1969) Effectiveness of a cryotherapy technique on spasticity. Phys Ther, 49: 349–353

Kinnman J, Andersson T, Andersson G (2000a) Effect of cooling suit treatment in patients with multiple sclerosis evaluated by evoked potentials. Scand J Rehab Med, 32: 16–19

Kinnman J, Andersson T, Wetterquist L, Kinnman Y, Andersson U (2000b) Cooling suit for multiple sclerosis: Functional improvement in daily living? Scand J Rehab Med, 32: 20–24

Kirk JA, Kersley GD (1968) Heat and cold in the physical treatment of rheumatoid arthritis of the knee. Ann Phys Med, 9: 270–274

Knight KL, Aquino J, Johannes SM, Urban CD (1980) A re-examination of Lewis' cold-induced vasodilation in the finger and the ankle. J Athl Train, 15: 238–250

Knight KL, Brucker JB, Stoneman PD, Rubley MD (2000) Muscle injury management with cryotherapy. Athl Ther Today, 5: 26–30

Knight KL, Elam JF (1981) Rewarming of the ankle, finger, and forearm after cryotherapy: Further investigation of Lewis' cold-induced vasodilation. J Can Athl Ther Assoc, 8: 17–18

Knight KL, Ingersoll CD, Trowbridge CA, Connolly TA, Cordovia ML, Hyink LL, Welch SM (1994) The effects of cooling the ankle, the triceps surae, or both on functional agility. J Athl Train, 29: 165–169

Knutsson E (1970a) On effects of local cooling upon motor functions in spastic paresis. Prog Phys Ther, 1: 124–131

Knutsson E (1970b) Topical cryotherapy in spasticity. Scand J Rehab Med, 2: 159–163

Konrath G, Lock T, Goitz H, Scheider J (1996) The use of cold therapy after anterior cruciate ligament reconstruction. A prospective, randomized study and literature study. Am J Sports Med, 24: 629–633

Kraus H (1941) The use of surface anesthesia in the treatment of painful motion. JAMA, 16: 2582–2583

Landen BR (1967) Heat or cold for the relief of low back pain? Phys Ther, 47: 1126–1128

Lane LE (1971) Localized hypothermia for the relief of pain in musculoskeletal injuries. Phys Ther, 51: 182–183

La Riviere J, Osternig LR (1994) The effect of ice on joint position sense. J Sports Rehab, 3: 58–67

Lavelle BE, Snyder M (1985) Differential conduction of cold through barriers. J Adv Nurs, 10: 55–61

Leblanc J, Cote J, Dulac S, Dulong-Turcot F (1978) Effects of age, sex, and physiological fitness on responses to local cooling. J Appl Physiol, 44: 813–817

Lessard LA, Scudds RA, Amendola A, Vaz AA (1997) The efficacy of cryotherapy following arthroscopic knee surgery. J Orthop Sports Phys Ther, 26: 14–22

Leutz DW, Harris H (1995) Continuous cold therapy in total knee arthroplasty. Am J Knee Surg, 8: 121–123

Levy AS, Marmar E (1993) The role of cold compression dressings in the postoperative treatment of total knee arthroplasty. Clin Orthop, 297: 174–178

Lewis T (1930) Observations upon the reactions of the vessels of the human skin to cold. Heart, 15: 177–208

Long BC, Cordova ML, Brucker JB, Demchak TJ, Stone MB (2005) Exercise and quadriceps muscle cooling time. J Athl Train, 40: 260–263

Lorenze EJ, Caroutonis G, DeRosa AJ (1960) Effect on coronary circulation of cold packs to hemiplegic shoulders. Arch Phys Med Rehab, 41: 394–399

Lowden BJ, Moore RJ (1975) Determinants and nature of intramuscular temperature changes during cold therapy. Am J Phys Med, 54: 223–233

Malone TR, Englehardt DL, Kirkpatrick JS, Basset FH (1992) Nerve injury in athletes caused by cryotherapy. J Athl Train, 27: 235–237

Martin SS, Spinder KP, Tarter JW, Detwiler K, Petersen HA (2001) Cryotherapy: An effective modality for decreasing intra-articular temperature after knee arthroscopy. Am J Sports Med, 29: 288–291

McGuire DA, Hendricks SD (2006) Incidences of frostbite in arthroscopic knee surgery postoperative cryotherapy rehabilitation. J Arthros Relat Surg, 22: 1141–1146

Melzack R, Gutte S, Gonshor A (1980a) Relief of dental pain by ice massage of the hand. Can Med Assoc J, 122: 189–191

Melzack R, Jeans ME, Stratford JG, Monks RC (1980b) Ice massage and transcutaneous electrical stimulation: Comparison of treatment for low-back pain. Pain, 9: 209–217

Mennel J (1976) Spray-stretch for the relief of pain from muscle spasm and myofascial trigger points. J Am Podiatr Assoc, 66: 873–876

Merrick MA, Jutte LS, Smith ME (2003) Cold modalities with different thermodynamic properties produce different surface and intramuscular temperatures. J Athl Train, 38: 28–33

Merrick MA, Knight KL, Ingersoll CD, Potteiger JA (1993) The effects of ice and compression wraps on intramuscular temperatures at various depths. J Athl Train, 28: 236–245

Metzman L, Gamble JG, Rinsky LA (1996) Effectiveness of ice packs in reducing skin temperatures under casts. Clin Orthop, 330: 217–221

Michlovitz S, Smith W, Watkins M (1988) Ice and high voltage pulsed stimulation in the treatment of acute lateral ankle sprains. J Orthop Sports Phys Ther, 9: 301–304

Miglietta O (1964) Electromyographic characteristics of clonus and influence of cold. Arch Phys Med Rehab, 45: 508–512

Miglietta O (1973) Action of cold on spasticity. Am J Phys Med, 52: 198–205

Modell W, Travel J, Kraus H (1952) Relief of pain by ethyl chloride spray. N Y State J Med, 52: 1550–1558

Moeller JL, Monroe J, McKeag DB (1997) Cryotherapy-induced common peroneal nerve palsy. Clin J Sports Med, 7: 212–216

Moore CD, Cardea JA (1977) Vascular changes in leg trauma. South Med J, 70: 1285–1286

Morsi E (2002) Continuous-flow cold therapy after total knee arthroplasty. Arthroplasty, 17: 718–722

Myrer JW, Measom G, Fellingham GW (1998) Temperature changes in the human leg during and after two methods of cryotherapy. J Athl Train, 33: 25–29

Myrer JW, Measom G, Fellingham GW (2000) Exercise after cryotherapy greatly enhances intramuscular rewarming. J Athl Train, 35: 412–416

Myrer JW, Myrer KA, Measom GJ, Fellingham GW, Evers SL (2001) Muscle temperature is affected by overlying adipose when cryotherapy is administered. J Athl Train, 36: 32–36

Nadler SF, Prybicien M, Malanga GA, Sicher D (2003) Complications from therapeutic modalities: Results of a national survey of athletic trainers. Arch Phys Med Rehab, 84: 849

Nielson AJ (1978) Spray and stretch for myofascial pain. Phys Ther, 58: 567–569

Nielson AJ (1981) Case study: Myofascial pain of the posterior shoulder relieved by spray and stretch. J Orthop Sports Phys Ther, 3: 21–26

Ohkoshi Y, Ohkoshi M, Nagasaki S, Ono A, Hashimoto T, Yamane S (1999) The effect of cryotherapy on intra-articular temperature and postoperative care after anterior cruciate ligament reconstruction. Am J Sports Med, 27: 357–362

Okcu G, Yercan HS (2006) Is it possible to decrease skin temperature with ice packs under cast and bandages? A cross-sectional, randomized trial on normal and swollen ankles. Arch Orthop Trauma Surg, 126: 668–673

O'Toole G, Rayatt S (1999) Frostbite at the gym: A case report of an ice pack burn. Br J Sports Med, 33: 278–279

Otte JW, Merrick MA, Ingersoll CD, Cordova ML (2002) Subcutaneous adipose tissue thickness alters cooling time during cryotherapy. Arch Phys Med Rehabil, 83: 1501–1505

Palmieri RM, Garrison JG, Leonard JL, Edwards JE, Weltman A, Ingersoll CD (2006) Peripheral ankle cooling and core body temperature. J Athl Train, 41: 185–188

Parker JT, Small NC, Davis PG (1983) Cold-induced nerve palsy. Athl Train, 18: 76

Pincivero D, Gieck J, Saliba E (1993) Rehabilitation of a lateral ankle sprain with cryokinetic and functional progressive exercise. J Sport Rehab, 2: 200–207

Post JB, Knight KL (1992) Ankle skin temperature changes with a repeated ice pack application. J Athl Train, 27: 136–140

Price R, Lehmann JF, Boswell-Bessette S, Burleigh S, de Lateur BJ (1993) Influence of cryotherapy on spasticity at the human ankle. Arch Phys Med Rehab, 74: 300–304

Quist LH, Peltier G, Lundquist KJ (1996) Frostbite of the eyelids following inappropriate applications of ice compresses. Arch Ophthalmol, 114: 226

Rembe EC (1970) Use of cryotherapy on the postsurgical rheumatoid hand. Phys Ther, 50: 19–23

Robbins LD (1989) Cryotherapy for headache. Headache, 29: 598–600

Rubley MD, Denegar CR, Buckley WE, Newell KM (2003) Cryotherapy, sensation and isometric-force variability. J Athl Train, 38: 113–119

Ruiz DH, Myrer J, Durrant E, Fellingham GW (1993) Cryotherapy and sequential exercise bouts following cryotherapy on concentric and eccentric strength in the quadriceps. J Athl Train, 28: 320–323

Saito N, Horiuchi H, Kobayashi S, Nawata M, Takaoka K (2004) Continuous local cooling for pain relief following total hip arthroplasty. J Arthroplasty, 19: 334–337

Sanchez-Inchausti G, Vaquero-Martin J, Vidal-Fernandez C (2005) Effect of arthroscopy and continuous cryotherapy on the intramuscular temperature of the knee. Arthroscopy, 21: 552–556

Scarcella JB, Cohn BT (1995) The effect of cold therapy on the postoperative course of total hip and knee arthroplasty patients. Am J Orthop, 24: 847–852

Schaubel HJ (1946) The local use of ice after orthopedic procedures. Am J Surg, 72: 711–714

Scheffler NM, Sheitel PL, Lipton MN (1992) Use of Cryo/Cuff for the control of postoperative pain and edema. J Foot Surg, 31: 141–148

Schroder D, Passler HH (1994) Combination of cold and compression after knee surgery. A prospective randomized study. Knee Surg Sports Traumatol Arthrosc, 2: 158–165

Shelbourne KD, Rubinstein RA, McCarrol JR, Weaver J (1994) Postoperative cryotherapy for the knee in ACL reconstruction surgery. Orthop Int Ed, 2: 165–170

Showman J, Wedlick LT (1963) The use of cold instead of heat for the relief of muscle spasm. Med J Aust, 50: 612–614

Singh H, Osbahr DC, Holovacs TF, Cawley PW, Speer KP (2001) The efficacy of continuous cryotherapy on the postoperative shoulder: A prospective, randomized investigation. J Shoulder Elbow Surg, 10: 522–525

Sloan JP, Hain R, Pownall R (1989) Clinical benefits of early cold therapy in accident and emergency following ankle sprain. Arch Emerg Med, 6: 1–6

Speer KP, Warren RF, Horowitz L (1996) The efficacy of cryotherapy in the postoperative shoulder. J Shoulder Elbow Surg, 5: 62–68

Starkey JA (1976) Treatment of ankle sprains by simultaneous use of intermittent compression and ice packs. Am J Sports Med, 41: 142–144

Stockle U, Hoffmann R, Schultz M, von Fournier C, Sudkamp NP, Haas N (1997) Fastest reduction of posttraumatic edema: Continuous cryotherapy or intermittent impulse compression? Foot Ankle Int, 18: 432–438

Thieme H, Ingersoll C, Knight K, Ozmun JC (1996) Cooling does not affect knee proprioception. J Athl Train, 31: 8–11

Travell J (1949) Rapid relief of acute stiff neck by ethyl chloride spray. J Am Med Wom Assoc, 4: 89–95

Travell J (1952) Ethyl chloride for painful muscle spasm. Arch Phys Med Rehab, 32: 291–298

Tremblay F, Estephan L, Legendre M, Sulpher S (2001) Influence of local cooling on proprioceptive acuity in the quadriceps muscle. J Athl Train, 36: 119–123

Tsang KKW, Buxton BP, Guion WK, Joyner AB, Browder KD (1997) The effects of cryotherapy applied over various barriers. J Sports Rehab, 6: 343–354

Uchio Y, Ochi M, Fujihara A, Adachi N, Iwasa J, Sakai Y (2003) Cryotherapy influences joint laxity and position sense on healthy knee joint. Arch Phys Med Rehab, 84: 131–135

Walker RH, Morris BA, Angulo DL, Scheinder J, Colwell CW (1991) Postoperative use of continuous passive motion, transcutaneous electrical nerve stimulation and continuous cooling pad following total knee arthroplasty. J Arthroplasty, 6: 151–156

Webb JM, Williams D, Ivory JP, Day S, Williamson DM (1998) The use of cold compression dressings after total knee replacement: A randomized controlled trial. Orthopedics, 21: 59–61

Weresh MJ, Bennett GL, Njus G (1996) Analysis of cryotherapy penetration: A comparison of the plaster cast, synthetic cast, Ace wrap dressing, and Robert-Jones dressing. Foot Ankle Int, 17: 37–40

Weston M, Taber C, Casgranda L, Cornwall M (1994) Changes in local blood volume during cold gel pack application to traumatized ankles. J Orthop Sports Phys Ther, 19: 197–199

Whitelaw GP, DeMuth KA, Demos HA, Schepsis A, Jacques E (1995) The use of Cryo/Cuff versus ice and elastic wrap in the postoperative care of knee arthroscopy patients. Am J Knee Surg, 8: 28–30

Wilkerson GB (1991) Treatment of the inversion ankle sprain through synchronous application of focal compression and cold. J Athl Train, 26: 220–237

Wilkerson GB, Horn-Kingery HM (1993) Treatment of the inversion ankle sprain: Comparison of different modes of compression and cryotherapy. J Orthop Sports Phys Ther, 17: 240–246

Williams J, Harvey J, Tannenbaum H (1986) Use of superficial heat and ice for the rheumatoid arthritic shoulder: A pilot study. Physiother Can, 38: 3–13

Yackzan L, Adams C, Francis KT (1984) The effects of ice massage on delayed muscle soreness. Am J Sports Med, 12: 159–165

Zaffagnini S, Iacono F, Petito A, Loreti I, Fu FH, Marcacci M (1998) Cryo/Cuff use after arthroscopic surgery: Effect on knee joint temperature. Am J Knee Surg, 11: 203–207

Zemke JE, Anderson JC, Guion WK (1998) Intramuscular temperature responses in the human leg to two forms of cryotherapy: Ice massage and ice bag. J Orthop Sports Phys Ther, 27: 301–307

Review Articles

Airhihenbuwa C, St Pierre R, Winchell D (1987) Cold vs. heat therapy: A physician's recommendations for first aid treatment of strain. Emergency, 19: 40–43

Allen RJ (2006) Physical agents used in the management of chronic pain by physical therapists. Phys Med Rehabil Clin N Am, 17: 315–345

Bleakley C, McDonough S, MacAuley D (2004) The use of ice in the treatment of acute soft-tissue injury. Am J Sports Med, 32: 251–261

Chapman CE (1991) Can the use of physical modalities for pain control be rationalized by the research evidence? Can J Physiol Pharmacol, 69: 704–712

Cook D, Georgouras K (1994) Complications of cutaneous cryotherapy. Med J Aust, 161: 210–213

Daanen HA (2003) Finger cold-induced vasodilation: A review. Eur J Appl Physiol, 89: 411–426

Ernst E, Fialka V (1994) Ice freezes pain? A review of the clinical effectiveness of analgesic cold therapy. J Pain Symptom Manage, 9: 56–59

French SD, Cameron M, Walker BF, Reggars JW, Esterman AJ (2006) A Cochrane review of superficial heat and cold for low back pain. Spine, 31: 998–1006

Halvorson GA (1990) Therapeutic heat and cold for athletic injuries. Physician Sportsmed, 18 (5): 87–94

Hardy M, Woodall W (1998) Therapeutic effects of heat, cold, and stretch on connective tissue. J Hand Ther, 11 (4–5): 148–156

Hayes K (1993) Heat and cold in the management of rheumatoid arthritis. Arthritis Care Res, 6: 156–166

Hocutt JE (1981) Cryotherapy. Am Fam Physician, 23: 141–144

Hubbard TJ, Aronson SL, Denegar CR (2004a) Does cryotherapy hasten return to participation? A systematic review. J Athl Train, 39: 88–94

Hubbard TJ, Denegar CR (2004b) Does cryotherapy improve outcomes with soft tissue injury? J Athl Train, 39: 278–279

Kellett J (1986) Acute soft tissue injuries: A review of the literature. Med Sci Sports Exerc, 18: 489–500

Kerr KM, Daley L, Booth L (1999) Guidelines for the management of soft tissue (musculoskeletal) injury with Protection, Rest, Ice, Compression and Elevation (PRICE) during the first 64 hours. Chartered Society of Physiotherapy, London

Kowal MA (1983) Review of physiological effects of cryotherapy. J Orthop Sports Phys Ther, 5: 66–73

MacAuley D (2001a) Do textbooks agree on their advice on ice? Clin J Sport Med, 11: 67–72

MacAuley D (2001b) Ice therapy: How good is the evidence? Int J Sports Med, 22: 379–384

McDowell J, McFarland E, Nalli B (1994) Use of cryotherapy for orthopedic patients. Orthop Nurs, 13: 21–30

McLean DA (1989) The use of cold and superficial heat in the treatment of soft tissue injuries. Br J Sports Med, 23: 53–54

McMaster WC (1982) Cryotherapy. Physician Sportsmed, 10: 112–119

Meeusen R, Lievens P (1986) The use of cryotherapy in sports injuries. Sports Med, 3: 398–414

Merrick MA (2002) Secondary injury after musculoskeletal trauma: A review and update. J Athl Train, 37: 209–217

Nanneman D (1991) Thermal modalities: Heat and cold. A review of physiologic effects with clinical applications. Am Assoc Occup Health Nurs J, 39: 70–75

Rivenburgh DW (1992) Physical modalities in the treatment of tendon injuries. Clin Sports Med, 11: 645–659

Swenson C, Sward L, Karlsson J (1996) Cryotherapy in sports medicine. Scand J Med Sci Sports, 6: 193–200

Tepperman PS, Devlon M (1983) Therapeutic heat and cold: A practitioner's guide. Postgrad Med, 73: 69–76

Chapters of Textbooks

Bell GW, Prentice WE (2002) Infrared modalities. In: Therapeutic Modalities for Physical Therapists, 2nd ed. Prentice WE (Ed). McGraw-Hill, New York, pp 202–270

Cameron MH (2003) Thermal Agents: Cold and heat. In: Physical Agents in Rehabilitation: From Research to Practice, 2nd ed. WB Saunders Co., Philadelphia, pp 133–158

Hayes KW (2000) Cryotherapy. In: Manual for Physical Agents, 5th ed. Hayes KW (Ed). Prentice-Hall Health, Upper Saddle River, pp 57–70

Hecox B, Sanko JP (2006) Cryotherapy. In: Integrated Physical Agents in Rehabilitation, 2nd ed. Hecox B, Mehreteab TA, Weisberg J, Sanko J (Eds). Pearson Prentice Hall. Upper Saddle River, pp 167–178

Knight KL, Draper DO (2008a) Cryotherapy beyond immediate care. In: Therapeutic Modalities: The Art and Science. Lippincott Williams & Wilkins, Philadelphia, pp 215–237

Knight KL, Draper DO (2008b) Application procedures: Post-immediate care cryotherapy. In: Therapeutic Modalities: The Art and Science. Lippincott Williams & Wilkins, Philadelphia, pp 238–253

Lehmann JF, DeLateur BJ (1990) Cryotherapy. In: Therapeutic Heat and Cold, 4th ed. Lehmann JF (Ed). Williams and Wilkins, Baltimore, pp 590–632

Low J, Reed A (1990) Cold therapy. In: Electrotherapy Explained. Principles and Practice. Butterworth Heinemann, London, pp 202–220

Michlovitz SL (2005) Cold Therapy Modalities: Frozen Peas and More. In: Modalities for Therapeutic Interventions, 4th ed. Michlovitz SL, Nolan TP (Eds). FA Davis Co., Philadelphia, pp 43–60

Michlovitz SL, von Nieda K (2006) Therapeutic Heat and Cold. In: Physical Agents Theory and Practice, 2nd ed. Behrens BJ, Michlovitz SL (Eds). FA Davis Co., Philadelphia, pp 37–53

Sekins KM, Emery AF (1990) Thermal science for physical medicine. In: Therapeutic Heat and Cold, 4th ed. Lehmann JF (Ed). Williams and Wilkins, Baltimore, pp 62–112

Starkey C (2004) Thermal Modalities. In: Therapeutic Modalities, 3rd ed. FA Davis Co., Philadelphia, pp 110–123

Textbooks

Knight KL (1995) Cryotherapy in Sports Injury Management. Human Kinetics, Champaign

Travell JG, Simons DG (1999a) Myofascial Pain and Dysfunction: The Trigger Point Manual. Volume 1: Upper Half of Body, 2nd ed. Williams & Wilkins, Philadelphia

Travell JG, Simons DG (1999b) Myofascial Pain and Dysfunction: The Trigger Point Manual. Volume 2: The Lower Extremity. Williams & Wilkins, Philadelphia

Commentary Letters

Proulx RP (1976) South California frostbite. J Am Coll Emerg Phys, 5: 618

Simons DG, Travell JG, Simons LS (1989) Suggestions: Alternate spray; alternative treatments. Progress report. Am Phys Ther Assoc, 18: 2

Stevens DM, D'Angelo JV (1978) Frostbite due to improper use of frozen gel pack. N Engl J Med, 299: 1415

Vallentyne SW, Vallentyne JR (1988) The case of the missing ozone: Are physiatrists to blame? Arch Phys Med Rehab, 69: 992–993

9 | CHAPTER

Hydrotherapy

Chapter Outline

Learning Objectives

Knowledge: List and describe the three common delivery methods for hydrotherapy.

Comprehension: Describe the intrinsic, thermal, and mechanical properties of water.

Application: Illustrate how, and for what pathological conditions, you would apply hydrotherapy using a bath, a tub, and a tank.

Analysis: Compare the three water immersion methods.

Synthesis: Explain how the sanitary and mechanical properties of water play a key role in wound management.

Evaluation: Discuss the electrical safety and water contamination issues associated with the practice of hydrotherapy.

I. RATIONALE FOR USE

A. DEFINITION AND DESCRIPTION

Hydrotherapy is broadly defined as the use of water (*hydro*) for therapeutic purposes. Because water that is warmer or colder in relation to the patient's immersed neutral skin temperature is used therapeutically, hydrotherapy is further classified in this chapter as the application of *neutro-hydrotherapy* (water at skin temperature), *thermo-hydrotherapy* (water above skin temperature), and *cryo-hydrotherapy* (water below skin temperature).

B. DELIVERY MODES

Hydrotherapy is delivered in three modes: *bath/tub/tank therapy*, *pool/aquatic therapy*, and *spa/balneotherapy*. **Table 9-1** lists the key characteristics of each mode. The main difference between these three modes of hydrotherapy is the *type of water* used: tap water with or without therapeutic additives for bath/tub/tank therapy, tap water with chlorine alone for pool/aquatic therapy, and natural waters and muds for spa/balneotherapy.

C. FOCUS ON BATH/TUB/TANK MODE

The focus of this chapter is on the delivery of hydrotherapy using the classic bath/tub/tank mode found in most clinical settings around the world. The pool/aquatic therapy mode is beyond the scope of this chapter because the main therapeutic effects come from physical exercises, and not from the effect of water per se. In other words, pool/aquatic therapy is basically an exercise-based treatment, rather than a water-based or hydrotherapy-type treatment. The spa/balneotherapy mode is also beyond the scope of this chapter because the water type and mud used for therapy are found only in oceans or natural springs, and thus are not commonly available in traditional clinical settings.

D. HYDROTHERAPY EQUIPMENT AND ACCESSORIES

Clinical hydrotherapy is commonly delivered using various immersion baths, tubs, and tanks as well as nonimmersion manual water irrigators. Immersion equipment may be movable or stationary and is fitted with drains and thermostatically controlled water valves. Nonimmersion equipment is portable and manually operated. **Figure 9-1** shows common types of baths (**A**), tubs (**B**, **C**, and **D**), tanks (**E**, **F**), and manual water irrigator (**G**) used today to deliver hydrotherapy in clinical settings. This figure also shows key accessories, namely, electrical turbines mounted on tubs and tanks (**B**, **C**, **D**, **E**, and **F**) as well as patient-lifting systems (**H**, **I**) facilitating access to hydrotherapy tubs and tanks.

E. RATIONALE FOR USE

The rationale for the use of tap water for therapeutic purposes rests with its intrinsic sanitary, thermal, and mechanical properties and with the fact that tap water is cheap and readily available in all clinical settings. Hydrotherapy, using baths, tubs, tanks, and water irrigators, is applied for several pathologies, particularly for the management of burn wounds. It is also used to facilitate therapeutic exercise programs for those unable to perform them on land because of the gravity force acting on their body, by providing buoyancy and drag forces, which may be used to induce weightlessness and either assist or resist therapeutic movements.

II. HISTORICAL PERSPECTIVE

A. WATER HEALING

Historical accounts suggest that hydrotherapy began in the era of *water healing*, which existed in Greece from 500 to 300 BC, during which time Hippocrates himself is reported

TABLE 9-1	HYDROTHERAPY MODES AND THEIR KEY CHARACTERISTICS	
TUB/TANK/BATH THERAPY	**POOL/AQUATIC THERAPY**	**SPA/BALNEOTHERAPY**
Tap water mixed with therapeutic additives	Tap water mixed with chlorine	Natural waters and mud with their own minerals
Bath, tub, and tank	Full-size pool, customized pool	Ocean water and mud
Single patient only	Single, and group of patients	Single, and group of patients
Water-based treatment	Exercise-based treatment	Water-based treatment
Normal and damaged skin	Normal skin only	Normal skin only

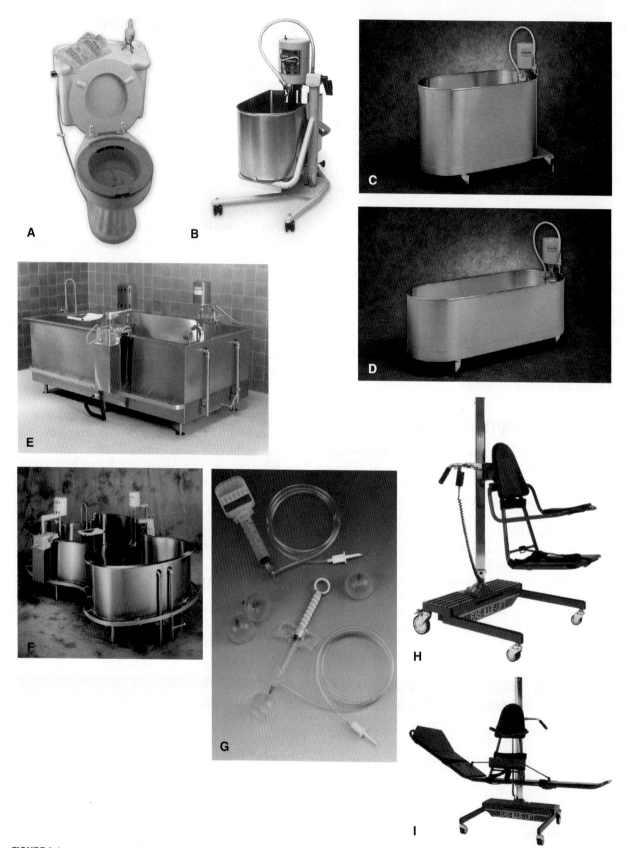

FIGURE 9-1 Common types of immersion baths, tubs, tanks, and nonimmersion irrigators, with accessories. (**A**) hip/buttock sitz bath, (**B**) extremity tub with turbine, (**C**) partial-body immersion High-Boy tub with turbine, (**D**) partial-body immersion Low-Boy tub with turbine, (**E**) full-body immersion tank with turbines, (**F**) full-body immersion Hubbard tank with turbines, (**G**) nonimmersion manual pressured-water irrigator, (**H**) motorized patient-handling system mounted with a chair, (**I**) a stretcher used for partial and full-body immersion tubs and tanks. (A: Courtesy of Invacare Corporation; B: Courtesy of Alimed Inc.; C–F: Courtesy of Whitehall Manufacturing; G: Courtesy of Alimed Inc.; H and I: Courtesy of Ferno Performance Pools.)

to have used hot and cold water immersion baths to treat a wide variety of diseases (Baruch, 1920; Jackson, 1990; Irion, 1997). Sir John Floyer is reported to have written, in the seventeenth century, the first treatise on hydrotherapy, entitled *An Inquiry into the Right Use and Abuse of Hot, Cold and Temperate Baths* (Irion, 1997). The eighteenth through twentieth centuries saw a major increase in the use of water for therapeutic purposes. Hydrotherapy evolved from its traditional mode of body immersion in baths, tubs, and tanks to include two other modes known as pool/aquatic therapy and spa/balneotherapy.

B. PRACTICE SURVEYS

Studies indicate that the use of bath/tub/tank therapy is a common practice in most clinical settings (Toomey et al., 1986a, 1986) and burn centers (Thomson et al., 1990; Shankowsky et al., 1994) in Canada, the United States, and elsewhere in the world (Whitelock, 1990; Smith, 1997).

C. BODY OF LITERATURE

The topic of tub, bath, and tank hydrotherapy has been the subject of several *articles* (see References), *review articles* (Jackson, 1990; Whitelock, 1990; McCulloch, 1995, 1998; Walsh, 1996; Smith, 1997; Rodeheaver, 1999; Cochrane, 2004; Hess et al., 2004), and *chapters of textbooks* (Sekins et al., 1990; Low et al., 1994; Babb et al., 1996; Kreighbaum et al., 1996; Walsh, 1996; Clement, 1997; Irion, 1997; Bell et al., 1998; Cameron, 2003; Bukowski et al., 2005; Hall, 2006; Hecox et al., 2006; Stowers et al., 2006). As stated above, the coverage of the other two modes of hydrotherapy, that is, aquatic/pool therapy and spa/balneotherapy, is beyond the scope of this chapter.

III. BIOPHYSICAL CHARACTERISTICS

A. WATER PROPERTIES

The biophysics of hydrotherapy is based on the intrinsic, thermal, and mechanical properties of tap water.

1. Intrinsic Properties
The intrinsic properties of water refer to its density, specific gravity, and viscosity.

2. Thermal Properties
The thermal properties relate to its specific heat and thermal conductivity.

3. Mechanical Properties
The mechanical properties of water refer to its buoyancy force, hydrostatic pressure, and drag force.

B. DENSITY

The density (designated by the Greek letter ρ) of a substance, such as water, is the measure of how compactly its atoms and molecules are arranged together (Kreighbaum et al., 1996). Density is defined as mass (m) over volume (v), that is, $\rho = m/v$. The more compactly arranged the molecules, the denser the substance is.

1. Weight Density (ρ_w)
Because weight (w) is directly proportional to mass (weight = mass × gravity) and the measurement of weight is more readily available than that of mass, the concept of weight density can be substituted for density, such that weight density (ρ_w) equals weight (w) over volume (v).

2. Unit and Value
Common units of ρ_w are Newtons per liter (N/L), where 1 liter equals 1,000 cubic centimeters, or pounds per cubic foot (lb/ft^3). The ρ_w of fresh water is 9.8 N/L or 62.4 lb/ft^3 (Kreighbaum et al., 1996).

C. SPECIFIC GRAVITY

The specific gravity (S_g) of a substance is the ratio of its weight density to the weight density of water (Kreighbaum et al., 1996).

1. Unit and Value
The specific gravity (S_g) of water is unity, or 1, because its weight density, as a fluid, equals 9.8 N/L or 62.4 lb/ft^3, as stated above (S_g = 9.8 N/L / 9.8 N/L = 1; 62.4 lb/ft^3 / 62.4 lb/ft^3 = 1).

2. Flotation
The flotation of a substance depends on its specific gravity (S_g). For example, if the weight density (ρ_w) of an object or body segment is *less than or equal* to the ρ_w of water (i.e., $S_g \leq 1$), that object or body segment will float. In contrast, if its ρ_w is *greater* than the ρ_w of water (i.e., $S_g > 1$), then that object or body segment will sink. This is why a piece of wood (S_g = 0.79) will float, but a piece of aluminum (S_g = 2.65) will sink if immersed in water.

3. Human Body
The S_g of the human body, which varies depending on the individual's somatotype and residual air volume in the lungs at immersion, is *less than one*. As a result, the human body generally floats when totally immersed in water. The S_g of the human body is 0.97, which means that approximately 97% of the body surface is totally submerged in water and the remaining 3% is exposed to air.

D. VISCOSITY

The viscosity (designated by the Greek letter ν) of a fluid refers to the ease with which it flows (Low et al., 1994).

Viscosity is caused by the chemical binding forces holding the fluid molecules together, such as the forces binding hydrogen (H_2) to oxygen (O) molecules to form water (H_2O). The stronger these chemical binding forces are, the more viscous the substance is.

1. Temperature
Viscosity (v) is inversely influenced by temperature. The lower a fluid's temperature, the higher its viscosity will be (Low et al., 1994).

2. Coefficient of Viscosity (η)
The viscous state of a fluid is commonly represented by its coefficient of viscosity (designated by the Greek letter η [eta]) and is expressed in units of Pascal-second (Pa.s). The coefficient of viscosity of tap water at 20°C is 1.0×10^{-3} Pa.s

E. SPECIFIC HEAT

The specific heat (designated by the letter c) of a fluid or material refers to its capacity to hold (store) heat (Sekins et al., 1990). Heat is defined as the total kinetic energy, or molecular motion, of a substance. Readers may refer to Chapter 5, titled *Illustrated Glossary of Electrophysical Terminology*, for more details on the concepts of heat and specific heat.

1. Unit
Specific heat values may be expressed in different units. The values presented in this textbook are expressed in calories (cal) per gram (g) degree Celsius (cal/g°C).

2. Water Specific Heat Value
The specific heat value (c) of water is 1 cal/g°C because a heat input of 1 calorie is needed to increase the temperature of 1 g of pure water at 15°C by 1°C.

3. Comparative c Values
At any given temperature, water (c = 1.00) holds approximately 2 times more heat than paraffin oil (c = 0.45) and 4 times more than air (c = 0.24). In other words, a paraffin mixture contains approximately 50% less heat than water at the same temperature, which explains why humans can tolerate paraffin bath therapy at a much higher temperature than they can hydrotherapy (see comparative values in Table 5-3).

F. THERMAL CONDUCTIVITY

Thermal conductivity (designated by the letter k) refers to the rate at which a substance conducts heat (Sekins et al., 1990). The higher the thermal conductivity of a substance, the better this substance performs as a heat conductor. Readers may refer to Chapter 5 for more details on the concepts of thermal conductivity.

1. Unit
Thermal conductivity values (k) may be expressed in different units. The values presented in this textbook are expressed in calories (cal) per second centimeter degree Celsius (cal/sec-cm°C).

2. Water Thermal Conductivity Value
The thermal conductivity value of water at 15°C is 1.42 cal/sec-cm°C.

3. Comparative k Values
Water (k = 1.42) conducts heat approximately 70 times more rapidly than air (k = 0.02) and 2.5 times more rapidly than paraffin oil (k = 0.59). This explains why humans feel the heat contained in water much more rapidly than that in air or paraffin oil when all three elements are at the same temperature (see comparative values in Table 5-3).

4. Heat Conductor
The thermal conductivity of subcutaneous fat (k = 0.45) is approximately 50% that of the skin (k = 0.90) and approximately 30% that of skeletal muscle (k = 1.53). This makes subcutaneous fat a less effective heat conductor, or a better heat insulator, than skin and muscle. Thus, the thicker the layer of subcutaneous fat between skin and muscle, the lesser the amount of heat that can be conducted from the skin to the deeper tissues during thermotherapy.

G. HYDROSTATIC PRESSURE

Hydrostatic pressure (P) is the pressure exerted by water on a submerged object or body part (Kreighbaum et al., 1996). According to *Pascal's law*, hydrostatic pressure is applied from all directions on the surface of the immersed object or body part and varies directly in relation to the depth of immersion. In other words, this law stipulates that the deeper an object is immersed in water, the greater the water pressure exerted on it. Thus, the deeper the immersion, the greater the hydrostatic pressure exerted on the object or body part.

1. Formula and Units
Hydrostatic pressure (P) equals the amount of force (F) acting over a given area (A), or P = F/A. It is commonly expressed as Newton per square meter (N/m^2), pound per square inch (lb/in^2 or psi), or millimeter of mercury (mm Hg).

2. Magnitude of Hydrostatic Pressure
Figure 9-2 shows the magnitude of hydrostatic pressure exerted on a potential body part in relation to various water immersion depths. For example, an ankle joint immersed in water at a depth of 1.2 m (4 ft) theoretically experiences hydrostatic pressure of approximately 89.6 mm Hg (1.73 lb/in^2). To understand what these various pressures would feel like on the body, imagine how you feel when your

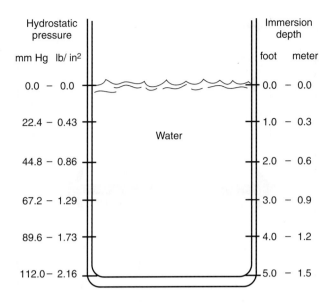

Hydrostatic pressure

mm Hg	lb/ in²
0.0	0.0
22.4	0.43
44.8	0.86
67.2	1.29
89.6	1.73
112.0	2.16

Water

Immersion depth

foot	meter
0.0	0.0
1.0	0.3
2.0	0.6
3.0	0.9
4.0	1.2
5.0	1.5

1 foot of water = 0.8826 inch of mercury (Hg) = 22.4 mm Hg

1 mm Hg = 0.0193 lb/ inch²; 1 psi = 51.8 mm Hg

FIGURE 9-2 Relationship between hydrostatic pressure and immersion depth.

arm is squeezed by the blood pressure cuff to have your diastolic and systolic blood pressure taken. Remember, as a reference point, that normal blood pressure values, are approximately 80 over 120 mm Hg.

H. BUOYANCY FORCE

Buoyancy is a fluid force, as illustrated in **Figure 9-3**, that always acts vertically upward (Hall, 2006). This force generated by water is based on *Archimedes' principle*, which states that an object or body part, totally or partially immersed in a fluid, experiences an upward, buoyant force equal to the weight of the volume of fluid displaced by that object or body part (Kreighbaum et al., 1996).

1. Buoyancy Calculation

Buoyancy force (B_f) is calculated as the product of the displaced volume (V_d) and the fluid's weight density (ρ_w), that is, $B_f = V_d \times \rho_w$ (Hall, 2006). For example, if a patient's upper limb has a volume of 0.3 L and that limb is completely submerged in water at 20°C, the buoyant force (B_f) acting on it is equal to 2.94 N (2.94 N = 0.3 L × 9.8 N/L).

2. Weightlessness

Buoyancy force is an antigravitational force and, as such, induces a state of relative body weightlessness. The percentage of the body immersed in water directly affects the magnitude of the buoyancy force that induces this relative weightlessness. This explains why a patient suffering from a hip disorder may experience hip pain while standing on land (no buoyancy force acting) but much less pain when standing in water with approximately 70% of his or her body submerged (with buoyancy force acting) in water during hydrotherapy.

3. Center of Buoyancy

Gravitational force (G_f) acts at the center of gravity (C_g), which is the center at which the object or body mass is concentrated (Kreighbaum et al., 1996; Hall et al., 1996). Buoyancy force (B_f), on the other hand, acts at the center of buoyancy (C_b). The center of buoyancy is the center of volume of the body displacing water, which is the point around which the body's volume is equally distributed (Hall, 2006).

4. Rotational Effect

In humans, the volume centers (C_b) of the body and of each of its segments are not located at the same place as their mass centers (C_g), because the density related to each body part varies from one part to the next (Kreighbaum et al., 1996). Because weight acts at the center of gravity and buoyancy acts at the center of volume, a rotational effect, or torque, is created that rotates the body until it is positioned so that these two acting forces are vertically aligned (Hall, 2006). For example, if the body is positioned in water such that both centers are not vertically aligned, the body will rotate until both centers become vertically aligned with each other, at which point the body resumes a balanced position at rest.

5. Vertical Alignment

Figure 9-3A shows, from left to right, the vertical alignment of the C_g with the C_b of an upper limb immersed in water as the limb is gradually pushed upward and rotated by the B_f until both centers coincide. If B_f equals G_f when both centers coincide, then this upper limb will reach a balanced position and float near the surface.

6. Assistive Versus Resistive Force

Figure 9-3B shows, from left to right, that the buoyancy force can be *assistive*, if acting in the same direction as the desired body movement, or *resistive*, if acting in the opposite direction from the desired movement.

I. DRAG FORCE

The force exerted by water on a submerged and moving object or body segment is defined as the drag force. Drag is the force parallel to the direction of motion, but in the opposite direction. Drag force resists the movement of an object or body part in water. There are three different drag forces: surface drag, profile drag, and wave drag (Kreighbaum et al., 1996; Hall, 2006). They act together to exert a total drag force on the moving object or body part. **Figure 9-4** illustrates these three drag forces acting together to resist the adduction movement of a lower limb, using as an example the sole of the foot of a patient floating supine near the surface of the water.

1. Surface Drag

Surface drag (S_d) force, also known as skin friction and viscous drag, is caused by friction between adjacent layers of water near the body part moving through water (Hall, 2006). One important factor that may increase

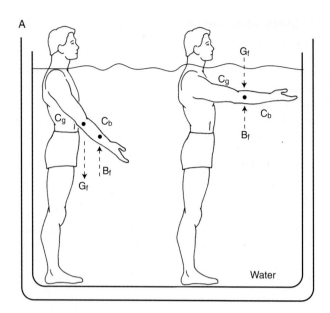

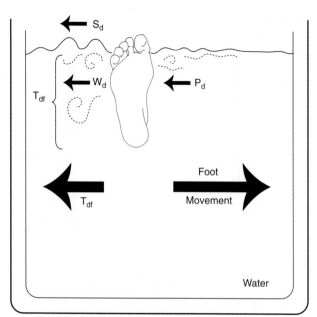

FIGURE 9-4 Surface drag (S_d), profile drag (P_d), and wave drag (W_d) force, which together form the total drag force (T_{df}) resisting the lower limb movement of a subject lying supine in the water. Shown is the front view of the lower limb (sole of the foot) performing an adduction movement near the surface of the water.

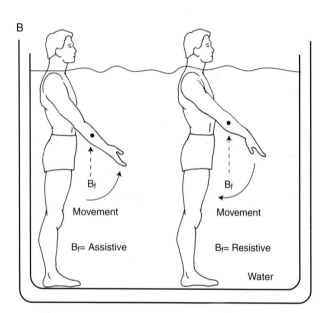

FIGURE 9-3 Buoyancy force (B_f) acting on its center of buoyancy (C_b) to lift or move upward the upper limb, which is itself pulled down by the gravitational force (G_f) acting on its center of gravity (C_g). **A:** When the two centers are vertically aligned with each other, and if B_f equals G_f, the upper limb will resume a stable resting position near the surface of the water. **B:** The buoyancy force may be resistive or assistive, depending on which direction the limb movement is taking place in the water.

or decrease this drag force is the relative degree of roughness of the moving body surface. The smoother the surface, the lesser the surface drag exerted on the moving body part.

2. Profile Drag

Profile drag (P_d) force, also known as form drag or pressure drag, is created by a pressure differential between the lead and rear sides of a body moving in water (Hall, 2006).

This force is the major contributor to overall drag during most human and projectile motion in water (Hall, 2006). Two important factors that may increase or decrease this force are the body part's relative velocity with respect to water and the amount of the body part's surface area that is aligned perpendicular to the flow (Hall, 2006). Doubling the velocity of movement in water will quadruple the magnitude of the profile drag force. Doubling the surface area of the moving object or body part will also quadruple the magnitude of the profile drag.

3. Wave Drag

Wave drag (W_d) force is created by the generation of waves at the interface between two different fluids, such as water and air (Hall, 2006). W_d increases with the proximity of the moving body part from the water surface and with the velocity of that moving body part. Thus, the closer the body part from the surface of the water, and the faster the displacement of this body part in water, the greater the wave drag force exerted on that body part.

4. Total Drag Force

As shown in **Figure 9-4**, the total drag force (T_{df}) opposing the lower limb movement results from the grouped drag action exerted by the surface (S_d), profile (P_d), and wave (W_d) drag forces, where $T_{df} = S_d + P_d + W_d$.

J. ENERGY TRANSFER MODE

Thermal energy transfer between water and skin is achieved through conduction and convection (see Chapter 5). Thermal transfer by convection far exceeds that achieved by conduction, because in most hydrotherapeutic applications, water always circulates around the treated body area as a result of passive and/or active movements and the use of electric turbines.

1. Immersion in Still Water: Conduction

A thin layer of insulation around and next to the skin, called *thermopane*, is formed when the immersed body part and the water stay still during treatment (Bell et al., 1998). In such cases, thermal energy transfer happens by conduction only.

2. Immersion in Turbulent Water: Convection

The thermopane is lost when body movement, use of electric turbines, or both create water agitation or turbulence around the immersed body part. In such cases, the thermal energy transfer occurs primarily by convection.

K. CONTROL OVER WATER PROPERTIES

Practitioners have *no control* over the density, specific gravity, specific heat, and thermal conductivity of tap water used to deliver bath/tub/tank hydrotherapy. They have, however, *some control* over the following properties of water. Viscosity can be increased or decreased by varying water temperature. Hydrostatic pressure can be increased or decreased by varying the depth of immersion. Buoyancy force can be increased or decreased by varying the percentage of body immersion. Finally, total drag force can be increased or decreased by varying body movement velocity and body surface area or by the usage of an electrical turbine. The setting of these water properties will establish the dosimetry that will be delivered to the patient in order to achieve the therapeutic goals.

IV. PHYSIOLOGICAL AND THERAPEUTIC EFFECTS

A. THERMOMECHANICAL, CLEANSING, AND DEBRIDEMENT EFFECTS

Figure 9-5 summarizes the proposed physiological and therapeutic effects associated with the practice of bath,

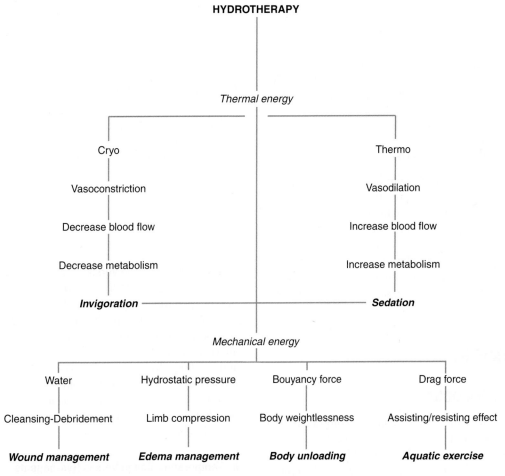

FIGURE 9-5 Proposed physiological and therapeutic effects of hydrotherapy.

tub, and tank hydrotherapy, which are thermomechanical, cleansing, and debridement in nature.

B. CLEANSING AND DEBRIDEMENT EFFECTS

Still and turbulent water, when in contact with a wound surface, have a cleansing effect on it by removing unwanted substances, such as dirt and residual therapeutic cream, which may delay or prevent healing. Turbulent water, created by the use of manual irrigators or electrical turbines, has also a debridement effect on an open wound. Debridement is the excision or removal of contused or devitalized tissues (debris) from a wound surface. To sum up, hydrotherapy has a cleansing effect on normal, closed, and open wounds, as well as a debridement effect (when turbulent water is used) on an open wound (**Fig 9-5**). These two effects are beneficial to the management of open wounds.

C. THERMAL EFFECTS

The cooling or heating effects induced by hydrotherapy may have a sedative (warm water: thermo-hydrotherapy) or invigorating (cold water: cryo-hydrotherapy) effect on patients, depending on the water temperature used (**Fig 9-5**). These thermal effects are similar to, *but much less pronounced than*, those induced by dedicated thermo- (see Chapter 6) and cryoagents (see Chapter 8)) covered in this textbook. This is because lower agent–skin temperature differentials (T°_{ag-s}) are used in hydrotherapy, especially when a significant percentage of the body is immersed in water.

D. MECHANICAL EFFECTS

The mechanical effects of hydrotherapy manifest themselves by exerting hydrostatic pressure, buoyancy, and drag forces on the immersed body part. Hydrostatic pressure (Pascal's law) may be used for the management of edema. Buoyancy force (Archimede's principle) may be beneficial for body unloading in cases of difficult and painful weight bearing. Finally, drag forces (surface, profile, and wave) may be called upon to either assist or resist tub- and tank-water-based therapeutic exercises.

V. DOSIMETRY

A. CLEANSING DOSAGE

There is a consensus in the field of hydrotherapy that tap water used to cleanse wounds should be employed alone, without any other additives. If additive solutions or products are used (e.g., therapeutic soap, antimicrobial, or antibacterial solutions), careful monitoring of the concentrations of such agents is recommended in order to prevent any cytotoxic reaction.

B. DEBRIDEMENT DOSAGE

Open wounds, in their inflammatory phase of healing, need debridement in order to facilitate healing. Wound debridement can be done *on land* with tweezers and scalpels or water-pressured irrigation systems or *under water*, also with tweezers and scalpels, and electric turbines.

1. Water-Pressured Irrigation System
Practitioners should use only certified systems, able to deliver water pressure doses within the recommended pressure range (207 to 777 mm Hg—4 to 15 psi).

2. Electrical Turbine
The turbine rate of airflow set within the water will determine the water turbulence dose needed over and around the open wound to cause debridement. The practitioner should remember that electricity and water do not mix well together and make sure to always plug the line-activated electrical turbine into a ground fault circuit interrupter (GFCI) receptacle to avoid electrical macroshock or any risk of electrocution (see Chapter 27).

C. THERMAL DOSAGE

Three parameters must be considered in order to set the thermal dose needed: water temperature, body immersion level, and immersion duration.

1. Water Temperature
Water temperature is critical in hydrotherapy because it determines the types of treatment (i.e., cryo-, neutro-, or thermo-hydrotherapy) used. Choice of water temperature determines the thermal potential of the hydrotherapeutic application; that is, the greater the temperature differential between the agent and the skin (T°_{ag-s}), whether it is below (cryo-) or above (thermo-) normal or neutral skin temperature, the more severe the thermal dose received.

a. Temperature Range Versus Types of Hydrotherapy
Shown in **Figure 9-6** is a thermal scale indicating the temperature ranges normally associated with each type of hydrotherapy. In this textbook, the neutral range falls between 32°C and 34°C (90°F–93°F). Temperatures above and below this neutral range will cause heating and cooling effects on soft tissues. Water temperature level is described, from the coldest to the hottest level, as *very cold, cold, cool, tepid, neutral, warm, hot, and very hot*. A temperature range is presented for each of these levels.

b. Temperature Range Versus Hydroagents
Figure 9-7 shows a thermal scale indicating the ranges of temperature normally associated with the use of baths, tubs, and tanks. Contrast baths may be used at extreme

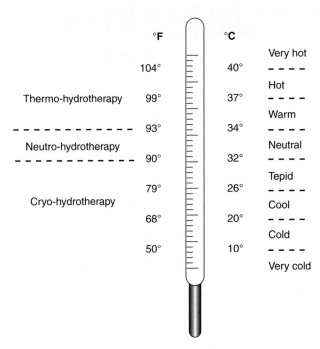

FIGURE 9-6 Thermal scale showing the ranges of temperature associated with the use of cryo-, thermo-, and neutro-hydrotherapeutic agents. Water temperature ranges from very cold to very hot.

temperature ranges (over 40°C [104°F], very hot water, and below 20°C [68°F], very cold water). Such extreme water temperatures can be sustained by patients because the immersion is cyclic, its duration is short (only a few minutes) in each bath, and the body immersion level (see below) is low (only a small percentage of body surface—hands and feet). Tubs (whirlpools), for the immersion of

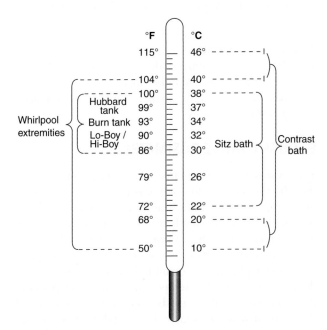

FIGURE 9-7 Thermal scale showing the ranges of temperature normally associated with the use of hydro agents.

the upper or lower extremities (wrist/hands, ankle/feet), may be filled with water at a temperature within the range of 10–40°C (50–104°F). Water temperature in sitz bath (perineal and genital area) is usually within the range of 22–38°C (72–100°F). Finally, water temperatures usually associated with the use of larger tubs (Lo- and Hi-Boy), burn tanks, and Hubbard tanks fall within the narrowest range immediately above and below the neutral range (30–38°C [86–100°F]). This narrower temperature range is due to the fact that body immersion levels are the highest with the use of tanks. The larger the percentage of body immersion, the closer the water temperature range should be to the neutral range. Water temperatures outside these ranges increase the risk of the patient's intolerance to treatment, as well as the severity of systemic effects (see below).

2. Body Immersion Level

The level of body immersion, whether it is partial or full, is also important to dosimetry because it determines whether the thermal effects are local (restricted primarily to the treated area) or systemic (spread to the entire body) in nature.

a. Partial Versus Full Body Immersion

There are two levels of immersion practitioners can choose from: partial-body and full-body immersion. *Partial-body immersion* refers to the immersion of one or more body parts. *Full-body immersion*, on the other hand, refers to the immersion of the entire body, that is, from the neck down.

b. Local Versus Systemic Effects

The larger the temperature differential between water (ag) and the exposed skin ($T°_{ag-s}$), and the greater the level or percentage of body immersion in water, the greater the chance to induce systemic thermal reaction during hydrotherapy. Summarized in **Table 9-2** are some potential systemic reactions that may occur if thermo- or cryo-hydrotherapy is delivered using a high $T°_{ag-s}$, combined with full-body immersion. The practitioner should note that the sedative (thermo) and invigorating (cryo) effects attributed to hydrotherapy (see **Fig 9-5**) are caused by the induction of those systemic reactions.

3. Immersion Duration

Generally speaking, the longer the immersion period or duration, given a similar water temperature, the greater the desired local or systemic effects on the patient will be. Immersion durations may vary from 10 to 45 minutes, depending on the treated condition and the patient's overall health status.

D. MECHANICAL DOSAGE

Hydrotherapy can induce three mechanical effects on the immersed body part: hydrostatic pressure, buoyancy force, and drag forces.

TABLE 9-2	SYSTEMIC PHYSIOLOGIC EFFECTS OF HYDROTHERAPY[a]	
CRYO-HYDROTHERAPY	**NEUTRO-HYDROTHERAPY**	**THERMO-HYDROTHERAPY**
Decreases core temperature	Resting core temperature	Increases core temperature
Decreases pulse rate	Resting pulse rate	Increases pulse rate
Increases blood pressure	Resting blood pressure	Decreases blood pressure
Decreases respiratory rate	Resting respiration rate	Increases respiratory rate
Increase muscle tone	Resting muscle tone	Decreases muscle tone
Invigorating/stimulating effect	Neutral effect	Relaxing/sedative effect
Induces shivering response	Basal response	Induces sweating response

[a]The magnitude of these physiological effects vary relative to the patient's physical health status, the temperature gradient between the agent and the treated body part, the percentage or level of body immersion, and the total immersion duration.

1. Hydrostatic Pressure

The magnitude of this pressure (P) is set, as illustrated in **Figure 9-2**, by the depth at which the affected body part is immersed (see Pascal's law above). The deeper the immersion, the greater the compressive effect caused by the hydrostatic pressure exerted on the immersed body part.

2. Buoyancy Force

The magnitude of this force (B_f) is set, as illustrated in **Figure 9-3**, by the level or percentage (%) of body immersion in water. For example, a patient standing still and upright in a pool will experience a much greater buoyancy force (effect of weightlessness) if his or her body is immersed fully, as opposed to partially. This is explained by Archimedes's principle, which states that the larger the weight of the volume of water displaced by the immersed body, the larger the buoyancy force acting on this body.

3. Drag Forces

The magnitude of each of the three drag forces (surface, profile, and wave) on the immersed body part, as illustrated in **Figure 9-4**, depends on the following elements.

a. Surface Roughness

The magnitude of the surface drag force (S_d) can be increased by augmenting the roughness of the immersed body part. This can be done by dressing (shirt, pants) the immersed body part. In other words, the smoother the immersed body part (bare skin), the smaller the surface drag force acting on it.

b. Displacement Velocity and Body Part Surface Area

The magnitude of the profile drag force (P_d) can be increased by (1) augmenting the body part's relative displacement velocity with respect to water and (2) enlarging the body part's surface area that is aligned perpendicular to the flow (Hall, 2006). The patient is asked to move his immersed limb faster to augment the displacement velocity. Floats are attached to the extremities of the immersed moving body part to increase the body surface area. Recall that when either the velocity of movement in water or the surface area of the moving body part is *doubled*, the magnitude of the profile drag force is *quadrupled*.

c. Proximity to Water Surface

The magnitude of wave drag force (W_d) can be increased by positioning the immersed limb close to the surface of water while causing waves. The closer the immersed body part to the water surface, the greater the wave drag force acting on it.

d. Combined Elements

The effects of the elements described above on each of the three drag forces will either increase or decrease the total drag force (T_{df}) acting on the immersed and displaced body part during therapy.

E. QUANTITATIVE DOSIMETRY

The evidence-based practice of hydrotherapy requires that the therapeutic dose administered to a patient during therapy be *quantitatively* assessed. To *qualitatively* assess dosage level by simply asking the patient about his or her perception of heat during treatment, as done routinely in today's practice, is not enough. A simple, practical, and rapid way of quantitatively assessing thermal dosage is to measure two temperature differentials, namely, the temperature difference between the agent (ag) and the exposed skin (s) surface ($T°_{ag-s}$) and the temperature differential between the exposed skin surface before (b) and after (a) treatment ($T°_{b-a}$). Chapter 26 shows the practitioner how to take these two measurements using a portable infrared surface thermometer.

1. Case Example

The water temperature inside a Lo-Boy tub is measured (read from the tub thermometer) at 37°C (99°F) and the exposed skin surface at 30°C (86°F), with an infrared portable thermometer. The thermal dose delivered ($T°_{ag-s}$) equals 7°C (13°F), which represents its *potential* heating effect. Immediately after treatment, the exposed skin temperature is measured at 34°C (93°F); the *actual* skin heating effect ($T°_{b-a}$) of this dosage was +4°C (+7°F).

2. Recap

In the context of evidence-based practice, it is good sense to ask the patient how warm the thermal agent feels during and after the treatment, but it is even better to supplement this qualitative information with actual temperature measurements, as shown above. This textbook strongly encourages practitioners to supplement their qualitative approach with the suggested quantitative approach. It is easy and practical, and not time-consuming, to take these temperature measurements, using an infrared portable thermometer.

VI. EVIDENCE FOR INDICATIONS

A. GUIDED BY EVIDENCE

Dictionaries generally define *evidence* as anything that establishes a fact or gives reason to believe something.

The aim of this textbook is to present scientific evidence for the use of therapeutic EPAs. To be guided by evidence is the process of integrating the evidence from research, however imperfect or scarce this evidence may be, with clinical experience and patients' values. In other words, the *evidence-based practice* of EPA requires practitioners to consider the evidence from research, in addition to their own clinical experience and the patient's own preference and beliefs, when the time comes to justify, prescribe, and apply the therapeutic agent. To be guided by the evidence is a process, not a search for the absolute truth. Finally, a lack of evidence from research behind any given EPA does not mean that this EPA should never be used. What it means is that no statement can be made on its therapeutic effectiveness and that until more evidence from research is presented, its routine use cannot be recommended.

B. EVIDENCE FROM HUMAN RESEARCH

Box 9-1 provides evidence for bath, tub, and tank hydrotherapy based on an exhaustive search of published English-language, peer-reviewed literature on human research. The term *indication* in the title refers to the list of pathologies for which hydrotherapy is used. Ratings of therapeutic benefit (Yes or No) and grading of strength of scientific evidence (I, II, or III), including the reference, are included for each pathological condition.

1. Rating Therapeutic Benefit

The rating, expressed as Yes or No, is based on the overall conclusion(s) reached on the issue of therapeutic

Box 9-1	Research-Based Indications for the Use of Hydrotherapy

PATHOLOGY	BENEFIT	GRADE	REFERENCE
Rheumatoid arthritis	Yes	II	Ahern et al., 1995
	Yes	II	Hall et al., 1996
	Yes	II	Curkovic et al., 1993
	No	II	Fricke et al., 1952
Delayed-onset muscle soreness	Yes	I	Kuligowski et al., 1998
	Yes	I	Vaile et al., 2007b
	Yes	I	Eston et al., 1999
	Yes	II	Vaile et al., 2007a
Osteoarthritis of the hip	Yes	II	Sylvester, 1990
	No	II	Green et al., 1993
	Yes	II	Sterner-Victorin et al., 2004
Labor pain	Yes	I	Rush et al., 1996
	No	I	Cammu et al., 1994

(Continued)

Box 9-1 **Continued**

PATHOLOGY	BENEFIT	GRADE	REFERENCE
Multiple sclerosis	Yes	II	Boynton et al., 1959
	No	II	Chiara et al., 1988
Ankle sprain	Yes	II	Cote et al., 1988
Atopic dermatitis causing itch	Yes	II	Frushtorfer et al., 1986
Clonus	Yes	II	Miglietta, 1964
Soft-tissue wounds complicated by fractures	Yes	II	Abraham et al., 1974
Open wound	Yes	III	Gogia et al., 1988
Postoperative abdominal pain (surgical wound healing)	Yes	II	Juve Meeker, 1998
Osteoarthritis of the knee	Yes	II	Silva et al., 2007
Postoperative knee pain	Yes	II	Barber, 2000
Traumatic hand injury	Yes	II	Hoyrup et al., 1986
Grades III and IV pressure ulcers	Yes	II	Burke et al., 1998
Varicose veins	Yes	I	Ernst et al., 1990, 1992
Anal pain	Yes	I	Dodi et al., 1986
Post-anal sphincterotomy	No	II	Gupta, 2007
Acute anal fissures	No	I	Gupta, 2006
Postpartum perineal pain	Yes	II	Ramler et al., 1986
Postpartum hemorrhoids	No	I	Thomas et al., 1993
Post-episiotomy laceration	No	II	Hill, 1989
Perineal pain	Yes	II	Droegemeuller, 1980
Colles' fracture	No	II	Toomey et al., 1986b
Stings from Bluebottle jellyfish	Yes	II	Loten et al., 2006
Exercise induced hyperthermia	Yes	II	Clements et al., 2002
Anal sphincter relaxation	No	II	Pinho et al., 1993
Hamstring lengthening	No	II	Burke et al., 2001
Type II diabetes	No	I	Petrofsky et al., 2007

effectiveness by the author(s) who conducted the peer-reviewed study.

2. Grading Strength of Evidence

The grading, numerically classified as I, II, and III, is based on the type of research methodology, or research-design used by the author(s). All the studies listed are human studies published in English-language, peer-reviewed journals. It follows that the strength of evidence in studies graded I is stronger than that in those graded II, which itself is stronger than in those graded III.

a. Grade I

Evidence based on human *controlled* studies, regardless of their level of randomization and blindness.

b. Grade II

Evidence based on human *noncontrolled* studies, regardless of their level of randomization and blindness.

c. Grade III

Evidence based on human *case* studies, regardless of their level of randomization and blindness.

3. Strength of Evidence Behind the Agent

The strength of evidence in favor of the agent, as presented in the research-based indication box, is arbitrarily assessed in this textbook as being *weak*, *moderate*, or *strong*. For example, the larger the number of studies graded I, regardless of therapeutic benefit, the stronger the scientific evidence behind the agent.

4. Strength for Justification of Usage of the Agent

The strength of evidence justifying usage of the agent for individual pathologies or groups of pathologies, as listed in the research-based indication box, is arbitrarily assessed in this textbook as being *poor*, *fair*, *good*, or *conflicting*. For example, when a larger number of studies on an agent show therapeutic benefit (Yes) and are graded I, for any given pathology, the justification for usage of this agent for this pathology is assessed as good. A *conflicting justification* is reported when a similar number of studies, with similar grades, show both therapeutic benefit (Yes) and no benefit (No).

C. STRENGTH OF EVIDENCE AND JUSTIFICATION FOR USAGE OF HYDROTHERAPY

The results gathered in **Box 9-1** show *moderate* strength of evidence behind the use of hydrotherapy, with the majority of studies graded as II. These results also show that the body of research on the effectiveness of hydrotherapy has been concentrated on the management of three conditions: rheumatoid arthritis, osteoarthritis, and delayed-onset muscle soreness. Together these results show that justification for usage is *fair to good* for delayed-onset muscle soreness, and *poor to fair* for rheumatoid arthritis and osteoarthritis. Interestingly, no studies could be found on the use of hydrotherapy for open wounds despite the fact that this EPA has been used for decades in rehabilitation centers and burn units around the world. The justification for the usage of hydrotherapy for the remaining pathologies listed in **Box 9-1** is found to be *weak*. Until more evidence from research is provided with regard to those remaining pathologies, or any other pathology, the routine use of hydrotherapy for such pathologies *cannot be recommended*.

VII. CONTRAINDICATIONS

Table 9-3 lists the contraindications for hydrotherapy. Skin status, incontinence, allergy, pregnancy, and overall health status are key elements to be considered among the contraindications for bath, tub, and tank hydrotherapy.

TABLE 9-3	CONTRAINDICATIONS TO HYDROTHERAPY
CONTRAINDICATIONS	**RATIONALE**
Over skin areas where cold/hot sensation discrimination is severely impaired	Risk of thermal skin damage.
Over macerated tissues surrounding a wound	Risk of further tissue maceration with prolonged and repeated immersion.
Over a bleeding surface area	Risk of increased bleeding with prolonged and repeated immersion.
Patients who have fecal and/or urinary incontinence	Risk of auto- and cross-contamination with partial- to full-body immersion.
Patients with fever	Risk of increased core temperature, with thermo-hydrotherapy.
Multiple sclerosis patients	Risk of increasing fatigue and muscle weakness, with thermo-hydrotherapy.

(Continued)

TABLE 9-3	CONTINUED

CONTRAINDICATIONS	RATIONALE
Patients who are allergic to additive solutions	Risk of inducing unnecessary skin and/or systemic reactions. Carefully monitor the patient's overall response during the first treatment session.
Women in the first trimester of pregnancy	Risk of fetal teratogenic effects, with thermo-hydrotherapeutic agents capable of increasing the basal temperature of a pregnant woman above 39°C (102.6°F) (Sedgwick Harvey et al., 1981). Healthy, *nonpregnant* women can remain in a thermal tub at 39°C (102°F) for at least 15 min and at 41°C (106°F) for at least 10 min without risk of reaching a core temperature of 39°C (102°F) or above (Sedgwick Harvey et al., 1981).
Patients suffering from severe cardiac and/or respiratory disorders	Risk of unduly stressing and overloading the diseased heart-lung system and organs if partial- to full-body immersion is used. Patients will not be able to adapt to the induced systemic effects caused by thermo- and/or cryo-hydrotherapy. There is no justification for refusing hydrotherapy to ankylosing spondylitis patients with vital lung capacity less than 1,500 cc (Harrison, 1981).
Confused and unreliable patients	Risk of complications during therapy, such as accidental drowning if full-body immersion is used.

VIII. RISKS, PRECAUTIONS, AND RECOMMENDATIONS

The practice of hydrotherapy is not without risks for both patients and practitioners. The main risks associated with this EPA, as well as some precautions and recommendations designed to improve safety and effectiveness, are listed in **Table 9-4**. Issues related to electrical safety (when turbines are used) and auto- and cross-contamination with bacteria are key elements to be considered by practitioners when using hydrotherapy.

IX. CONSIDERATIONS FOR APPLICATION AND DOCUMENTATION

A. BASIC CONSIDERATIONS

The safe and effective practice of hydrotherapy requires that consideration be given to the following parameters: water temperature setting, patient's skin and health status, selection of equipment and accessories, and application methods.

1. Water Temperature Setting

This parameter is critical in the practice of hydrotherapy. Shown in **Figures 9-6** and **9-7** are *recommendations* with regard to the ranges of temperature practitioners can use to deliver hydrotherapy, using different hydroagents. These temperature ranges suggest that the greater the percentage of body immersion in water, the smaller the temperature range fluctuates above and below the neutral temperature range. Before initiating hydrotherapy, practi-

tioners must consider the possible systemic body effects that both cryo- and thermo-agents can induce in patients, especially if both the percentage of body immersion is high and water temperatures are set further away from the neutral range. **Table 9-2** lists systemic body reactions commonly induced in humans under cryo-, neutral-, and thermo-hydrotherapy conditions. It is strongly recommended that practitioners record the *patient's vital signs* before, during, and after such hydrotherapeutic immersions in order to prevent, monitor, or detect these systemic body reactions.

2. Skin and Health Status Assessment

The patient's skin status is crucial in hydrotherapy because it affects many other aspects of therapy. For example, immersing an open and infected wound in water clearly has greater practical (cleaning and disinfection of equipment and accessories) and clinical (auto- and cross-contamination) consequences than immersing intact skin. This assessment is also important because it determines the patient's overall risk (i.e., unwanted systemic reactions—see **Table 9-2**) in receiving hydrotherapy. For example, a patient with poor-to-fair physical and/or mental health requires much more body monitoring and visual surveillance from the clinician during therapy than a patient in good-to-excellent mental and physical health.

3. Selection of Equipment and Accessories

Hydrotherapy is delivered using tap water, with or without additives, and also using a variety of baths, tubs, tanks, and accessories. The most common equipment and accessories used to deliver bath, tub, and tank hydrotherapy are described in **Box 9-2**. The selection is guided

TABLE 9-4	RISKS, PRECAUTIONS, AND RECOMMENDATIONS FOR HYDROTHERAPY

RISKS	RATIONALE
Macroshock and electrocution	Risk of severe tissue burns and possible death by electrocution, for both patients and practitioners, when electrical-line-powered devices and accessories are used because wet skin offers less impedance to current flow. Failure to plug line-powered equipment into GFCI receptacles also increase this risk.
Falling	Risk for patients and practitioners of falling while walking on slippery floors in hydrotherapy rooms.
Fainting and drowning	Risk for patients of fainting during full-body immersion in warm to hot water, leading to the risk of drowning
Pathogen transmission and contamination	Risk of pathogenic transmission and contamination caused by the proliferation of microbes, such as *Pseudomonas aeruginosa, Staphylococcus aureus,* and *Candida* on the surfaces of hydrotherapy baths, tubs, and tanks, and accessories (McManus et al., 1985; Taddonio et al., 1990; Tredget et al., 1992; Richard et al., 1994; Shandowsky et al., 1994; Hollyoak et al., 1995a, 1995b). These microbes often originate from open wounds, skin surfaces, and fecal flora, and tend to proliferate in warm, moist environments outside the host. Contamination of water, equipment, and accessories can lead to minor skin irritation (folliculitis) and sometimes to local or systemic infection (Berger et al., 1990; McGuckin et al., 1981).

PRECAUTIONS	RATIONALE
Body systemic reactions	Adequate monitoring of vital signs, including heart rate, blood pressure, ventilation rate, and mouth body temperature, should be conducted when systemic reactions are anticipated after cryo-/thermo-hydrotherapy using both partial- and full-body immersion.
Fear of water	Gradually increasing the percentage of the body immersed from one treatment session to the next should allow most patients to gain adequate control over their fear of water.
Patients with cervical cord injuries and cryo-hydrotherapy	These patients cannot adapt to cold stress as much as healthy subjects; this adaptive response appears to decrease with time (Claus-Walker et al., 1974).
Burn patients and adding salt to water	Severe hyponatremia (i.e., low concentration of sodium in the blood) can be prevented if a proper amount of salt is added to the tap water before treatment (Said et al., 1987). Consult the treating dermatologist if needed.
Patients with postmyocardial infarction and a work capacity of ≈4.0 METs	Resume bathing in cold and warm water only after careful consideration (Kawamura et al., 1997). Consult the treating cardiologist if needed.
Usage of silver-copper disinfectant system	Effective in purifying water, the silver-copper disinfectant system has been shown to corrode stainless-steel pipes. The corroded steel has a black deposit that readily adheres to the burned patient's skin (Nguyen et al., 1995). Use caution with such water disinfectant systems.

(Continued)

TABLE 9-4	CONTINUED

RECOMMENDATIONS	RATIONALE
Disrobe the treated body areas and remove all objects, such as jewelry	Maximize heat transfer and avoid cutaneous burn due to heating of metal objects.
Inspect the exposed skin area before each treatment	Assure close monitoring of potential side effects, such as skin irritation and burn caused by the agent.
Conduct skin thermal sensory discrimination testing—**mandatory**	Minimize risk of cutaneous burn (see Chapter 25 for details).
Wash and dry treated body areas before therapy (pb)	Minimize the risk of contaminating water and optimize heat transfer.
Check on patient regularly during therapy	Prevent complications and assure maximum safety during therapy.
Plug all line-powered devices and accessories into GFCI receptacles—**mandatory**	Prevent macroshock and electrocution (see Chapter 27).
Conduct regular visual inspection of electrical cables, plugs, and chassis	Prevent macroshock and electrocution (see Chapter 27).
Wipe floors regularly and install anti-slippery mats in strategic areas	Prevent from slipping and falling.
Keep patients alert during treatment and keep constant visual monitoring of patients during full-body immersion	Prevent from fainting and drowning.
Apply a regular and rigorous regimen of cleansing, rinsing, and disinfecting procedures after usage, and conduct routine culture tests on all equipment and accessories used for therapy	Prevent pathogenic contamination and transmission.
Cardiopulmonary resuscitation (CPR) certification for all staff working in hydrotherapy	Minimize the risk associated with electrocution and drowning by allowing for quick CPR maneuvers on the victim.
Always use protective equipment, i.e., gown, gloves, mask, and goggles	Minimize the risk of infection when treating cases of open wounds (infected or not) with turbulent water induced by turbines or water irrigation devices. Risk stems primarily from inhalation/contact with water-borne bacteria, aerosolized mist, and blood-borne pathogens (Cameron, 2003).
Regulate hydrotherapy room temperature, ventilation, and humidity	Eliminate any aerosol, mist, or vapor from turbulent water and their additives. A room temperature of 25–30°C (77–86°F), with a relative humidity of 50%, is recommended for most hydrotherapeutic applications (Atkinson et al., 1981).
Use cartoon viewings with burn children	Can substantially decrease children's pain and fear during therapy (Kelly et al., 1984).
Use toe/finger neoprene caps with severe cryo-hydrotherapy	Reduce cold-induced pain associated with the immersion in cold to very cold water (Nimchick et al., 1983; Misasi et al., 1995).
Assess muscle force *before* hydrotherapy	Body immersion in either cold or hot water alters the intrinsic muscle force capacity for up to 3 hr after therapy (Cornwall, 1994).

(Continued)

TABLE 9-4	CONTINUED

RECOMMENDATIONS	RATIONALE
Inform patients fully about sensations felt during cryotherapy	Decreases the perceived pain associated with cryo-immersion in healthy subjects (Misasi et al., 1995; Streator et al., 1995).
Avoid positioning the treated body part in the dependent position (parallel to the line of gravity)	Minimize limb volume increase during therapy (Magness et al., 1970; McCulloch et al., 1992). No significant difference in limb volume has been observed between the relaxed versus actively mobilized limb during therapy (Hoyrup et al., 1986).
Set the water irrigation device at pressures in the range of 207–777 mm Hg or 4–15 psi	This pressure range is safe and effective in removing bacteria from wounds (Agency for Health Care Policy and Research, 1994; Luedtke-Hoffmann et al., 2000).
Monitor water additive concentration	Use of clean tap water, without any antimicrobial agent, is recommended (Cameron, 2003). If additives are used, such as antimicrobial or antiseptic agents, their concentration (ppm) in water must be carefully monitored and adjusted to prevent cytotoxic reactions that may alter wound healing (Cameron, 2003). Refer to the manufacturer's recommendations when using therapeutic additive solutions, and never hesitate to ask the opinion of a pharmacist.
Orient turbine jets away from newly grafted tissues and use neutral water temperature	Newly grafted tissue may not tolerate the turbulent action as well as the high thermal effect of water. Orient the turbine jets away from the graft tissue, and use a neutral (32–34°C [90–93°F]) to warm (35–37°C [94–99°F]) water temperature (Cameron, 2003).
Measure temperature differential between the agent and the skin ($T°_{ag-s}$) before treatment—**mandatory**	The taking of this measurement is a must in the context of evidence-based practice because it provides quantitative assessment of the thermal dose delivered to the soft tissues (see Chapter 26).
Measure skin temperature differential before and after treatment ($T°_{b-a}$) treatment—**mandatory**	The taking of this measurement is a must in the context of evidence-based practice because it reveals the extent of soft-tissue heating caused by the thermal agent at the end of treatment (see Chapter 26).
Conduct regular maintenance and calibration procedures	Ensure optimal therapeutic efficacy and effectiveness. Follow the recommended maintenance schedules outlined by manufacturers.
Implement a risk management program and litigation	To prepare for and minimize the risk of litigation, clinicians who administer hydrotherapy should have in place both a comprehensive risk-management program and an emergency action plan in case of accidents such as drowning and electrocution (Clement, 1997).

primarily by the body part(s) under treatment, which may require partial- or full-body immersion as well as nonimmersion.

4. Application Methods

Hydrotherapy is delivered using nonimmersion and immersion methods. **Box 9-3** describes the most common application methods.

5. Contrast Immersion

This method has traditionally been used to enhance peripheral blood flow (Cochrane, 2004). The first published

article on the physiological effects of contrast immersion appears to be that of Woodmansey et al. (1938), who observed alterations in blood flow through recording surface skin temperatures in healthy subjects versus rheumatic patients after various periods of immersion in cold versus hot water. Because blood vessels dilate in hot water and constrict in cold water, and considering the results of Woodmansey et al. (1938), the contrast immersion method was seen by many practitioners as a means of passive vascular exercise similar to the active vascular exercise induced by voluntary contraction. In other words, it was believed that this passive method triggered a *peripheral and deep vascular pumping*

Box 9-2   Common Hydrotherapy Equipment and Accessories

Baths

Common Bath

Commercial plastic container used primarily to bathe the extremities, that is, ankle/foot and wrist/hand.

Contrast Bath

Commercial dual plastic container, filled with cold water on one side and warm water on the other, is known as a contrast bath. Two individual common baths are often used as a substitute for the dual plastic container. This type of bath is also used to bathe the extremities.

Sitz Bath

Commercially designed plastic or stainless steel bath, used to bathe the hip and buttock areas. The word *sitz* comes from the German verb *sitzen*, meaning to sit. Shown in **Figure 9-1A** is a plastic sitz bath fitted with a gravity water irrigation system.

Tubs

Extremity Tub

Commercially designed stainless steel tub fitted with a drain valve, a thermometer, and an electric turbine (see **Fig 9-1B**). The turbine can be adjusted to the desired pressure, height, and direction in relation to the treated body part. A tub of this type, commercially and clinically known as an *extremity tub*, is used to bathe the extremities, including the elbows and knees.

Partial-Body Tub

Commercially designed stainless steel tub fitted with a drain valve, a thermometer, and an electric turbine. The turbine can be adjusted to the desired pressure, height, and direction, in relation to the treated body part. Tubs of this type, commercially and clinically known as *high-boy* (Hi-Boy) and *low-boy* (Lo-Boy) tubs, are used for partial-body immersion (see **Fig 9-1C** and **D**). The term *whirlpool* is also frequently used in clinical settings to designate such tubs.

Full-Body Tank

Commercially designed stainless steel tanks fitted with a drain valve, a thermometer, and one or more electric turbines. These turbines can be adjusted to the desired pressure, height, and direction, in relation to the treated body part. These tanks, commercially and clinically known as burn (**Fig 9-1E**) and Hubbard (**Fig 9-1F**), are larger in size and volume than the partial-body immersion Hi-Boy and Lo-Boy tubs, and are used for full-body immersion.

Irrigation System

Pressured Water Irrigation System

Commercial system used for pressured water irrigation, or lavage, of wounds. Used when it is impossible, or not required, to immerse the body part treated. The irrigation pressure delivered by the device should range between 4 and 15 pounds per square inch (psi) because pressures below 4 psi (207 mm Hg) may not cleanse the wound adequately, and pressures greater than 15 psi (777 mm Hg) may cause trauma and drive bacteria in the wound tissue (Agency for Health Care Policy and Research, 1994; Luedtke-Hoffmann et al., 2000). Shown in **Figure 9-1G** is a single-patient, reusable manual irrigation system, which meets the AHCPR pressure recommendations.

Patient-handling System

Manually operated hydraulic commercial system, used to safely and comfortably transfer patients to partial-body immersion tubs and full-body immersion tanks. The handling system may be fitted with a chair (**Fig 9-1H**) or a stretcher if the patient needs to lie down during treatment. (**Fig 9-1I**)

Water Additives

Commercial solutions, added to tap water, with one or several of the following properties: bactericidal, fungicidal, virucidal, odoricidal, and antifoam. The purposes of these additives are to enhance wound healing and facilitate treatment application. The concentrations of these various additives in water must be carefully graded and monitored for each patient to prevent cytotoxic reactions.

---

action similar to that documented experimentally during voluntary muscle contractions. It follows that for those patients who have difficulty with voluntary joint movement because of pain or trauma, the use of contrast immersion appears as an ideal substitute for voluntary contractions to enhance blood flow and decrease residual edema in traumatized soft tissues (Cooper, et al., 1979). Is there scientific evidence to suggest that contrast immersion does trigger a peripheral and deep vascular pumping effect similar to that induced during voluntary muscle contraction?

a. Evidence From the Literature

Results of recent experimental studies involving healthy individuals have raised serious doubts about the deep vascular pumping effect traditionally attributed to contrast immersion (Myrer et al., 1994, 1997; Benoit et al., 1996; Higgins et al., 1998). Together, the results of these recent studies indicate that contrast immersion, when applied passively on the limbs of healthy individuals, fails to produce any significant intramuscular temperature changes, meaning that this method of water immersion has no

Box 9-3   Application Methods

Nonimmersion

The affected body area is treated with a pressured water irrigation system.

Immersion

The affected body part is immersed in water. Body immersion may be full (from neck down) or partial in nature. Immersion may also be passive (no body movement) or active (body movement from water turbulence caused by electric turbine).

Contrast immersion

Alternating immersion of the affected body part in water with contrasting temperature. Common dual-plastic containers are used: one is filled with ice-cold water, the other with hot water. Recommended temperature ranges for cold and hot water are as follows: 5–20°C (41–68°F);

and 37–43°C (99–110°F). Heat-to-cold ratio of immersion (H:C ratio) could fluctuate between a wide range of values. H:C ratios are commonly expressed in *minutes of immersion;* for example, a ratio of 4:1 is interpreted as meaning 4 min of immersion in hot water, followed by 1 min of immersion in cold water. These H:C time ratios may be kept constant or made variable during therapy. An example of a constant H:C time ratio might be 4:2, 4:2, 4:2, and 4:2, yielding a total of four cycles of immersion lasting 24 minutes, total. An example of a variable H:C time ratio might be 5:3, 4:2, and 3:1, for a total of three cycles of immersion lasting 18 minutes in total. No scientific evidence suggests that one specific H:C time ratio is therapeutically more beneficial than another for a given condition, or that the immersion cycle should begin or end with either a hot- or a cold-water immersion. The recommended application duration for contrast immersion is 20–30 minutes. The contrast immersion method can be delivered passively (i.e., no voluntary body movement) or actively (i.e., with voluntary body movement).

---

significant vasodilation/vasoconstriction effect on the larger and deeper blood vessels. It appears, therefore, that if passive application of contrast immersion is to cause a vascular pumping effect, then this exercise is limited to the peripheral blood vessels only.

b. Active Contrast Immersion

Research has shown that vascular as well as lymphatic pumping is best achieved by cycles of voluntary muscle contractions and joint motions that we all do on a daily basis. Thus active, as opposed to passive, contrast immersion, wherein the patient performs short bouts of exercise, may be the best method for obtaining the peripheral and deep vascular pumping effect. In other words, adding an active component (voluntary muscle contractions) to the passive effect of contrast immersion on peripheral blood flow should result in the desired therapeutic vascular and lymphatic therapeutic pumping action.

c. Transition Method

Because it exposes the body part to cryotherapeutic and thermotherapeutic effects, the contrast immersion method appears to be one of the best methods for transitioning the patient from cryotherapy to thermotherapy for the management of most soft-tissue disorders.

B. PROCEDURES

Safe, effective, and optimal application of hydrotherapy requires that clinicians go through a systematic set of procedures for each and every application. Presented below is a list of such procedures.

1. Checklists

Before proceeding with treatment, always go through the list of contraindications (see **Table 9-3**) and list of risks, precautions, and recommendations (see **Table 9-4**).

2. Thermal Sensory Discrimination

Always assess the patient's thermal sensory discrimination, that is, his or her ability to sense heat and cold on the skin in contact with the agent (see Chapter 25). Document the result of this test in the patient's file (see Section C, Documentation).

3. Skin Inspection and Preparation

Undress and inspect the body part to be treated, and remove any jewelry.

4. Hydroagent Preparation

Follow the manufacturer's recommendations with regard to the preparation of sitz baths, tubs, tanks, and water irrigators. If one or more electrical turbines are used, make sure that all of them are plugged into *GFCI receptacles* in order to eliminate the risk of electrocution.

5. Practitioner's Preparation

For the treatment of open wounds (infected, noninfected, and burns), practitioners must have adequate body protection (gown, gloves, and mask or goggles).

6. During Treatment

Ensure that the patient is comfortably positioned. Instruct the patient not to touch the electrical turbine (when applicable).

7. Cleansing and Debridement

Monitor water content (additives or not) and irrigation pressure from manual irrigator and electrical turbine.

8. Thermal Effect

Set the desired thermal dose by monitoring the water temperature. Measure the temperature differential between the agent and the skin (T°_{ag-s}) before application and the skin temperature differential before and after (T°_{b-a}) treatment, using an infrared thermometer (see Chapter 26). Water temperature is obtained from the tub's or tank's built-in thermometer. These temperature differentials will reveal how hot or cold the hydroagent was before application and how hot or cold the skin was at the end of treatment, thus providing objective dosimetry. Select dosage levels (T°_{ag-s}) that are able to induce heating or cooling changes (T°_{b-a}) that will best meet the therapeutic goals.

9. Mechanical Effect

When applicable, set and monitor the desired hydrostatic pressure, buoyancy force, and drag forces (discussed earlier).

10. End of Treatment

Always inspect the exposed skin surface for signs of damage. Question the patient on the level of heat or cold he or she has perceived during treatment; the answers will give an indication of the qualitative dose received. Any unusual sensation felt by the patient during treatment should be documented in the patient's file.

11. Maintenance and Calibration

Optimal functioning of hydrotherapy equipment and accessories can only be obtained through adequate maintenance and calibration. Lack of maintenance can lead to safety issues (see Chapter 27) and increase the risk of auto- and cross-contamination. Lack of periodic calibration can lead to inadequate dosimetry. Follow the manufacturer's recommendation with regard to the agent's maintenance (cleaning and disinfection) and calibration issues.

12. Auto- and Cross-Contamination Issues

Patients requiring hydrotherapy can contaminate the water with bacteria from infected ulcers or wounds, from surfaces of the skin, and from fecal flora. A critical consideration in the practice of hydrotherapy is the prevention of auto- and cross-contamination of patients from the growth of pathogens, such as the opportunistic *Pseudomonas aeruginosa*, on equipment and accessories. Such pathogens may cause urinary tract infections, respiratory system infections, dermatitis, and folliculitis, in addition to a variety of soft tissue and systemic infections. Prevention is best achieved through a rigid and complete maintenance program and schedule for cleaning, rinsing, and disinfecting all equipment and accessories after each use or between patients.

C. DOCUMENTATION

All health practitioners are expected to record adequate information in the patient's file. **Table 9-5** shows the key parameters to be documented in the patient's file following hydrotherapy.

TABLE 9-5	KEY TREATMENT PARAMETERS TO BE DOCUMENTED IN PATIENT'S FILE AFTER HYDROTHERAPY

- *Patient's skin thermal sensory discrimination testing:* record the result (see Chapter 25)
- *Skin status:* description
- *Health and mental status:* description
- *Hydro equipment:* description
- *Accessories:* description
- *Water temperature:* °C or °F
- *Water additives (when applicable):* name of solution and concentration per volume of water
- *Body part treated:* description
- *Treating method:* nonimmersion; immersion; contrast immersion
- *If immersion:* level—partial or full body
- *If immersion:* duration (min)
- *If contrast immersion:* H:C time ratio
- *Temperature differential between the agent (ag) and the skin surface (s) before application (T°_{ag-s}):* °C or °F
- *Temperature differential between skin surface before (b) and after (a) treatment (T°_{b-a}):* °C or °F

Case Study 9-1   Burn Wounds

A 55-year-old woman, hospitalized for 5 days for multiple burn injuries to her lower limbs after a home fire, is referred for hydrotherapy in preparation for plastic surgery. The physical examination reveals the presence of partially infected large burn wounds over the soles of her feet and over the left lateral side of her trunk, hip, and thigh. She reports that her wounds are very sensitive and that dry debridement and wound-dressing changes, done at bedside, are extremely painful. She reports increasing pain when she tries to adopt a sitting position. Her plastic surgeon is concerned that her wounds may get more infected, and healing delayed, if adequate wound care is inadequate at bedside. The surgeon's therapeutic objectives are to have all wounds cleaned and completely debrided, with adequate granulation tissue present, before he proceeds with his corrective dermatological surgical interventions. The patient spends a large portion of her day lying in bed and is unable to walk because of her painful wounds. Her immediate goals are better pain relief during wound-dressing changes and optimal wound preparation for surgery.

Evidence-Based Steps Toward the Resolution of This Case

1. **List medical diagnosis.**
   Multiple first-, second-, and third-degree burn wounds

2. **List key impairment(s).**
   - Severe pain
   - Multiple burn wounds

3. **List key functional limitation(s).**
   - Unable to sit
   - Unable to walk

4. **List key disability/disabilities.**
   - Unable to work

5. **Justification for hydrotherapy.**
   Is there justification for the use of hydrotherapy in this case? This chapter has established that the strength of evidence behind hydrotherapy is *moderate* and that the justification for its usage is *poor to fair*, for soft-tissue pathology (see Section VI). It has also revealed the *absence* of clinical trials on the effect of hydrotherapy on burn wounds, although many centers regularly use hydrotherapy for the management of open and burn wounds. Despite this absence of scientific evidence for burn wounds, this textbook, nonetheless, recommends the use of this agent for the following reasons. First, the current wound care for this patient is not acceptable because debridement and dressing changes, done at bedside, are too painful. Second, these partially infected wounds, spread over the foot, thigh, hip, and trunk areas, need thorough cleansing

and debridement for optimal wound healing. These findings thus justify the application of hydrotherapy for its cleansing and debridement effects, using full-body immersion in a burn or Hubbard tank. Another justification for hydrotherapy is that it makes wound-dressing changes (soaking in water) less painful. In other words, full-body immersion into water is expected to provide adequate cleansing and debridement of this patient's wounds. It is also expected to make dressing changes much less painful and psychologically distressing by having them thoroughly soaked before slow and gentle removal by the treating hydrotherapy clinician (i.e., from dry to wet dressing changes). The selection of hydrotherapy is also based on the body of evidence found in the following articles: McCulloch 1995, 1998; Burke et al., 1998; Rodeheaver, 1999; Hess et al., 2004. Because EPAs should never be used in isolation or as a sole intervention, hydrotherapy is used here concomitantly with hospital-based medical and nursing wound care.

6. **Search for contraindications.**
   None is found.

7. **Search for risks and precautions.**
   Because systemic body reactions are very likely to occur with full-body immersion in the thermo-hydrotherapy mode, vital signs are monitored. The treating dermatologist recommends that salt be added to water to prevent hyponatremia (low concentration of sodium in blood) in this burn patient.

8. **Outline the therapeutic goal(s) you and your patient wish to achieve.**
   - Decrease pain during wound care (cleansing, debridement)
   - Decrease pain during wound-dressing changes
   - Achieve complete cleansing and debridement of all wounds
   - Eliminate wound infection
   - Improve sitting and walking
   - Accelerate return to work

9. **For each therapeutic goal, list which outcome measurement(s) you will use to assess treatment effectiveness.**
   - Pain during cleansing, debridement, and dressing change: Visual Analog Scale (VAS)
   - Wound scar monitoring: Sussman Wound Healing Tool (SWHT)

10. **Instruct your patient about what he or she should experience, do, and not do during the application of hydrotherapy.**
    - Feel moderate warm sensation
    - Feel light sensation of weightlessness

(Continued)

- Feel moderate pain during debridement and dressing removal
- Feel fatigued at the end of treatment

11. Outline your therapeutic prescription based on the evidence available.

There is no evidence from research (**Box 9-1**) on which to rely for establishing the prescription of hydrotherapy in this case. The following prescription, therefore, is based in part on the literature (McCulloch 1995, 1998; Burke et al., 1998; Rodeheaver, 1999; Hess et al., 2004). The full-body immersion technique is preferred over the nonimmersion technique because multiple wounds are present. The Hubbard tank is preferred over the burn tank because it provides the clinician more space to deliver treatment. The partial-immersion Lo-Boy tub is not indicated because the patient is unable to adopt a sitting position. Finally, this prescription is also based on clinical experience with this agent and pathology.

- *Hydrotherapy mode:* thermo-hydrotherapy
- *Water temperature:* 38°C (100°F)
- *Water additive:* salt as prescribed by the treating dermatologist
- *Tank type:* Hubbard
- *Level of immersion:* full-body
- *Wound debridement method:* under water, using an electrical turbine. The jet stream pressure and direction, in relation to the surface of each wound, are carefully adjusted to reduce the risk of granulation tissue damage with progressive wound debridement.
- *Application duration:* between 30 and 40 minutes
- *Total number of treatments:* 12 treatments, one treatment per day
- *Wound dressing management:* dressings are soaked in water and then removed

12. Analyze outcome measurements.

Pre- and posttreatment comparison:

- Pain during cleansing, debridement: decreased VAS score from 7 to 2
- Pain during wound dressing change: decreased VAS score from 9 to 3
- Wound care: improved SWHT score; complete cleansing and debridement of all wound condition achieved; no infection after the sixth treatment.

13. Assess therapeutic effectiveness based on outcome measures.

The results show that 12 consecutive and daily hydrotherapy treatments, combined with hospital-based medical and nursing care, led to the complete cleansing and debridement of all wounds, in addition to significantly reduced pain during wound-dressing changes and debridement. Wounds were free of infection after the sixth treatment. All wounds are now ready for surgical intervention. The patient is very pleased with the therapeutic progress made and is looking forward to the upcoming surgical and rehabilitation phases of her treatment. Overall, the hydrotherapy treatment had a beneficial effect on the patient's disablement status created by the pathology, as illustrated in the **figure below**.

14. Outline the prognosis.

The prognosis is excellent considering that all wounds are now free of infection and show nice granulation tissue in preparation for surgical corrections. Full healing is expected. It is too soon to predict, however, whether ideal healing will occur for all the wounds. If the therapeutic plan progresses as expected over the next few weeks, full weight-bearing capacity and mobility will return. This patient will eventually resume her activities of daily living and her work as a lawyer.

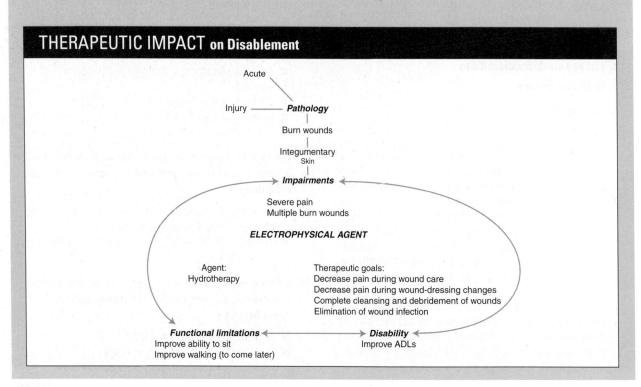

THERAPEUTIC IMPACT on Disablement

Acute

Injury —— *Pathology*

Burn wounds

Integumentary
Skin

Impairments

Severe pain
Multiple burn wounds

ELECTROPHYSICAL AGENT

Agent:
Hydrotherapy

Therapeutic goals:
Decrease pain during wound care
Decrease pain during wound-dressing changes
Complete cleansing and debridement of wounds
Elimination of wound infection

Functional limitations
Improve ability to sit
Improve walking (to come later)

Disability
Improve ADLs

CRITICAL THINKING QUESTIONS

Clarification: What is meant by hydrotherapy and by modes of hydrotherapy?

Assumptions: You have assumed that as a treating clinician you can exert control (i.e., increase or decrease the effects) over many properties of water. How do you justify that assumption?

Reasons and evidence: By what reasoning did you come to the conclusion that the larger the percentage of body immersion in water, the smaller the temperature differential between the water and the skin, and the greater the possibility of inducing systemic effects?

Viewpoints or perspectives: You are convinced that the buoyancy and drag forces associated with hydrotherapy can play a significant role in some pathological conditions. What would you say to a colleague who disagrees with you?

Implications and consequences: Knowing that there is poor-to-fair evidence to justify the use of hydrotherapy for soft-tissue pathology, what might that imply in terms of its current and future use?

About the question: Is it really important to clean, rinse, and disinfect hydrotherapy equipment and accessories after each use or between each patient? Why do you think I ask this question?

References

Articles

Abraham E, McMaster WC, Krijger M, Waugh TR (1974) Whirlpool therapy for the treatment of soft-tissue wounds complicated by extremity fractures. J Trauma, 14: 222–226

Ahern M, Nicholls E, Simionata E, Clark M, Bond M (1995) Clinical and psychological effects of hydrotherapy in rheumatic diseases. Clin Rehab, 9: 204–212

Atkinson G, Harrison A (1981) Implications of the health and safety at work act in relation to hydrotherapy department. Physiotherapy, 67: 263–265

Barber FA (2000) A comparison of crushed ice and continuous flow of cold therapy. Am J Knee Surg, 13: 97–101

Benoit TG, Martin DE, Perrin DH (1996) Hot and cold whirlpool treatments of knee joint laxity. J Athl Train, 31: 242–244, 286–287

Berger RS, Seifert MR (1990) Whirlpool folliculitis: A review of its cause, treatment and prevention. Cutis, 45: 97–98

Boynton BL, Garramore PM, Buca JT (1959) Observation of the effect of cold baths for patients with multiple sclerosis. Phys Ther Rev, 39: 297–299

Burke DG, Holt LE, Rasmussen R, MacKinnon NC, Vossen JF, Pelham TW (2001) Effects of hot and cold water immersion and modified proprioceptive neuromuscular facilitation flexibility exercise on hamstring length. J Athl Train, 36: 16–19

Burke DT, Ho CH, Saucier MA, Stewart G (1998) Effects of hydrotherapy on pressure ulcer healing. Am J Phys Med Rehab, 77: 394–398

Cammu H, Clasen K, van Wettere L, Derde MP (1994) To bathe or not to bathe during the first stage of labor. Acta Obstet Gynecol Scand, 73: 468–472

Chiara T, Carlos J, Martin D, Miller R, Nadeau S (1998) Cold effect on oxygen uptake, perceived exertion and spasticity in patients with multiple sclerosis. Arch Phys Med Rehab, 79: 523–528

Claus-Walker J, Halstead LS, Carter RE, Campos RJ, Spencer WA, Canzoneri J (1974) Physiological responses to cold stress in healthy subjects and in subjects with cervical cord injuries. Arch Phys Med Rehab, 55: 485–490

Clements JM, Casa DJ, Knight JC, McClung JM, Blake AS, Meenen PM, Gilmer AM, Caldwell KA (2002) Ice-water immersion and cold-water immersion provide similar cooling rates in runners with exercise-induced hyperthermia. J Athl Train, 37: 146–150

Cooper Dl, Fair J (1979) Contrast baths and pressure treatment for ankle sprains. Physician Sportsmed, 7: 143

Cornwall MW (1994) Effect of temperature on muscle force and rate of muscle force production in men and women. J Orthop Sports Phys Ther, 20: 74–80

Cote DJ, Prentice WE, Hooker D, Shields EW (1988) Comparison of three treatment procedures for minimizing ankle sprain swelling. Phys Ther, 68: 1072–1076

Curkovic B, Vitulic V, Babic-Naglic D, Durrigl T (1993) The influence of heat and cold on the pain threshold in rheumatoid arthritis. Z Rheumatol, 52: 289–291

Dodi G, Bogoni F, Infantino A, Pianon P, Mortellaro LM, Lise M (1986) Hot and cold in anal pain. A study of the changes in internal anal sphincter pressure profiles. Dis Colon Rectum, 29: 248–251

Droegemueller W (1980) Cold sitz baths for relief of perineal pain. Clin Obstet Gynecol, 23: 1039–1043

Ernst E, Saradeth T, Resh KL (1990) A single blind randomized, controlled trial of hydrotherapy for varicose veins. Vasa, 20: 147–152

Ernst E, Saradeth T, Resh KL (1992) Hydrotherapy for varicose veins: A randomized controlled trial. Phlebology, 7: 154–157

Eston R, Peters D (1999) Effects of cold water immersion on the symptoms of exercise-induced muscle damage. J Sports Sci, 17: 231–238

Fricke FJ, Gersten JW (1952) Effect of contrast baths on the vasomotor response of rheumatoid arthritis patients. Arch Phys Med Rehab, 33: 210–216

Fruhstorfer H, Hermanns M, Latzke L (1986) The effects of thermal stimulation on clinical and experimental itch. Pain, 24: 259–269

Gogia PP, Hurt BS, Zirn TT (1988) Wound management with whirlpool and infrared cold laser treatment. A clinical report. Phys Ther, 1239–1242

Green J, McKenna F, Redfern EJ, Chamberlain MA (1993) Home exercises are as effective as outpatient hydrotherapy for osteoarthritis of the hip. Br J Rheumatol, 32: 812–815

Gupta P (2006) Randomized, controlled study comparing sitz-bath and no-sitz bath treatments in patients with acute anal fissures. ANZ J Surg, 76: 718–721

Gupta PJ (2007) Effects of warm water sitz on symptoms in post-anal sphincterotomy in chronic anal fissure—a randomized and controlled study. World J Surg, 31: 1480–1484

Hall J, Skevington SM, Maddison PJ, Chapman K (1996) A randomized and controlled trial of hydrotherapy in rheumatoid arthritis. Arthritis Care Res, 9: 206–215

Harrison RA (1981) Tolerance of pool therapy by ankylosing spondylitis patients with low vital capacity. Physiotherapy, 67: 296

Higgins D, Kaminski TW (1998) Contrast therapy does not cause fluctuations in human gastrocnemius intramuscular temperature. J Athl Train, 33: 336–340

Hill PD (1989) Effects of heat and cold on the perineum after episiotomy/laceration. J Obstet Gynecol Neonatal Nurs, 18: 124–129

Hollyoak V, Allison D, Summers J (1995a) Pseudomonas aeruginosa wound infection associated with a nursing home's whirlpool bath. Commun Dis Rep CDR Rev, 23: R100–R102

Hollyoak V, Boyd P, Freeman R (1995b) Whirlpool baths in nursing homes: Use, maintenance and contamination with Pseudomonas aeruginosa. Commun Dis Rep CDR Rev, 23: R102–R104

Hoyrup G, Kjorvel L (1986) Comparison of whirlpool and wax treatment for hand therapy. Physiotherapy, 38: 79–82

Juve Meeker B (1998) Whirlpool therapy on postoperative pain and surgical wound healing: An exploration. Pat Educ Couns, 33: 39–48

Kawamura K, Ozawa M, Sorimachi M, Ueda H, Ebato S, Ando H, Hasegawa M, Matsuzaki A, Katagiri T (1997) Hemodynamic effects of warm bathing in a Hubbard tank and exercise loading in patients after myocardial infarction. J Cardiol, 30: 231–239

Kelly ML, Jarvie GL, Middlebrook JL, McNeer MF, Drabman RS (1984) Decreasing burned children's pain behavior: Impacting the trauma of hydrotherapy. J Appl Behav Anal, 17: 147–158

Kuligowski LA, Lephart SM, Giannantonio FP, Blanc RO (1998) Effect of whirlpool therapy on signs and symptoms of delayed-onset muscle soreness. J Athl Train, 33: 222–228

Loten C, Stokes B, Worsley D, Seymour JE, Jiang S, Isbistergk GK (2006) A randomized controlled trial of hot water (45 degrees C) immersion versus ice packs for pain relief in bluebottle stings. Med J Aust, 184: 329–333

Luedtke-Hoffmann KA, Schader DS (2000) Pulsed lavage in wound cleansing. Phys Ther, 80: 292–300

Magness JL, Garret TR, Erickson DJ (1970) Swelling of the upper extremity during whirlpool baths. Arch Phys Med Rehab, 51: 297–299

McCulloch J, Boyer Boyd A (1992) The effects of whirlpool and the dependent position on lower extremity volume. J Orthop Sports Phys Ther, 16: 169–173

McGuckin M, Thorpe R, Abrutyn E (1981) Hydrotherapy: An outbreak of Pseudomonas aeruginosa wound infections related to Hubbard tank treatments. Arch Phys Med Rehab, 62: 283–285

McManus AT, Mason AD, McManus WF, Pruitt BA (1985) Twenty-five year review of Pseudomonas aeruginosa bacteremia in a burn center. Eur J Clin Microbiol, 4: 219–223

Miglietta O (1964) Electromyographic characteristics of clonus and influence of cold. Arch Phys Med Rehab, 45: 508–512

Misasi S, Morin G, Kemler D, Olmstead PS, Pryzgocki K (1995) The effect of toe cap and bias on perceived pain during cold water immersion. J Athl Train, 30: 49–52

Myrer JW, Draper DO, Durrant E (1994) Contrast therapy and intramuscular temperature in the human leg. J Athl Train, 29: 318–322

Myrer JW, Measom G, Durrant E, Fellingham GW (1997) Cold and hot-pack contrast therapy: Subcutaneous and intramuscular temperature change. J Athl Train, 32: 238–241

Nguyen ND, Wadley HN, Edlich RF (1995) Corrosion of stainless steel pipes in a hydrotherapy pool by a silver-copper disinfection system. J Burn Care Rehab, 16: 280–283

Nimchick PS, Knight KL (1983) Effects of wearing a toe cap or a sock on temperature perceived during ice water immersion. J Athl Train, 18: 144–147

Petrofsky J, Lohman E, Lee S, de la Cuesta Z, Labial L, Iouciulescu R, Moseley B, Korson R, Al Malty A (2007) Effects of contrast bath on skin blood flow on the dorsal and plantar foot in people with type 2 diabetes and aged matched controls. Physioth Theory Pract, 23: 189–197

Pinho M, Correa JC, Furtado A, Ramos JR (1993) Do hot baths promote anal sphincter relaxation? Dis Colon Rectum, 36: 273–274

Ramler D, Roberts J (1986) A comparison of cold and warm sitz baths for relief of perineal pain. J Obstet Gynecol Neonatal Nurs, 15: 471–474

Richard P, LeFoch R, Chamoux C, Pannier M, Espaze E, Richet H (1994) Pseudomonas aeruginosa outbreak in a burn unit: Role of antimicrobials in the emergence of multiple resistant strains. J Infect Dis, 170: 377–383

Rush J, Burlock S, Lambert K, Loosley-Millman M, Hutchison B, Enkin M (1996) The effects of whirlpools baths in labor: A randomized controlled trial. Birth, 23: 136–143

Said RA, Hussein MM (1987) Severe hyponatremia in burn patients secondary to hydrotherapy. Burns Incl Therm Inj, 13: 327–329

Sedgwick Harvey MA, McRorie M, Smith DW (1981) Suggested limits to the use of the hot tub and sauna by pregnant women. Can Med Assoc J, 125: 50–53

Shankowsky HA, Cailloux LS, Tredget EE (1994) North American survey of hydrotherapy in modern burn care. J Burn Care Rehab, 15: 143–146

Silva LE, Valim V, Passenha AP, Oliveira LM, Myamoto S, Jones A, Natour J (2007) Hydrotherapy versus conventional land-based exercise for the management of patient with osteoarthritis of the knee: A randomized clinical trial. Phys Ther, 88: 12–21

Sterner-Victorin E, Kruse-Smidje C, Jung K (2004) Comparison between electro-acupuncture and hydrotherapy, both in combination with patient education and patient education alone, on the symptomatic treatment of osteoarthritis of the hip. Clin J Pain, 20: 179–185

Streator S, Ingersoll CD (1995) Sensory information can decrease cold-induced pain perception. J Athl Train, 30: 293–296

Sylvester KL (1990) Investigation of the effect of hydrotherapy in the treatment of osteoarthritic hips. Clin Rehab, 4: 223–228

Taddonio TE, Thomson PD, Smith DJ, Prasad JK (1990) A survey of wound monitoring and topical antimicrobial therapy practices in the treatment of burn therapy. J Burn Care Rehab, 11: 423–427

Thomas IL, Erian M, Sarson D, Yan L, White S, Battistutta D (1993) Postpartum hemorrhoids—evaluation of a cooling device (Anorex) for relief of symptoms. Med J Aust, 159: 459–640

Thomson PD, Bowden MS, McDonald K, Smith DJ, Prasad JK (1990) A survey of burn hydrotherapy in the United States. J Burn Care Rehab, 11: 151–155

Toomey R, Grief-Schwartz R (1986a) Extent of whirlpool use in Canadian physiotherapy departments: A survey. Physiother Can, 38: 277–278

Toomey R, Grief-Schwartz R, Piper MC (1986b) Clinical evaluation of the effects of whirlpool on patients with Colles' fractures. Physiother Can, 38: 280–284

Tredget EE, Shankowsky HA, Joffe AM, Inkson TI, Volpel K, Paranchych W, Kibsey PC, Alton JD, Burke JF (1992) Epidemiology of infections in Pseudomonas aeruginosa in burn patients: The role of hydrotherapy. Clin Infect Dis, 15: 941–949

Vaile JM, Gill ND, Blazevich AJ (2007a) The effect of contrast water therapy on symptoms of delayed onset muscle soreness. J Strength Cond Res, 21: 697–702

Vaile J, Halson S, Gill N, Dawson B (2007b) Effects of hydrotherapy on the signs and symptoms of delayed onset muscle soreness. Eur J Appl Physiol, 102: 447–455

Woodmansey A, Collins DH, Ernst MM (1938) Vascular reactions to the contrast bath in health and in rheumatic arthritis. Lancet, 2: 1350–1353

Review Articles

Cochrane DJ (2004) Alternating hot and cold water immersion for athlete recovery: A review. Phys Ther Sports, 5: 26–32

Hess CL, Howard MA, Attinger CE (2004) A review of mechanical adjuncts in wound healing: Hydrotherapy, ultrasound, negative pressure therapy, hyperbaric oxygen, and electrostimulation. Ann Plast Surg, 51: 210–218

Jackson R (1990) Waters and spa in the classical world. Med Hist Suppl, 10: 1–13

Luedtke-Hoffmann KA, Shafer DS (2000) Pulsed lavage in wound cleansing. Phys Ther, 80: 292–300

McCulloch J (1995) Physical modalities in wound management: Ultrasound, vasopneumatic devices and hydrotherapy. Ostomy Wound Manage, 41: 21–37

McCulloch JM (1998) The role of physiotherapy in managing patients with wounds. J Wound Care, 7: 241–244

Rodeheaver GT (1999) Pressure ulcer debridement and cleansing: A review of current literature. Ostomy Wound Manage, 45: 80S–85S

Smith R (1997) Hydrotherapy around the globe. Rehabilitation Int, Fall: 25–27

Whitelock H (1990) Hydrotherapy in the 1990s. Aust J Physiother, 36: 144–145

Chapters of Textbooks

Babb R, Muntzer E (1996) Hydrotherapy: Whirlpools to aquatic pools. In: Physical Agents: Theory and Practice for the Physical Therapists Assistant. Behrens BJ, Michlovitz, SL (Eds). FA Davis, Philadelphia, pp 135–158

Bell GW, Prentice WE (1998) Infrared modalities. In: Therapeutic Modalities for Allied Health Professionals. Prentice WE (Ed). McGraw-Hill Health Professions Division, New York, pp 201–262

Bukowski EL, Nolan TP (2005) Hydrotherapy: The Use of water as a Therapeutic Agent. In: Modalities for Therapeutic Intervention, 4th ed. Michlovitz SL, Nolan TP (Eds). FA Davis Co, Philadelphia, pp 123–140

Cameron MH (2003) Hydrotherapy. In: Physical Agents in Rehabilitation. From Research to Practice, 2nd ed. WB Saunders Co., Philadelphia, pp 261–305

Clement A (1997) Risk management. In: Aquatic Rehabilitation. Ruoti RG, Morris DM, Cole AJ (Eds). Lippincott, Philadelphia, pp 375–390

Hall SJ (2006) Human movement in a fluid medium. In: Basic Biomechanics, 5th ed. McGraw-Hill, New York, pp 479–510

Hecox B, Leinanger PM (2006) Hydrotherapy. In: Integrated Physical Agents in Rehabilitation, 2nd ed. Hecox B, Mehreteab TA, Weisberg J, Sanko J (Eds). Pearson Prentice Hall, Upper Saddle River, pp 397–426

Irion JM (1997) Historical overview of aquatic rehabilitation. In: Aquatic Rehabilitation. Ruoti RG, Morris DW, Cole AJ (Eds). Lippincott, Philadelphia, pp 3–14

Kreighbaum E, Barthels KM (1996) Biomechanics: A Qualitative Approach to Studying Human Movement. Allyn and Bacon, Boston, pp 98–99, 104, 414–446, 451–492

Low J, Reed A (1994) Thermal energy. In: Physical Principles Explained. Butterworth-Heinemann, London, pp 148–176

Sekins KM, Emery AF (1990) Thermal science for physical medicine. In: Therapeutic Heat and Cold, 4th ed. Lehmann JF (Ed). Williams & Wilkins, Baltimore, pp 62–112

Stowers R, Babb R (2006) Aquatics and Hydrotherapy. In: Physical Agents: Theory and Practice, 2nd ed. Behrens BJ, Michlovitz SL (Eds). FA Davis Co, Philadelphia, pp 80–97

Walsh MT (1996) Hydrotherapy: The use of water as a therapeutic agent. In: Thermal Agents in Rehabilitation, 3rd ed. Michlovitz SL (Ed). FA Davis, Philadelphia, pp 139–167

Textbook

Baruch S (1920) An Epitome of Hydrotherapy. WB Saunders, Philadelphia, pp 45–99, 151–198

Clinical Practice Guideline

Agency for Health Care Policy and Research (1994) Treatment of Pressure Ulcers: Clinical Practice Guideline No. 15. AHCPR Publication No. 95–0625. U.S. Department of Health and Services, Rockville, pp 6–7, 47–53

Shortwave Diathermy Therapy

Chapter Outline

Learning Objectives

Knowledge: List and describe the rationale behind the contraindications, risks, and precautions associated with shortwave diathermy (SWD) therapy.
Comprehension: Compare the capacitive and inductive methods of SWD delivery.
Application: Illustrate how to apply capacitive and inductive applicators over various body areas, using various applicator arrangements.

Analysis: Explain how the application of SWD induces heat in deep soft tissues.
Synthesis: Explain the rationale for using the capacitive method over the inductive one, and vice versa, and discuss the importance of subcutaneous fat tissue overlying the treated tissue.
Evaluation: Discuss the research-based evidence behind the application of therapeutic SWD.

I. RATIONALE FOR USE

A. DEFINITION AND DESCRIPTION

The term *shortwave diathermy* (SWD) is defined as the use of shortwave electromagnetic energy for the purpose of heating deep soft tissues. The word *shortwave* refers to the shortwave electromagnetic band, or region, of the electromagnetic spectrum, and the word *diathermy* means "through heat" (*dia-* = through; *thermy* = heat). The resistance offered by soft tissues to the passage of this electromagnetic energy causes them to heat up.

B. SHORTWAVE DIATHERMY DEVICES

Shown in **Figure 10-1** are typical portable (**A**) and cabinet-type (**B**) devices used today to deliver SWD therapy. The portable model (**A**) is shown with a pair of capacitive flexible pad applicators. The cabinet model (**B**) is presented with its articulated arms to which capacitive applicators are attached. Both types of devices are line powered.

C. CAPACITIVE AND INDUCTIVE APPLICATORS

Shown in **Figure 10-2** are typical capacitive plate and inductive coil applicators. They come in different sizes and shapes to accommodate the treated body area. Capacitive plate applicators are made of rubber and glass (*bottom half of figure*) material. Inductive drum applicators, on the other hand, are made of one or more flat spiral copper coils mounted and hidden in a rigid hard plastic casing (*upper half of figure*).

D. RATIONALE FOR USE

The rationale behind the development and use of SWD therapy lies in the demand for an electrotherapeutic agent capable of *deep* heating of *large* surface areas of soft tissues, such as muscle and joint structures, while minimally heating superficial tissues, such as skin and subcutaneous fat, exposed to the radiating energy.

II. HISTORICAL PERSPECTIVE

A. DISCOVERY

During the late 1800s, Jacques-Arsène d'Arsonval, a French physician and physiologist, observed that high-frequency electromagnetic currents applied over soft tissues produced perceptible warming without muscle contraction (Kloth et al., 1984; Guy, 1990). This observation led German physician Carl Franz Nagelschmidt to coin the term *diathermy,* meaning "through heating," in 1907. Three generations of SWD devices have been developed and commercialized over the past 80 years: *longwave, shortwave,* and *microwave diathermy.*

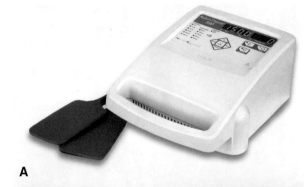
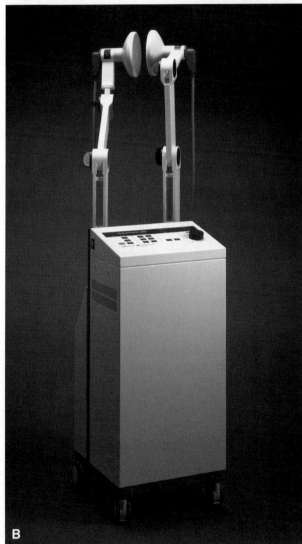

FIGURE 10-1 Typical portable (**A**) and cabinet-type (**B**) shortwave diathermy devices. (Courtesy of Mettler Electronics.)

B. LONGWAVE DIATHERMY

The *first* generation of diathermy devices, designed during the 1920s and termed *longwave diathermy* (LWD), was built to emit electromagnetic waves at frequencies ranging from 500 KHz to 10 MHz. Historical accounts indicate that the clinical use of LWD devices diminished during the 1930s and 1940s with the arrival of the second

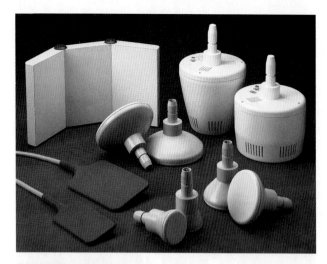

FIGURE 10-2 Typical capacitive and inductive applicators. (Courtesy of Mettler Electronics.)

generation of diathermy devices, which allowed electromagnetic energy to be delivered to soft tissues across an air space (as opposed to a wet pad, used with LWD devices), thus greatly facilitating clinical applications (Kloth et al., 1984; Low 1988).

C. SHORTWAVE DIATHERMY

The *second* generation of diathermy devices, termed *shortwave diathermy* (SWD), was built to emit electromagnetic waves within the *shortwave region* of the electromagnetic spectrum. Frequencies approved by the Federal Communication Commission (FCC) for SWD devices used in clinical practice are 13.56, 27.12, and 40.68 MHz. SWD devices emitting at a frequency of 27.12 MHz are technically easier and less expensive to manufacture. Consequently, this is the most commonly found frequency in therapeutic SWD devices manufactured today around the world.

1. Continuous Shortwave Diathermy

The first model of SWD devices was designed to deliver continuous (C) electromagnetic radiation to cause deep heating of soft tissues. This type of application is known clinically as *continuous shortwave diathermy* (CSWD).

2. Pulsed Shortwave Diathermy

The second model of SWD devices differs from the original model in that the delivery of electromagnetic radiation is periodically interrupted, or pulsed. This type of application is known clinically as *pulsed SWD* (PSWD). The first commercialized PSWD devices were marketed under the name *Diapulse*, meaning pulsed diathermy. The use of PSWD should not be confused with the use of pulsed electromagnetic fields (PEMFs) therapy, also known as *magnetotherapy*. The key difference between the two is that the latter is characterized by a magnetic current only (magnetic versus electromagnetic), delivered at low carrier frequencies (kilohertz versus megahertz). PEMF therapy is beyond the scope of this chapter.

3. Modern SWD

During the 1970s, a third model of SWD devices, capable of producing both continuous (CSWD) and pulsed (PSWD) electromagnetic waves, was developed and marketed worldwide. The SWD devices shown in **Figure 10-1** are examples of this third model, the modern type of SWD devices. The scope of this chapter is on the use and application of both CSWD and PSWD therapy.

D. MICROWAVE DIATHERMY

Concurrent with the development of SWD, a *third* generation of through-heating devices for what is known as *microwave diathermy* (MWD) was introduced. The FCC-approved frequency for MWD devices in clinical practice is 2450 MHz. Compared with SWD, the main advantage of MWD is that it is much easier to focus on the body, thus providing a much more localized heating effect. The main disadvantage of MWD, compared with SWD, is that penetration of electromagnetic energy in the tissues decreases as the frequency increases, thus providing shallower tissue heating in the deeper tissues (Cameron et al., 2003). This fact explains why MWD has been gradually abandoned over the past 20 years in favor of SWD. Therefore, MWD is beyond the scope of this chapter.

E. TODAY'S SHORTWAVE DIATHERMY PRACTICE

The survey-based literature on the practice of SWD in the field of physical therapy reveals a relatively high level of ownership combined with a declining level of use (see Shields et al., 2002). The declining use of SWD therapy may be attributed to several reasons, the key one being linked to safety concerns. Emission of *unwanted stray radiation* during therapy, which affects patients, operators, and other personnel in the vicinity of the device, is likely the main reason for the decline in SWD therapy in the latter half of the 20th century (Shields et al., 2002; see also VIII. Risks, Precautions, and Recommendations).

F. BODY OF LITERATURE

SWD therapy has been the subject of several *articles* (see References), *review articles* (Hayne, 1984; Delpizzo et al., 1989; Goats, 1989; Martin et al., 1991; Weinberger et al., 1991; Kitchen et al., 1992; Marks et al., 1999; Shields et al., 2001a,b; Shields et al., 2002; Shields et al., 2004), *chapters of textbooks* (Guy, 1990; Lehmann et al., 1990; Low et al., 1988; Low et al., 1990, 1994; Michaelson, 1990; Kloth et al., 1996; Prentice et al., 1998; Khan, 2000; Scott, 2002; Cameron et al., 2003; Starkey, 2004a,b; Day et al., 2006; Knight et al., 2008), and *specialized documents* (Ruggera, 1980; American National Standards

Institute, 1982; Health and Welfare Canada, 1983, 2002; Kloth et al., 1984; Food and Drug Code of Federal Regulations, 1995; Australian Physiotherapy Association, 2001; Medtronic, 2001; Food and Drug Administration, 2002).

III. BIOPHYSICAL CHARACTERISTICS

A. SHORTWAVES

The biophysics of SWD therapy, as its name implies, center on the production of short electromagnetic waves, delivered at 27.12 MHz. Before considering the following material, readers are urged to review the section on *Electromagnetic Terminology* in Chapter 5, which provides an illustrated glossary of terms and concepts related to the delivery of electromagnetic energy to soft tissues. The shortwave region of the EM spectrum (see **Table 5-2**) corresponds to those waves delivered at frequencies ranging between 3 and 30 MHz.

B. NONIONIZING RADIATION

Shortwave radiation is *nonionizing* in nature, meaning that the level of electromagnetic energy generated per photon (eV) is negligible, and thus not sufficient to separate, dislodge, or strip an electron from its atom (see **Table 5-2** and **Figure 5-2**).

C. ELECTROMAGNETIC WAVE

Shown in **Figure 10-3** are electromagnetic waves generated from a typical SWD device. An electromagnetic wave is defined as the interaction between an electric (E) and a magnetic (M) field, with each field oriented perpendicular to the other (Low et al., 1994). Electromagnetic (EM) waves travel freely in space at a constant velocity equivalent to the speed of light, or 300 million meters per second (300×10^6 m/s).

D. SWD WAVELENGTH

Biophysics has established that electromagnetic wavelength is inversely related to frequency on the basis of the formula $\lambda = c / f$, where λ is the wavelength, c is the speed of light (300×10^6 m/s), and f is the frequency. Considering the fact that the speed of light is constant, it follows that the wavelength of an SWD device emitting at the frequency of 27.12 MHz is 11 meters, or 3.5 feet, in length (11 m = $300 \times 10^6 / 27.12 \times 10^6$).

E. ELECTROMAGNETIC RESONANCE

A key biophysical phenomenon associated with SWD therapy is electromagnetic resonance. Also known as *tuning*, resonance occurs when the patient circuit (i.e., ions

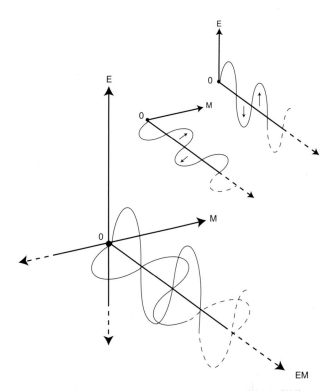

FIGURE 10-3 Schematic representation of electromagnetic (EM) waves generated by a typical SWD device. The electric (E) and magnetic (M) fields are at a right angle (90°) to each other. The variations of amplitude in both fields are sinusoidal and transverse to the direction of travel of the waves.

and dipoles in exposed biological tissues) oscillates at the same frequency as the device circuit (i.e., oscillating current generator), which is 27.12 MHz in most devices. Electromagnetic energy is fully delivered to the tissues only when complete resonance occurs between the two circuits.

1. Resonance Indicator

Resonance occurs automatically in most devices. When it does, a signal, such as a flashing light, appears on the console to inform the operator that full resonance has been achieved. The final power output of the device is always adjusted after resonance is achieved.

2. Loss of Resonance

Resonance between the patient and the device circuit can be lost during a treatment session because of movement at the applicator/skin surface interface. Thus, patients should be instructed to remain still or minimize all body movements to avoid disturbing the applicator arrangement during treatment.

3. Regular Monitoring

It is strongly recommended that the device resonance indicator be checked periodically to make sure full resonance is maintained through the entire treatment session, thus maximizing the flow of electromagnetic radiation in the soft tissues.

F. ENERGY TRANSFER MODE

SWD uses *radiation* as its mode of energy transfer. Radiation implies the transmission of energy through space. The electromagnetic energy generated at the applicator's surface travels through an air space before being absorbed by the exposed tissues.

IV. PHYSIOLOGICAL AND THERAPEUTIC EFFECTS

A. THERMAL VERSUS NONTHERMAL

When soft biological tissues are exposed to the electromagnetic energy generated by SWD, part of this energy is absorbed, which triggers a cascade of atomic and molecular reactions responsible for the observed physiological and therapeutic effects. There is general consensus in the literature that SWD induces both thermal and nonthermal effects within soft tissues. A popular view associates the application of pulsed shortwave diathermy (PSW) delivered at a low power output, with nonthermal effects in soft tissues. A nonthermal effect is by definition an effect caused by means other than heat. In other words, the term *nonthermal* implies the absence of heat. The evidence presented below indicates that the nonthermal effect commonly associated with PSWD should be seriously questioned.

B. PSWD AND THERMAL EFFECTS

There is scientific evidence, as summarized in **Box 10-1**, to support the claim that PSWD can induce significant soft-tissue heating in healthy subjects (Draper et al., 1999, 2002, 2004; Garrett et al., 2000; Peres et al., 2002; Brucker et al., 2005). The experimental work conducted by two of these authors demonstrates that PSWD using an inductive drum applicator, applied over a period of 20 minutes at an average rms power output as low as 48 W, led to heating human muscles by approximately 4°C at a depth of 3 cm below the skin surface (Draper et al., 1999; Garrett et al., 2000). Four of these authors further demonstrated that the combination of PSWD and stretching, as opposed to stretching alone, can significantly increase joint flexibility because of the heating of the deeper musculotendinous area (Peres et al., 2002; Draper et al., 2002, 2004; Brucker et al., 2005).

C. HYPOTHETICAL NONTHERMAL EFFECTS

No scientific evidence could be found in published English-language, peer-reviewed studies on humans to support the view that SWD, delivered in its continuous or pulsed mode, induces in situ or in vivo nonthermal effects in soft tissues. Until some evidence is provided, the nonthermal effects associated with PSWD therapy can only be hypothetical. Moreover, the body of scientific evidence summarized in **Box 10-1** seriously questioned the view, raised by Kloth et al. (1996), that PSWD administered at low dosage (i.e., less than 38 W) will induce maximum nonthermal and minimal thermal effects. This view should also be considered as hypothetical, considering the fact that PSWD administered with a mean power output of only 10 W above the threshold value (48 W versus 38 W) proposed by Kloth et al. (1996) led to an important muscle-heating effect (i.e., an increase of approximately 4°C) at a depth of

Box 10-1	Physiological Effects of PSWD in Healthy Subjects

SOURCE	EXPERIMENTAL RESULTS
Draper et al., 1999	PSWD, applied with an average rms power output of 48 W for 20 min, increased gastrocnemius muscle temperature by 3.5°C 3 cm below the skin surface.
Garrett et al., 2000	PSWD, applied with an average rms power output of 48 W for 20 min, increased triceps surae muscle temperature by 4.5°C 3 cm below the skin surface.
Peres et al., 2002	PSWD, applied with an average rms power output of 48 W for 20 min before a prolonged static stretch was found more effective in increasing triceps surae elasticity than stretching alone.
Draper et al., 2002	PSWD (unspecified power output) application plus short-duration stretching for 15 min was found more effective in increasing hamstring elasticity than short-duration stretching alone.
Draper et al., 2004	PSWD, applied with an average rms power output of 48 W for 20 min, plus low-load and long-duration stretching for 15 min, were found more effective in increasing hamstring elasticity than low-load long-duration stretching alone.
Brucker et al., 2005	PSWD, applied with an average rms power output of 48 W for 20 min during stretching did not improve long-term retention (3 weeks later) of triceps surae muscle elasticity gained.

3 cm below the skin surface. To sum up, the current body of scientific evidence (**Box 10-2**) indicates that both CSWD and PSWD, delivered at an average rms power output as low as 48 W, are capable of inducing very important thermal effects in human deep soft tissues.

D. CSWD VERSUS PSWD

There is growing evidence to suggest that over the past two decades the use of PSWD may have surpassed CSWD as the mode of delivery of choice. A possible explanation for this shift may be that the application of PSWD, associated with less stray radiation, is safer for the operator (Tzima et al., 1994). Another likely reason the use of PSWD is on the increase is the fact that a much greater number of clinical studies have been published over the past years showing that low-wattage PSWD can induce a significant deep-heating response in human soft tissues.

E. PROPOSED MECHANISMS BEHIND THERMAL EFFECTS

There is a theoretical consensus in the literature (see Scott, 2002) that the thermal effects induced by the application of SWD, as illustrated in **Figure 10-4**, are primarily caused by two mechanisms: *ionic oscillation* and *dipole rotation*.

1. Ionic Oscillation

Soft tissues contain billions of charged particles or ions, such as sodium (Na^+), potassium (K^+) and chloride (Cl^-). When these ions are exposed to the high-frequency oscillating current generated by the device, they are presumed to move to and fro, or oscillate, in response to the oscillating electric field (Scott, 2002).

2. Dipole Rotation

Soft tissues also contain billions of dipolar, or water, molecules—hydrogen (H^+) and oxygen (O^-). When these dipoles are exposed to this same high-frequency oscillating current, these bipolar molecules are presumed to rotate in response to the oscillatory field (Scott, 2002).

F. CONVERSION OF KINETIC ENERGY INTO HEAT

The combined effect of these microscopic oscillatory and rotational movements of particles is the production of kinetic energy, which is then converted into thermal or heat energy within the exposed tissues (**Fig 10-4**). Kinetic energy is that energy associated with movement. Thus, the more electromagnetic energy absorbed by a biological tissue, the greater the ionic oscillatory and dipole rotational movements and, therefore, the greater the heating of deep tissues.

G. PROPOSED THERAPEUTIC EFFECTS

The deep-tissue heating effect resulting from the application of SWD is associated, as shown in **Figure 10-4**, with increased blood flow, increased cell metabolism, increased tissue elasticity, and decreased joint viscosity.

V. DOSIMETRY

A. SCALES

Dosimetry associated with SWD therapy can be described, as presented in **Table 10-1**, using two scales: *qualitative* and *quantitative*. The qualitative scale describes the dosage in terms of the level of thermal heat sensation the patient

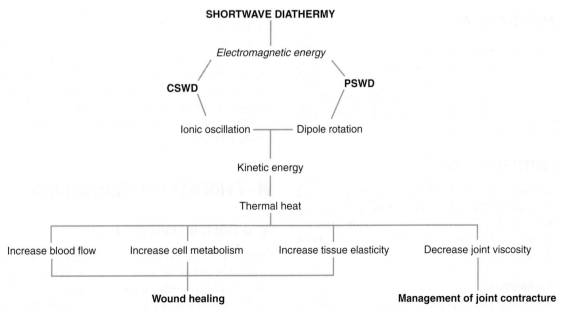

FIGURE 10-4 Proposed physiological and therapeutic effects of SWD therapy.

TABLE 10-1	SWD QUALITATIVE AND QUANTITATIVE DOSIMETRIC SCALES

QUALITATIVE SCALE

Dose I	No perception of heat
Dose II	Mild perception of heat
Dose III	Comfortable perception of heat
Dose IV	Maximum tolerable perception of heat

QUANTITATIVE SCALE

	DOSIMETRIC EXAMPLES	
PARAMETERS	**CSWD**	**PSWD**
Peak power (P_p):	500 W	500 W
Pulse frequency (f):	N/A	200 Hz
Pulse duration (PD):	N/A	400 μs
Mean power (P_m):	N/A	40 W
Application duration (T):	20 min (1200 s)	20 min (1200 s)
Dose (D):	600 kJ	48 kJ

perceives during treatment. The quantitative scale, on the other hand, describes the dosage in terms of the amount of energy actually delivered at the applicator/skin interface.

B. QUALITATIVE SCALE

In the qualitative scale, the patient's perception of heat during treatment is ranked according to a four-level dose system (dose I, II, III, or IV). Heat perception is recorded as *none* (dose I), *mild* (dose II), *comfortable* (dose III), or *maximum tolerable* (dose IV). The more heat perceived, the higher the dose number.

C. QUANTITATIVE SCALE

The quantitative scale takes into account the amount of heat, measured in joules (J), that the device generates at the applicator/skin interface. Shown in **Table 10-1** are the key dosimetric parameters, formulas, and calculations for both CSWD and PSWD.

1. Key Parameters

Quantitative dosimetry depends on four key parameters: power, pulse frequency, delivery mode, and application

duration. Power is the rate of energy delivered expressed in watts (W). Peak power (P_p) generated during the continuous mode (CSWD) may be as high as 800 W in most modern SWD units. If the device is used in its pulsed mode (PSWD), mean power (P_m) is calculated on the basis of the peak power (P_p), measured in W, pulse duration (PD), measured in seconds, and pulse frequency (f), measured in Hz, used. It is calculated as follows: ($P_m = P_p \times PD \times f$).

2. Dose

The dose (D), or energy, delivered at the applicator level is expressed in Joules (J) and results from the product of power (P), measured in W, multiplied by the application duration (T), measured in seconds. If CSWD is used, the dose is calculated as follows: $D = P_p \times T$. If PSWD is used, the dose is calculated on the basis of mean power: $D = P_m \times T$.

3. Dosimetric Examples

Shown in **Box 10-1** are examples of those key parameters using both CSWD and PSWD mode of delivery. For the CSWD mode, power is set at 500 W and application duration at 20 minutes. The dose delivered at the applicator level is 600 kJ: ($D= P_p \times T$; 600000 J = 500 W $\times$ 1200 s). For the PSWD mode, pulse frequency is set at 200 Hz, pulse duration at 400 μs, and application duration at 20 minutes; mean power (P_m) is thus equal to 40 W (40 W = 500 W $\times$ 0.0004 s $\times$ 200 Hz). The resulting dose equals 48 kJ (D = $P_m \times$ T; 48000 J = 40 W $\times$ 1200 s).

D. USE OF BOTH SCALES

There is no linear relationship between one scale and the other. For example, a relatively small amount of electromagnetic energy (e.g., 100 kJ) may be perceived by the patient as a comfortable dose (Dose III), whereas a greater amount of heat (e.g., 500 kJ) may be perceived by another patient as a mild dose (Dose II), depending on which body area was exposed and what methods and types of applicator are used. Consequently, it is strongly recommended that practitioners use both scales in determining the dosage to be delivered to their patients during therapy.

VI. EVIDENCE FOR INDICATIONS

A. GUIDED BY EVIDENCE

Dictionaries generally define "evidence" as anything that establishes a fact or gives reason to believe something. The aim of this textbook is to present scientific evidence behind therapeutic EPAs. To be guided by the evidence is the process of integrating the evidence from research, however imperfect or scarce this evidence may be, with clinical experience and patients' values. In other words, *evidence-based practice* of EPA requires that practitioners consider the evidence from research, as well as their own clinical experience and the patient's preference and beliefs about a given EPA, when the time comes to justify, prescribe, and apply the therapeutic agent. To be guided by evidence is a process, not a search for the absolute truth. Finally, a lack of evidence from research in favor of any given EPA does not mean that this EPA should never be used. What it means is that no statement can be made on its therapeutic effectiveness and that until more evidence from research is presented, its routine use cannot be recommended.

B. EVIDENCE FROM HUMAN RESEARCH

Box 10-2 provides evidence for SWD therapy based on an exhaustive search of published English-language, peer-reviewed studies on humans. The term *indication* is used in reference to a list of pathologies for which SWD therapy is applied. Ratings of therapeutic benefit (Yes or No) and a grading of the strength of scientific evidence (I, II, or III), as well as the reference, are included for each pathological condition.

1. Rating Therapeutic Benefit

The rating, expressed in Yes or No, is based on the overall conclusion(s) reached on the issue of therapeutic

Box 10-2	Research-Based Indications for the Use of Shortwave Diathermy		
PATHOLOGY	**BENEFIT**	**GRADE**	**REFERENCE**
Osteoarthritis	Yes	I	Hamilton et al., 1959
	Yes	I	Wright, 1964
	Yes	I	Jan et al., 2006
	Yes	II	Quirk et al., 1985
	Yes	II	Chamberlain et al., 1982
	Yes	II	Valtonen et al., 1975
	Yes	II	Bansil et al., 1975
	Yes	II	Lankhorst et al., 1982
	No	I	Callaghan et al., 2005
	No	I	Klaber-Moffett et al., 1996
	No	I	Clarke et al., 1974
	No	I	Svarcova et al., 1988
	No	II	Sylvester, 1990
	No	II	Jan et al., 1991
Ankle sprains—fractures	Yes	II	Wilson, 1972
	Yes	II	Wilson, 1974
	Yes	II	Pennington et al., 1993
	Yes	III	Seiger et al., 2006
	No	I	Pasila et al., 1978
	No	I	Barker et al., 1985
	No	I	McGill, 1988
Pressure sores	Yes	I	Comorosan et al., 1993
	Yes	II	Itoh et al., 1991
	Yes	II	Seaborne et al., 1996
Foot postoperative symptoms	Yes	I	Kaplan et al., 1968
	Yes	I	Santiesteban et al., 1985
Temporomandibular disorders	Yes	I	Gray et al., 1994
	Yes	II	Selby, 1985
Low-back pain	Yes	II	Wagstaff et al., 1986
	No	I	Gibson et al., 1985
Algoneurodystrophy	Yes	II	Comorosan et al., 1991

(Continued)

Box 10-2   Continued

PATHOLOGY	BENEFIT	GRADE	REFERENCE
Subdeltoid calcified bursitis	Yes	II	Ginsberg, 1961
Chronic neck pain	Yes	I	Foley-Nolan et al., 1990
Acute whiplash	Yes	I	Foley-Nolan et al., 1992
Wound healing	Yes	II	Cameron, 1964
Wound healing after blepharoplasty	Yes	II	Nicolle et al., 1982
Postsurgical dental symptoms	Yes	I	Aronofsky, 1971
Neck and back trigger points	Yes	II	McCray et al., 1984
Cutaneous graft healing	Yes	I	Goldin et al., 1981
Pelvic inflammation	Yes	III	Balogun et al., 1988
Hand lesions	Yes	I	Barclay et al., 1983
Ligamentous lesions	Yes	III	Wright, 1973
Herpes zoster	Yes	II	Allberry et al., 1974
Neck disorders	No	II	Dziedzic et al., 2005
Post inguinal herniorrhaphy pain	No	I	Reed et al., 1987
Perineal lesions after childbirth	No	I	Grant et al., 1989

effectiveness by the author(s) who conducted the peer-reviewed study.

2. Grading Strength of Evidence

The grading, numerically classified as I, II, and III, is based on the type of research methodology or experimental design used by the author(s). All those listed are studies on humans published in English-language, peer-reviewed journals. It follows that the strength of evidence in studies graded I is stronger than that in those graded II, which itself is stronger than in those graded III.

a. Grade I

Evidence based on *controlled* studies on humans, regardless of their level of randomization and blindness.

b. Grade II

Evidence based on *noncontrolled* studies on humans, regardless of their level of randomization and blindness.

c. Grade III

Evidence based on *case* studies on humans, regardless of their level of randomization and blindness.

3. Strength of Evidence Behind the Agent

The strength of evidence behind the agent, as presented in the research-based indication box, is arbitrarily assessed in this textbook as *weak, moderate,* or *strong*. For example, the larger the number of studies graded I, regardless of therapeutic benefit, the stronger the scientific evidence in support of the agent.

4. Strength of Justification for Usage of Agent

The strength of evidence justifying usage of the agent for an individual pathology or groups of pathologies, as listed in the research-based indication box, is arbitrarily assessed in this textbook as being *poor, fair, good,* or *conflicting*. For example, where a larger number of grade- studies on an agent, for any given pathology, show therapeutic benefit (Yes), compared to similar studies that report no benefit, the justification for the use of this agent to treat this pathology is assessed as *good*. *Conflicting* usage is reported when an equal number of studies with similar grades show both therapeutic benefit (Yes) and no benefit (No).

C. STRENGTH OF EVIDENCE AND JUSTIFICATION FOR USAGE

The results presented in **Box 10-2** show *moderate-to-strong* strength of evidence for the use of SWD, with most of the studies graded in a similar proportion as I and II. These results suggest *conflicting* justification for usage of this EPA for osteoarthritis and ankle sprain/fractures. They also show *poor* justification for all the remaining pathologies listed, with only a few studies showing benefits for each of them. Until more evidence from research is available with regard to the therapeu-

tic effectiveness of this EPA, its routine use *cannot be recommended*.

VII. CONTRAINDICATIONS

Table 10-2 outlines the contraindications associated with the practice of SWD therapy. Note that the contraindications listed apply to both delivery modes, that is, continuous (CSWD) and pulsed (PSWD), considering that PSWD, contrary to common belief, is also capable of significant and deep thermal effects on soft tissues.

TABLE 10-2	CONTRAINDICATIONS TO SHORTWAVE DIATHERMY THERAPY
CONTRAINDICATIONS	**RATIONALE**
Over body areas where sensation to heat is severely impaired	Risk of over dosage, leading to tissue burn.
Over patients with electronic implants	Risk of electronic interference with the implant caused by the electromagnetic field (Valtonen et al., 1975; Jones, 1976; Medtronic Ltd, 2001; FDA, 2002; Health and Welfare Canada, 2002).
Over patients with implanted electrical leads, *even if these leads are no longer connected to an implanted device or the device is not turned on*	Risk of excessive heating in the tissues surrounding the lead electrodes (Medtronic Ltd, 2001; FDA, 2002; Health and Welfare Canada, 2002).
Over surgically implanted metals, such as plates, rods, pins, and nails	Risk of tissue burn surrounding the implant caused by heating of implant (Kitchen et al., 1992; Kloth et al., 1996; Shields et al., 2004). A study on four patients with surgically implanted metals showed that the application of PSWD, with a mean power of 48 W, may be safe (Seiger et al., 2006). This result needs to be replicated on larger populations before surgically implanted metals can be removed from the contraindication list.
Over metallic objects externally worn by patients and other metallic objects, such as a table or chair, used to deliver the treatment	Risk of skin burn if these objects come in contact with the skin, as surface temperatures of metallic objects increases during therapy.
Over carcinogenic lesion	Risk of enhanced proliferation of cancer cells.
Over abdominal and pelvic areas of pregnant women	Risk of embryonic or fetal congenital malformations if uterine temperature exceeds 39°C (Lary et al., 1987; Docker et al., 1992).
Over abdominal and pelvic areas of women who are actively menstruating	Risk of inducing a hemorrhagic response.
Over hemorrhagic areas	Risk of enhancing a hemorrhagic response.
Over ischemic areas	Risk of tissue necrosis due to the fact that poor peripheral circulation associated with the ischemic disorder may lead to an inadequate thermoregulatory reaction to the thermal effect induced.
Over the testes	Risk of infertility due to the increased testicular temperature.
Over the eyes	Risk of eye damage due to the increased ocular temperature.
Over epiphyses of growing children	Risk of interfering with normal bone growth.

VIII. RISKS, PRECAUTIONS, AND RECOMMENDATIONS

The practice of SWD is not without risks. A female operator of the device is at risk of miscarriage and congenital abnormalities in offspring if she remains in the vicinity of the functioning device repetitively and for a relatively long period of time during therapy. The main risks associated with this EPA, as well as some precautions and recommendations designed to improve safety and effectiveness, are listed in **Table 10-3**. A recent study conducted in England by Shah et al. (2007) reveals that while departments report good practices and procedures regarding the use of therapeutic SWD devices, field observations have identified issues with potential to create health and safety problems.

IX. CONSIDERATIONS FOR APPLICATION AND DOCUMENTATION

A. CONSIDERATIONS AND PROCEDURES

The safe, effective, and optimal application of this EPA requires that clinicians go through a systematic set of considerations and procedures for each and every application. Presented below is a list of such considerations and procedures.

TABLE 10-3	RISKS, PRECAUTIONS, AND RECOMMENDATIONS FOR SHORTWAVE DIATHERMY THERAPY
RISKS	**RATIONALE**
Operator's overexposure* to electromagnetic field during treatment. * **Overexposure** is defined as an almost daily utilization of SWD devices during which the operator spends a few hours per day working/walking/standing between functioning devices.	Risk of miscarriage and higher incidence of congenital malformations in offspring due to stray (unwanted leakage) radiation generated at the applicator and chassis, as well as at the cable level. Current body of evidence indicates that this risk is small (Ouellet-Hellstrom et al., 1993) and not statistically significant (Källen et al., 1982; Logue et al., 1985; Taskinen et al., 1990; Larsen, 1991; Larsen et al., 1991; Guberan et al., 1994).
Over copper-bearing intrauterine devices	Risk of thermal damages to the lining of the uterus (Neilson et al., 1979; Heick et al., 1991).
PRECAUTIONS	**RATIONALE**
Functioning SWD device near other functioning EPA devices	May cause electronic interference (see recommendation below).
Operator's proximity to functioning SWD devices, cables, and applicators	May be overexposed to stray radiation (see recommendation below).
Neighboring patients and personnel wearing implanted electronic devices	May be exposed to stray radiation (see recommendation below).
Patients with mental confusion	May lead to improper dosimetry.
RECOMMENDATIONS	**RATIONALE**
Check device functioning prior to treatment using a neon tube	Because shortwave radiation is invisible to the human eye, the use of a neon tube is necessary to ascertain that electromagnetic radiation is emitted.
Keep the functioning SWD devices at least 5 m (15 ft) from all other functioning therapeutic EPA devices.	Minimize electronic interference.
Remain at least 1 m (3 ft) from any functioning SWD devices and 0.5 m (1.5 ft) from their cables and applicators.	Minimize operator's body exposure to stray radiation (Stuchly et al., 1982; Health and Welfare Canada, 1983; Martin et al., 1990; Docker et al., 1992). Tzima et al. (1994) specifically recommend that the operator remain 1 m (3 ft)

(Continued)

TABLE 10-3	CONTINUED

RECOMMENDATIONS	RATIONALE
	from functioning CSWD devices and 0.5–0.8 m (1.5–2 ft) from PSWD devices.
Keep neighboring staff and patients at least 5 m (15 ft) from any functioning SWD device	Minimize body exposure to stray radiation (Docker et al., 1992; Kitchen et al., 1992).
Pregnant operators **must avoid overexposure** to SWD devices	Overexposure to the electromagnetic field generated by SWD devices (see contraindication above) may be potentially harmful, causing miscarriage and congenital malformations (Martin et al., 1990; Taskinen et al., 1990; Docker et al., 1992; Ouellet-Hellstrom et al., 1993; Lerman et al., 2001). Occasional exposure poses no risk.
Use adequate layers of toweling at the applicator/skin interface	Will absorb the sweat during treatment. Sweat bubbles on the skin act as a lens, focusing the beam of radiation and leading to potential skin burn.
Avoid contact between the applicator and the exposed skin surface	Prevent any contact skin burn.
Avoid touching the chassis, cables, and applicators of a functioning SWD device	Clearly instruct the patient not to touch, thus preventing electrical shock if the integrity of electric isolation is lost (see Chapter 27).
Plug line-powered SWD device into GFCI receptacles	Prevent the occurrence of macroshocks (see Chapter 27).
Conduct regular maintenance and calibration procedures	Ensure optimal therapeutic efficacy and effectiveness. Follow the recommended maintenance schedules outlined by manufacturers.

1. Checklists

Before proceeding with treatment, always go through the list of contraindications (**Table 10-2**) and list of risks, precautions, and recommendations (**Table 10-3**).

2. Thermal Sensory Discrimination

Always assess the patient's capacity for thermal sensory discrimination (see Chapter 25 for details) and record the result in the patient's chart.

3. Skin Preparation

Clean the skin area under the applicators by rubbing the skin with alcohol. Ensure that the radiated body part is free of externally worn metal, such as jewelry, and that the table and chair used for therapy are free of metal.

4. Delivery Modes

Select between the continuous (CSWD) and pulsed (PSWD) mode of delivery. Recall that the application of PSWD, even at low power outputs, can induce significant and deep thermal effects in soft tissues.

5. Device Testing

Prior to each treatment, test whether the SWD device is functioning by turning on the power output while moving,

in front of the applicator, the neon test tube provided by the manufacturer. If the device is functioning, the neon gas within the tube will glow under the effect of electromagnetic radiation. The rationale behind such testing is that SWD devices generate invisible rays.

6. Application Methods

SWD, whether in CSWD or PSWD mode, is applied in either of two methods: capacitive and inductive. The *capacitive* method is delivered using two types of applicators: rigid plates, which are encased in plastic housing, and flexible pads. The *inductive* method is also delivered using two types of applicators: rigid coils encased in plastic housing, also called drums, and flexible cables. Shown in **Figure 10-5** are clinical applications of capacitive (**A**) and inductive (**B**) applicators. These applicators come in various shapes and sizes to fit the part of the body being treated.

a. Capacitive Method

This method is called capacitive because the applicator arrangement is similar to that of a *capacitor*, meaning two metallic plates (i.e., a pair of rigid or flexible applicators) separated by a dielectric (i.e., the treated body segment). In this method, two capacitive-type electrodes are positioned on either side of the body segment being treated, as

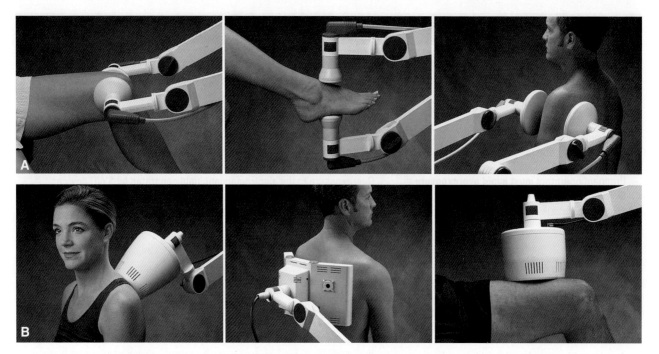

FIGURE 10-5 Typical applications of capacitive (**A**) and inductive (**B**) applicators. (Courtesy of Mettler Electronics.)

illustrated in **Figure 10-5A** concerning cases of the knee, foot, and shoulder areas.

i. Electrical Field. The high-frequency alternating current (27.12 MHz) flowing between the two plates and through the patient's body area being treated produces a strong *electrical field,* which induces ionic oscillatory and dipole rotational movements. These microscopic movements cause kinetic energy, which is then converted into thermal (heat) energy in the exposed tissues (see **Fig 10-4**).

ii. Heat Absorption and Distribution. When SWD is delivered using the capacitive method, the heat will mainly be absorbed and distributed in soft tissues with low electrolyte levels, low water content, or high electrical impedance, such as skin and subcutaneous fat. With this method of delivery, therefore, the greater the thickness of subcutaneous fat in the treated body segment, as illustrated in **Figure 10-6A** (left), the more superficial the heat absorption and distribution will be.

iii. Using SWD on Body Areas With Low Subcutaneous Fat. The rationale for using SWD rather than other thermal agents is that this agent helps to heat soft tissues such as muscles, tendons, ligaments, and joint capsules. Skin can be heated with any thermal agent, and subcutaneous fat is very rarely a tissue one wants to heat for therapeutic reasons. Where, then, on the body should the capacitive method be used? This method should be used on body areas with low subcutaneous fat, such as the knee, foot, and shoulder (see **Fig 10-5A**). It can also be used over other body areas like thighs, arms, and the back if the patient has a low body fat index, as illustrated in **Figure 10-6A**. This method should not be used on overweight and obese patients.

b. Inductive Method

This method is called inductive because the application involves the use of an inductor, that is, a coil of metal wire housed in a plastic case (drum). **Figure 10-6B** shows the use of three different inductive drum-type applicators over the upper back, lower back, and thigh, respectively.

i. Magnetic Field and Eddy Currents. The flow of a high-frequency alternating current in the coil generates a changing magnetic field, which interacts with the treated body segment to then induce eddy currents in the exposed tissues. The flow of these eddy currents in the exposed tissues causes ionic and dipole movements, which produce heat in the exposed tissues (see **Fig 10-4**).

ii. Heat Absorption and Distribution. When SWD is delivered using the inductive method, the heat will mainly be absorbed and distributed in soft tissues with either high electrolyte levels and high water content or low electrical impedance, such as muscle and the synovial fluid of joint capsules.

iii. Using SWD on Body Areas With High Water Content. The inductive method should be used if the purpose is to heat the deepest layers of soft tissues, regardless of the thickness of the subcutaneous fat covering them, as illustrated in **Figure 10-6B**.

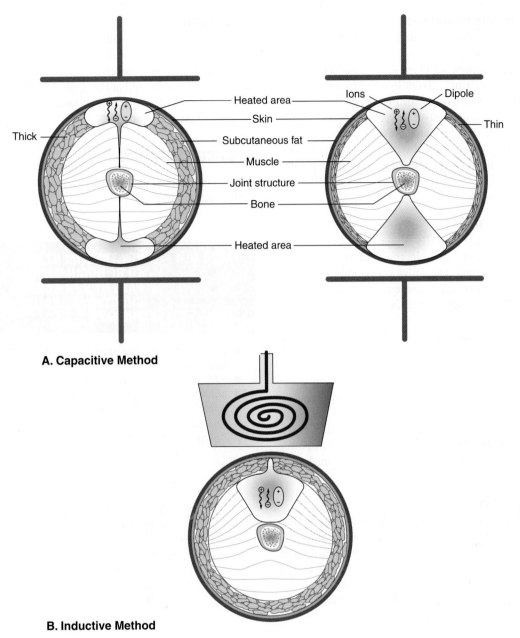

A. Capacitive Method

B. Inductive Method

FIGURE 10-6 Schematic representation of heat distribution patterns, with ions and dipoles, in the exposed soft tissues during SWD therapy. (**A**) The theorized heat distribution pattern achieved using a pair of capacitive applicators over a body segment (cross-sectional view) with a thicker (left) and thinner (right) layer of subcutaneous fat. (**B**) The theorized heat distribution pattern achieved using an inductive drum applicator.

c. Review

The capacitive method is used over body areas with minimal subcutaneous fat (shoulder, elbow, wrist, hand; knee, ankle, foot) because energy absorption occurs mostly in subcutaneous fat tissue. The inductive method is applied over the remaining body areas (neck, back, hip, thigh, leg) because energy absorption occurs mostly in tissues with large water content, such as muscles.

7. Coupling Medium: Air Space

Electromagnetic waves travel well in space, and consequently no direct contact is needed between the applica-tor and the skin surface. An air space, however, is needed because the applicator's surface should *never* come in contact with bare skin during therapy (risk of skin burn). This air space is the coupling medium. A layer of dry toweling is used to absorb the buildup of sweat from the exposed skin during treatment in order to prevent direct contact between the applicator's surface and the skin.

8. Applicator/Skin Surface Distance

The applicators should be positioned at a distance of approximately 2–3 cm from the skin surface.

9. Laws Governing Application

Four laws govern the application of SWD: Grotthus-Draper, Arnd-Schultz, inverse square, and Lambert's cosine laws (see Chapter 5). These laws stipulate that for SWD to induce thermal effects in soft tissues, electromagnetic energy must first be absorbed (Grotthus-Draper law), that a certain amount of energy is needed (Arnd-Schultz law), that the applicator must be positioned relatively close to the skin surface (the inverse square law), and that the applicator surface must be positioned parallel to the treated skin surface to minimize beam reflection (Lambert's cosine law).

10. Device Preparation

Ensure that the SWD device is kept at least 3 m (10 feet) from any other functioning electrical EPAs. Determine the application method (capacitive versus inductive), and select the appropriate applicator type and applicator arrangement. Position each applicator while assuring an air space of 2–3 cm at the applicator–skin surface interface. Cover the exposed skin area with a layer of dry towel to absorb sweat.

11. Dosimetry

Select dosages, using both the qualitative and quantitative scales, that will best meet the severity of the pathological condition and the desired therapeutic goals. Remember that PSWD, delivered at a relatively low power output, can induce important thermal effects in deeper soft tissues.

12. During Treatment

Ensure that the patient is comfortably positioned so that continuous electronic resonance is maintained throughout treatment. Instruct the patient to minimize movement of the exposed body segment. Inform the patient that if something were to go wrong during treatment, he or she can immediately stop the device simply by pulling on the rope attached to the device's operating switch.

13. End of Treatment

Inspect the exposed skin surface and question the patient on the level of heat he or she has perceived during treatment (qualitative dose received). Also, record the quantitative dose (kJ) delivered at the applicator/skin surface. In the patient's file, document any unusual sensation that the patient felt during treatment.

B. DOCUMENTATION

Table 10-4 shows the key parameters to be documented in the patient's file.

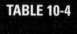 TABLE 10-4	KEY TREATMENT PARAMETERS TO BE DOCUMENTED IN PATIENT'S FILE AFTER SHORTWAVE DIATHERMY THERAPY

- *Skin sensory thermal discrimination testing:* result (see Chapter 25)
- *SWD device type:* portable or cabinet
- *Mode of delivery:* CSWD or PSWD
- *Application method:* capacitive or inductive
- *Applicator:* plate or drum
- *Dosage:* qualitative: Dose I, II, III, or IV

    Quantitative:
    For CSWD:
    - Peak power: W
    - Duration of application: S
    - Dose: kJ

    For PSWD:
    - Mean power: W
    - Duration of application: S
    - Dose: kJ

Case Study 10-1   Ankle Joint Stiffness

A 48-year-old man, the victim of a baseball-related ankle injury, is referred for treatment by his orthopedic surgeon, who has just removed his patient's 6-week-old cast. No surgical intervention was needed; the severe ankle sprain was treated with cast immobilization. The patient's main complaints are right ankle stiffness and difficulty walking. Physical examination reveals no sign of inflammation, no swelling, and a lack of ankle dorsiflexion (–18 degrees) caused by triceps surae contracture and ankle joint ankylosis. There is also marked plantiflexor and dorsiflexor muscle atrophy (–2 cm) and weakness (35% force deficit). The patient has difficulty walking, as well as climbing and descending stairs. He is pain-free when at rest and when he bears weight on his injured right ankle. The patient's goals are to resume normal activities of daily living (ADLs) and return to play baseball as soon as possible. The treating practitioner, who operates the SWD device, is 5 months pregnant.

Evidence-Based Steps Toward the Resolution of This Case

1. List medical diagnosis.

Third-degree ankle sprain.

2. List key impairment(s).
- Triceps surae contracture
- Ankle joint ankylosis
- Plantarflexor/dorsiflexor muscle atrophy
- Ankle muscle weakness

3. List key functional limitation(s).
- Difficulty walking
- Difficulty climbing and descending stairs
- Difficulty with ADLs

4. List key disability/disabilities.
- Unable to play baseball

5. Justification for SWD Therapy.

Is there justification for the use of SWD therapy in this case? This chapter has established that there is *moderate* strength and *conflicting* justification for the use of SWD for ankle pathology (see Section VI. Evidence for Indications). So where is the justification for using SWD? It is justified because this agent can induce significant and deep muscle heating in healthy human muscles, as well as increase elasticity in the triceps surea muscles (Wilson, 1972, 1974; Draper et al., 1999; Garrett et al., 2000; Draper et al., 2002; Peres et al., 2002; Draper et al., 2004; Brucker et al., 2005). In this case, the decrease in dor-

siflexion ankle range of motion and ankle joint stiffness are primarily caused by the triceps surea contracture (reduced muscle elasticity) induced by the 6-week cast period. The application of CSWD is expected to induce significant heating at the calf musculotendinous area and at the ankle joint periarticular structures. This deep-heating effect is expected to increase calf muscle tendon elasticity and decrease joint viscosity. Together, these effects are expected to reduce contracture and joint stiffness, thus leading to a more functional ankle joint. SWD therapy is preferred to hot pack therapy (Chapter 6) because it induces deeper thermal effects with minimal skin heating. SWD therapy is also preferred to ultrasound therapy (Chapter 20) because the treated surface area is much larger than the maximum ultrasound applicator surface area. In other words, ultrasound therapy is not suitable for this condition because multiple or longer applications will be needed, adding unacceptable additional time to the delivery of therapy. PSWD is used here, but CSWD could be used as well. Because EPAs should never be used in isolation or as a sole intervention, a regimen of passive and active ankle stretching and plantiflexor/dorsiflexor muscles strengthening is used here concomitantly with SWD therapy.

6. Search for contraindications.

None are found.

7. Search for risks and precautions.

The treating practitioner, who operates the SWD in this case, is 5 months pregnant. Is she at risk? No, because she seldom (3–5 applications per week) uses SWD therapy in her daily workload. In other words, the use of SWD therapy poses negligible risk to her pregnancy because her work organization shows that she is **not** overexposed to it (see **Table 10-3**).

8. Outline the therapeutic goal(s) you and your patient wish to achieve.
- Decrease triceps surea contracture
- Increase ankle joint dorsiflexion
- Improve gait
- Improve ability to climb and descend stairs
- Accelerate return to normal ADLs
- Accelerate return to playing baseball

9. List the outcome measurement(s) used to assess treatment effectiveness.
- Ankle range of motion: goniometry
- Gait/stair/ADL performance: Patient-Specific Functional Scale (PSFS)

(Continued)

Case Study 10-1 Continued

10. **Instruct the patient about what he/she should experience, do, or not do during the SWD treatment.**
    - Sensation: comfortable heat (dose III)
    - Do not move your affected lower limb during treatment

11. **Outline the prescription of SWD based on the evidence available.**

    The prescription below is partly based on studies on healthy subjects (Draper et al., 1999; Garrett et al., 2000; Draper et al., 2002; Peres et al., 2002; Draper et al., 2004; Brucker et al., 2005) and patients affected with an ankle pathology (Wilson, 1972, 1974; Pennington et al., 1993; Seiger et al., 2006).

    - *SWD device:* 27.12 MHz; cabinet type
    - *Delivery mode:* CSWD
    - *Peak power:* 200 W
    - *Pulse duration:* 400 μsec
    - *Pulse frequency:* 800 Hz
    - *Resulting mean power:* 64 W
    - *Application duration:* 20 min
    - *Dose delivered at the applicator–skin interface:* 76.8 kJ
    - *Application site:* Over the triceps surae musculotendinous area
    - *Applicator type and surface area of applicator:* Inductive drum; 200 cm^2
    - *Spacing between applicator and skin surface:* 2 cm air space with one layer of dry towel

    - *Number and frequency of treatments:* 9, delivered 3 times a week for 3 weeks.

12. **Analyze outcome measurements.**

    Pre- and posttreatment comparison:
    - Right ankle ROM: gain of 22 degrees dorsiflexion (from –18 to –4 degrees)
    - Walk/stair/ADL performance: PSFS score improved by 100%
    - Leisure: accelerated return to baseball

13. **Assess treatment effectiveness based on outcome measures.**

    The results show that nine PSWD treatments applied over the triceps surea's musculotendinous area, immediately followed by a regimen of ankle-stretching and strengthening programs, delivered over a 3-week period, led to a 22 degrees improvement in ankle dorsiflexion, which translated to a normal ability to walk, climb, and descend stairs, as well as do all ADLs. This treatment approach has also accelerated his return to his favorite sport, baseball. Overall, this therapeutic approach had a beneficial effect on the patient's disablement status created by the pathology, as illustrated in the **figure below**.

14. **State the prognosis.**

    The prognosis is excellent if the patient further strengthens his right ankle before returning to baseball.

THERAPEUTIC IMPACT on Disablement

CRITICAL THINKING QUESTIONS

Clarification: What is meant by shortwave diathermy (SWD) therapy?

Assumptions: You have assumed that the inductive method may be superior to the capacitive method for inducing heat in deeper soft tissues. How do you justify making that assumption?

Reasons and evidence: What led you to believe, contrary to common belief in the field, that the application of PSWD at a relatively low dose is capable of inducing significant thermal effect in deeper tissues such as muscle?

Viewpoints or perspectives: How would you respond to a pregnant colleague who says that working regularly with SWD devices poses no risk to her and her unborn child?

Implications and consequences: What are the implications, and possible consequences, of treating a patient who reports having worn an implantable electronic device a few years ago?

About the question: Is there any scientific evidence in studies on humans that PSWD induces nonthermal effects in soft tissues? Why do you think I ask this question?

References

Articles

Allberry J, Manning FR, Smith EE (1974) Shortwave diathermy for herpes zoster. Physiotherapy, 60: 386

Aronofsky DH (1971) Reduction of dental post-surgical symptoms using non thermal pulsed high-peak-power electromagnetic energy. Oral Surg, 32: 688–696

Balogun JA, Okonofua FE (1988) Management of chronic pelvic inflammation disease with shortwave diathermy. A case report. Phys Ther, 68: 1541–1545

Bansil CK, Joshi JB (1975) Effectiveness of shortwave diathermy and ultrasound in the treatment of osteoarthritis of the knee joint. Med J Zambia, 9: 138–139

Barclay V, Collier R, Jones A (1983) Treatment of various hand injuries by pulsed electromagnetic energy (Diapulse). Physiotherapy, 69: 186–188

Barker AT, Barlow PS, Porter J, Smith ME, Clifton S, Andrews L, O'Dowd WJ (1985) A double-blind clinical trial of low-power pulsed shortwave therapy in the treatment of a soft tissue injury. Physiotherapy, 71: 500–504

Brucker JB, Knight KL, Rubley MD, Draper DO (2005) An 18-day stretching regimen, with or without pulsed, shortwave diathermy, and ankle dorsiflexion after 3 weeks. J Athl Train, 40: 276–280

Callaghan MJ, Whittaker PE, Grimes S, Smith L (2005) An evaluation of pulsed shortwave diathermy on knee osteoarthritis using radioleucoscintigraphy: A randomized, double blind, controlled trial. Joint Bone Spine, 72: 150–155

Cameron BM (1964) A three-phase evaluation of pulsed, high frequency, radio short waves (Diapulse) on 646 patients. Am J Orthop, 6: 72–78

Chamberlain MA, Care G, Harfied B (1982) Physiotherapy in osteoarthrosis of the knees. A controlled trial of hospital versus home exercises. Int Rehab Med, 4: 101–106

Clarke GR, Willis LA, Stenners L, Nichols PJ (1974) Evaluation of physiotherapy in the treatment of osteoarthrosis of the knee. Rheum Rehab, 13: 190–197

Comorosan S, Pana L, Pop L, Cracium C, Cirlea AM, Paslarv L (1991) The influence of pulsed high peak power electromagnetic energy (Diapulse) treatment on posttraumatic algoneurodystrophies. Rev Roum Physiol, 28: 77–81

Comorosan S, Vasilco R, Arghiropol M, Paslaru L, Jieanu V, Stelea S (1993) The effect of diapulse therapy on the healing of decubitus ulcer. Rom J Physiol, 30: 41–45

Docker M, Bazin S, Dyson M, Kirk DC, Kitchen S, Low J, Simpson G (1992) Guidelines for the safe use of continuous shortwave therapy equipment. Physiotherapy, 78: 755–757

Draper DO, Castro JL, Feland B, Schulties S, Egget D (2004) Shortwave diathermy and prolonged stretching increase hamstring flexibility more than prolonged stretching alone. J Orthop Sports Phys Ther, 34: 13–30

Draper DO, Knight K, Fujiwara T, Castel JC (1999) Temperature change in human muscle during and after pulsed shortwave diathermy. J Orthop Sports Phys Ther, 29: 13–22

Draper DO, Miner L, Knight KL, Ricard MD (2002) The carry-over effects of diathermy and stretching in developing hamstring flexibility. J Athl Train, 37: 37–42

Dziedzic K, Hill J, Lewis MS, Sim J, Daniels J, Hay EM (2005) Effectiveness of manual therapy or pulsed shortwave diathermy in addition to advice and exercise for neck disorders: A pragmatic randomized controlled trial in physical therapy clinics. Arthritis Rheum, 53: 214–222

Foley-Nolan D, Barry C, Coughlan RJ, O'Connor P, Roden D (1990) Pulsed high frequency (27 MHz) electromagnetic therapy for persistent neck pain. A double blind, placebo-controlled study of 20 patients. Orthopedics, 13: 445–451

Foley-Nolan D, Moore K, Codd M, Barry C, O'Connor P, Coughlan RJ (1992) Low energy high frequency pulsed electromagnetic therapy for acute whiplash injuries. Scand J Rehab Med, 24: 51–59

Garrett CL, Draper DO, Knight KL, Durrant E (2000) Heat distribution in the lower leg from pulsed short wave diathermy and ultrasound treatments. J Athl train, 35: 50–55

Gibson T, Grahame R, Harkness J, Woo P, Blagrave P, Hills R (1985) Controlled comparison of shortwave diathermy treatment with osteopathic treatment in non-specific low back pain. Lancet, 1 (8440): 1258–1261

Ginsberg AJ (1961) Pulsed shortwave in treatment of bursitis with calcification. Int Rec Med, 174: 71–75

Goldin JH, Broadbent NR, Nancarrow JD, Marshall T (1981) The effects of Diapulse on the healing of wounds: A double blind randomized controlled trial in man. Br J Plast Surg, 34: 267–270

Grant A, Sleep J, McIntosh M, Ashurst H (1989) Ultrasound and pulsed electromagnetic energy treatment for the perineal trauma: A randomized placebo-controlled trial. Br J Obstet Gynaecol, 96: 434–439

Gray RJ, Quayle, AA, Hall CA, Schofield MA (1994) Physiotherapy in the treatment of temporomandibular joint disorders: A comparative study of four treatment methods. Br Dent J, 176: 257–261

Guberan E, Campana A, Faval P, Guberan M, Sweetnam PM, Tuyn JW, Usel M (1994) Gender ratio of offspring and exposure to shortwave radiation among female physiotherapists. Scand J Work Environ Health, 20: 345–348

Hamilton DE, Bywaters EG, Please NW (1959) A controlled trial of various forms of physiotherapy in arthritis. Br Med J, 2: 542–545

Heick A, Esperson T, Pedersen HL, Raahauge J (1991) Is diathermy safe in women with copper-bearing IUDs? Acta Obstet Gynecol Scand, 70: 153–155

Itoh M, Montemayor JS, Matsumoto E, Eason A, Lee MH, Folk FS (1991) Accelerated wound healing of pressure ulcers by pulsed high peak power electromagnetic energy (Diapulse). Decubitus, 4: 24–25

Jan MH, Lai JS (1991) The effect of physiotherapy on osteoarthritic knees of females. J Formos Med Assoc, 90: 1008–1013

Jan MH, Chai HM, Wang CL, Lin YF, Tsai LY (2006) Effects of repetitive shortwave diathermy for reducing synovitis in patients with knee osteoarthritis: An ultrasonic study. Phys Ther, 86: 236–244

Jones SL (1976) Electromagnetic field interference and cardiac pacemakers. Phys Ther, 56: 1013–1018

Klaber-Moffett JA, Richardson PH, Frost H, Osborn A (1996) A placebo-controlled double-blind trial to evaluate the effectiveness of pulsed shortwave therapy for osteoarthritic hip and knee pain. Pain, 67: 121–127

Källen B, Malmquist G, Moritz U (1982) Delivery outcome among physiotherapists in Sweden. Is nonionizing radiation a fetal hazard? Arch Environ Health, 37: 81–85

Kaplan EG, Weinstock RE (1968) Clinical evaluation of Diapulse as adjunctive therapy following foot surgery. J Am Podiatr Assoc, 58: 218–221

Lankhorst GJ, van de Stadt RJ, van der Korst JK, Hinlopen-Bonrath E, Griffioen FM, de Boer W (1982) Relationship of isometric knee extension torque and functional variables in osteoarthrosis of the knee. Scand J Rehab Med, 14: 7–10

Larsen AI (1991) Congenital malformations and exposure to high-frequency electromagnetic radiation among Danish physiotherapists. Scand J Work Environ Health, 17: 318–323

Larsen AI, Olsen J, Svane O (1991) Gender-specific reproductive outcome and exposure to high-frequency electromagnetic radiation among physiotherapists. Scand J Work Environ Health, 17: 324–329

Lary J, Conover D (1987) Teratogenic effects of radiofrequency radiation. IEEE Eng Med Biol Mag, 6: 42–46

Lerman Y, Jacubovich R, Green MS (2001) Pregnancy outcome following exposure to shortwaves among female physiotherapist in Israel. Am J Ind Med, 39: 499–504

Logue JN, Hamburger S, Silverman PM, Chiacchierini RP (1985) Congenital anomalies and paternal occupational exposure to shortwave, microwave, infrared and acoustic radiation. J Occup Med, 27: 451–452

Martin CJ, McCallum HM, Heaton B (1990) An evaluation of radiofrequency exposure from therapeutic diathermy equipment in the light of current recommendations. Clin Phys Physiol Meas, 11: 53–63

McCray RE, Patton NJ (1984) Pain relief at trigger points: A comparison of moist heat and shortwave diathermy. J Orthop Sports Phys Ther, 51: 175–178

McGill SN (1988) The effect of pulsed shortwave therapy on lateral ligament sprain of the ankle. N Z J Physiother, 10: 21–24

Neilson NC, Hansen R, Laesen T (1979) Heat induction in copper-bearing IUDs during shortwave diathermy. Acta Obstet Gynecol Scand, 58: 495

Nicolle FV, Bentall RM (1982) The use of radiofrequency pulsed energy in the control of postoperative reaction to blepharoplasty. Aesthetic Plast Surg, 6: 169–171

Ouellet-Hellstrom R, Stewart WF (1993) Miscarriages among female physical therapists who report using radio-and microwave-frequency electromagnetic radiation. Am J Epidemiol, 138: 775–786

Pasila M, Visuri T, Sundholm A (1978) Pulsating shortwave diathermy: Value in the treatment of recent ankle and foot sprains. Arch Phys Med Rehab, 59: 383–386

Pennington GM, Danley DL, Sumko MH, Bucknell A, Nelson JH (1993) Pulsed, non-thermal, high-frequency electromagnetic energy (DIAPULSE) in the treatment of grade I and II ankle sprains. Mil Med, 158: 101–104

Peres SE, Draper DO, Knight KL, Ricard MD (2002) Pulse shortwave diathermy and prolonged long-duration stretching increase dorsiflexion range of motion more than identical stretching without diathermy. J Athl Train, 37: 43–50

Quirk AS, Newman RJ, Newman KJ (1985) An evaluation of interferential therapy, shortwave diathermy and exercise in treatment of osteoarthritis of the knee. Physiotherapy, 71: 55–57

Reed MW, Bickerstaff DR, Hayne CR, Wyman A, Davies J (1987) Pain relief after inguinal herniorrhaphy. Ineffectiveness of pulsed electromagnetic energy. Br J Clin Pract, 41: 782–784

Santiesteban AJ, Grant C (1985) Post-surgical effect of pulsed shortwave therapy. J Am Podiat Med, 75: 306–309

Seaborne D, Quirion-De Girardi C, Rousseau M, Rivest M, Lambert J (1996) The treatment of pressure sores using pulsed electromagnetic energy (PEME). Physiother Can, 48: 131–137

Seiger C, Draper DO (2006) Use of pulsed shortwave diathermy and joint mobilization to increase ankle range of motion in the presence of surgical implanted metal: A case series. J Orthop Sports Phys Ther, 36: 669–677

Selby A (1985) Physiotherapy in the management of temporomandibular joint disorders. Austr Dent J, 30: 273–280

Shah SG, Farrow A (2007) Investigation of practices and procedures in the use of therapeutic diathermy: A study from the physiotherapist's health and safety perspectives. Physioth Res Int, 12: 228–241

Shields N, Gormley J, O'Hare N (2004) Short-wave diathermy: Current clinical and safety practices. Physioth Res Int, 7: 191–202

Stuchly MA, Repacholi MH, Lecuyer DW, Mann RD (1982) Exposure to the operator and patient during shortwave diathermy treatments. Health Physics, 42: 341–366

Svarcova J, Trnavsky K, Zvarova J (1988) The influence of ultrasound, galvanic currents and shortwave diathermy on pain intensity in patients with osteoarthritis. Scand J Rheumatol (Suppl), 67: 83–85

Sylvester KL (1990) Investigation of the effect of hydrotherapy in the treatment of osteoarthritic hips. Clin Rehab, 4: 223–228

Taskinen H, Kyyronen P, Hemminki K (1990) Effects of ultrasound, shortwave, and physical exertion on pregnancy outcome in physiotherapists. J Epidemiol Community Health, 44: 196–201

Tzima E, Martin CJ (1994) An evaluation of safe practices to restrict exposure to electric and magnetic fields from therapeutic and surgical diathermy equipment. Physiol Meas, 15: 201–206

Valtonen EJ, Alaranta H (1971) Comparative clinical study of the effect of shortwave and longwave diathermy on osteoarthritis of the knee and hip. Scand J Rehab Med, 3: 109–112

Valtonen EJ, Lilius HG, Tiula C (1975) Disturbances in the function of cardiac pacemakers by shortwave and microwave diathermies and pulsed high frequency currents. Ann Clin Gynaecol Fenn, 64: 284–287

Wagstaff P, Wagstaff S, Downey M (1986) A pilot study to compare the efficacy of continuous and pulsed magnetic energy (shortwave diathermy) on the relief of low back pain. Physiotherapy, 72: 563–566

Wilson DH (1972) Treatment of soft tissue injuries by pulsed electrical energy. Br Med J, 2: 269–270

Wilson DH (1974) Comparison of shortwave diathermy and pulsed electromagnetic energy in treatment of soft tissue injuries. Physiotherapy, 60: 309–310

Wright GG (1973) Treatment of soft tissue and ligamentous injuries in professional footballers. Physiotherapy, 59: 385–387

Wright V (1964) Treatment of osteoarthritis of the knees. Ann Rheum Dis, 23: 389–391

Review Articles

Delpizzo V, Joyner KH (1989). On the safe use of microwave and shortwave diathermy units. Austr J Physiother, 33: 152–162

Goats GC (1989) Continuous shortwave (radio-frequency) diathermy. Br J Sports Med, 23: 123–127

Hayne CR (1984) Pulsed high frequency energy: Its place in physiotherapy. Physiotherapy, 70: 459–466

Kitchen S, Partridge C (1992) Review of shortwave diathermy continuous and pulsed patterns. Physiotherapy, 78: 243–252

Marks R, Ghassemi M, Duarte R, van Nguyen JP (1999) A review of the literature on shortwave diathermy as applied to osteoarthritis of the knee. Physiotherapy, 85: 304–316

Martin CJ, McCallum HM, Strelley S, Heaton B (1991) Electromagnetic fields from therapeutic diathermy equipment: A review of hazards and precautions. Physiotherapy, 77: 3–7

Shields N, Gormley J, O'Hare N (2001a) Short-wave diathermy: A review of existing clinical trials. Phys Ther Rev, 6: 1001–118

Shields N, Gormley J, O'Hare N (2001b) Short-wave diathermy in Irish physiotherapy departments. Br J Ther Rehab, 8: 331–339

Shields N, Gormley J, O'Hare N (2002) Short-wave diathermy: Current clinical and safety practice. Physioth Res Int, 7: 191–2002

Shields N, O'Hare N, Gormley J (2004) Contra-indications to shortwave diathermy: Survey of Irish physiotherapists. Physiotherapy, 90: 42–53

Weinberger A, Lev A (1991) Temperature elevation of connective tissue by physical modalities. Crit Rev Phys Med Rehab Med, 3: 121–146

Chapters of Textbooks

Cameron MH, Perez D, Otano-Lata S (2003) Electromagnetic radiation. In: Physical Agents in Rehabilitation: From Research to Practice, 3rd ed. Cameron MH (Ed). WB Saunders Co., Philadelphia, pp 369–413

Day MJ, Katz, JS (2006) Diathermy. In: Integrating Physical Agents in Rehabilitation, 2nd ed. Hecox B, Mehreteab TA, Weisberg J, Sanko J (Eds). Prentice Hall, Upper Saddle River, pp 215–238

Guy AW (1990) Biophysics of high-frequency currents and electromagnetic radiation. In: Therapeutic Heat and Cold, 4th ed. Lehmann JF (Ed). Williams & Wilkins, Baltimore, pp 179–236

Khan J (2000) High-frequency currents—Shortwave diathermy. In: Principles and Practice of Electrotherapy, 4th ed. Churchill Livingstone, New York, pp 5–19

Kloth LC, Ziskin MC (1996) Diathermy and pulsed radio frequency radiation. In: Thermal Agents in Rehabilitation, 3rd ed. Michlovitz SL (Ed). FA Davis Co., Philadelphia, pp 213–254

Knight KL, Draper DO (2008) Diathermy. In: Therapeutic Modalities: The Art and Science. Lippincott Williams & Wilkins, Philadelphia, pp 284–300

Lehmann JF, De Lateur BJ (1990) Therapeutic heat. In: Therapeutic Heat and Cold, 4th ed. Lehmann JF (Ed). Williams & Wilkins, Baltimore, pp 417–581

Low J (1988) Shortwave diathermy, microwave, ultrasound and interferential therapy. In: Pain Management in Physical Therapy. Wells PE, Frampton V, Bowsher D (Eds). Appleton & Lange, Norwalk, pp 113–132

Low J, Reed A (1990) Electromagnetic fields: Shortwave diathermy, pulsed electromagnetic energy and magnetic therapies. In: Electrotherapy Explained: Principles and Practice. Butterworth-Heinemann, London, pp 221–254

Low J, Reed A (1994) Waves. In: Physical Principles Explained. Butterworth-Heineman, London, p 33

Michaelson SM (1990) Bioeffects of high-frequency currents and electromagnetic radiation. In: Therapeutic Heat and Cold, 4th ed. Lehmann JF (Ed). Williams & Wilkins, Baltimore, pp 237–361

Prentice WE, Draper DO (1998) Shortwave and microwave diathermy. In: Therapeutic Modalities for Allied Health Professionals. Prentice WE (Ed). McGraw-Hill, New York, pp 169–200

Scott S (2002) Diathermy. In: Electrotherapy Evidence-Based Practice, 11th ed. Kitchen S, Bazin S (Eds). Churchill Livingstone, London, pp 145–165

Starkey C (2004a) Shortwave diathermy. In: Therapeutic Modalities, 3rd ed. FA Davis Co, Philadelphia, pp 184–191

Starkey C (2004b) Clinical application of shortwave diathermy. In: Therapeutic Modalities, 3rd ed. FA Davis Co, Philadelphia, pp 192–202

Specialized Documents

American National Standards Institute (ANSI) (1982) Safety levels with respect to human exposure to radio frequency electromagnetic fields, 300 KHz to 100 GHz. ANSI, Washington, DC

Australian Physiotherapy Association (2001) Guidelines for the Clinical Use of Electrophysical Agents—2001.

Food and Drug Administration (FDA) (2002) Public Health Notification: Diathermy interaction with implanted leads and implanted systems with leads.

Food and Drug Code of Federal Regulations (1995) 21 Parts 800 to 1299. Office of the Federal National Archives and Records, Washington, DC, 890.5290, 428–429

Health and Welfare Canada (1983) Safety Code 25—Shortwave diathermy guidelines for limited radiofrequency exposure. Publication 83-EHD-98

Health and Welfare Canada (2002) Health Canada is advising Canadians of a dangerous interaction between diathermy therapy and implanted metallic leads.

Kloth L, Morrison MA, Ferguson BH (1984) Therapeutic microwave and shortwave diathermy: A review of thermal effectiveness, safe use, and state of the art. U.S. Food and Drug Administration, U.S. Department of Health and Human Services, HHS Publication FDA 85-8237

Medtronic Ltd. (2001) Medtronic Safety Reminder. Contraindication to diathermy for patients implanted with any type of Medtronic neurostimulation system. May 2001.

Ruggera PS (1980) Measurement of emission levels during microwave and shortwave diathermy treatments. Bureau of Radiological Health Report, HHS Publication (FDA), 80–8119

Low-Level Laser Therapy

Learning Objectives

Knowledge: State the fundamental properties of a laser light and the key physical components of a laser device.

Comprehension: Distinguish between the process of spontaneous and stimulated emission of photons.

Application: List the parameters that must be considered when determining laser dosage.

Analysis: Explain how laser energy induces photobiomodulation effects in soft tissues.

Synthesis: Explain the optical and therapeutic window of laser light used in low-level laser therapy.

Evaluation: Discuss the concepts of absorption and scattering in relation to laser penetration depth.

I. RATIONALE FOR USE

A. DEFINITION AND DESCRIPTION

The term *laser* is the acronym for *Light Amplification by Stimulated Emission of Radiation*. Light is broadly defined as the emission of electromagnetic waves, made of photons, traveling in space. A laser light, in comparison with all other forms of light such as incandescent (a light bulb) and luminescent (a fluorescent tube), is monochromatic, collimated, and coherent. A laser is a device that produces such a light.

1. Phototherapy

The use of lights, or photons, for therapeutic purposes is known as phototherapy. Common lights used for phototherapy are in the infrared, visible, and ultraviolet band of the electromagnetic spectrum. Laser devices used in rehabilitation generate lights within the visible and infrared spectra. Lasers in the infrared band produce beams of light that are invisible to the human eye.

2. Laser Classification

Practically all international standards divide lasers into four major hazard classes—Class I, II, IIIa, IIIb, and IV—based on the power outputs and exposure time of the device [see Occupational Safety and Health Administration (OSHA, 2007) and www. osha.gov for details]. Hazard refers to the potential risk of the laser's causing biological damage to the skin and eye. Class I, II, and IIIa lasers have low power outputs (less than 5 mW) and are not used for therapeutic purposes.

a. Class IIIb—Power and Hazard

All lasers with power outputs ranging between 5 and 500 mW are grouped in this class. These lasers pose eye hazards, such as damage to the retina, if their beams of energy are focused on the human eye. They pose no hazard to the skin.

b. Class IV

All lasers with power outputs greater than 500 mW are grouped in this class. These lasers pose eye (damage to retina) and skin (cell destruction) hazards, if their beams of energy are focused on such tissues.

c. Low- Versus High-Level Laser

Lasers with power outputs less than 500 mW are labeled as low-level laser (LLL) and are used for therapy (T). Lasers with power outputs greater than 500 mW, on the other hand, are labeled as high-level laser (HLL) and are used for surgery (S).

3. LLLT Versus HLLS

Shown in **Table 11-1** is a comparison between class IIIb and class IV lasers used in health care. Class IIIb lasers are used to deliver low-level laser therapy, known by the acronym LLLT (Baxter, 1994; Calderhead, 1988; Oshiro et al., 1998; Schindl et al., 2000). The word therapy is used in reference to the improved cell function achieved through laser-induced photobiomodulation effects. Class IV lasers, because of their high power level, are used in surgery; this application is known under the acronym HLLS. The term surgery is used in reference to the cell destruction due to laser-induced photothermal effects.

4. Focus on LLLT

This chapter focuses on the use of low-level laser devices to treat soft-tissue pathologies in the field of physical rehabilitation.

B. LLLT DEVICES

Shown in **Figure 11-1** are typical line-powered cabinet-type (**A**) and battery-powered portable-type (**B**) lasers used to deliver LLLT. Today's devices are built using two lasing media: inert gases and semiconductor materials or diodes (see below). A complete laser device consists of a console to which a probe is attached.

TABLE 11-1	COMPARISON OF LASER TYPES USED IN HEALTH CARE	
	LOW-LEVEL LASER THERAPY (LLLT)	**HIGH-LEVEL LASER SURGERY (HLLS)**
OSHA CLASSIFICATION	**CLASS IIIB**	**CLASS IV**
Power level	Low power (≤500 mW)	High power (>500 mW)
Usage	Therapy	Surgical therapy
Method of action	Photobiomodulation	Photothermal
Physiological effect	Enhance cellular function	Cellular destruction

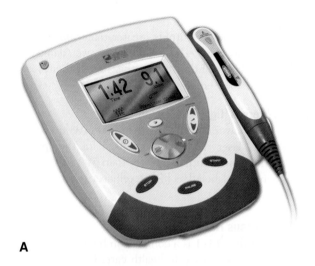

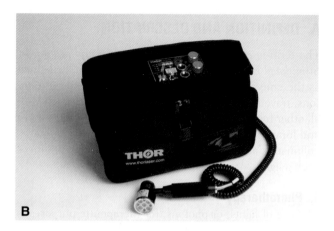

FIGURE 11-1 Typical cabinet (**A**) and portable (**B**) diode-type LLLT devices. (A: Courtesy of Chattanooga Group; B: Courtesy of THOR Laser, Inc.)

1. Probes

Figure 11-2 shows the two types of laser probes commonly used to deliver LLLT. The key difference between the single (**A**) and cluster (**B**) probe is that the former contains only one laser diode, whereas the latter contains a group, or a cluster, of laser diodes. Practically speaking, a single probe is used to deliver a low dosage over small areas, while cluster probes are used to deliver a higher dosage over larger treatment areas.

2. Protective Eyewear

The use of class IIIb lasers requires *both* the patient and the operator to wear eye protection goggles during therapy (see www.osha.gov). **Figure 11-3** shows a typical pair of laser safety goggles (**A**) worn by both the patient and the treating clinician (**B**). These goggles filter out the wavelength(s) generated by the LLLT device, while allowing maximum visible light transmission to the clinician during therapy. For a pair of goggles to be effective, its filter must match the photonic wavelength generated by the laser device being used.

C. RATIONALE FOR USE

The use of LLLT arose from pioneering studies on animals and humans performed in the 1960s and 1970s by the Hungarian Endre Mester, who is regarded by many in the field as the *therapeutical father* of LLLT (Calderhead, 1988; Baxter, 1994, Tuner et al., 2002). More specifically, Mester et al. (1970, 1971, 1985, 1989) claimed that by using a ruby-type laser of low-level power, a therapeutic response rate of approximately 90% was obtained after treating more than 1000 patients with various chronic and recalcitrant wounds and ulcers. Global recognition of these findings spurred researchers and clinicians to further explore the photobiological effects induced by LLLT in humans. The rationale for inducing photobiomodulation using LLLT is based on its

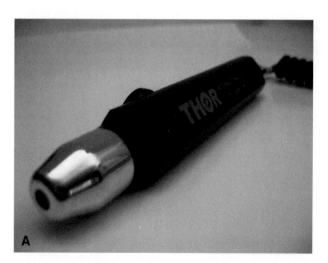

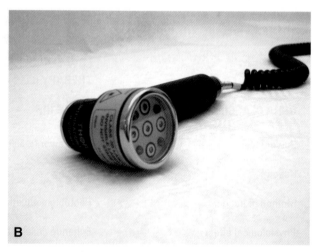

FIGURE 11-2 Typical single (**A**) and cluster (**B**) probes used to deliver LLLT. (Courtesy of THOR Laser, Inc.)

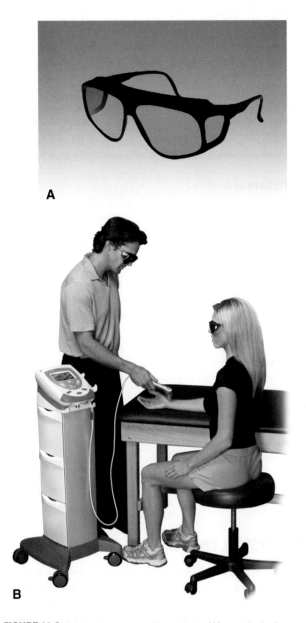

A

B

FIGURE 11-3 Typical laser protective goggles (**A**) worn by both patient and treating clinician (**B**) during treatment (A: Courtesy of THOR Laser, Inc.; B: Courtesy of Chattanooga Group, Inc.)

ability to affect cellular function using a nonthermal, nondestructive source of energy with no known side effects.

II. HISTORICAL PERSPECTIVE

A. THEORETICAL FOUNDATIONS

In 1917, Albert Einstein proposed the theoretical biophysical concept of stimulated (*S*) emission (*E*) of radiation (*R*), which became the central process underlying the production of a la*SER* light. Einstein is thus considered to be the *biophysical father* of all lasers.

B. FIRST LASERS

In 1960, American physicist Theodore Maiman developed and manufactured the first laser, using a solid ruby crystal as the lasing medium (Calderhead, 1988; Baxter, 1994). A year later another American physicist, Ali Javan, constructed the first helium-neon (HeNe) gas laser.

C. DIODE LASERS

The invention of diodes, or semiconductors, in the 1970s led to the development of lower-cost, more powerful lasers. Today, the majority of lasers used for LLLT are diode-type lasers. Modern diode-type lasers are made of gallium-arsenide (GaAs) and gallium-aluminum-arsenide (GaAlAs) used as semiconductor substrates.

D. FIRST EVIDENCE OF PHOTOBIOSTIMULATION

A few years after the first working laser was invented, Endre Mester wanted to test whether laser radiation might cause cancer in animals (Mester et al., 1968). He shaved the dorsal hair of mice, divided them in two groups, and exposed one group to a low-power ruby laser. The results were spectacular. Mester showed not only that ruby laser radiation caused no cancer in the skin of the irradiated mice but also that the hair of the treated group of mice grew more quickly than the hair of the untreated group. This was the first demonstration that laser energy can induce photobiostimulation effects on in vivo mammalian soft tissues (Hamlin et al., 2006).

E. FIRST HUMAN APPLICATIONS

Mester is credited with the first human applications of LLLT conducted in patients with various chronic and recalcitrant wounds and ulcers (Mester et al., 1971, 1985, 1989).

F. AMERICAN FDA APPROVAL

In 2002, the U.S. Food and Drug Administration (FDA) approved the use of LLLT (diode laser; 830 nm) for the treatment of carpal tunnel syndrome (Department of Health and Services, FDA, 2002). This first FDA approval of LLLT is seen by many in the field as the first step in this electrophysical agent's (EPA) march toward recognition for other pathologies.

G. TODAY'S LLLT PRACTICE

Recent studies on the practice of LLLT in the field of physical therapy reveal a wide variability in its availability and frequency of use (Robertson et al., 1998; Shields et al., 2002; Nussbaum et al., 2007). In Australia, the finding that lasers were useful only for treating lesions less than a few millimeters deep was consistent with its limited availability (Robertson et al., 1998). In Ireland, laser availability was measured at 62%, with frequency of use at 57% (Shields et al., 2002). In Canada, the availability of lasers was measured at 57%, and percentage of usage at 30%. No studies could be found on the use of LLLT in the United States.

H. BODY OF LITERATURE

Over the past two decades, LLLT has been the subject of numerous *articles* (see References), *review articles* (Basford, 1986; Enwemeka, 1988; Basford, 1989a,b; King, 1989; Kitchen et al., 1991; Oshiro et al., 1991; Beckerman et al., 1992; Basford, 1993, 1995; Dreyfuss et al., 1993; Gam et al., 1993; Laakso et al., 1993a,b; Tuner et al., 1998; Flemming et al., 1999; Marks, 1999; Brosseau et al., 2000; Schindl et al., 2000; Lucas et al., 2000; Bjordal et al., 2001; Bjordal et al., 2003; Nussbaum et al., 2003; Enwemeka et al., 2004; Reddy, 2004; Woodruff et al., 2004; Bjordal et al., 2005; Brosseau et al., 2005a,b; Hawkins et al., 2005; Posten et al., 2005; Stasinopoulos et al., 2005; Hamlin et al., 2006; Maher, 2006; Bjordal et al., 2007; Naeser, 2006; Lopes-Martins et al., 2007; Parker, 2007; Bjordal et al., 2008), *chapters of textbooks* (Calderhead, 1988; Low et al., 1990; Seichert, 1991; Khan, 1999; Baxter, 2002; Saliba et al., 2002; Karu, 2003; Weisberg et al., 2006, Knight et al., 2008), and a few *textbooks* (Oshiro et al., 1988; Baxter, 1994; Kamami, 1997; Karu, 1989, 1998; Niems, 1996; Tuner et al., 2002).

III. BIOPHYSICAL CHARACTERISTICS

A. KEY ELEMENTS

The biophysics of lasers is a very complex subject (Nolan, 1987; Karu, 1989, 1988; Baxter, 1994; Kamami, 1997; Knappe et al., 2004) and addressing its full complexity is beyond the scope of this chapter. Nonetheless, readers must consider *three key elements* in order to understand the basis of laser therapy: the fundamental properties of light, the physical components of a laser, and the process of laser light emission.

B. FUNDAMENTAL PROPERTIES OF LIGHT

The *first* element refers to the properties of a laser light. This light differs from all other lights, whether incandescent or luminescent, on the basis of three properties: (1) monochromacity, (2) collimation, and (3) coherence (Baxter, 1994; Knappe et al., 2004).

1. Monochromacity

Monochromacity implies that all photons accounting for the laser light have a single wavelength, and thus a single color. The therapeutic advantage of monochromatic light is that its absorption can be targeted at specific, wavelength-dependent photoacceptor molecules, called chromophores, buried within soft tissues.

2. Collimation

Collimation refers to the ability of a laser beam not to diverge, or spread, significantly with distance. The advantage of a collimated beam of light is its ability to be focused precisely on a very small target area.

3. Coherence

Coherence refers to the fact that the photons that make up a laser light travel in phase, in both time and space, with each other. In other words, it means that all photons travel in the same direction at the same time. This property does not appear to present any therapeutic advantage, however, because evidence shows that laser beam coherence is lost almost immediately after the light is absorbed by the skin, due to refraction and scattering (Nussbaum et al., 2003; Enwemeka, 2006).

4. Laser Light

A light amplified by stimulated emission of radiation, or a laser light, is thus characterized as being monochrome, collimated, and coherent. All other lights are polychrome, uncollimated, and incoherent, meaning that their photons travel in all directions from the source and contain multiple wavelengths of light of various colors and intensities. Biophysical literature indicates that of all lights, a laser light is the closest to perfect monochromacity, collimation, and coherence.

C. PHYSICAL COMPONENTS

The *second* element that differentiates a laser light from all other light sources, as illustrated in **Figure 11-4** and described in **Table 11-2**, relates to the three basic physical components of a laser device: *active medium, resonance chamber*, and *power source* (Knappe et al., 2004). Two types of laser are commonly used today in the field of LLLT: gaseous and diode lasers. The active medium, resonance chamber, and power source associated with these two types of laser are described below.

1. Active Medium

The active medium corresponds to the material used to emit a laser light, for which the laser is named.

a. Helium-Neon (HeNe)

Gaseous lasers used for LLLT, as shown in **Figure 11-4A**, are made of a mixture of two inert gases, helium (He) and neon (Ne), and are called HeNe lasers.

b. Galium-Aluminum-Arsenide (GaAlAs)

As shown in **Figure 11-4B**, diode lasers are constructed using semiconductors (two slabs of material separated by a junction) made of different chemical elements. The three

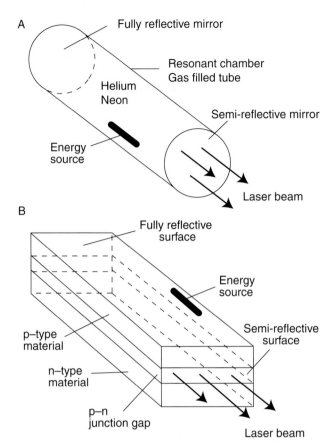

FIGURE 11-4 Schematic physical representation of a helium-neon (**A**) and diode-type (**B**) laser device. The active medium, resonance chamber, and power source are shown for each laser type. The laser beam (shown by *arrows*) for both lasers escapes through the semi-reflective mirror of the resonance chamber.

main active media used to construct a diode laser are gallium (Ga), aluminum (Al), and arsenide (As). These lasers are thus called GaAs lasers, or GaAlAs lasers.

2. Resonance Chamber

The resonance, or optical, chamber of a laser is the cavity within the laser device that contains the active medium. In this chamber the active medium is activated or lased, leading to the production of a beam of laser light.

a. Sealed Glass Tube

The resonance chamber of a HeNe laser is made of a sealed glass tube, housing the active medium (**Fig 11-4A**). This

tube is mounted with a fully reflective mirror at one end and a semi-reflective mirror at the other. The beam of laser light is emitted through the semi-reflective mirror.

b. The p-n Junction Gap

The resonance chamber of a diode laser corresponds to the p-n junction gap between two slabs of semiconductor material sandwiched together. This gap is commonly referred to as a diode (**Fig 11-4B**). The p-n junction is created by placing a p-type semiconductor material (p for positively charged, because it has a deficit of free electrons and therefore contains holes that accept free electrons) in contact with an n-type semiconductor material (n for negatively charged, because it has a surplus of electrons). The chamber's parallel reflecting mirrors are obtained by cleaving along the natural planes of the semiconductor materials used to make the diode.

3. Power Source

Gaseous and diode-type lasers used in the field of LLLT, as illustrated in **Figure 11-4A-B**, are all powered by an electrical source of energy. An electrical current passing through the resonance chamber powers the laser; that is, it stimulates (or lases) the laser's active medium (**Table 11-2**).

D. PROCESS OF LASER LIGHT EMISSION

The *third* and final element that one needs to know in order to understanding the nature of laser is the *process of light emission*, which results from activation of the active medium, housed in the resonance chamber. The sequential biophysical steps leading to emission of a laser light are described below. These biophysical steps are the same, regardless of the laser type. Illustrated in **Figure 11-5** is a simple atomic model to help visualize the complex fundamental steps needed to create a laser light. This model presupposes the use of an active medium with a population of five atoms, all shown resting (i.e., power OFF) at their ground level (**Fig 11-5A**). In reality, any given active medium has a population of millions of molecules and billions of atoms.

1. First Step: Pumping of Active Medium

This step involves the activation, or pumping, of the active medium caused by an electrical current (i.e., power ON)

TABLE 11-2	PHYSICAL COMPONENTS OF LASERS USED FOR LOW-LEVEL LASER THERAPY			
TYPE		**COMPONENT**		
	ACTIVE MEDIUM		**RESONANCE CHAMBER**	**POWER SOURCE**
Gaseous	Helium-neon		Sealed glass cylinder	Electrical
Diode	Gallium-arsenide; gallium-aluminumarsenide		p-n junction gap (diode)	Electrical

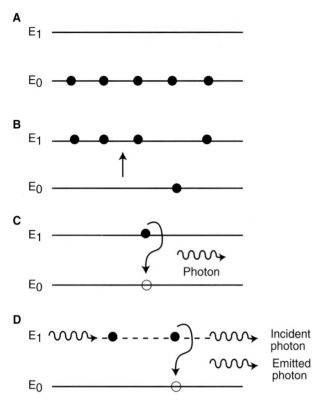

FIGURE 11-5 Schematic sequences of key atomic states and processes leading to emission of a laser beam of light. For simplicity, an active medium population of only five atoms is presented in a system with two energy levels. **A:** Active medium in its resting or ground state. **B:** Pumping of active medium causes the majority of atoms to jump to their metastable energy level, thus causing a population inversion. **C:** Spontaneous emission of a photon traveling parallel to the lateral wall of the resonance chamber. **D:** An incident photon striking an electron in its metastable energy level, thus causing the process of stimulated emission, which corresponds to the release of a newly emitted photon perfectly identical to the incident photon. E_0, ground energy state; E_1, metastable energy state.

passing into the resonance chamber. To pump the active medium is to energize it. It is the process of moving atoms, and therefore their electrons, from their resting ground state (E_0) to their excited state (E_1). This means that in the resonance chamber there are now a growing number of atoms whose electrons have been excited.

2. Second Step: Population Inversion

This step is achieved when a majority of atoms are in their excited state. **Figure 11-5B** illustrates this population inversion by showing electrons of four of the five atoms (80%) in their excited state.

3. Third Step: Spontaneous Emission

This step corresponds to the emission of a photon caused by the spontaneous drop of an electron from its excited state to its ground state, as illustrated in **Figure 11-5C**. As more and more electrons spontaneously drop from their higher energy level, more and more spontaneous photons are emitted in the resonance chamber. All photons not traveling

parallel to the wall of the resonance chamber are absorbed by the lining of the wall and cease to exist. These three first steps are common to the production of all light sources.

4. Fourth Step: Stimulated Emission

This fourth step is critical to the creation of a laser light. Remember that the term *laser* stands for *light amplification by stimulated emission of radiation*. This process corresponds to the emission of a photon caused by an incident photon striking an atom's electron into its metastable energy state, which is defined as an excited state that has a long lifetime (i.e., a state that lasts long enough for the incident photon to strike the excited atom before it spontaneously de-excites itself by dropping to its ground state). This striking action, as illustrated in **Figure 11-5D**, causes the electron to drop from its metastable energy level to its resting energy level, releasing a new photon that is identical to the incident photon. Physics has shown that only one spontaneously emitted photon, traveling parallel to the lateral wall of the resonance chamber, is needed to trigger the process of stimulated emission. Both the incident and the newly emitted photons now travel together and in phase with each other in the resonance chamber (**Fig 11-5D**). This process of stimulated emission is self-perpetuating in that these 2 traveling photons will later strike 2 other excited electrons, leading to the emission of 4 photons, and later to 8, 16, 32, 64 photons, and so on.

5. Fifth and Final Step: Amplification

The final step, amplification, is achieved through the back-and-forth movements of incident and newly emitted photons traveling parallel to the lateral wall of the resonance chamber as they are reflected between the parallel reflective and semi-reflective mirrors forming the end walls of the chamber. Physics has shown that the back-and-forth passing of these photons through the active medium dramatically amplifies the process of stimulated emission, triggering a chain reaction as more and more perfectly identical photons fill the resonance chamber (see above).

E. LASER BEAM EMISSION

The ultimate emission of a beam of laser light through the laser's probe occurs when the amplification process is maximal, that is, when the resonance chamber has reached its maximum capacity to store photons. At this point, and as long as pumping continues (i.e., the laser device is turned ON), a percentage of photons escapes the chamber through the semi-reflective mirror to form an *almost perfect monochromatic, collimated, and coherent beam of light* at the tip of the probe. This laser beam is then used to deliver LLLT.

F. OPTICAL AND THERAPEUTIC WINDOW

Photons emitted by LLLT lasers have different wavelengths, which are determined by the nature and specific composition of their active medium. Shown in **Table 11-3** is the optical spectrum and therapeutic window occupied by LLLT lasers. The *visible band* of the electromagnetic spectrum rests between the infrared and ultraviolet bands; its optical and therapeutic window range is between 750 and 400 nm. Visible light is made of six different lights (from violet to red). The *infrared band* is within an optical and therapeutic window adjacent to the visible band, ranging between 1 mm to 750 nm. Infrared light is invisible to the human eye.

1. Red-Light Lasers

The gaseous HeNe laser emits a light in the visible red band (750–600 nm); this red light is made of photons having a wavelength of 632.8 nanometers (10^{-9} m). Within the red band of visible light can be found Mester's original ruby laser, which emitted photons with a wavelength of 694 nm (**Table 11-3**). These lasers are referred to as red-light lasers.

2. Infrared-Light Laser

The diode-type lasers used to deliver LLLT emit lights within the infrared (IR) band (1 mm to 750 nm). Shown in **Table 11-3** are the GaAlAs laser, emitting photons of 820 nm, and the GaAs laser, emitting photons of 904 nm. These lasers are commonly referred to as infrared or IR lasers.

a. Visible Red Light—Probe Tip

Why do we see a red beam of light at the tip of an IR laser probe, although infrared light is invisible to the human eye? What is the purpose of this red light? The red light comes from a light-emitting diode, or LED, embedded in the laser probe, which contains the laser diode (LD). This visible light has two purposes: (1) it serves as a safety measure, to remind both patient and operator that an invisible therapeutic laser beam is being emitted from the probe; and (2) it serves as a visual aid, to help in guiding the therapeutic beam of invisible light over the area being treated.

3. Recap

Lasers used to deliver LLLT generate, as illustrated in **Table 11-3**, visible red (HeNe) and invisible infrared (GaAlAs; GaAs) lights within an optical window ranging between 904 and 600 nm. All laser lights within this optical window are presumed to trigger photobiomodulation effects on soft tissues though energy absorption by chromophores buried in these tissues (see below).

G. FINITE LASER DEVICE LIFE

The useful life of a laser is predetermined and specified by the manufacturer. The laser's active medium has a finite number of hours, which can vary between 5,000 and 20,000 hours, during which it can be optimally stimulated.

TABLE 11-3	LOW-LEVEL LASER THERAPY OPTICAL SPECTRUM AND WINDOW

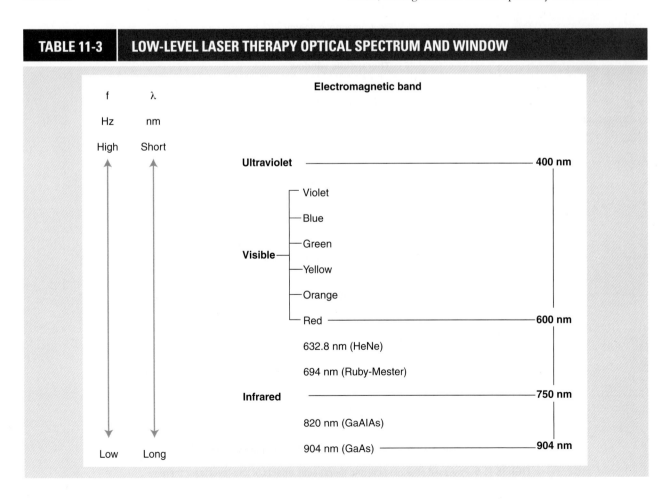

IV. PHYSIOLOGICAL AND THERAPEUTIC EFFECTS

A. PHOTOBIOMODULATION

The exact physiological and therapeutic effects of LLLT on human soft tissues are, unfortunately, far from well established or understood. There is a strong consensus in the scientific literature, however, that LLLT induces photobiomodulation effects through photochemical interactions between photons and the healthy cells within and surrounding the soft-tissue pathology (Calderhead, 1988; Baxter, 1994; Kamami, 1997, Schindl et al., 2000; Knappe, 2004; Reddy, 2004; Bjordal et al., 2006; Hamlin et al., 2006; Lopes-Martins et al., 2007). Shown in **Figure 11-6** are the proposed physiological and therapeutic effects of LLLT. Biomodulation is defined as the process of modulating (stimulating or inhibiting) the biochemical responses or functions of a cell.

1. Photobiostimulation

If the biomodulation process increases cellular function, the laser light is said to have *stimulated* the exposed tissue, creating a photobiostimulation effect.

2. Photobioinhibition

In contrast, if the biomodulation decreases cellular function, it is said to have *inhibited* the exposed tissue, creating a photobioinhibition effect.

3. Terminology

The physiological and therapeutic effects of LLLT rest on several biophysical concepts and laws related to the electromagnetic field. In order to facilitate learning, readers are *urged to review* the illustrated glossary of terms presented in Chapter 5 before considering the following material.

4. Dose Response

The photobiomodulation effect on soft tissues triggered by LLLT is believed to be dosage-dependent. It is presumed to follow the *Arndt-Schultz law* (see Chapter 5), which states that lower dosages trigger photobiostimulation, and higher dosages trigger photoinhibition (Baxter, 1994; Bjordal et al., 2001, 2006, 2008).

5. Optimal Dose

Recent studies indicate that there may be optimal doses of laser light for a particular soft tissue, meaning that doses

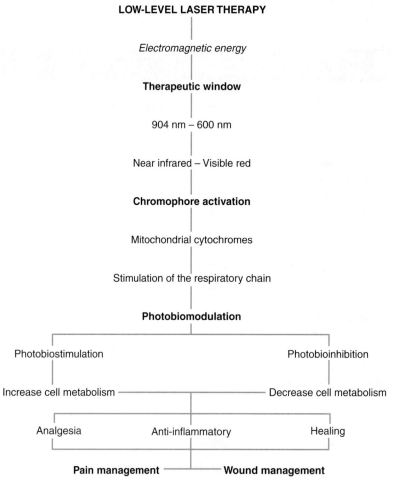

FIGURE 11-6 Proposed physiological and therapeutic effects of low-level laser therapy.

lower or higher than those optimal levels will have a diminished therapeutic outcome (Bjordal et al., 2006, 2008; Hamlin et al., 2006).

B. PHOTOCHEMICAL MECHANISMS

LLLT works by stimulating a cell's innate metabolism through a series of photochemical effects (Hamlin et al., 2006). Photochemistry, a subdiscipline of chemistry, is the study of interactions between light and atoms.

1. Photonic Absorption

The first law of photobiology, known as the *Grotthus-Draper law* (see Chapter 5), states that for photobiostimulation to occur, photonic energy must first be absorbed by the exposed soft tissue.

2. Chromophores

Research has shown that photobiomodulation results from the transfer of energy from a photon, in this case a laser photon, to a photon acceptor molecule within the cell (Karu, 1989, 1998). These photo-acceptor molecules, found in biological tissues, are called *chromophores*, meaning "color lover" (*chromo* = color; *phore* = lover). Melanin (skin darkening), hemoglobin (red blood), and retinal rhodopsin (color vision) are among the best-known chromophores, or pigments, found in human tissues.

a. Mitochondrial Cytochromes

There is a solid body of evidence to suggest that mitochondrial cytochromes (see below) are among the most important chromophores, as shown in **Figure 11-6**, involved in the photobiomodulation effects caused by LLLT on soft tissues (Karu, 1989; 1998; Hamlin et al, 2006).

b. Chromophore's Wavelength Window

Studies in photobiology have revealed that every chromophore has its own wavelength window for accepting photons, meaning that only photons that have wavelengths corresponding to the chromophore's wavelength window will be absorbed. For example, photons with wavelengths shorter than 600 nm are readily absorbed by melanin and hemoglobin, whereas photons with wavelengths longer than 904 nm are readily absorbed by water (Nussbaum et al., 2003).

c. LLLT Spectrum and Therapeutic Window

Lasers used for therapy emit photons within two bands of the electromagnetic spectrum: the visible red and the invisible near infrared. This means that such lasers have a therapeutic optical window ranging between 904 and 600 nm (**Table 11-3**).

d. Respiratory Chain Enzymes

Research on LLLT has revealed that the respiratory chain enzymes, or cytochromes, within the mitochondria are particularly sensitive to photons emitted in the 904–600 nm window range, which makes them the prime chromophores that cause the photobiomodulation effect of LLLT (Oshiro et al., 1988; Karu, 1989, 1998; Karu et al., 1989; Tiphlova et al., 1989, Smith, 1991; Laakso et al., 1993a).

e. Key Fundamental Property for Photobiomodulation

Which of the three fundamental properties of a laser light— monochromacity, collimation, and coherence—is the key to the photobiomodulation effects of LLLT? The body of evidence gathered so far indicates that *monochromacity may be the key property* because both coherence and collimation properties are practically lost as soon as the photons are absorbed by the exposed tissues (Enwemeka, 2006). This significant loss of coherence and collimation is due to the effects of refraction and scattering (see Chapter 5 and Section V. Dosimetry) that take place between the beam of laser light and the exposed biological tissues.

f. Recap

Mechanisms of LLLT at the cellular level, illustrated in **Figure 11-6**, are based on the absorption of monochromatic visible (>600 nm) and near-infrared (<904 nm) radiation by components of the cellular respiratory chain or mitochondrial cytochrome (Karu, 1989, 1998; Hamlin et al., 2006). This absorption of light energy then triggers a series of biochemical reactions that eventually increases (biostimulation) or decreases (bioinhibition) cellular metabolism and function.

C. PENETRATION DEPTH

For any laser light to physiologically and therapeutically affect tissue, it must first be able to penetrate the skin and underlying targeted soft tissue before being absorbed by the wavelength-specific chromophores buried in the layers of this tissue (see above).

1. Scattering

When a laser beam of light hits soft tissues, a significant portion of its photons is scattered, or deflected, in various directions away from the original direct path to the targeted lesion (see Chapter 5). The biophysics of laser indicates that the degree of scattering is wavelength-dependent. It is greatest at short wavelengths and gradually decreases at longer wavelengths (Houza et al., 1993; Nussbaum et al., 2003). This means that photons of red lasers (632.8 nm) will experience more scattering than those of IR lasers (904–820 nm) when penetrating soft tissues.

2. Penetration

The depth to which a laser beam of light can penetrate soft tissues depends on two factors: absorption and scattering.

a. Absorption

The greater the absorption of photons by superficial tissues, the fewer the number of photons the deeper tissues can absorb. In other words, penetration depth (P) is inversely related to absorption (A), meaning the greater the absorption superficially, the lesser the penetration depth (P = 1/A). Biophysics indicates that red visible laser light (HeNe) is absorbed much more by superficial tissues (skin and blood) than is IR invisible light (Nussbaum et al., 2003).

b. Scattering

Biophysics has established that penetration depth (P) is inversely related to scattering (S), meaning that P decreases as S increases (P = 1/S). As stated above, scattering is more pronounced with shorter-wavelength lasers (red) than with longer-wavelength lasers (IR).

c. IR lasers Penetrate Deeper

Table 11-4 compares the relative amounts of absorption and scattering (i.e., more or less) associated with both red and infrared lasers. Because photons from red-light lasers (HeNe) are absorbed more superficially and present more scattering than photons from infrared-light laser (GaAs and GaAlAs), it follows that IR lasers penetrate soft tissues more deeply than red-light lasers.

3. Penetration Depth Value

Penetration depth value is defined (Low et al., 1990; Baxter, 1994) as the tissue depth, measured in centimeters, at which the laser beam energy is reduced to 37% of its original value (100%). This reduced value is derived from the following formula: penetration depth value = 1/e, where e is a constant value of 2.718. According to Kolari et al. (1993) and as illustrated in **Table 11-4**, the penetration depth values in human skin are approximately 0.5 cm for HeNe lasers and 1.0 cm for diode lasers.

4. Primary Versus Secondary Action

How can photobiomodulation effects be triggered in deeper tissues, such as muscles and tendons, when we know that no more than 37% of the original laser energy will directly reach depths greater than 0.5–1.0 cm? For photobiomodulation to occur in these deeper tissues, one has to postulate the presence of a powerful indirect, or secondary, light-dependent or non-light-dependent intermolecular mechanism in the superficial layers of tissues, which transmits to deeper cells the primary light-dependent activity occurring in superficial chromophores (Saliba et al., 2002; Nussbaum et al., 2003; Hamlin et al., 2006). To what extent each of these two mechanisms of action are responsible for the global photobiostimulation effect induced by LLLT remains unknown.

D. THERAPEUTIC EFFECTS

LLLT is used today, as illustrated in **Figure 11-6**, for the management of pain and open dermal wounds. The exact mechanisms by which red and IR lasers trigger these therapeutic effects in humans remain unknown. The broad mechanism is that red and IR laser lights trigger chromophore activity, which in turn activates cell metabolism, leading to optimal cell function (Bjordal et al., 2003; 2006, 2008; Hamlin et al., 2006).

V. DOSIMETRY

A. DIODE LASERS

Present-day LLLT practice, as evidenced by the body of literature found in this chapter, is mainly based on diode-type lasers (i.e., GaAs and GaAlAs). Usage of gaseous lasers, such as the HeNe lasers, has *declined* over the past years because diode lasers are cheaper to manufacture, more powerful, and offer a much broader array of laser lights. The following dosimetry, therefore, addresses *only* the usage of diode- or semiconductor-type lasers.

B. KEY PARAMETERS

The dosimetry of LLLT depends on five key parameters: power (P), power density (P_d), energy density (E_d), dose per diode (D_p), and dose tissue (D_t). The synonyms, formulas, and units for each of these parameters are sum-

TABLE 11-4	RED AND INFRARED LASER PENETRATION DEPTHS	
	RED HeNe GASEOUS	**INFRARED GaAs—GaAlAs DIODE**
WAVELENGTH (λ)	SHORTER	LONGER
Absorption (A)	More	Less
Scattering (S) (S=1/λ)	More	Less
Penetration (P) (P=1/S)	Less	More
Penetration (P) (P=1/A)	Less	More
Penetration depth value	~0.5 cm	~1.0 cm

marized in **Table 11-5**. Dosimetry also depends on two additional parameters, the application mode and the type of laser used, as discussed below.

1. Power (P)

Power is the rate of energy delivered, expressed in watts, where 1 watt = 1 Joule per second. Because the power of all LLLT devices is less than 500 mW (see **Table 11-1**), P is commonly expressed in milliwatts (mW); it can also be expressed in Joules per second (J/s). For example, a laser with a power of 40 mW delivers 40 mJ/s or 0.04 J/s.

2. Power Density (P_d)

Power density is the power (P) delivered per diode's beam area (A), measured in square centimeters (cm^2). P_d is thus expressed in milliwatts per square centimeter (mW/cm^2).

3. Energy Density (E_d)

Energy density, expressed in joules per square centimeters (J/cm^2), is the energy delivered per diode's beam area multiplied by the time of radiation (T). E_d is calculated by multiplying power density (P_d), where P is expressed in J/s and A in square centimeters, by the time of radiation (T), i.e. application duration or exposure time, expressed in seconds ($E_d = P_d \times T$ or P/A $\times$ T).

4. Dose per Diode (D_d)

The dose per diode is the amount of laser energy delivered to the tissue by each diode, expressed in Joules (J). This dose (D_d) corresponds to the power (P) of the diode, expressed in J/s, multiplied by the time of radiation (T),

expressed in seconds ($D_d = P \times T$). The dose per diode corresponds to the *dose per point* of application because each diode has its own point of application.

5. Dose Tissue (D_t)

The dose tissue (D_t) is the total amount of laser energy delivered to the exposed tissue, expressed in Joules (J). This dose (D_t) is equal to the sum of all the doses per diode(s) multiplied by the number of points of applications during a single treatment session.

C. APPLICATION MODES

LLLT may be delivered using two application modes: continuous or pulsed.

1. Continuous

This mode consists of applying laser power output continuously, or without interruption, for the entire time of radiation. Full or peak power (P) is thus delivered to the exposed tissue using this mode.

2. Pulsed

This mode consists of interrupting, or pulsating, the laser power output during the time of radiation. The resulting mean or average power (P_m) is calculated using the following formula: P_m = peak power (P) $\times$ pulse duration (PD) $\times$ frequency (f), where P is expressed in watts, PD in seconds, and f in Hertz. For example, if P = 0.02 W, PD = 0.0002 s, and f = 3000 Hz, then P_m = 0.012 W = 12 mW.

TABLE 11-5	LOW-LEVEL LASER THERAPY DOSIMETRIC PARAMETERS, FORMULAS, AND UNITS		
PARAMETER	**SYNONYM**	**FORMULA**	**UNITS**
Power (P)	Radiant power	NA	mW
Power density (P_d)	Irradiance	$P_d = P/A$ $mW/cm^2 = mW/cm^2$	mW/cm^2
Energy density (E_d)	Fluence	$E_d = P_d \times T$ $P_d = P/A$, thus $E_d = P/A \times T$ $J/cm^2 = (J/s/cm^2) \times T$ $J/cm^2 = (J/s) \times (1/cm^2) \times s$	J/cm^2
Dose per diode (D_d)	Dose per point of application	$D_d = P \times T$ $J = (J/s) \times s$	J
Dose tissue (D_t)	Total dose to tissue	D_t = Sum of each $D_d \times$ nb of applications $J = (J/s) \times s$	J

A, diode radiating beam area; T, time of radiation per diode or point.

D. INFRARED LASER

As stated previously, the current body of literature (see References) indicates that diode-type lasers emitting in the *infrared (IR) band* of the electromagnetic spectrum are by far the most popular lasers used today to deliver LLLT. Today's IR lasers are made with either a single diode embedded in a single probe (**Fig 11-2A**) or multiple diodes embedded in a cluster probe (**Fig 11-2B**).

1. Diode Types: Laser Versus Nonlaser

Although a single-diode laser always includes one laser diode (LD), multiple-diode lasers may or may not include, in addition to their LDs, other nonlaser diodes, called superluminous diodes (SLDs). These LDs and SLDs are embedded in the cluster probe, which may contain several diodes (**Fig 11-2B**).

2. Superluminous Diode

Biophysics has revealed that a SLD produces a monochromatic, collimated, and *incoherent* light; therefore, the light emitted by an SLD is *not* a laser light because of its incoherent property. Because lights from SLDs are not laser lights, they *should not* be considered in the calculation of laser dosage. The power and wavelength of each of these SLDs, however, should be documented in the patient's file because they are part of the total photobiological effects induced in the exposed soft tissues.

E. DOSIMETRIC CALCULATIONS

Shown in **Table 11-6** and **Table 11-7** are *examples* of calculations needed to obtain the dose of laser energy

TABLE 11-6	DOSIMETRIC CALCULATIONS FOR CONTINUOUS MODE USING SINGLE AND MULTIPLE LASER DIODES	
	LASER TYPE	
PARAMETER	**SINGLE DIODE**	**MULTIPLE DIODES**
Laser diode (LD)	1	4
Probe type	Handheld	Cluster
P and wavelength	20 mW–820 nm	1°: 10 mW – 820 nm 2°: 20 mW – 820 nm 3°: 20 mW – 904 nm 4°: 10 mW – 904 nm
Diode beam area (A)	0.5 cm^2	0.5 cm^2
P_d	40 mW/ cm^2	1°: 20 mW/cm^2 2°: 40 mW/cm^2 3°: 40 mW/cm^2 4°: 20 mW/cm^2
T	120 s	120 s
E_d	4.8 J/cm^2	1°: 2.4 J/cm^2 2°: 4.8 J/cm^2 3°: 4.8 J/cm^2 4°: 2.4 J/cm^2
D_d	2.4 J	1°: 1.2 J 2°: 2.4 J 3°: 2.4 J 4°: 1.2 J
Nb of application	2	1
D_t	4.8 J	7.2 J

$P_d = P/A$; $E_d = P_d \times T$; $D_d = P \times T$; $D_t =$ sum of each $D_d \times$ nb of applications; T, duration of radiation per application

TABLE 11-7	DOSIMETRIC CALCULATIONS FOR PULSED MODE USING SINGLE AND MULTIPLE LASER DIODES	

	LASER TYPE	
PARAMETER	**SINGLE DIODE**	**MULTIPLE DIODES**
Laser diode (LD)	1	4
Probe type	Handheld	Cluster
Pulsation	P_m = P (W) $\times$ PD (s) $\times$ f (Hz) Pulse duration (PD) for both lasers: 200 microseconds or 0.0002 seconds Frequency (f) for both lasers: 3000 Hz	
P and wavelength	20 mW–820 nm	1°: 10 mW–820 nm 2°: 20 mW–820 nm 3°: 20 mW–904 nm 4°: 10 mW–904 nm
Mean power (P_m)	12 mW	1°: 6 mW 2°: 12 mW 3°: 12 mW 4°: 6 mW
Diode beam area (A)	0.5 cm^2	0.5 cm^2
P_d	24 mW / cm^2	1°: 12 mW/cm^2 2°: 24 mW/cm^2 3°: 24 mW/cm^2 4°: 12 mW/cm^2
T	120 s	120 s
E_d	2.88 J/cm^2	1°: 1.44 J/cm^2 2°: 2.88 J/cm^2 3°: 2.88 J/cm^2 4°: 1.44 J/cm^2
D_d	1.44 J	1°: 0.72 J 2°: 1.44 J 3°: 1.44 J 4°: 0.72 J
Nb of application	2	1
D_t	2.88 J	4.32 J

P_d = P/A; E_d = $P_d \times$ T; D_d = $P_m \times$ T; D_t = sum of each $D_d \times$ nb of applications; T, duration of radiation per application

delivered to the pathological tissue, or the dose tissue (D_t), after treatment, using a single-diode and multiple-diode laser, each programmed for *continuous mode* (**Table 11-6**) and *pulse mode* (**Table 11-7**). These tables show that the diode's peak power (P; continuous mode) or mean power (P_m; pulsed mode), diode beam radiating area (A), time of radiation per point (T), and the number of applications per treatment session are key factors that significantly influence the therapeutic laser dose.

1. Examples of Continuous Mode

Table 11-6 shows examples of lasers with one LD (handheld probe) and four LDs (cluster probe) programmed to deliver in the *continuous* mode.

a. Single Diode

This single-diode laser has a power of 20 mW and emits photons all having 820 nm in length. The diode has a beam-radiating area of 0.5 cm^2. The time of radiation per point of application is 120 seconds; there are 2 points of application. This laser has a power density (P_d) of 40 mW/cm^2 (20 mW/ 0.5 cm^2) and an energy density (E_d) of 4.8 J/cm^2 (0.04J/s × 120 s). The dose per diode (D_d) (or per point of application) is 2.4 J (0.02 J/s × 120 s). The dose tissue is 4.8 J because there are two applications (2.4 J × 2). To sum up, the exposed tissue in this example has received a dose of 4.8 J of infrared laser light, emitted at one wavelength (820 nm), distributed over a total area of 1 cm^2 (2 side by side applications × 0.5 cm^2).

b. Multiple Diodes

This multi-diode laser is made of four laser diodes, each diode with a different power and wavelength. Each diode has a beam radiating area of 0.5 cm^2 and the time of radiation per point is 120 seconds. The power density values (P_d) for the four diodes are 20, 40, 40, and 20 mW/cm^2. The energy density (E_d) and dose per diode (D_d), corresponding to the four diodes, are equal to 2.4, 4,8, 4.8, and 2.4 J/cm^2 and 1.2, 2,4, 2.4, and 1.2 J, respectively. Because there is only one application of these four diodes embedded in the cluster probe, the dose tissue (D_t) is equal to the sum of the four doses per diode, that is 7.2 J. To sum up, the exposed tissue in this example has received a dose of 7.2 J of infrared laser light, emitted at two wavelengths (820 and 904 nm), distributed over a total area of 2 cm (4 diodes × 0.5 cm^2).

2. Examples of Pulsed Mode

Table 11-7 shows examples of lasers with one LD (handheld probe) and four LDs (cluster probe) programmed to deliver in the *pulsed* mode. The power, wavelength, beam radiating area, and time of radiation are the same as in the example shown in **Table 11-6**.

a. Single Diode

This laser is programmed to emit pulsed laser light, with each pulse of 200 microseconds delivered at a frequency of 3000 pulses per seconds (Hz). The mean power (P_m) resulting from this pulsation regimen is 12 mW (0.020W × 0.0002 s × 3000 Hz, where power is expressed in watt and pulse duration in second). This example shows that if the laser beam is pulsated while all the other parameters are kept constant the dose tissue decreases by 40% (from 4.8 to 2.88 J).

b. Multiple Diodes

This laser is also programmed to emit pulsed light with the same pulsation regimen. As in the example of continuous mode, pulsating laser energy, while all the other parameters are kept constant, leads to a 40% decrease of the dose tissue (from 7.2 to 4.32 J).

F. RECOMMENDED DOSAGE

The exact dose per diode (D_d) and dose tissue (D_t) that trigger optimal photobiomodulation effects in pathological

soft tissues are unknown. There is today a consensus that expressing dosage in terms of energy density (E_d), in J/cm^2, as recommended in the past (see previous edition of this textbook), may be *misleading* (see below). The current recommendation is to express dosage in terms of *energy delivered*, in joules (Bjordal et al., 2006). Dosage may therefore be expressed either as dose per diode (D_d), or per point, or as dose tissue (D_t), as exemplified in this chapter.

1. Rationale for Change

To express dosage in terms of energy density (E_d = power/ beam area × time) is misleading for the following reasons. For example, suppose we have two 1-diode lasers in continuous mode lasers: one with parameters of 20 mW, 0.5 cm^2, and 50 s and the other with parameters of 10 mW, 0.25 cm^2, and 50 s. Both lasers have the same energy density: E_d = 2 J/cm^2. However, the *energy delivered by the two lasers (D_d) is quite different*: 1 J for the first laser and 0.5 J for the second laser.

2. Energy Over Energy Density

Considering that it is the amount of laser energy delivered to, and absorbed by, the chromophores buried in the exposed soft tissues that modulates the photobiomodulation effects of LLLT, the optimal way to express the therapeutic dose delivered is, therefore, in terms of energy (joules), calculated as dose diode (D_d) or dose tissue (D_t).

3. Trial and Error

The current body of evidence suggests that selecting one dose (diode or tissue) over the other, for any given pathology, is still based on trial and error, despite the efforts made by the *World Association for Laser Therapy* (WALT) to standardize LLLT dosages for some pathological conditions (see www.walt.nu).

VI. EVIDENCE FOR INDICATIONS

A. GUIDED BY EVIDENCE

Dictionaries generally define *evidence* as anything that establishes a fact or gives reason to believe something. The aim of this textbook is to present scientific evidence on therapeutic EPAs. To be guided by the evidence is the process of integrating the evidence from research, however imperfect or scarce this evidence may be, with clinical experience and patients' values. In other words, the *evidence-based practice* of EPA requires that practitioners consider the evidence from research, in addition to their own clinical experience and patient's own preference and beliefs about therapy, when the time comes to justify, prescribe, and apply the therapeutic agent. To be guided by evidence is a process, not a search for the absolute truth. Finally, a lack of evidence from research in support of any given EPA does not mean that this EPA should never be used. What it means is that no statement can be made on its therapeutic effectiveness and that until more evidence from research is presented, its routine use cannot be recommended.

B. EVIDENCE FROM HUMAN RESEARCH

Box 11-1 provides evidence for LLLT based on an exhaustive search of published English-language, peer-reviewed studies on humans. The term *indication* is used in reference to a list of pathologies for which LLLT is used. Ratings of therapeutic benefit (Yes or No) and grading of strength of scientific evidence (I, II, or III), including the reference, are included for each pathological condition.

Box 11-1	Research-Based Indications for the Use of Low-Level Laser Therapy		
PATHOLOGY	**BENEFIT**	**GRADE**	**REFERENCE**
Cutaneous wounds and ulcers	Yes	I	Schindl et al., 1998
	Yes	II	Robinson et al., 1991
	Yes	II	Bihari et al., 1989
	Yes	II	Sugrue et al., 1990
	Yes	II	Crous et al., 1988
	Yes	II	Mester et al., 1971
	Yes	II	Mester et al., 1985
	Yes	II	Mester et al., 1989
	Yes	II	Schindl, et al., 1999b
	Yes	III	Gogia et al., 1988
	Yes	III	Ashford et al., 1999
	Yes	III	Khan, 1984
	Yes	III	Lagan et al., 2000
	No	I	Kopera et al., 2005
	No	I	Lucas et al., 2003
	No	I	Santoianni et al., 1984
	No	I	Lundeberg et al., 1991
	No	I	Kokol et al., 2005
	No	I	Lagan et al., 2002
	No	II	Nussbaum et al., 1994
Epicondylitis	Yes	I	Vasseljen et al., 1992
	Yes	I	Lam et al., 2007
	Yes	I	Simunovic et al., 1998
	Yes	I	Lam et al., 2007
	Yes	I	Logdberg-Andersson et al., 1997
	Yes	II	Stergioulas, 2007
	Yes	II	Oken et al., 2008
	Yes	II	Palmieri, 1984
	No	I	Lundeberg et al., 1987
	No	I	Krasheninnikoff et al., 1994
	No	I	Haker et al., 1990
	No	I	Papadopoulos et al., 1996
	No	I	Haker et al., 1991
	No	I	Basford et al., 2000
	No	II	Konstantinovic et al., 1997
Rheumatoid arthritis	Yes	I	Palmgren et al., 1989
	Yes	I	Goldman et al., 1980
	Yes	I	Walker, et al., 1987b
	Yes	I	Goats et al., 1996
	Yes	II	Fulga, 1998
	Yes	II	Fulga et al., 1994

(Continued)

Box 11-1   Continued

PATHOLOGY	BENEFIT	GRADE	REFERENCE
	Yes	II	Asada et al., 1989
	Yes	II	Obara et al., 1987
	No	I	Heussler et al., 1993
	No	I	Johannsen et al., 1994
	No	I	Hall et al., 1994
	No	II	Bliddal et al., 1987
Osteoarthritis	Yes	I	Lonauer, 1986
	Yes	I	Willner et al., 1985
	Yes	I	Jensen et al., 1987
	Yes	I	Walker, 1983
	Yes	I	Stelian et al., 1992
	Yes	I	Gur et al., 2003a
	Yes	I	Ozdemir et al., 2001
	Yes	I	Lewith et al., 1981
	Yes	II	Trelles et al., 1991
	No	I	Bulow et al., 1994
	No	I	Basford et al., 1987
	No	I	Brosseau et al., 2005
Myofascial pain	Yes	I	Ceccherelli et al., 1989
	Yes	I	Ilbuldu et al., 2004
	Yes	I	Gur et al., 2004
	Yes	II	Hakguder et al., 2003
	No	I	Altan et al., 2005
	No	I	Thorsen et al., 1992
	No	I	Thorsen et al., 1991
	No	I	Waylonis et al., 1988
Postherpetic pain	Yes	I	Schindl et al., 1999a
	Yes	I	Moore et al., 1988
	Yes	II	McKibben et al., 1990
	Yes	II	Kemmotsu et al., 1991
	Yes	II	Yaksish, 1993
	Yes	I	Ohtsuka et al., 1992
Temporomandibular disorders	Yes	I	Mazzetto et al., 2007
	Yes	I	Kulekcioglu et al., 2003
	Yes	I	Cetiner et al., 2006
	Yes	II	Fikackova et al., 2007
	Yes	II	Nunez et al., 2006
	No	I	Conti, 1997
Tendinopathies	Yes	I	Bjordal et al., 2006a
	Yes	I	England et al., 1989
	No	I	Siebert et al., 1987
	No	I	Vecchio et al., 1993
	No	I	Darre et al., 1994
Carpal tunnel syndrome	Yes	I	Naeser et al., 2002
	Yes	I	Evcik et al., 2007
	Yes	II	Weintraub, 1997
	No	I	Irvine et al., 2004
	No	II	Ekim et al., 2007

(Continued)

Box 11-1   Continued

PATHOLOGY	BENEFIT	GRADE	REFERENCE
Chronic pain from various conditions	Yes	I	Walker, 1983
	Yes	I	Atsumi et al., 1987
	Yes	I	Emmanoulidis et al., 1986
	Yes	II	Shiroto et al., 1989
Low-back pain	Yes	I	Basford et al., 1999
	Yes	II	Djavid et al., 2007
	Yes	II	Gur et al., 2003b
	No	I	Klein et al., 1990
Trigger points	Yes	I	Snyder-Mackler et al., 1989
	Yes	I	Olavi et al., 1989
	Yes	I	Simunovic, 1996
Orofacial pain	Yes	I	Ong et al., 2001
	No	I	Hansen et al., 1990
Trigeminal pain	Yes	I	Eckerdal et al., 1996
	Yes	I	Walker et al., 1987a
Maxillofacial disorders	Yes	II	Pinheiro et al., 1997
	Yes	II	Pinheiro et al., 1998
Muscle soreness	No	I	Craig et al., 1996
	No	I	Craig et al., 1999
Mixture of soft-tissue disorders	Yes	II	Li, 1990
	No	I	Mulcahy et al., 1995
Mixture of ankylosing spondylitis, low-back pain, and periarthritic conditions	Yes	II	Gartner et al., 1987
	Yes	II	Tam, 1999
Ankle pain	Yes	II	Stergioulas, 2004
	No	I	De Bie et al., 1998
Recalcitrant radiation ulcers	Yes	III	Schindl et al., 2000
	Yes	III	Schindl et al., 1997
Postmastectomy lymphedema	Yes	I	Catari et al., 2003
	Yes	I	Kaviani et al., 2006
Fibromyalgia	Yes	I	Gur et al., 2002
	Yes	II	Matsutani et al., 2007
Clonus	Yes	I	Walker, 1985
De Quervain disease	Yes	II	Terashima et al., 1990
Dermatitis	Yes	II	Morita et al., 1993

(Continued)

Box 11-1   Continued

PATHOLOGY	BENEFIT	GRADE	REFERENCE
Epitrochleitis	No	I	Papadopoulous et al., 1996
Plantar fasciitis	No	I	Basford et al., 1998
Scar tissue	Yes	III	Ohshiro et al., 1992
Postsurgical abdominal pain	Yes	I	Moore et al., 1992
Neurogenic pain	Yes	I	Kreczi et al., 1986
Herpes zoster	Yes	III	Matsumura et al., 1993
Herpes simplex	Yes	I	Schindl et al., 1999a
Fibrotic lumps - mammoplasty	Yes	III	Nussbaum, 1999
Diabetic neuropathic foot	Yes	III	Schindl et al., 1999
Fibromyositic rheumatism	Yes	II	Longo et al., 1997
Chondromalacia patella	No	I	Rogvi-Hansen et al., 1991
Episiotomies	Yes	I	Kymplova et al., 2005
Raynaud's phenomenon	Yes	I	Hirschl et al., 2004
Shoulder pain	No	I	Bingol et al., 2005
Diabetic microangiopathy	Yes	I	Schindl et al., 2002
Minor surgical wounds	No	II	Lagan et al., 2001
Postoperative aseptic wounds	Yes	III	Herascu et al., 2005
Induced superficial wound	Yes	I	Hopkins et al., 2004

1. Rating Therapeutic Benefit

The rating, expressed as Yes or No, is based on the overall conclusion(s) reached on the issue of therapeutic effectiveness by the author(s) who conducted the peer-reviewed study.

2. Grading Strength of Evidence

The grades, numerically assigned as I, II, and III, are based on the type of research methodology or research design used by the author(s). All those listed are studies on humans published in English-language, peer-reviewed journals. It follows that the strength of evidence in studies graded I is higher than that in studies graded II, which is higher than the strength of evidence in those graded III.

a. Grade I

Evidence based on *controlled* studies on humans, regardless of their level of randomization and blindness.

b. Grade II

Evidence based on *noncontrolled* studies on humans, regardless of their level of randomization and blindness.

c. Grade III

Evidence based on *case* studies on humans, regardless of their level of randomization and blindness.

3. Strength of Evidence Behind the Agent

The strength of evidence in support of the agent, as presented in each research-based indication box, is arbitrarily assessed in this textbook as being *weak, moderate,* or *strong.* For example the larger the number of studies graded I, regardless of therapeutic benefit, the stronger the scientific evidence in support of the agent.

4. Strength of Justification for Usage of the Agent

The strength of evidence justifying the usage of an agent for an individual pathology or groups of pathologies, as listed in the research-based indication box, is arbitrarily assessed in this textbook as being *poor, fair, good,* or *conflicting*. For example, where the number of grade I studies showing therapeutic benefit (Yes), for any given pathology, is larger than that of similar studies showing no benefit, the justification for the usage of this agent for that pathology is assessed as *good*. A *conflicting* usage is reported when an equal number of studies with similar grades show therapeutic benefit (Yes) and no benefit (No).

C. STRENGTH OF EVIDENCE AND JUSTIFICATION FOR USAGE

The results gathered in **Box 11-1** show *moderate-to-strong* strength of evidence for the indications, with the majority of studies graded I or II. They also show *conflicting* justification for the use of this agent for cutaneous wounds and ulcers, epicondylitis, myofascial pain, and tendinopathies with a relatively equal number of grade I and II studies showing benefit and no benefit. These results, however, show *fair-to-good* justification for the use of LLLT for rheumatoid osteoarthritis and postherpetic pain with a majority of grade I studies demonstrating therapeutic benefits. Finally, the results presented in **Box 11-1** show that LLLT has been used to treat a variety of other pathologies, but until more evidence from research is provided, the routine use of LLLT *cannot be recommended for such group of pathologies*.

D. CONTROVERSY

As is often the case with emerging therapies, one should not be surprised to discover that LLLT is still the topic of a major controversy regarding its therapeutic effectiveness for soft-tissue pathologies, as indicated in recent publications by Maher (2006) and Bjordal (2007). The body of evidence (**Box 11-1**) shown in this chapter suggests that

it is *still much too soon* to draw any *definitive* conclusions about the therapeutic effectiveness of LLLT for the treatment of soft-tissue pathologies.

VII. CONTRAINDICATIONS

Table 11-8 lists the contraindications associated with the practice of LLLT. Direct application over the eyes may cause severe damage, because the eye itself will further focus the laser beam of photons over the retina.

VIII. RISKS, PRECAUTIONS, AND RECOMMENDATIONS

The practice of LLLT is not without risks for the patient. The key risks associated with this EPA, along with some precautions and recommendations designed to improve safety and effectiveness, are listed in **Table 11-9**.

IX. CONSIDERATIONS FOR APPLICATION AND DOCUMENTATION

A. CONSIDERATIONS AND PROCEDURES

The safe, effective, and optimal application of this EPA requires that clinicians go through a systematic set of considerations and procedures for each and every application. Presented below is a list of such considerations and procedures.

1. Checklists
Before proceeding with treatment, always go through the list of contraindications (**Table 11-8**) and the list of risks, precautions, and recommendations (**Table 11-9**).

TABLE 11-8	CONTRAINDICATIONS TO LOW-LEVEL LASER THERAPY
CONTRAINDICATIONS	**RATIONALE**
Over the eye	Risk of damaging the retina.
Over a malignant lesion	Risk of further enhancing and spreading the lesion.
Over the abdominal and pelvic area of pregnant women	Risk of interfering with normal development and growth of the fetus.
Over a hemorrhagic area	Risk of exacerbating the condition by laser-induced vasodilation (Baxter, 2002).
Over thyroid gland	Risk of interfering with the thyroid gland normal function (Navratil et al., 2002).
With epileptic patients	Risk of inducing an epileptic seizure (Navratil et al., 2002).

TABLE 11-9	RISKS, PRECAUTIONS, AND RECOMMENDATIONS FOR LOW-LEVEL LASER THERAPY

RISKS	RATIONALE
Over an infected area	Risk of stimulating or inhibiting bacterial activity.
Over testicular region	Risk of affecting fertility.
Over sympathetic ganglia, vagus nerve, and cardiac region in patients with heart disease	Risk of adverse heart effects (Baxter, 2002).
Over photosensitive skin areas	Risk of adverse reaction—a test dose is recommended before regular application (Baxter, 2002).
Over bone epiphysial region in growing children	Risk of affecting bone growth.

PRECAUTIONS	RATIONALE
Over bruised muscle	May enhance bruising (Gabel, 1995).
Patients with mental confusion	May lead to misunderstanding affecting treatment safety.

RECOMMENDATIONS	RATIONALE
Use closed rooms to deliver therapy	Avoid unnecessary exposure of surrounding staff and patients.
Wearing of protective eye glasses or goggles by both patient and practitioner—**mandatory**	Avoid eye damage. Make sure the goggles are of the right type, i.e., designed to block the specific wavelength emitted by the device used.
Increase energy density with specific patients	Ensure adequate energy absorption when treating overweight or obese patients with red or infrared light and patients with dark skin using red light (Nussbaum et al., 2007b).
Apply handheld laser probe with a light pressure (contact technique)	Increases light energy transmission (Nussbaum et al., 2007).
Clean exposed skin surface with alcohol before treatment	Avoid mechanical obstruction to the flow of the laser beam.
Keep the laser device under lock and key	Ensure that **only** clinicians have access to the device.
Plug line-powered device into a GFCI receptacle	Prevent the occurrence of macroshocks (see Chapter 27).
Conduct regular maintenance and calibration	Assure optimal device function. True power outputs specified by some manufacturers may be much less than advertised, leading to improper dosimetry (Nussbaum, 1999).

2. Skin Preparation

Before each application, the area of the exposed skin to be treated is inspected and cleaned with water and soap, or rubbing alcohol, to remove impurities.

3. Skin Sensory Discrimination Testing

In contrast to many EPAs covered in this textbook, there is no need to conduct skin sensory discrimination testing on the patient before use of LLLT, because this agent triggers no tissue heating during application.

4. Laser Selection

Practitioners can choose between red-light gaseous (HeNe) and infrared-light diode or semiconductor (GaAs; GaAlAs) lasers. Infrared-light lasers are made of one or more diodes. Multidiode lasers offer a wider range of wavelengths. Infrared lasers are more penetrating than gaseous lasers.

5. Mode of Delivery

LLLT can be delivered using the continuous or pulsed mode.

6. Device Testing

Prior to each treatment, test whether the laser device is functioning by applying the probe over the test photoelectrical cell mounted on the device console. The rationale behind such testing is that IR lasers generate invisible light and exposure to the laser beam generates no sensation. Recall that the red light seen at the tip of the probe is not a laser light.

7. Probe Type

Single (handheld) and *cluster* (mechanically mounted on the laser device) probes of different shapes and radiating beam areas may be used (**Fig 11-2**). Selection is based on the size of the treatment surface area; larger surface areas will require cluster probes in order to minimize the number of applications.

8. Application Methods

LLLT may be administered using two methods: *point by point* and *scanning*. With the point-by-point method, a handheld single probe is used; this method has three different techniques of application (contact, noncontact, and grid). With the *scanning* method, either a single probe or cluster probes are used. Scanning of the treated area may be manual or automatic.

a. Point by Point

This method refers to the application of a single diode over the surface overlying the pathological lesion. This single laser beam thus makes one point of contact with the skin. To treat a given surface area, the single probe is manually moved from one point to the next; hence, the term *point by point*. This method may be applied using two techniques: contact or noncontact.

i. Contact. This technique involves making a light contact between the tip of the probe and the skin surface. Contact with and without pressure can be used. The probe is held perpendicular to the skin surface. This technique eliminates photonic reflection off the skin surface and minimizes beam divergence because of the probe's proximity to the area being treated.

ii. Noncontact. This technique consists in keeping a distance, or gap, of a few millimeters between the probe tip and the skin surface overlying the treatment area. The laser probe is held perpendicular to and within a few millimeters (approximately 2–4 mm) of the skin surface to reduce wave reflection and beam divergence (Baxter, 1994). This technique is recommended when patients cannot tolerate the pressure exerted by the laser probe on the surface of the area being treated, as with the contact technique described later.

iii. Grid. This technique consists in making a grid by mapping the entire treatment surface area with 1-cm^2 squares to guide point-by-point application. Each cm^2 corresponds to one point. The grid can be made either visually or with a plastic sheet and a pen. The application can be done with the probe in contact or further away from the skin (noncontact).

b. Scanning

This method refers to the scanning of the entire treatment surface area. This scanning action may be done by manipulating the single probe (up-and-down and side-to-side movements) so as to cover the entire treatment surface area. It can also be done automatically by means of robotic displacements of the diodes within the cluster probe, or of the cluster probe itself, over the treatment area.

9. Protective Eyewear

Patients and clinicians *must* wear protective glasses or goggles, which filter the wavelengths emitted by the laser device during therapy (**Fig 11-3B**).

10. End of Treatment

Always inspect the exposed skin surface after treatment. Wipe the probe tip clean, using rubbing alcohol swab, if the contact method was used. Lock the laser device, and store the key in a safe place for further use.

B. DOCUMENTATION

Table 11-10 shows the key parameters to be documented in the patient's file.

TABLE 11-10	KEY TREATMENT PARAMETERS TO BE DOCUMENTED IN PATIENT'S FILE AFTER LOW-LEVEL LASER THERAPY

- *Laser type:* HeNe, GaAs, or GaAlAs
- *Number of laser diodes (LD):* Number
- *Number of nonlaser diode (SLD, when applicable):* Number
- *Wavelength:* Single diode: nm; Multiple diodes: list each wavelength (nm)
- *Delivery mode:* Continuous; Pulsed: pulse duration (PD): s; Frequency (f): Hz
- *Probe type:* Single (I LD); cluster (multiple LD and SLD, when applicable)
- *Application method and technique:* Point by point: contact, noncontact, grid; Scanning: manual or automatic
- *Diode beam radiating area:* cm^2
- *Power:* If continuous mode, peak power (P): mW; If pulsed mode, mean power (P_m): mW
- *Power density:* W/cm^2
- *Energy density:* J/cm^2
- *Application duration:* s
- *Dose per diode or per point:* J
- *Number of applications or points of application:* Number
- *Dose tissue:* J

Case Study 11-1   Cervical Osteoarthritis

A 62-year-old taxi driver, diagnosed with chronic cervical osteoarthritis, consults about his condition. His main complaint is severe neck pain during head movement, particularly when driving his car for a relatively long period of time without rest periods. Physical and radiographic examinations suggest that pain may be caused by bilateral osteoarthritic changes affecting facet joints (zygapophyseal joint) at the C2–C5 level. Physical examination also reveals a loss of 20° of flexion and 10° of extension. There is also a loss of 15° of right head rotation and 25° of left rotation. The patient is looking for an alternative to his current cocktail of analgesic and anti-inflammatory drugs that, in addition to not giving him adequate pain relief, is adding to his gastric problems. He fervently wants to reduce the number of pills he is currently taking. A few months ago he tried TENS therapy for a period of 6 weeks but got no satisfactory pain relief. He also tried hot pack therapy, but that did not provide lasting pain relief either. Surgery is not indicated. The patient's goals are to reduce his pain level when driving at work for long hours and improve his head mobility

Evidence-Based Steps Toward the Resolution of This Case

1. **List medical diagnosis.**
   - Osteoarthritis

2. **List key impairment(s).**
   - Pain
   - Decrease cervical range of motion

3. **List key functional limitation(s).**
   - Difficulty with head movements

4. **List key disability/disabilities.**
   - Difficulty with driving car at work

5. **Justification for low-level laser therapy.**

   Is there justification for use of LLLT in this case? This chapter has established that there is *fair-to-good justification* for the use of LLLT for osteoarthritis with a majority of grade I studies demonstrating therapeutic benefits (see Section VI). Recent review articles by Bjordal et al. (2003, 2006, 2007) further support the justification for using LLLT in the present case of cervical osteoarthritis. Still further justification stems from the fact that none of his previous therapies (drugs, TENS, and hot pack) has given him adequate pain relief. It is hypothesized that LLLT will decrease pain by modulating the inflammatory process affecting the facet joints. Because EPAs should never be used in isolation or as a sole intervention, a regimen of manual spinal mobilization is added.

6. **Search for contraindications.**
   None is found.

7. **Search for risks and precautions.**
   None is found.

8. **Outline the therapeutic goal(s) you and your patient wish to achieve.**
   - Decrease pain
   - Reduce drug consumption
   - Improve cervical range of motion (ROM)
   - Improve ability to drive car at work

9. **List the outcome measurement(s) used to assess treatment effectiveness.**
   - Pain: Visual Analog Scale (VAS)
   - Drug intake: pill count in personal diary
   - Neck ROM: cervical range of motion goniometer (CROM)
   - Car driving performance: Neck Disability Index (NDI)

10. **Instruct the patient about what he/she should experience, do, or not do during the LLLT treatment.**
    - Feel no sensation under the probe during therapy
    - Do not remove protective glasses/goggles during therapy

11. **Outline the prescription of LLLT based on the evidence available.**

    The prescription is based on published articles (Lewith et al., 1981; Walker, 1983; Willner et al., 1985; Lonauer, 1986; Jensen et al., 1987; Stelian et al., 1992; Gur et al., 2003a). It is also based on the dosage recommendations made by Bjordal et al. (2003, 2006, 2007), as well as on those listed on the Web site of the World Association for Laser Therapy (www.walt.nu). A single diode (mono-wavelength) is used, allowing the point-by-point method of application to be administered. In order to obtain the dosimetric prescriptive values presented below, readers may refer to the dosimetric calculations presented in **Table 11-8.**

    - *Laser device:* infrared GaAs
    - *Number of diode(s):* one (mono-wavelength)
    - *Wavelength:* 904 nm
    - *Application mode:* continuous
    - *Probe type:* single probe (handheld)
    - *Probe beam area (A):* 0.5 cm^2
    - *Power (P):* 50 mW
    - *Power density (P_d):* 100 mW/cm^2
    - *Method of application:* point by point
    - *Technique of application:* contact, over facet joint
    - *Application duration per point (T):* 90 s

- *Energy density (E_d): 9 J/cm²*
- *Dose per diode (D_d) or per point:* 4.5 J
- *Number of applications per treatment:* 6 points (3 points to left and right C3, C4, and C5)
- *Dose tissue (D_t) per treatment:* 27 J
- *Number of treatment sessions per day:* one
- *Total number of treatments:* 15, that is, 5 per week over the course of 3 consecutive weeks

12. **Analyze outcome measurements.**

Pre- and posttreatment comparison:

- Pain: decreased VAS score from 7 to 2
- Drug intake: decreased number of pills by 50%
- Cervical ROM:
  - Flexion and extension: both increased by 20°
  - Left rotation: increased by 4°
  - Right rotation: increased by 8°
- Ability to drive car at work (taxi): Improved NDI score by 60%

13. **Assess treatment effectiveness on the basis of outcome measures.**

The results show that 15 applications of LLLT, delivered over 3 consecutive weeks, used concomitantly with a regimen of therapeutic neck manual mobilization, led to a significant decrease in pain, which correlated well with his decreased drug intake. This therapeutic regimen also improved the patient's neck mobility and ability to drive his car for longer periods of time without rest as a taxi driver. The patient, although symptomatic, is very pleased with the results, particularly with the decrease in his daily intake of pills. Overall, LLLT had a beneficial impact on the patient's disablement status created by the pathology, as illustrated in the **figure below**.

14. **State the prognosis.**

There is, unfortunately, no curative treatment for osteoarthritis. The prognosis is good if the patient keeps mobilizing his head daily and within the pain-free range. It is more than likely that this patient may have to be treated again with LLLT over the next months and years in order to maintain the fragile balance between neck pain and neck or head mobility.

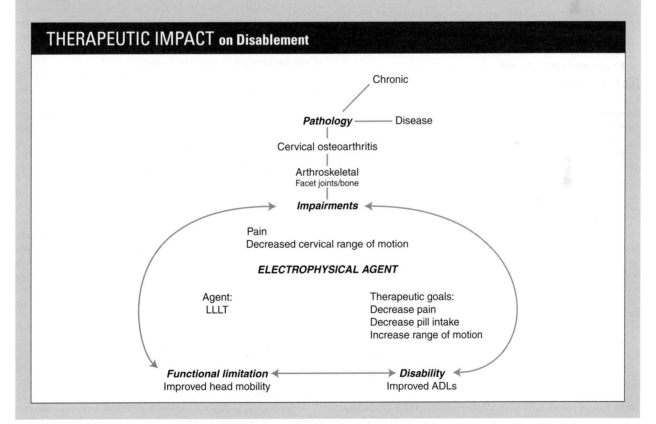

CRITICAL THINKING QUESTIONS

Clarification: What is meant by low-level laser therapy (LLLT)?

Assumptions: You have assumed that the therapeutic optical window of LLLT is within the visible red and invisible near-infrared band of the electromagnetic spectrum. How do you justify making that assumption?

Reasons and evidence: What led you to believe that monochromacity may be the key property behind the therapeutic effects of LLLT?

Viewpoints or perspectives: How would you respond to a colleague who says that the use of LLLT is well justified today for the treatment of cutaneous wounds and tendinopathies?

Implications and consequences: What are the implications and consequences of using a single handheld probe instead of a cluster probe? What are the implications and consequences if neither the operator nor the patient wears protective goggles when delivering or receiving LLLT?

About the question: What is the estimated penetration depth of HeNe and diode-type lasers used to deliver LLLT to soft tissues? Why do you think I ask this question?

References

Articles

Altan L, Bibgol U, Aykac M, Yurtkuran M (2005) Investigation of the effect of GaAs laser therapy on cervical myofascial pain syndrome. Rheumatol Int, 25: 23–27

Asada K, Yutani Y, Shimazu A (1989) Diode laser therapy for rheumatoid arthritis. A clinical evaluation of 102 joints treated with low reactive-level laser therapy (LLLT). Laser Ther, 1: 147–151

Ashford R, Lagan K, Brown N, Howell C, Nolan C, Brady D, Walsh M (1999) Low-intensity laser therapy for chronic venous leg ulcers. Nurs Stand, 14: 66–70, 72

Atsumi K, Fijumasa I, Abe Y (1987) Biostimulation effect of low-power energy of diode laser for pain relief. Lasers Surg Med, 7: 77–82

Basford JR, Malanga GA, Krause DA, Harmsen WS (1998) A randomized controlled evaluation of low-intensity laser therapy: Plantar fasciitis. Arch Phys Med Rehabil, 79: 249–254

Basford JR, Sheffield CH, Cieslak KR (2000) Laser therapy: A randomized, controlled trial of the effects of low power intensity Nd:Yag laser irradiation on lateral epicondylitis. Arch Phys Med Rehabil, 81: 1504–1510

Basford JR, Sheffield CG, Harmsen WS (1999) Laser therapy: A randomized, controlled trial of the effects of low-intensity Nd·YAG laser irradiation on musculoskeletal back pain. Arch Phys Med Rehabil, 80: 647–652

Basford JR, Sheffield CG, Mair SD, Ilstrup DM (1987) Low-energy helium-neon laser of thumb ostearthritis. Arch Phys Med Rehabil, 68: 794–797

Bihari I, Mester AR (1989) The biostimulative effects of low-level laser therapy of long-standing crural ulcers using helium-neon laser, helium-neon plus infrared lasers, and noncoherent light: Preliminary reports of a randomized double-blind comparative study. Laser Ther, 1: 75–78

Bingol U, Altan L, Yurtkuran M (2005) Low-power laser treatment for shoulder pain. Photomedicine Laser Surg, 23: 459–464

Bjordal JM, Lopes-Martins RA, Iversen VV (2006a) A randomized placebo controlled trial of low level laser therapy for activated Achilles tendonitis with microdialysis measurement of peritendinous prostaglandin E2 concentration. Br J Sports Med, 40: 76–80

Bliddal H, Hellesen C, Ditlevsen P, Asselberghs J, Lyager L (1987) Soft-laser therapy of rheumatoid arthritis. Scand J Rheumatol, 16: 225–228

Brosseau L, Wells G, Marchand S, Gaboury I, Stokes B, Morin M, Casimiro L, Yonge K, Tugwell P (2005) Randomized controlled trial on lower laser therapy (LLLT) in the treatment of osteoarthritis (OA) on the hand. Lasers Surg Med, 36: 210–219

Bülow PM, Jensen H, Danneskiold-Samsoe B (1994) Low-power Ga-Al-As laser treatment of painful osteoarthritis of the knee. Scand J Rehab Med, 26: 155–159

Catari CJ, Anderson SN, Gannon BJ, Piller NB (2003) Treatment of postmastectomy lymphedema with low-level laser therapy: A double blind, placebo-controlled trial. Cancer, 98: 1114–1122

Ceccherelli F, Altafini L, Lo Castro G, Avila A, Ambrosio F, Giron GP (1989) Diode laser in cervical myofascial pain: A double-blind study versus placebo. Clin J Pain, 5: 301–304

Cetiner S, Kahraman SA, Yucetas S (2006) Evaluation of low-level laser therapy in the treatment of temporomandibular disorders. Photomedicine Laser Surg, 24: 637-641

Conti PC (1997) Low-level laser therapy in the treatment of temporomandibular disorders (TMD): A double-blind pilot study. Cranio, 15: 144–199

Craig JA, Barlas P, Baxter GD, Walsh DM, Allen JM (1996) Delayed-onset of muscle soreness: Lack of effect of combined phototherapy/low-intensity laser therapy at low pulse repetition rates. J Clin Laser Med Surg, 14: 375–380

Craig JA, Barron J, Walsh DM, Baxter GD (1999) Lack of effect of combined low-intensity laser therapy/phototherapy (CLILT) on delayed onset muscle soreness in humans. Lasers Surg Med, 24: 223–230

Crous LC, Malherbe CP (1988) Laser and ultraviolet light irradiation in the treatment of chronic ulcers. S Afr J Physiother, 44: 73–77

Darre EM, Klokker M, Lund P, Rasmussen JD, Hansen K, Vedtoffe PE (1994) Laser therapy of Achilles tendonitis. Ugeskr Laeger, 156: 6680–6683

De Bie RA, de Vet HC, Lenssen TF, van den Wildenberg FA, Kootstra G, Knispschild PG (1998) Low-level laser therapy in ankle sprains. A randomized clinical trial. Arch Phys Med Rehabil, 79: 1415–1420

Djavid GE, Mehrdad R, Ghasemi M, Hasan-Zedeh H, Sotoodeh-Manesh A, Pouryaghoub G (2007) In chronic low-back pain, low-level laser therapy combined with exercise is more beneficial than exercise alone in the long term: A randomized trial. Aust J Physiother, 53: 155–160

Eckerdal A, Bastian HL (1996) Can low reactive–level laser therapy be used in the treatment of neurogenic facial pain? A double-blind, placebo-controlled investigation of patients with trigeminal neuralgia. Laser Ther, 8: 247–252

Ekim A, Armagan O, Tascioglu F, Oner C, Colak M (2007) Effect of low-level laser therapy in rheumatoid patients with carpal tunnel syndrome. Swiss Med Wkly, 137: 347–352

Emmanoulidis O, Diamantopoulos C (1986) CW IR low-power laser application significantly accelerates chronic pain rehabilitation of professional athletes. A double-blind study. Lasers Surg Med, 6: 173–178

England S, Farrell AJ, Coppock JS, Struthers G, Bacon PA (1989) Low-power laser therapy of shoulder tendonitis. Scand J Rheumatol, 18: 427–431

Evcik D, Kavuncu V, Cakir T, Subasi V, Yaman M (2007) Laser therapy in the treatment of carpal tunnel syndrome: A randomized controlled trial. Photomed Laser Surg, 25: 34–39

Fikackova H, Dostalova T, Navratil L, Klaschka J (2007) Effectiveness of low-level laser therapy in temporomandibular joint disorders: A placebo-controlled study. Photomed Laser Surg, 25: 297–303

Fulga C (1998) Anti-inflammatory effect of laser therapy in rheumatoid arthritis. Rom J Inter Med, 36: 273–279

Fulga C, Fulga IC, Prodescu M (1994) Clinical study of the effect of laser therapy in rheumatic degenerative diseases. Rom J Intern Med, 32: 227–233

Gabel P (1995) Does laser enhance bruising in acute sporting injuries? Aust J Physiother, 41: 273–275

Gartner CH, Becker M, Dusoir T (1987) Pain control in spondyloarthritis with infrared laser. Lasers Surg Med, 7: 79–81

Goats GC, Flett E, Hunter JA, Stirling A (1996) Low-intensity laser and phototherapy for rheumatoid arthritis. Physiotherapy, 82: 311–320

Gogia PP, Hurt BS, Zirn TT (1988) Wound management with whirlpool and infrared cold laser treatment. Phys Ther, 68: 1239–1242

Goldman JA, Chiapella J, Casey H, Bass N, Graham J, McClatchey W, Dronavalli RV, Brown R, Bennet WJ, Miller SB, Wilson CH, Pearson B, Haun C, Persinski L, Huey H, Muckerheide M (1980) Laser therapy in rheumatoid arthritis. Laser Surg Ther, 1: 93–101

Gur A, Cosut A, Sarac AJ, Cevik R, Nas K, Uyar A (2003a) Efficacy of different therapy regimes of low-power laser in painful osteoarthritis of the knee: A double-blind and randomized-controlled trial. Lasers Surg Med, 33: 330–338

Gur A, Karakoc M, Cevik R, Nas K, Sarac AJ, Karakoc M (2003b) Efficacy of low power laser therapy and exercise on pain and functions in chronic low back pain. Lasers Surg Med, 32: 233–238

Gur A, Kakaroc M, Nas K, Cevik R, Sarac J, Ataoglu S (2002) Effects of low power laser and low dose amitriptyline therapy on clinical symptoms and quality of life in fibromyalgia: A single-blind, placebo-controlled trial. Rheumatol Int, 22: 188–193

Gur A, Sarac AJ, Cevik R, Altindag O, Sarac S (2004) Efficacy of 904 nm Gallium Arsenide Low level laser therapy in the management of chronic myofascial pain in the neck: A double-blind and randomized-controlled trial. Lasers Surg Med, 35: 229–235

Haker E, Lunderberg T (1990) Laser treatment applied to acupuncture points in lateral humeral epicondylalgia. A double-blind study. Pain, 43: 243–247

Haker EH, Lundeberg TC (1991) Lateral epicondylalgia: Report of non-effective midlaser treatment. Arch Phys Med Rehabil, 72: 984–988

Hakguder A, Birtane M, Gurcan S, Kokino S, Turan FN (2003) Efficacy of low level laser therapy in myofascial pain syndrome: An algometric and thermographic evaluation. Lasers Surg Med: 33: 339–343

Hall J, Clarke AK, Elvins DM, Ring EF (1994) Low-level laser therapy is ineffective in the management of rheumatoid arthritic finger joints. Br J Rheumatol, 33: 142–147

Hansen HJ, Thoroe U (1990) Low-power laser biostimulation of chronic oro-facial pain. A double-blind, placebo-controlled cross-over study in 40 patients. Pain, 43: 169–179

Herascu N, Velciu B, Calin M, Savastru D, Talianu C (2005) Low-level laser therapy (LLLT) efficacy in post-operative wounds. Photomed Laser Surg, 23: 70–73

Heussler JK, Hinchey G, Margiotta E, Quinn R, Butler P, Martin J, Sturgess AD (1993) A double-blind, randomized trial of low-power laser treatment in rheumatoid arthritis. Ann Rheum Dis, 52: 703–706

Hirschl M, Katsenschlager R, Francesconi C, Kundi M (2004) Low level laser therapy in primary Raynaud's phenomenon—results of a placebo controlled, double blind intervention study. J Rheumatol, 31: 2408–2412

Hopkins JT, McLoda TA, Seegmiller JG, Baxter GD (2004) Low-level laser therapy facilitates superficial wound healing in humans: A triple-blind, sham-controlled study. J Athl Training, 39: 223–229

Houza G, Gerenemus R, Dover J, Arndt K (1993) Lasers in dermatology. Arch Dermatol, 129: 1026–1035

Ilbuldu E, Cakmak A, Disci R, Aydin R (2004) Comparison of laser, dry needling, and placebo laser treatments in myofascial pain syndrome. Photomed Laser Surg, 22: 306–311

Irvine J, Chong SL, Amirjani N, Chan KM (2004) Double-blind randomized controlled trial on low-level laser therapy in carpal tunnel syndrome. Muscle & Nerve, 30: 182–187

Jensen H, Herreby M, Kjer J (1987) Infrared laser-effect in painful arthrosis of the knee? Ugeskr Laeger, 149: 3104–3106

Johannsen F, Hauschild B, Remvig L, Johnsen V, Petersen M, Bieler T (1994) Low-energy laser therapy in rheumatoid arthritis. Scand J Rheumatol, 23: 145–147

Karu TI, Ryabykh TP, Fedoseyeva GE, Puchkova NI (1989) Helium-neon laser-induced respiratory burst of phagocytotic cells. Lasers Surg Med, 9: 585–588

Kaviani A, Fateh M, Nooraie RY, Alinagi-Zadeh MR, Ataie-Fashtami L (2006) Low-level laser therapy in management of postmastectomy lymphedema. Lasers Med Sci, 21: 90–94

Kemmotsu O, Sato K, Furumido H, Harada K, Takigawa C, Kaseno S, Yokota S, Hanaoka Y, Yamamura T (1991) Efficacy of low reactive-level laser therapy for pain attenuation of postherpetic neuralgia. Laser Ther, 3: 71–76

Khan J (1984) Case reports: Open wound management with the HeNe (632.8 nm) cold laser. J Orthop Sports Phys Ther, 6: 203–204

Klein RG, Eek BC (1990) Low-energy laser treatment and exercise for chronic low back pain: Double-blind controlled trial. Arch Phys Med Rehabil, 71: 34–37

Knappe V, Frank F, Rohde E (2004) Principles of lasers and biophotonics effects. Photomedicine and Laser Surg, 22: 411-417

Kokol R, Berger C, Haas J, Kopera D (2005) Venous leg ulcers: No improvement of wound healing with 685-nm low level laser therapy. Randomized, placebo-controlled, double blind study. Hautarzt, 56: 570–575

Kolari PJ, Airaksinen O (1993) Penetration of infrared and helium-neon laser light into the tissue. Acupuncture and Electro Therapeutics Research Journal, 13: 232–233

Konstantinovic L, Antonic M, Badareski Z (1997) Combined low-power laser therapy and local infiltration of corticosteroids in the treatment of radial humeral epicondylitis. Vojnosanit Pregl, 54: 489–463

Kopera D, Kokol R, Berger C, Haas J (2005) Does the use of low-level laser influence wound healing in chronic venous leg ulcers? J Wound, 14: 391–394

Krasheninnikoff M, Ellitsgaard N, Rogvi-Hansen B, Zeuthen A, Harder K, Larsen R, Gaardbo H (1994) No effect of low-power laser in lateral epicondylitis. Scand J Rheumatol, 23: 260–263

Kreczi T, Klinger D (1986) A comparison of laser acupuncture versus placebo in radicular and pseudoradicular pain syndromes as recorded by subjective responses of patients. Acupunct Electrother Res, 11: 207–216

Kulekcioglu S, Sivrioglu K, Ozcan O, Parlak M (2003) Effectiveness of low-level laser therapy in tempomandibular disorders. Scan J Rheumatol, 32: 114–118

Kymplova J, Navratil L, Knizek J (2003) Contribution of phototherapy to the treatment of episiotomies. J Clin Laser Med Surg, 21: 35–39

Lagan KM, McDonough SM, Clements BA, Baxter GD (2000) A case report of low intensity laser therapy (LILT) in the management of venous ulceration: Potential effects of wound debridement upon efficacy. J Clin Laser Med Surg, 18: 15–22

Lagan KM, Clements BA, McDonough S, Baxter GD (2001) Low intensity laser therapy 9830nm) in the management of minor postsurgical wounds: A controlled clinical study. Lasers Surg Med, 28: 27–32

Lagan KM, McKenna T, Witherow A, Johns J, McDonough SM, Baxter GD (2002) Low-intensity laser therapy/combined phototherapy in the management of chronic venous ulceration: a placebo-controlled study. J Clin Laser Med Surg, 20: 109–116

Lam KL, Cheing GL (2007) Effects of 904-nm low-level laser therapy in the management of lateral epicondylitis: A randomized controlled trial. Photomed Laser Surg, 25: 65–71

Lewith GT, Machin D (1981) A randomized trial to evaluate the effects of infrared stimulation on local trigger points, versus placebo, on the pain caused by cervical osteoarthritis. Acup Electroth Res Int J, 6: 277–284

Li XH (1990) Laser in the department of traumatology: With a report of 60 cases of soft tissue injury. Laser Ther, 2: 119–122

Logdberg-Andersson M, Mutzell S, Hazel A (1997) Low level laser therapy of tendinitis and myofascial pain: A randomized double-blind controlled study. Laser Therapy, 9: 79–86

Lonauer G (1986) Controlled double-blind study on the efficacy of HeNe laser beams versus HeNe infrared laser beams in the therapy of activated osteoarthritis of finger joints. Lasers Surg Med, 6: 172–175

Longo L, Simunovic Z, Postiglione M, Postiglione M (1997) Laser therapy for fibromyositic rheumatisms. J Clin Laser Med Surg, 15: 217–220

Lucas C, van Gemet MJ, de Haan RJ (2003) Efficacy of low-level laser therapy in the management of stage III decubitus ulcers: A prospective, observer-blinded multicenter randomized clinical trial. Lasers Med Sci, 18: 72–77

Lundeberg T, Haker E, Thomas M (1987) Effect of laser versus placebo in tennis elbow. Scand J Rehab Med, 19: 135–138

Lundeberg T, Malm M (1991) Low-power HeNe laser treatment of venous leg ulcers. Ann Plastic Surg, 27: 537–539

Matsumura C, Ishikawa F, Imai M, Kemmotsu O (1993) Useful effect of application of helium-neon LLLT on an early stage of case of herpes zoster: A case report. Laser Ther, 5: 43–46

Matsutani LA, Marques AP, Ferreira EA, Assumpcao A, Lage LV, Casarotto RA, Pereira CA (2007) Effectiveness of muscle stretching exercises with and without laser therapy at tender points for patients with fibromyalgia. Clin Exp Rheumatol, 25: 410–415

Mazzetto MO, Carasco TG, Bidinelo EF, de Andrade Pizzo RC, Mazetto RG (2007) Low intensity laser application in temporomandibular disorders: A phase I double-blind study. Cranio, 25: 186–192

McKibben LS, Downie R (1990) Treatment of postherpetic pain using a 904 nm low-energy infrared laser. Laser Ther, 2: 20–25

Mester E, Korenyi-Both A, Spiry T, Tisza S (1970) The effect of laser irradiation on the regeneration of muscle fibres (preliminary report). Z Exp Chirurg, 8: 258–262

Mester E, Mester A (1989) Wound healing. Laser Ther, 1: 7–15

Mester E, Mester AF, Mester A (1985) The biomedical effect of laser application. Lasers Surg Med, 5: 31–39

Mester E, Spiry T, Szende B, Tota JG (1971) Effect of laser rays on wound healing. Am J Surg, 122: 532–535

Mester E, Szende B, Gartner P (1968) The effect of laser beams on the growth of hair in mice. Radiobiol Radiother, 9: 621–626

Moore KC, Hira N, Broome IJ, Cruikshank JA (1992) The effect of infrared diode laser irradiation on the duration and severity of postoperative pain. A double-blind trial. Laser Ther, 4: 145–150

Moore KC, Hira N, Kumar PS, Jayakumar CS, Oshiro T (1988) A double-blind crossover trial of low-level laser therapy in the treatment of post herpetic neuralgia. Laser Ther, 1: 7–9

Morita H, Kohno J, Hori M, Kitano Y (1993) Clinical application of low reactive–level laser therapy (LLLT) for atopic dermatitis. Keio J Med, 42: 174–176

Mulcahy D, McCormack D, McElwain J, Wagstaff S, Conroy C (1995) Low-level laser therapy: A prospective double-blind trial of its use in an orthopedic population. Injury, 26: 315–317

Naeser MA, Han KA, Lieberman BE, Branco KF (2002) Carpal tunnel syndrome pain treated with low-level laser and microamperes transcutaneous electric nerve stimulation: A controlled study. Arch Phys Med Rehabil, 83: 978–988

Navratil L, Kymplova J (2002) Contraindications in non-invasive laser therapy: Truth and fiction. J Clin Laser Med Surg, 20: 341–343

Nolan LJ (1987) Laser physics and safety. Clin Podiatr Med Surg, 4: 777–786

Nunez SC, Garces AS, Suzuki SS, Ribeiro MS (2006) management of mouth opening in patients with temporomandibular disorders through low-level laser therapy and transcutaneous electrical nerve stimuloution. Photomed Laser Surg, 24: 45-49

Nussbaum EL (1999) Low-intensity laser therapy for benign fibrotic lumps in the breast following reduction mammaplasty. Phys Ther, 79: 691–698

Nussbaum EL, Biemann I, Mustard B (1994) Comparison of ultrasound/ ultraviolet-C and laser for treatment of pressure ulcers in patients with spinal cord injury. Phys Ther, 74: 812–823

Nussbaum EL, Burke S, Johnstone L, Lahiffe G, Robitaille E, Yoshida K (2007a) Use of electrophysical agents: Findings and implications of a survey of practice in Metro Toronto. Physioth Can, 59: 118–131

Nussbaum EL, Van Zuylen J, Baxter GD (1999) Specification of treatment dosage in laser therapy: Unreliable equipment and radiant power determination as confounding factors. Physiother Can, 51: 159–167

Nussbaum EL, Van Zuylen J, Jing F (2007b) Transmission of light through human skin folds during phototherapy: Effects of physical characteristics, irradiation wavelength, and skin-diode coupling. Physioth Can, 59: 194–207

Obara J, Yanase M, Motomura (1987) The pain relief of low-energy laser irradiation on rheumatoid arthritis. Pain Clinic, 8: 18–22

Ohshiro T, Maeda T (1992) Application of 830-nm diode laser LLLT as successful adjunctive therapy of hypertrophic scars and keloids. Laser Ther, 4: 155–168

Ohtsuka H, Kemnotsu O, Doazaki S, Imai I (1992) Low reactive–level laser therapy near the stellate ganglion for postherpetic facial neuralgia. Masui, 91: 1809–1813

Oken O, Kahraman Y, Ayhan F, Canpolat S, Yorgancioglu ZR, Oken OF (2008) The short-term efficacy of laser, brace, and ultrasound treatment in lateral epicondylitis: A prospective, randomized, controlled trial. J Hand Ther, 21: 63–67

Olavi A, Pekka R, Pertti K (1989) Effects of the infrared laser therapy at treated and non-treated trigger points. Acupunct Electrother Res, 14: 9–14

Ong KS, Ho VC (2001) Pain reduction by low-level laser therapy: A double-blind, controlled, randomized study in bilaterally symmetrical oral surgery. Am J Pain Manage, 11: 12–16

Ozdemir F, Birtane M, Kokino S (2001) The clinical efficacy of low-power laser therapy on pain and function in cervical osteoarthritis. Clin Rheumatol, 20: 181–184

Palmgren N, Jensen GF, Kaa K, Windelin M, Colov HC (1989) Low-power laser therapy in rheumatoid arthritis. Laser Med Sci, 4: 193–196

Palmieri B (1984) Stratified double blind crossoever study on tennis elbow in young amateur athletes using infrared lasertherapy. Med Laser Report, 1–7

Papadopoulos ES, Smith RW, Cawley MI, Mani R (1996) Low-level laser therapy does not aid the management of tennis elbow. Clin Rehab, 10: 9–11

Pinheiro AL, Cavalcanti ET, Pinheiro TI, Alves MJ, Manzi CT (1997) Low-level laser therapy in the management of disorders of the maxillofacial region. J Clin Laser Med Surg, 15: 181–183

Pinheiro AL, Calvalcanti ET, Pinheiro TI, Alves MJ, Miranda ER, De Quevedo AS, Manzi CT, Vieira AL, Rolim AB (1998) Low-level laser therapy is an important tool to treat disorders of the maxillofacial region. J Clin Laser Med Surg, 16: 223–226

Robinson B, Walters J (1991) The use of low laser therapy in diabetic and other ulcerations. J Br Pod Med, 46: 10–14

Robertson VJ, Spurritt D (1998) Electrophysical agents: implications of their availability ans use in undergraduate clinical placements. Physiotherapy, 84: 335–344

Rogvi-Hansen B, Ellitsgaard N, Funch M, Dall-Jensen M, Prieske J (1991) Low-level laser treatment of chondromalacia patellae. Int Orthop, 15: 359–361

Santoianni P, Monfrecola G, Martellota D, Ayala F (1984) Inadequate effect of helium-neon laser on venous leg ulcers. Photodermatology, 1: 245–249

Schindl A, Heinze G, Schindl M, Pernerstorfer-Schon H, Schindl L (2002) Systemic effects of low-intensity laser irradiation on skin microcirculation in patients with diabetic microangiopathy. Microvasc Res, 64: 240-246

Schindl A, Neumann R (1999a) Low-intensity laser therapy is an effective treatment for recurrent herpes simplex infection. Results from a randomized, double-blind, placebo-controlled trial. J Invest Med, 113: 221–223

Schindl A, Schindl M, Pernerstorfer-Schon H, Kerschan K, Knobler R, Schindl L (1999b) Diabetic neuropathic foot ulcer: Successful treatment by low-intensity laser therapy. Dermatology, 198: 314–316

Schindl A, Schindl M, Pernerstorfer-Schon H, Mossbacher U, Schindl L (2000) Low-intensity laser irradiation in the treatment of recalcitrant radiation ulcers in patients with breast cancer—long-term results of three cases. Photodermatol Photoimmunol Photomed, 16: 34–37

Schindl A, Schindl M, Schindl L (1997) Successful treatment of persistent radiation ulcer by low-power laser therapy. J Am Acad Dermatol, 37: 646–648

Schindl A, Schindl M, Schon H, Knobler R, Havelec L, Schindl L (1998) Low-intensity laser irradiation improves skin circulation in patients with diabetic microangiopathy. Diabetes Care, 21: 580–584

Schindl M, Kerschan K, Schindl A, Schon H, Heinzl H, Schindl L (1999) Induction of complete wound healing in recalcitrant ulcers by low-intensity laser irradiation depends on ulcer cause and size. Photodermatol Photoimmunol Photomed, 15: 18–21

Shields N, Gormley J, O'Hare N (2002) Short-wave diathermy: current clinical and safety practices. Physiother Res Int, 7: 191–202

Shiroto C, Ono K, Onshiro T (1989) Retrospective study of diode laser therapy for pain attenuation in 3635 patients: Detailed analysis by questionnaire. Laser Ther, 1 : 41–48

Siebert W, Seichert N, Seibert B, Wirth CJ (1987) What is the efficacy of "soft" and "mild" lasers in therapy of tendinopathies? A double-blind study. Arch Orthop Trauma Surg, 106: 358–363

Simunovic Z (1996) Low-level laser therapy with trigger points technique: A clinical study of 243 patients. J Clin Laser Med Surg, 14: 163–167

Simunovic Z, Trobonjaca T, Trobonjaca Z (1998) Treatment of medial and lateral epicondylitis—tennis and golfer's elbow—with low-level laser therapy: A multicenter double-blind, placebo-controlled clinical study on 324 patients. J Clin Laser Med Surg, 16: 145–151

Smith KC (1991) The photobiological basis of low-level laser radiation therapy. Laser Ther, 3: 19–24

Snyder-Mackler L, Barry AJ, Perdins AI, Soucek MD (1989) Effects of helium-neon laser irradiation on skin resistance and pain in patients with trigger points in the neck or back. Phys Ther, 69: 336–341

Stelian J, Gil I, Habot B (1992) Improvement of pain and disability in elderly patients with degenerative osteoarthritis of the knee treated with narrow band light therapy. J Am Geriatr Soc, 40: 23–26

Stergioulas A (2004) Low-level laser treatment can reduce edema in second degree ankle sprains. J Clin Laser Med Surg, 22: 125–128

Stergioulas A (2007) Effects of low-level laser and plyometric exercises in the treatment of lateral epicondylitis. Photomed Laser Surg, 25: 205–213

Sugrue ME, Carolan J, leen EJ, feeley TM, Moore DJ, Shanik GD (1990) The use of infrared laser therapy in the treatment of venous ulceration. Ann Vasc Surg, 4: 179–181

Tam G (1999) Low-power laser therapy and analgesic action. J Clin Laser Med Surg 17: 29–33

Terashima H, Okajima K, Motegi M (1990) Low laser level irradiation for lateral humeral epicondylitis and De Quervain's disease. Laser Ther, 2: 27–32

Thorsen H, Gam AN, Jensen MK, Hojmark L, Wahlstrom L (1991) Low-energy laser treatment—Effect in localized fibromyalgia in the neck and shoulder regions. Ugeskr Laeger, 153: 1801–1804

Thorsen H, Gam AN, Svensson BH, Jess M, Jensen MK, Piculell I, Schack LK, Skjott K (1992) Low-level laser therapy for myofascial pain in the neck and shoulder girdle. A double-blind, cross-over study. Scand J Rheumatol, 21: 139–141

Tiphlova O, Karu T (1989) Role of primary photoacceptors in low-power laser effects: Action of HeNe laser radiation on bacteriophage T4-*Escherichia coli* interaction. Lasers Surg Med, 9: 67–69

Trelles MA, Rigau J, Sala P (1991) Infrared diode laser in low reactive–level laser therapy (LLCLT) for knee osteoarthritis. Laser Ther, 3: 198–153

Vasseljen O, Hoeg N, Kjelstad B, Johnsson A, Larsen S (1992) Low-level laser versus placebo in the treatment of tennis elbow. Scand J Rehab Med, 24: 37–42

Vecchio P, Cave M, King V, Adebajo AO, Smith M, Hazleman BL (1993) A double-blind study of the effectiveness of low-level laser treatment of rotator cuff tendonitis. Br J Rheumatol, 32: 740–742

Walker J (1983) Relief from chronic pain by low-power laser irradiation. Neurosci Lett, 43: 339–344

Walker JB (1985) Temporary suppression of clonus in humans by brief photostimulation. Brain Res, 340: 109–113

Walker JB, Akhanjee LK, Cooney MM (1987a) Laser therapy for pain of trigeminal neuralgia. Clin J Pain, 3: 183–187

Walker JB, Akhanjee LK, Cooney MM, Goldstein J, Tamayoshi S, Segal-Gidan F (1987b) Laser therapy for pain of rheumatoid arthritis. Clin J Pain, 3: 54–59

Waylonis GW, Wilke S, O'Toole D, Waylonis DA, Waylonis DB (1988) Chronic myofascial pain: Management by low-output helium-neon laser therapy. Arch Phys Med Rehabil, 69: 1017–102

Weintraub MI (1997) Noninvasive laser neurolysis in carpal tunnel syndrome. Muscle & Nerve, 20: 1029–1031

Willner R, Abeles M, Myerson G (1985) Low-power infrared laser biostimulation of chronic osteoarthritis in hand. Laser Surg Med, 5: 149–150

Yaksish I (1993) Low-energy laser therapy for treatment of post-herpetic neuralgia. Ann Acad Med Singapore, 22 (Suppl 3): 441–442

Review Articles

Basford JR (1986) Low-energy laser treatment of pain and wounds: Hype, hope or hokum? Mayo Clin Proc, 61: 671–675

Basford JR (1989a) The clinical and experimental status of low-energy laser therapy. Crit Rev Phys Rehab Med, 1: 1–9

Basford JR (1989b) Low-energy laser therapy: Controversies and new research findings. Lasers Surg Med, 9: 1–5

Basford JR (1993) Laser therapy: Scientific basis and clinical role. Orthopedics, 16: 541–547

Basford JR (1995) Low-intensity laser therapy: Still not an established clinical tool. Lasers Surg Med, 16: 331–342

Beckerman H, de Bie RA, Bouter LM, De Cuyper HJ, Oostendorp RA (1992) The efficacy of laser therapy for musculoskeletal and skin disorders. A criteria-based meta-analysis of randomized clinical trials. Phys Ther, 72: 413–491

Bjordal J, Couppé C, Ljunggren A (2001) Low-level laser therapy for tendinopathy. Evidence of a dose-response pattern. Phys Ther Rev, 6: 91–99

Bjordal JM, Couppé C, Chow RT, Tuner J, Ljunggren EA (2003) A systematic review of low level laser therapy with location-specific doses for pain from chronic joint disorders. Australian J Physiother, 49: 107–116

Bjordal JM, Bogen B, Lopes-Martin RA, Klovning A (2005) Can Cochrane reviews in controversial areas be biased? A sensitive analysis based on the protocol of a systematic Cochrane review on low-level laser therapy in osteoarthritis. Photomed Laser Surg, 23: 453–458

Bjordal JM, Johnson MI, Iversen VV, Aimbire FR (2006b) Low Level Laser Therapy (LLLT) in acute pain: A systematic review of possible mechanisms of action and clinical effects in randomized placebo-controlled trials. Photomed Laser Surg, 24: 158–168

Bjordal JM, Johnson MI, Lopes-Martins RA, Bogen B, Chow R, Ljunggren AE (2007) Short-term efficacy of physical interventions in osteoarthritic knee pain. A systematic review and meta-analysis of randomized placebo-controlled trials. BMC Musculoskelet Disord, 22: 8–51

Bjordal JM, Lopes-Martins RA, Joensen J, Couppe C, Ljunggren AE, Stergioulas A, Johnson MI (2008) A systematic review with procedural assessments and meta-analysis of Low Level Laser Therapy in lateral elbow tendinopathy (tennis elbow). BMC Musculoskeletal Dis, 9: 75–89)

Brosseau L, Robinson V, Wells G, De Bie R, Gam A, Harman K, Morin M, Shea B, Tugwell P (2005a) Low-level laser therapy (classes I, II, and III) for treating osteoarthritis. Cochrane Database Syst Rev, 2: CD002046

Brosseau L, Robinson V, Wells G, De Bie R, Gam A, Harman K, Morin M, Shea B, Tugwell P (2005b) Low-level laser therapy (classes I, II, and III) for treating rheumatoid arthritis. Cochrane Database Syst Rev, 2: CD002049

Brosseau L, Welch V, Wells G, Tugwell P, de Bie R, Gam A, Harman K, Shea B, Morin M (2000) Low-level laser therapy for osteoarthritis and rheumatoid arthritis: A meta-analysis. J Rheumatol, 27: 1961–1969

Dreyfuss P, Stratton S (1993) The low-energy laser, electro-acuscope and neuroprobe. Phys Sportsmed, 21 (8): 47–57

Enwemeka CS (1988) Laser biostimulation of healing wounds: Specific effects and mechanisms of action. J Orthop Sports Phys Ther, 9: 333–338

Enwemeka CS, Parker JC, Dowdy DS, Harkness EE, Sanford LE, Woodruff LD (2004) The efficacy of low-power laser in tissue repair and pain control: A meta-analysis study. Photomed Laser Surg, 22: 323–329

Flemming KA, Cullum NA, Nelson EA (1999) A systematic review of laser therapy for venous leg ulcers. J Wound Care, 8: 111–114

Gam AN, Thornsen H, Lonnberg F (1993) The effect of low-level laser therapy on musculoskeletal pain: A meta-analysis. Pain, 52: 63–66

Hamlin MR, Demidova TN (2006) Mechanisms of low level light therapy. Proc of SPIE, 6140: 1–12

Hawkins D, Houreld N, Abrahamse H (2005) Low level laser therapy (LLLT) as an effective therapeutic modality for delayed wound healing. Ann NY Acad Sci, 1056: 486–493

King PR (1989) Low-level laser therapy: A review. Laser Med Sci, 4: 141–150

Kitchen SS, Partridge CJ (1991) A review of low-level laser therapy. Physiotherapy, 77: 161–168

Laakso L, Richardson C, Cramond T (1993a) Quality of light—Is laser necessary for effective photobiostimulation? Aust J Physiother, 39: 87–92

Laakso L, Richardson C, Cramond T (1993b) Factors affecting low-level laser therapy. Aust J Physiother, 39: 95–99

Lopes-Martins R, penna SC, Joensen J, Iversen VV, Bjordal JM (2007) Low level laser therapy (LLLT) in inflammatory and rheumatic diseases: A review of therapeutic mechanisms. Cur Rheumatol Rev, 3: 147–154

Lucas C, Stanborough RW, Freeman CL (2000) Efficacy of low level laser therapy on wound healing in human subjects: A systematic review. Lasers Med Sci, 15: 83–94

Maher S (2006) Is low-level laser therapy effective in the management of lateral epicondylitis? Phys Ther, 86: 1161–1167

Marks R, de Palma F (1999) Clinical efficacy of low power laser therapy in osteoarthritis. Physiother Res Int, 4: 141–157

Naeser MA (2006) Photobiomodulation of pain in carpal tunnel syndrome: Review of seven laser therapy studies. Photomed Laser Surg, 24: 101–110

Nussbaum EL, Baxter GD, Lilge L (2003) A review of laser technology and light-tissue interactions as a background to therapeutic applications of low intensity lasers and other light sources. Phys Ther Rev, 8: 31–44

Oshiro T, Calderhaead RG (1991) Development of low reactive–level laser therapy and its present status. J Clin Laser Med Surg, 9: 267–275

Parker S (2007) Low-level laser use in dentistry. Br Dent J , 202: 131–138

Posten W, Wrone DA, Dover JS, Arndt KA, Silapunt S, Alam M (2005) Low-level laser therapy for wound healing: Mechanism and efficacy. Dermatol Surg, 31: 334–340

Reddy GK (2004) Photobiological basis and clinical role of low-intensity lasers in biology and medicine. J Clin Laser Med Surg, 22: 141–150

Schindl A, Schindl M, Pernerstorfer-Schon H, Schindl L (2000) Low-intensity laser therapy: A review. J Invest Med, 48: 312–326

Stasinopoulos DI, Johnson MI (2005) Effectiveness of low-level laser therapy for lateral elbow tendinopathy. Photomed Laser Surg, 23: 425–430

Tuner J, Hode L (1998) It's all in the parameters: A critical analysis of some well-known negative studies on low-level laser therapy. J Clin Laser Med Surg, 16: 245–248

Woodruff LD, Bounkeo JM, Brabbon WM, Dawes KD, Barham CD, Waddell DA, Enwemeka CS (2004) The efficacy of laser therapy in wound repair: A meta-analysis of the literature. Photomed laser Surg, 22: 241–247

Chapters of Textbooks

Baxter D (2002) Low-intensity laser therapy. In: Electrotherapy Evidence-Based Practice, 11th ed. Kitchen S, (Ed). Churchill Livingstone, Edinburgh, pp 171–189

Calderhead RG (1988) Basics. In: Low-Level Laser Therapy: A Practical Introduction. Ohshiro T, Calderhead RG (Eds). John Wiley & Sons, New York, pp 1–18

Karu TI (2003) Low-power laser therapy. In: Biomedical Photonics Handbook. Vo-Dinh T (Ed). CRC Press, Boca Raton, pp 1–25

Khan J (1999) Cold laser. In: Principles and Practice of Electrotherapy, 4th ed. Churchill Livingstone, New York, pp 33–47

Knight KL, Hopkins T (2008) Laser and Light Therapy. In: Therapeutic Modalities: The Art and Science. Knight KL, Draper DO (Eds). Lippincott Williams & Wilkins, Philadelphia, pp 334–349

Low J, Reed A (1990) Laser therapy. In: Electrotherapy Explained: Principles and Practice. Low J, Reed A (Eds), Butterworth Heinemann, London, pp 299–313

Saliba E, Foreman-Saliba S (2002) Low-power lasers. In: Therapeutic Modalities for Physical Therapists, 2nd ed. Prentice WE (Ed). McGraw-Hill, New York, pp 319–342

Seichert N (1991) Controlled trials of laser treatment. In: Physiotherapy: Controlled Trials and Facts, vol 14. Schlapbach P, Gerber NJ (Eds). Karger, Basel, pp 205–217

Weisberg J, Adams D (2006) Low-level laser therapy. In: Integrated Physical Agents in Rehabilitation, 2nd ed. Hecox B, Mehreteab TA, Weisberg J, Sanko J (Eds). Pearson Prentice Hall, Upper Saddle River, pp 447–455

Textbooks

Baxter GD (1994) Therapeutic Lasers: Theory and Practice. Churchill Livingstone, New York, pp 1–259

Kamami YV (1997) Le laser en pratique medicale. Masson, Paris, pp 1–189

Karu T (1989) Photobiology of Low-Power Laser Therapy. Hardwood, New York, pp 1–235

Karu T (1998) The Science of Low-Power Laser Therapy. Gordon & Breach Science, Amsterdam, pp 1–289

Niems M (1996) Laser-Tissue Interactions: Fundamentals and Applications. Springer. Berlin, pp 1–268

Ohshiro T, Calderhead RG (1988) Low-Level Laser Therapy: A Practical Introduction. John Wiley & Sons, New York, pp 1–143

Tuner J, Hode L (2002) Laser Therapy: Clinical Practice and Scientific Background. Prima Books, Grangesberg, p 1–570

Letters, Editorials, and Reports

Bjordal JM (2007) On: Is low-level laser therapy effective… . Phys Ther, 87: 224–226

Food and Drug Administration (FDA)—Department of Health & Human Services, (2002) Section 510K n.k0101175 Notification of Premarket Approval, February 6, 2002.

Enwemeka CS (2006) The place of coherence in light induced tissue repair and pain function. Letter to the Editor. Photomed Laser Surg, 24: 457

Occupational Safety and Health Hazard (OSHA)—US Department of Labor (2007): www.osha.gov

World Association for Laser Therapy (2006) Consensus agreement on the design and conduct of clinical studies with low-level laser therapy and light therapy for musculoskeletal pain and disorders. (Consensus Agreement Paper) Photomed Laser Surg, 24: 761–762

E-References

www.walt.nu/dosage-recommendations.html
www. osha.gov

Ultraviolet Therapy

Learning Objectives

Knowledge: State the physiological rationale behind the use of ultraviolet (UV) therapy for the management of dermatoses.

Comprehension: Distinguish between UVA, UVB, and UVC therapy.

Application: Show the steps required to conduct skin phototesting.

Analysis: Explain the proposed physiological and therapeutic effects of UVA, UVB, and UVC therapy

Synthesis: Formulate the dosimetric calculations a phototherapist needs to perform and consider to deliver safe and effective UV therapy.

Evaluation: Discuss the role of narrowband UVB relative to broadband UVB and psoralen UVA in the management of dermatoses.

I. RATIONALE FOR USE

A. DEFINITION AND DESCRIPTION

Sunlight is the greatest source of ultraviolet radiation on earth. *Ultraviolet* (UV) light is defined as electromagnetic radiation with wavelength shorter than that of visible light (thus invisible), but longer than x-ray. Ultraviolet radiation, as shown in **Table 12-1**, covers a small portion of the electromagnetic spectrum, spanning a wavelength region ranging from 400 to 100 nanometers (nm = 10^{-9} m). UV therapy is thus defined as the use of artificial UV light for therapeutic purposes. The main application of UV therapy is for the management of dermatoses (skin pathologies). Because the physiological and therapeutic effects caused by UV radiation vary enormously within wavelength, the therapeutic UV spectrum is further subdivided into three regions, as shown in **Table 12-1**: UVA (400–320 nm), UVB (320–290 nm), and UVC (290–100 nm). The UVA region is subdivided into two bands: psoralen UVA (PUVA; 400–320 nm) and UVA1 (400–340 nm). The UVB region is also subdivided into two bands: broadband (BBUVB; 320–290 nm) and narrowband (NBUVB; 313–309 nm).

B. THERAPEUTIC ULTRAVIOLET

Presented in **Table 12-2** are the key characteristics that distinguish the varieties of UV light therapy available today to treat skin pathologies: wavelengths, biological effects, sensitizing agent, skin penetration, erythemal response, carcinogenic risk, and popularity in current use.

1. UVA Therapy

Ultraviolet light A (UVA) is therapeutically delivered via two modes: Psoralen UVA or *PUVA*, and UVA1 (British Photodermatology Group, 1994; Halpern et al. 2000; Dawe, 2003).

a. PUVA

Psoralen UVA therapy (PUVA), introduced in the mid-1970s, requires the use of a natural photosensitizing agent, *psoralen*, combined with UVA light radiation (**Table 12-2**). It is necessary to use a photosensitizing agent prescribed by a dermatologist to enhance the patient's erythemal response, which would be weak if exposed to UVA light alone. Psoralen, a natural agent, may be administered orally (oral PUVA) or topically, either with a psoralen

TABLE 12-1	THE ULTRAVIOLET SPECTRUM

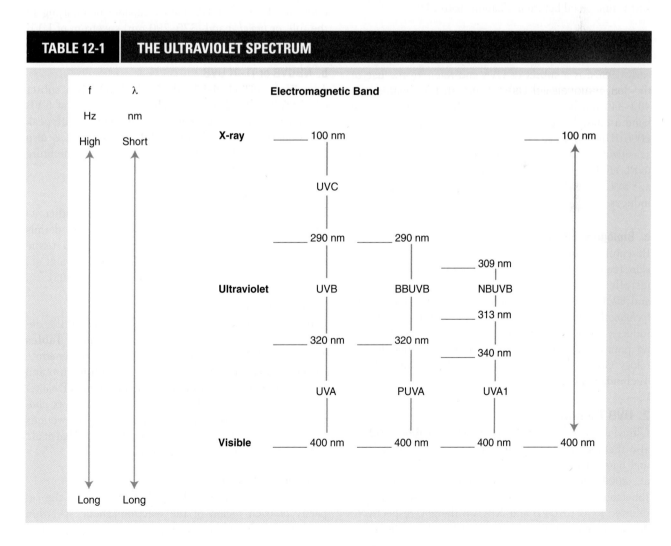

TABLE 12-2	CHARACTERISTICS OF ULTRAVIOLET LIGHT THERAPY				
	UVA		UVB		UVC
MODE	**PUVA**	**UVA1**	**BBUVB**	**NBUVB**	**UVC**
Wavelength	400–320 nm	400–340 nm	320–290 nm	313–309 nm	290–100 nm
Biological effect	Photochemical	Phototherapy	Phototherapy	Phototherapy	Photogermicidal
Sensitizing agent	Psoralen	None	None	None	None
Skin penetration	Hypodermis		Dermis		Epidermis
Erythemal response	Strong		Strong	Moderate	Not applicable
Carcinogenic risk	High		High	Moderate	Low
Popularity of use	Declining		Declining	Increasing	Sporadic

cream rubbed over the treated skin area (cream PUVA) or by means of a psoralen bath, in which the treated body part is immersed before irradiation (bath PUVA).

b. UVA1

Ultraviolet light A1 (UVA1) therapy, available since the early 1980s, is a subset of UVA and refers to the use of the longer wavelength UVA band, that is, within the 400–340 nm band, as opposed to the full 400–320 nm band used to deliver PUVA (Dawe, 2003; Tuchinda et al., 2006). This mode is easier to deliver than PUVA because a sensitizing agent is not required (**Table 12-2**). Compared to PUVA, UVA1 therapy is delivered at a much higher dosage to compensate for the weaker erythemal response it induces.

c. Biological Effect

Research has shown that PUVA penetrates deep into the skin, reaching the hypodermis, and induces a photochemical effect resulting from the interaction between psoralen and UVA light. PUVA is therefore categorized as a *photochemotherapy* agent. UVA1 therapy, on the other hand, induces only a *phototherapy* effect on the skin because no photosensitizing agent is used (British Photodermatology Group, 1994; Halpern et al., 2000; Dawe, 2003; Tuchinda et al., 2006).

2. UVB Therapy

Ultraviolet light B (UVB), as shown in **Table 12-2**, is also therapeutically delivered via two modes: broadband and narrowband UVB (Bilsland et al., 1997; Bandow et al., 2004; Dogra et al., 2004; Gambichler et al., 2005; Ibbotson et al., 2004). These two modes are clinically referred to as BBUVB and NBUVB therapy, respectively. No sensitizing agent is required to deliver UVB therapy.

a. BBUVB

This mode of therapy, introduced in the late 1970s, refers to the use of UV lamps capable of emitting in the full, or *broad*, band (320–290 nm) spectrum of UVB radiation.

b. NBUVB or TL-01 UVB

This mode, introduced in the early 1980s, is a subset of BBUVB and delivers a much narrower band of UVB wavelength, ranging between 313 and 309 nm, with peak emission at 311 nm (**Table 12-1**). This mode is also known as TL-01 UVB in the UV phototherapy literature (see Section III, Biophysical Characteristics).

c. Biological Effect

Research has shown that UVB light, within either its broad (B) or narrow (N) band, penetrates the dermis and induces a *phototherapy* effect on the skin tissue (Bilsland et al., 1997; Bandow et al., 2004; Dogra et al., 2004; Ibbotson et al., 2004; Gambichler et al., 2005).

3. UVC Therapy

Ultraviolet light C (UVC) therapy is defined as the delivery of UV light within the 290–100 nm range (**Tables 12-1** and **12-2**). UVC light has been shown to penetrate the epidermis and to deactivate or kill, both in vitro and in vivo, normal and antibiotic-resistant strains of bacteria and other families of germs, thus conferring its *photogermicidal* effect on dermatoses and cutaneous wounds (Conner-Kerr et al., 1998; Sullivan et al., 1999; Thai et al., 2002, 2005; Conner-Kerr et al., 2007).

4. Erythemal Response

The practice of UVA and UVB therapy relies on the capacity of each region of the electromagnetic spectrum to induce a skin erythemal response following exposure (see Section IV, Physiological and Therapeutic Effects). *Erythema* is defined as skin redness due to dilation of the superficial blood vessels. The erythemal response induced is controlled by determining the *minimal erythemal dose* (MED), in UVB therapy, and the *minimal phototoxic dose*, (MPD), in PUVA therapy (see Section V. Dosimetry). There is evidence to show (Bilsland et al., 1997; Cameron et al., 2002a) that the erythemal response induced, as shown in **Table 12-2**, is strong in both PUVA and BBUVB therapy, moderate in NBUVB therapy and absent in UVC therapy.

5. Carcinogenic Risk

It is scientifically established that prolonged or repeated skin exposure to either solar or artificial UV radiation may cause skin cancer (for a review, see Saladi et al., 2005). Unfortunately for patients, many dermatoses such as psoriasis and eczema require numerous treatment exposures before the condition will clear up, and lifetime treatment may be required because of the recurrent nature of these dermatoses. There is strong evidence to suggest that UVA therapy, particularly PUVA and BBUVB, have a much higher carcinogenic risk than NBUVB therapy, because their erythemal response, as shown in **Table 12-2**, is much stronger than that of NBUVB (see Stern et al. 1994; Saladi et al., 2005; Lee et al., 2005; Mann et al., 2005).

C. PHOTOTHERAPY USE TODAY

The practice of phototherapy using UVA and UVB has evolved over the past two decades, but UVC has remained rather stagnant, marginal, and sporadic. There is a clear trend in the current literature indicating that the practice of UVA (PUVA and UVA1) therapy is gradually declining in favor of UVB therapy. More precisely, the practice of BBUVB therapy is also slowly declining in favor of *NBUVB* therapy, which is today recognized as the first line of treatment for many of the most frequent dermatoses affecting humans (Bandow et al., 2004; Dogra et al., 2004; Gambichler et al., 2005; Ibbotson et al., 2004).

1. Decline of PUVA Therapy

Its high carcinogenic risk, combined with its other side effects such as increased skin phototoxicity with repeated treatments, led the British Photodermatology Group to recommend in 2000 that oral and topical PUVA treatments be kept to a minimum, only for dermatoses that do not respond to other treatments (Halpern et al., 2000).

2. Decline of BBUVB Therapy

Research on phototherapy has shown that the human skin's action spectrum for erythema is dominated by the *shorter UVB wavelength range* (305–290 nm). Conventional therapeutic BBUVB lamps, which emit radiation within the broad 320–290 nm range (**Table 12-1**), thus produce a large amount of light in this erythemogenic range. Because erythema leads to skin burning, which in turn further in-

creases the risk of skin cancer (carcinogenic risk), as discussed above, and because BBUVB was found to be less efficient than PUVA for treating dermatoses, BBUVB has never achieved therapeutical popularity (Dogra et al., 2004).

3. Decline of UVC Therapy

The body of scientific literature related to the practice of UVC, in contrast to UVA and UVB therapy, is limited (see References). This suggests that its practice today is sporadic although its carcinogenic risk is low.

4. Popularity of NBUVB Therapy

The practice of NBUVB therapy (313–309 nm band, with its peak spectra at 311 nm) is rapidly gaining in popularity among dermatologists and phototherapists around the world because it eliminates the strong erythemogenic effect caused by the shorter wavelength band (305–290 nm band) within the BBUVB range. Its popularity is also due to the fact that its narrow band corresponds to the core action spectrum for the treatment of psoriasis, one of the most common and disabling dermatoses affecting a fair percentage of the human population (Parrish et al., 1981; Fisher et al., 1984; Van Weelden et al., 1988).

D. SCOPE OF CHAPTER

Considering the facts presented above, the scope of this chapter is on the use of UVB and UVC light therapy. **Table 12-3** summarizes the main advantages of using UVB therapy over PUVA, where ease of application, absence of chemical agent, minimal patient side effects, and lower cost of delivery play a major role (see Bandow et al., 2004; Dogra et al., 2004; Ibbotson et al., 2004).

E. UV DEVICES

Shown in **Figure 12-1** are some common devices used today to deliver UV therapy: whole-body cubicule (**A**), hand/feet cabinet (**B**) and handheld lamp or wand (**C**). These devices are mounted with single or multiple UV lamps, or tubes, capable of emitting artificial UV light within the UVA, UVB, or UVC spectrum. These therapeutic devices are used to deliver whole-body (**B**), segmental-body (**B**), or localized-body or spot (**C**) exposures.

F. UV ACCESSORIES

The practice of UV therapy requires, as shown in **Figure 12-2**, protective goggles (A) to be worn during therapy and skin phototesting templates (B) to be used prior to therapy to determine the starting dose.

1. Protective Goggles

Because UV radiation is harmful to the eyes, protective UV goggles, such as those shown in **Figure 12-2A**, must be worn *at all times* by both patients and practitioners during skin phototesting and therapy sessions.

TABLE 12-3	COMPARISON OF PUVA VERSUS UVB THERAPY	
	PUVA	**UVB**
Carcinogenic risk	High	Moderate
Psoralen side effects	Present[a]	Absent
Ease of application	Complex[b]	Simple
Overall safety	Minimal	Maximal[c]
Psoralen cost	Present	Absent
Dermatologist's cost	Maximal	Minimal
Overall cost	High	Low

[a] Skin phototoxicity; nausea if oral PUVA used; eyewear protection for hours after therapy
[b] Application of cream over skin lesions; body parts soaking in psoralen bath solution
[c] Safe for children and pregnant women

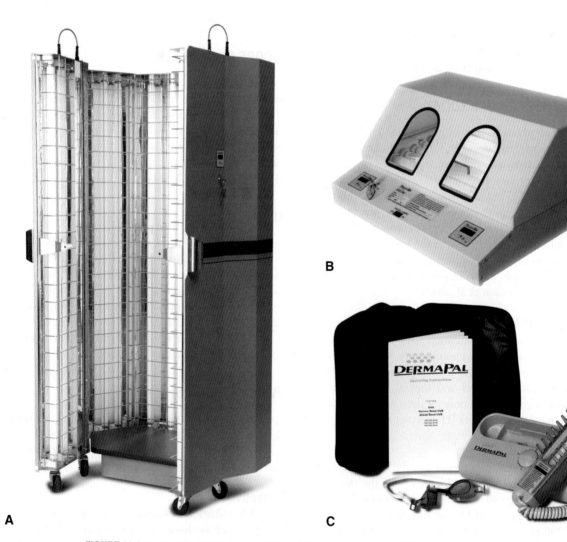

FIGURE 12-1 Typical ultraviolet therapy devices: (**A**) whole-body cubicle; (**B**) hands/feet cabinet; and (**C**) handheld lamp or wand. (Courtesy of Daavlin.)

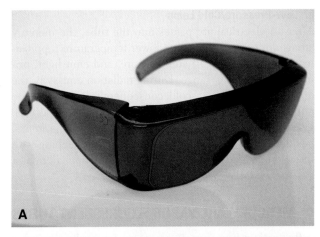

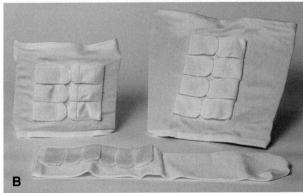

FIGURE 12-2 Typical ultraviolet accessories: (**A**) protective goggle; (**B**) skin phototesting templates. These commercial panels are made of UV-opaque fabrics and are completely washable. Each piece has several apertures or exposure ports that can be covered and uncovered during testing. Homemade templates or panels can also be used. (A: courtesy of Solarc Systems, Inc; B: courtesy of Daavlin.)

2. Skin Phototesting Template

A skin phototesting template, homemade or commercially made, is used to establish the patient's minimal erythemal dose (MED; see Section V, Dosimetry). This dose is used to establish the *starting* therapeutic dose. **Figure 12-2B** shows typical commercial testing templates, made of UV-resistant fabrics punctured with holes. Similar templates may be used to test for the patient's minimal phototoxic dose (MPD) when PUVA and UVA therapy is used.

G. RATIONALE FOR USE

Many people are affected over the course of their lives by a wide variety of skin pathologies or dermatoses, such as psoriasis, acne vulgaris, atopic dermatitis (eczema), and vitiligo, to name only a few. These skin disorders are traditionally treated by dermatologists using an array of oral drugs and topical creams (e.g., anti-inflammatory agents; antibiotics). Over the past decades, however, UV therapy has gained popularity as an alternative or complementary treatment for several dermatoses. UV therapy has evolved over the past 40 years from the use of PUVA to BBUVB, and from BBUVB to NBUVB therapy. Today UV therapy is

recognized, as shown in this chapter, as an important complementary therapy to conventional medical dermatological treatments in providing significant resolution of several dermatoses for periods lasting weeks to months.

II. HISTORICAL PERSPECTIVE

A. FOUNDATION

UV therapy arose from the pioneer work of the Danish physician Niels Finsen, who, in 1903, was awarded the Nobel Prize for Medicine for his successful treatment of lupus vulgaris using a carbon-arc UV lamp (Diffey et al., 2002; Roelandts, 2002; Dogra et al., 2004).

B. TECHNICAL DEVELOPMENTS

Over the years, significant technical developments led to the creation of various sources of artificial UV radiation, moving from Finsen's original carbon-arc-type lamp to today's mercury-arc lamps and fluorescent tubes (Diffey et al., 2002; Dogra et al., 2004).

C. CLINICAL LANDMARKS

In 1974, Parrish and colleagues reported the useful role of UVA radiation in combination with oral psoralen in the treatment of psoriasis; this application led to what is known as *PUVA therapy* (Parrish et al., 1974). A few years later, Wiskemann and colleagues introduced BBUVB therapy for the treatment of psoriasis and uremic pruritus (Dogra et al., 2004). A decade following the introduction of PUVA, Van Weelden et al. (1988) and Green et al. (1988) introduced NBUVB, also known as TL-01 UVB therapy, for the treatment of psoriasis.

D. THE TL-01 FLUORESCENT TUBE

Narrow band UVB (NBUVB) therapy came about after Philips Lighting, of the Netherlands, developed and manufactured the new TL-01 fluorescent tube capable of delivering UVB light in the narrower (N) band (range of 313–309 nm, with a peak at 311 nm) of the broad (B) band (320–290 nm) of UV light. With such a tube, the shorter and more-damaging wavelengths are absent during radiation thus minimizing the skin carcinogenic risk (**Table 12-2**). In today's literature and in this textbook, the terms NBUVB and TL-01 UVB therapy are used interchangeably.

E. BODY OF LITERATURE

Over the past two decades, UV therapy has been the subject of several *articles* (see References), *review articles* (Kitchen et al., 1991; British Photodermatology Group, 1994; Stern et al., 1994; Bilsland et al., 1997; Young,

1997; Njoo et al., 1999; Sarkany et al., 1999; Halpern et al., 2000; Krutmann, 2000; Honigsmann, 2001; Karrer et al., 2001; Wardin, 2001; Roelandts, 2002; Taylor et al., 2002; Dawe, 2003; Bandow et al., 2004; Dogra et al., 2004; Ibbotson et al., 2004; Gambichler et al., 2005; Kist et al., 2005; Lebwohl et al., 2005; Lee et al., 2005; Saladi et al., 2005; Su et al., 2005; Van der Leun et al., 2005; Amatiello et al., 2006; Koek et al., 2006; Tuchinda et al., 2006; Meduri et al., 2007), a few *chapters of textbooks* (Davis, 2002; Diffey et al., 2002; Cameron et al., 2003; Starkey, 2004; Weisberg et al., 2006; Conner-Kerr et al., 2007), and *textbooks* (Morison, 2005; Zanolli et al., 2005).

III. BIOPHYSICAL CHARACTERISTICS

A. UV LIGHT GENERATORS

Today's production of therapeutic artificial UV light comes from two types of light-emitting generators, called *UV lamps*, which are filled with mercury gas or vapor: mercury-arc gas lamp and mercury-arc vapor fluorescent lamp (see below). The term *arc* means that the lamps are powered by an electric arc. The process of UV light emission is based on the concept of *spontaneous emission* of photons, resulting from the sudden and spontaneous drop of electrons from their activated state to their resting state. This biophysical process is discussed at length in Chapter 11, which deals with the emission of laser light. To avoid duplication, we will not repeat the discussion here. Readers are requested to refer to Chapter 11, Section IV, Biophysical Characteristics, for full details of this concept and other biophysical processes leading to spontaneous emission of photons.

B. MERCURY-ARC GAS LAMP

A mercury-arc lamp consists of a small quantity of mercury gas sealed into a UV quartz transmitting tube. Two types of mercury-arc lamps are used in therapeutic UV devices today: high-pressure/hot lamps and low-pressure/cold lamps (Davis, 2002).

a. High-Pressure/Hot Lamp

After an electrical arc passes into the tube, the mercury atoms are excited, being heated up (the incandescence process) at a very high temperature (approximately 8,000°C or 14,432°F), and emit photons, primarily in the UVB spectrum (Davis, 2002). During radiation, the pressure inside the quartz tube is high, and the tube is hot. The hot tube must be cooled and this is done by means of a circulating air or water jacket. These lamps require a warm-up period before peak emission is achieved and a cool-down period, after being turned off, before they can be used again (Davis, 2002).

b. Low-Pressure/Cold Lamp

After an electrical arc passes into the tube, the mercury atoms are excited at a much lower temperature (approximately 60°C or 140°F) and pressure, and emit light, primarily in the UVC range. During radiation emission, the quartz tube is relatively cold; consequently, these lamps do not require warm-up or cool-down periods (Davis, 2002). Use of these lamps, known in Europe as *Kromayer lamps*, has declined significantly over the years, in keeping with the sporadic use of UVC therapy for infectious dermatoses and wounds.

C. MERCURY-ARC VAPOR FLUORESCENT TUBES

A fluorescent lamp or tube consists of a small quantity of mercury vapor sealed in a UV transmitting tube, mounted with an electrical filament and coated with phosphors. After an electrical current passes through the filament and into the tube, the mercury atoms are excited, and produce low-pressure photons in the full UV range (see Diffey et al., 2002). These tubes, sold in different sizes and lengths, are gradually replacing mercury-arc gas lamps in modern UV devices. Today, practitioners can choose from several types of fluorescent tubes with varying UV spectral emissions to deliver UV therapy.

D. TODAY'S UV DEVICES

Today, low-pressure mercury-arc vapor fluorescent tubes have replaced mercury-arc gas lamps in therapeutic UV devices designed for whole-body, segmental, or local exposure (see **Figure 12-1**). For example, a whole-body cubicle UV device, shown in **Figure 12-1A**, can hold a total of 50 tubes, in a combination of 30 BBUVB and 20 UVA tubes. Depending on which type of therapeutic UV radiation is indicated to treat a dermatologic condition, practitioners can turn on only the desired fluorescent tubes, leaving the other tubes turned off.

E. LAMP/TUBE LIFETIME

All UV lamps or tubes have a lifetime ranging between 5,000 and 10,000 hours (Diffey et al., 2002). Regular maintenance and prompt replacement of burnt-out lamps and tubes is mandatory to assure optimal irradiation and precise dosimetry.

IV. PHYSIOLOGICAL AND THERAPEUTIC EFFECTS

A. PHOTOTHERAPY

Research has demonstrated, as presented in **Table 12-2**, that photons within the A region of the UV spectrum can induce photochemical and phototherapy effects on the hypodermis, with those in the B and C regions inducing phototherapy effects on the dermis, and photogermicidal effects on the epidermis, respectively (Weichenthal et al., 2005). As was the case with low-level laser therapy (see Chapter 11), for physiological and therapeutic effects to occur, the energy contained in these UV photons must first be absorbed, as stipulated by the Grotthus-Draper law (see Chapter 5), by multiple chromophores buried within the skin layers. This energy is then released within the skin tissue, causing a cascade of therapeutic photobiological reactions.

B. PROPOSED MECHANISMS

The exact mechanisms behind the therapeutic effects of UV light remain obscure (Weichenthal et al., 2005). There is evidence, however, to support some of the proposed mechanisms of action, shown in **Figure 12-3**, which may partially explain the therapeutic effects of UV therapy. These mechanisms relate to the induction of erythema, local immunosuppression, cellular apoptosis, and bacterial suppression.

1. Induced Erythema
Induced UVA and UVB erythema are presumed to promote skin healing by increasing the blood supply to the treated area. A high enough dosage will induce an inflammatory response, which in turn stimulates the formation of granular tissue, leading to tissue repair (Weisberg et al., 2006).

2. Local Immunosuppression
The presumed local immunosuppressant effect is based on the fact that most of the UVA- and UVB-responsive dermatoses respond equally well to immunosuppressive drugs (Weichenthal et al., 2005).

3. Cellular Apoptosis
UVA- and UVB-induced cell death is presumed to be caused by direct activation of death receptors (Weichenthal et al., 2005). The fact that exposure of normal skin to erythemogenic doses of UVB radiation induces a hyperproliferative response, leading to thickening of the epidermis, argues *against* the assumption that UVB therapy improves psoriasis mainly by interfering with cell proliferation (Weichenthal et al., 2005).

4. Germicidal DNA–RNA Suppression
In vitro and *in vivo* studies have revealed that the photogermicidal effect associated with UVC therapy is caused by a DNA- and RNA-suppressive effect (Conner-Kerr et al., 1998; Sullivan et al., 1999; Conner-Kerr et al., 2007).

C. SKIN PATHOLOGY

UV therapy, unlike many EPAs covered in this textbook, is used solely for the management of dermatoses and infected dermal wounds (**Fig 12-3**).

V. DOSIMETRY

A. KEY PARAMETERS

Shown in **Table 12-4** are key parameters, with formulas and units, related to the dosimetry of UV therapy. These parameters are irradiance, exposure time, dose, and cumulative dose. Dosage of UV lights, as discussed below, is based on skin phototesting done *prior to treatment*. Phototesting is essential to allow practitioners to determine the starting UV dose.

1. Irradiance
The irradiance (I), or power density, of a UV device is measured in milliwatts per square centimeter (mW/cm²), by means of a UV sensor mounted on the device. The amount of irradiance of a given UV device is determined by the total number of lamps or tubes within the

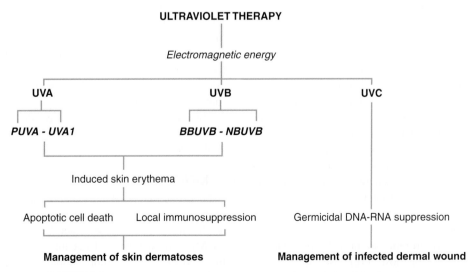

FIGURE 12-3 Proposed physiological and therapeutic effects of ultraviolet therapy.

TABLE 12-4	ULTRAVIOLET THERAPY DOSIMETRIC PARAMETERS		
PARAMETER	**SYNONYM**	**FORMULA**	**UNITS**
Irradiance (I)	Power density	$I = P/A$ Read from a UV sensor	mW/cm^2
Exposure time (T)	Time during which the skin is exposed to UV light	None	s
Dose (D)	Amount of UV energy delivered to the skin	$D = I \times T$ $mJ/cm^2 = mW/cm^2 \times s$ where $mW \times s = mJ$	mJ/cm^2
Cumulative dose (D_c)	Summation of all doses received within a treatment period or lifetime	$D_c = \Sigma D$	mJ/cm^2

device, each tube having its own irradiance. The greater the number of tubes within a device, the greater that device's total irradiance will be.

2. Exposure Time

This is the duration, or time (T), expressed in seconds (s), during which the skin is exposed to UV light. This duration varies in relation to the treatment dose used and the device's irradiance. Exposure time is synonymous to application duration.

3. Dose

The dose (D), or amount of UV energy delivered to the exposed skin tissue by a given UV device, is determined by the device's irradiance (I) multiplied by the exposition time (T), as shown by the formula $D = I \times T$ (Taylor et al., 2002; Van der Leun et al., 2005). The dose (D) is expressed in millijoules per square centimeter (mJ/cm^2) on the basis of the formula $D = I \times T$ ($mJ/cm^2 = mW/cm^2 \times s$, where 1 Joule = 1 W.s or 1000 mW.s). For example, a dose of 450 mJ/cm^2 will be delivered to a patient's skin if the phototherapist exposes a UV device with an irradiance of 3 mW/cm^2 for 150 s (450 mJ/cm^2 = 3 $mW/cm^2 \times$ 150 s). Dosage is in keeping with the *reciprocity law,* also known as the *Bunsen-Roscoe law,* which refers to the inverse relationship between irradiance and exposure time, meaning that a similar dose (D) can result from reducing exposure duration (T) or increasing irradiance (I), or vice versa (Van der Leun et al., 2005) For example, a dose of 400 mJ/cm^2 may be obtained as follows: 400 mJ/cm^2 = 2 $mW/cm^2 \times$ 200 s or 4 $mW/cm^2 \times$ 100 s. This means that the dose is similar if the irradiance is halved and the exposure time doubled, or if the irradiance is doubled while the exposure time is halved.

4. Cumulative Dose

Because several UV treatments are need for the management and maintenance of most dermatoses and because repeated exposure to UV lights over weeks, months, and

years present a greater *carcinogenic risk* for the skin, it is essential that the cumulative dose (D_c) received by the patient at the end of each treatment period be calculated and recorded in the patient's file (Taylor et al., 2002; Ibbotson et al., 2004). The *cumulative dose* is calculated by adding up each dose (D) the patient has received during the course of his treatment period, which may last weeks or months. The greater the cumulative dose per treatment period and the larger the number of treatment periods over time, the greater the risk of developing a skin cancer. Given that most dermatoses are recurrent, most patients will inevitably require repeated treatments over the course of their lifetime. Therefore, the ultimate goal of any phototherapist is to achieve optimal treatment outcomes with the smallest cumulative dose possible.

B. SKIN PHOTOTESTING

What UVB or UVC dose should the practitioner use to start therapy? Research on UV therapy has clearly established that a starting dose that is too low will not induce a therapeutic benefit, and a starting dose that is too high may induce serious side effects such as skin burning and pain, brought on by a strong skin erythemal response to too much UV energy (Lee et al., 2005; Weichenthal et al., 2005). There is consensus in the field of UVB phototherapy that skin phototesting, aimed at establishing the minimal erythemal dose or MED, *must* be conducted on all patients before UV therapy is started (Bisland et al., 1997; Halpern et al., 2000; Taylor et al., 2002; Ibbotson et al., 2004).

1. MED Testing

Exposure of human skin to UVB radiation induces an erythemal response, which can vary among people according to their skin phototype (see below). It is critical that an MED be determined because development of UVB-induced erythema in nonlesional, healthy skin surfaces will limit the UV dose that can be given at each treatment.

The ultimate therapeutic goal is to deliver an effective dose to the skin lesions while minimizing the erythemal effect on the surrounding healthy skin cells.

a. Erythemal Response

Erythema is skin redness caused by vascular dilation. The skin redness in UVB-induced erythema is also presumably mediated by prostaglandin release from the epidermis or by the DNA-damaging effect of UV radiation (Diffey et al., 2002; Cameron et al., 2003).

b. Skin Phototype

It is a common observation that human skin, depending on its color, responds differently to the sun's UV rays. Shown in **Table 12-5** is Fitzpatrick's empirical classification of human skin phototypes, which is based on his observation of the interaction between skin color and burning or tanning reaction to the sun (Fitzpatrick, 1988). This classification includes six skin types and shows that whiter skins (types I and II) are more likely to display a burning or erythemogenic reaction to UV radiation than are browner (types III, IV, and V) and blacker (type VI) skins. Assessing the patient's skin phototype prior to skin phototesting is useful when the time comes to determine the UV testing dose. For example, a higher dose is needed for a patient with a phototype IV skin compared to type II.

c. MED Definition

The effect of UV radiation on the skin is quantified on the basis of MED. As its name implies, this dose is defined as the lowest, or *minimal*, dose of UV radiation, measured in millijoules per square centimeter (mJ/cm^2), that will produce a barely detectable erythema 24 hours after exposure (Taylor et al., 2002). MED is commonly determined, as shown below, by adjusting the exposure time while keeping all other variables, such as lamp irradiance, distance from the patient, angle to the surface, and area of application, constant. MED is synonymous to an E-1, or first-degree erythemal dose (Conner-Kerr et al., 2007).

d. MED Conventional Testing Protocol

Illustrated in **Box 12-1** is an example of the *conventional protocol* (adapted from Taylor et al., 2002) that most practitioners use to determine MED or E-1 dose before administering UVB and UVC therapy.

i. Key parameters. In this example, phototesting is done on the skin over the lower back in a patient with phototype II skin (white skin, tans minimally, always burns easily; see **Table 12-5**). Testing may also be done over the buttocks, abdomen, or anterior forearm areas. The testing lamp's surface is positioned perpendicular to the lower back skin surface, in keeping with *Lambert's cosine law*, and is positioned at a fixed distance of 30 cm (12 in.) from the skin surface, according to the *inverse square law* (see Section IX, Considerations for Application and Documentation, and Chapter 5). The testing lamp emits light in the NBUVB range and has an irradiance value fixed at 3 mW/cm^2. A homemade UV-opaque flexible plastic template with eight apertures is used (**Box 12-1**). Only the bare skin areas exposed in each of these apertures are submitted to UV light. Practical commercial MED testing templates such as those shown in **Figure 12-2B** may also be used.

ii. Tested dosage. In the present example the phototherapist, guided by the patient's phototype (type II), *arbitrarily* chose eight testing doses, ranging from 124 to 1500 mJ/cm^2. The aperture exposure time ratio used is 1.41, or 0.70 or 70% (1/1.41) of the next in the sequence. This means that the exposure time for the second aperture, as noted in **Box 12-1**, was 70% of that of the first, and so on (500, 350, 245 seconds, etc.). Consequently, the manual aperture *uncovering sequence*, or *timeline*, done by the phototherapist during testing, from the second to the eighth aperture (the first aperture is uncovered for the full 500 seconds was as follows: the second aperture was uncovered after 150 seconds of irradiation, the third after 255 seconds, the fourth after 328 s, and so on, with the last, or eighth, aperture exposed for 41 seconds, as shown

TABLE 12-5	FITZPATRICK'S HUMAN SKIN PHOTOTYPE	
PHOTOTYPE	**SKIN COLOR**	**TANNING AND SUNBURNING HISTORY**
I	White	Never tans; always burns easily
II	White	Tans minimally; always burns easily
III	Light brown	Tans gradually; burns moderately
IV	Moderate brown	Tans well; burns minimally
V	Dark brown	Tans profusely; burns rarely
VI	Black	Deep pigmentation; never burns

Box 12-1   Sample Skin UVB Photosensitivity Testing Protocol

The following minimal erythemal dose (MED) phototesting protocol is done using a homemade template made of eight (8) apertures. In the present example, the minimal erythemal dose (MED) is found to be 516 mJ/cm^2 because it is at this dose that a just perceptible skin erythema, with no erythema visible on the adjacent lower dose aperture, was found (see criteria below).

Testing protocol:

Patient's skin phototype: II

Tested body region: lower back

Testing lamp model: 2-foot NBUVB Philips TL-01

Lamp irradiance at skin surface: 3 mW/cm^2

Distance of lamp from skin surface: 30 cm (12 in.)

Erythemal template: homemade thin opaque flexible plastic template, with eight 1 cm^2 apertures, affixed directly on the lower-back skin area

Covered skin area: the rest of the patient's skin was covered by a UV-protective sheet.

Aperture exposure time ratio: ratio of 1.41, or 70% of the next in sequence

Tested dose range: 123 to 1500 mJ/cm^2

Erythema: judged by eye in bright indoor lighting conditions after 24 hours

MED determination criteria: taken to the dose given to the aperture showing just perceptible erythema, with no erythema visible on the adjacent lower dose aperture

MED	Aperture	Dose (mJ/cm^2)	Exposure time (s)	Timeline (s)
	1	1500	500	0
	2	1050	350	150
	3	735	245	255
516 mJ/cm^2 ←	4	— 516	172	328
	5	360	120	380
	6	252	84	416
	7	177	59	441
	8	123	41	459
				500

in **Box 12-1**. Both the patient and the phototherapist wore protective UV goggles during the phototesting session.

iii. MED determination. At 24 hours after irradiation, the phototherapist visually establishes, in this example, an MED of 516 mJ/cm^2. This dose, for this patient, thus becomes the starting treatment dose (see below). This is the minimal dose capable of inducing an erythemal effect with the minimal erythemogenic side effect on the surrounding normal skin areas.

iv. Alternative and templates protocols. There is evidence in the literature that this testing protocol is not always followed because it is perceived by many practitioners as difficult to execute and time-consuming. One major difficulty is the precision required to gradually expose the apertures at specific times exactly, which requires good hand-eye coordination (i.e., precise timing, using a chronograph, combined with precise manual uncovering). To simplify skin phototesting, other protocols, using different erythemal templates, have been proposed (Gordon et al., 1998; Wishart, 2001; Otman et al., 2006).

v. Automated Tester. One such alternative testing protocol calls for the use of a perforated metal foil template affixed to the surface of the testing UV tube. The main difference here is that instead of the manual uncovering sliding motion to clock the exposure time of each aperture, the template, a perforated metal foil with different aperture sizes, is affixed to the surface of the UV tube. The perforations are made so that the aperture areas are reduced by a factor of X; thus, the testing dose delivered to each aperture is decreased by this same factor (see Gordon et al., 1998; Wishart, 2001; Otmann et al., 2006 for details). Using such a testing template eliminates the manual aperture uncovering sequence during MED testing

vi. PUVA skin phototesting. Readers need to recall that the focus of this chapter, as stated earlier, is on the practice of UVB and UVC therapy, not UVA therapy. The description of phototesting protocols used to determine the minimal phototoxic dose (MPD) before oral or topical (e.g., cream, bath, etc.) administration of psoralen UVA (PUVA) are thus beyond the scope of this chapter. Readers interested in such protocols may refer to the review articles by Halpern et al. (2000) and Dawe (2003) for details.

C. INCREMENTAL DOSAGE

Because the skin photo-adapts to repeated UV light exposures, the starting dose, which corresponds to the MED value, must be constantly increased during the entire course of therapy to induce a therapeutic erythemal response with each treatment (Davis, 2002; Diffey et al., 2002). Several incremental-dose regimens for delivering UVB therapy are proposed in the literature. One frequently recommended regimen is to increase the dose delivered during each treatment by 30 percent the weekly dose delivered, starting with the second week.

D. THERAPEUTIC DOSAGE CALCULATION

Box 12-2 presents an *example* of dosimetric calculations based on a treatment period lasting 8 weeks, where the patient was scheduled 3 times per week. Therapeutic dosage is calculated weekly, leading to the determination of the cumulative dose of UVB light received at the end of this 8-week treatment period. This example is based on an MED value of 300 mJ/cm^2 (i.e., 3 mW/cm^2 × 100 seconds). The total number of UV exposures/treatments is 24. As recommended in the literature, the starting UV dose is the MED value, and the incremental-dose regimen calls for a 30% increase per week from the 2nd through the 8th week (Dogra

---

Box 12-2	Therapeutic Dosage Calculation Example

MED: 300 mJ/cm^2

Irradiance at skin surface: 3 mW/cm^2

Exposure time: 100 s

Distance between lamp and skin surface: 30 cm (12 in)

Treatment frequency: 3 times per week

Starting dose and Week 1: MED or 300 mJ/cm^2

Week 2 to Week 8 incremental-dose regimen: MED increased by 30% over previous week

Treatment Schedule

	Monday	Wednesday	Friday	Weekly Dose
Week 1	300 (100 s)	300 (100 s)	300 (100 s)	900
Week 2	390 (130 s)	390 (130 s)	390 (130 s)	1170
Week 3	507 (169 s)	507 (169 s)	507 (169 s)	1521
Week 4	660 (220 s)	660 (220 s)	660 (220 s)	1980
Week 5	858 (286 s)	858 (286 s)	858 (286 s)	2574
Week 6	1115 (372 s)	1115 (372 s)	1115 (372 s)	3345
Week 7	1450 (483 s)	1450 (483 s)	1450 (483 s)	4350
Week 8	1885 (628 s)	1885 (628 s)	1885 (628 s)	5655

Cumulative dose: 21495 mJ/cm^2 or 21.5 J/cm^2

et al., 2004; Ibbotson et al., 2004; Gambichler et al., 2005). Each new dose is obtained by increasing the exposure time (T) by 30%, as shown in **Box 12-2**, while keeping the irradiance constant (I). In the example, the first treatment lasted 100 seconds, and the last one had a duration of 10 minutes and 28 seconds (628 seconds). Dose increment is necessary to account for the photo-adaptive nature of the skin. In the present example, the cumulative dose received by the patient during his 8-week treatment period was 21495 mJ/cm^2, or 21.5 J/cm^2. The therapist needs to know this cumulative dose, and all the subsequent ones for the patient, in order to assess the patient's overall carcinogenic risk associated with the management of his or her dermatosis using UV therapy.

VI. EVIDENCE FOR INDICATIONS

A. GUIDED BY EVIDENCE

Dictionaries generally define "evidence" as anything that establishes a fact or gives reason to believe something. The aim of this textbook is to present scientific evidence behind therapeutic EPAs. To be guided by evidence is the process of integrating the evidence from research, how-ever imperfect or scarce this evidence may be, with clinical experience and patients' values. In other words, when the time comes to justify, prescribe, and apply the therapeutic agent, the *evidence-based practice* of EPA requires that practitioners consider the evidence from research in addition to their own clinical experience and the patient's own preference and beliefs about therapy. To be guided by the evidence is a process, not a search for the absolute truth. Finally, a lack of evidence from research in support of any given EPA does not mean that this EPA should never be used. What it means is that no statement can be made about its therapeutic effectiveness and that until more evidence from research is presented, its routine use cannot be recommended.

B. EVIDENCE FROM HUMAN RESEARCH

Box 12-3 provides evidence for UVB and UVC therapy based on an exhaustive search of published English-language, peer-reviewed studies on humans. The term *indication* references a list of pathologies for which UVB and UVC agents are used. Ratings of therapeutic benefit ("Yes" or "No") and grading of strength of scientific evidence (I, II, or III), including the reference, are included for each pathological condition.

Box 12-3	Research-Based Indication for the Use of UVB and UVC Therapy

PATHOLOGY	BENEFIT	GRADE	REFERENCE
UVB Therapy			
Psoriasis	Yes	I	Boztepe et al., 2006
	Yes	I	Cameron et al., 2002a
	Yes	II	Kirke et al., 2007
	Yes	II	Dawe et al., 2003
	Yes	II	Dawe et al., 1998
	Yes	II	Gokdemir et al., 2005
	Yes	II	Picot et al., 1992
	Yes	II	Kollner et al., 2005
	Yes	II	Van Weelden et al., 1988
	Yes	II	Lim et al., 2006
	Yes	II	Leenutaphong et al., 2000
	Yes	II	Yones et al., 2006
	Yes	II	Van Weelden et al., 1990
	Yes	II	Parrish et al., 1981
	Yes	II	Fisher et al., 1984
	Yes	II	Hofer et al., 1998
	Yes	II	Coven et al., 1997
	Yes	II	Green et al., 1988
	Yes	II	Karvonen et al., 1989
	Yes	II	Larko, 1989
	Yes	II	Tanew et al., 1999
	Yes	II	Storbeck et al., 1993
	Yes	II	Gordon et al., 1999
	Yes	II	Ortel et al., 1993

(Continued)

Box 12-3 **Continued**

PATHOLOGY	BENEFIT	GRADE	REFERENCE
	Yes	II	Stern et al., 1986
	Yes	II	Yones et al., 2005
	Yes	II	Jury et al., 2006
	Yes	II	Sezer et al., 2007a
	Yes	II	Aydogan et al., 2006
	Yes	III	Wainwright et al., 1998
	Yes	III	Kaur et al., 2006
Atopic dermatitis	Yes	II	Clayton et al., 2006
	Yes	II	Valkova et al., 2004
	Yes	II	Hjerppe et al., 2001
	Yes	II	Grundmann-Kollmann et al., 1999
	Yes	II	George et al., 1993
	Yes	II	Reynolds et al., 2001
	Yes	II	Der-Petrossian et al., 2000
	Yes	II	Legat et al., 2003
	Yes	II	Jekler, 1992
	Yes	II	Sjovall et al., 1987
	Yes	II	Sezer et al., 2007b
Vitiligo	Yes	II	Yones et al., 2007
	Yes	II	Bhatnagar et al., 2007
	Yes	II	Westerhof et al., 1997
	Yes	II	Parsad et al., 2006
	Yes	II	Njoo et al., 2000
	Yes	II	Kanwar et al., 2005
	Yes	II	Scherschun et al., 2001
	Yes	II	Tjioe et al., 2002
	Yes	II	Don et al., 2006
	Yes	II	Hamzavi et al., 2004
	Yes	II	Yashar et al., 2003
	Yes	II	Natta et al., 2003
Mycosis fungoides	Yes	II	Ahmad et al., 2007
	Yes	II	Brazzelli et al., 2007
	Yes	II	Hofer et al., 1999
	Yes	II	Clark et al., 2000
	Yes	II	Gokdemir et al., 2006
	Yes	II	Gathers et al., 2002
	Yes	II	Diederen et al., 2003
Lichen planus	Yes	II	Taneja et al., 2002
	Yes	II	Saricaoglu et al., 2003
	Yes	II	Wakernagel et al., 2007
Pruritus	Yes	II	Seckin et al., 2007
	Yes	II	Baldo et al., 1996
	Yes	II	Baldo et al., 2002

(Continued)

Box 12-3 Continued

PATHOLOGY	BENEFIT	GRADE	REFERENCE
Chronic urticaria	Yes	II	Berroeta et al., 2004
Seborrheic dermatitis	Yes	II	Pirkhammer et al., 2000
Nodular prurigo	Yes	II	Tamagawa-Mineoka et al., 2007
Polymorphic eruption	Yes	II	Bilsland et al., 1993
Localized scleroderma	Yes	I	Kreuter et al., 2006
Pressure ulcers	Yes	I	Wills et al., 1983
Psoriasis with HIV	Yes	III	Fotiades et al., 1995
Mix of dermatoses	Yes	III	Tay et al., 1996
UVC Therapy Infected wounds	Yes	II	Taylor et al., 1972
	Yes	II	Thai et al., 2005
	Yes	III	Thai et al., 2002

1. Rating Therapeutic Benefit

The rating, expressed as *Yes* or *No*, is based on the overall conclusion(s) reached on the issue of therapeutic effectiveness by the author(s) conducting the peer-reviewed study.

2. Grading Strength of Evidence

The grading, numerically classified as I, II, and III, is based on the type of research methodology, or research design used by the author(s). All those listed are studies on humans published in English-language, peer-reviewed journals. It follows that the strength of evidence in studies graded I is stronger than that in those graded II, which itself is stronger than in those graded III.

a. Grade I

Evidence based on *controlled* studies on humans, regardless of their level of randomization and blindness.

b. Grade II

Evidence based on *noncontrolled* studies on humans, regardless of their level of randomization and blindness.

c. Grade III

Evidence based on *case* studies on humans, regardless of their level of randomization and blindness.

3. Strength of Evidence Behind the Agent

The strength of evidence behind an agent, as presented in the research-based indication box, is arbitrarily assessed in this textbook as *weak, moderate,* or *strong.* For example, the larger the number of studies graded I, regardless of therapeutic benefit, the stronger the scientific evidence behind the agent.

4. Strength for Justifying Usage of the Agent

The strength of evidence to justify the usage of an agent for an individual pathology or group of pathologies, as listed in the research-based indication box, is arbitrarily assessed in this textbook as *poor, fair, good,* or *conflicting.* For example, where a larger number of grade I studies show therapeutic benefit ("Yes") than no benefit, for any given pathology, the justification to use the agent for this pathology is assessed as *good. Conflicting* usage is reported when an equal number of studies with similar grades show therapeutic benefit ("Yes") and no benefit ("No").

C. STRENGTH OF EVIDENCE AND JUSTIFICATION FOR USAGE

The results accumulated in **Box 12-3** show *moderate* strength of evidence for the use of BBUVB and NBUVB therapy, with the majority of studies graded II, and *weak* evidence for UVC with only 3 studies. These results show *good* justification for the use of UVB therapy for psoriasis, atopic dermatitis (eczema), vitiligo, and mycosis fungoides with all published studies demonstrating therapeutic benefits. They also show *poor-to-fair* evidence for the use of UVC therapy for infected dermal wounds. Finally, the results presented in **Box 12-3** show that UVB therapy has been used to treat a variety of additional skin pathologies, and until more evidence can be provided by research, the routine use of UVB therapy *cannot be recommended for this group of pathologies.*

VII. CONTRAINDICATIONS

Table 12-6 presents the contraindications associated with the practice of UV therapy. Screening for a history of skin cancer as well as for the presence of some specific pathologies, such as diabetes and hyperthyroidism, is crucial.

VIII. RISKS, PRECAUTIONS, AND RECOMMENDATIONS

The practice of UVB therapy is not without risks for both patients and practitioners. The primary risks associated with this electrophysical agent, as well as some precautions and recommendations for improving safety and effectiveness, are listed in **Table 12-7**.

IX. CONSIDERATIONS FOR APPLICATION AND DOCUMENTATION

A. CONSIDERATIONS AND PROCEDURES

The safe, effective, and optimal application of this electrophysiological agent requires that clinicians go through a systematic set of considerations and procedures for each and every application. Presented below is a list of these considerations and procedures.

1. Checklists

Before proceeding with treatment, always go through the list of contraindications (**Table 12-6**), risks, precautions, and recommendations (**Table 12-7**).

2. Perform Skin Phototesting

Phototesting done on a healthy, nonlesion skin area establishes the minimal erythemal dose (MED or E-1), which is the starting therapeutic dose. If the patient's skin phototype is known (**Table 12-5**), it can help the phototherapist choose the appropriate dosage range for the test.

3. Skin Preparation

Most dermatoses involve several lesional plaques on the skin affecting a certain percentage of the body. Before each application, the exposed areas should be cleansed with water to remove all impurities, including any therapeutic cream or emollient. Theoretically speaking, only the lesions should be treated. Unfortunately, this is rarely entirely possible, considering the locations and extent of these lesional plaques in relation to normal skin. Normal skin areas in between lesional area(s) should be protected from UV radiation by means of UV-protective creams and materials such as goggles, a face shield, or other UV-blocking clothing such as shorts, gloves, and socks.

4. UV Device Selection

Select the most appropriate device according to the location of the lesions or plaques affecting the body. For example, a whole-body UV cubicle (**Fig 12-1A**) may be selected if a large proportion of the body is affected (i.e., covering several body segments). Conversely, a handheld UV wand (**Fig 12-1C**) may be used if the lesions are spread over a smaller are of the body (i.e., over the scalp).

TABLE 12-6	CONTRAINDICATIONS TO ULTRAVIOLET THERAPY
CONTRAINDICATIONS	**RATIONALE**
Over the eye	Risk of causing temporary damage to the conjunctiva (photoconjunctivitis) or to the cornea (photokeratitis), causing ocular pain, eye watering, and blurred vision.
Over a malignant skin lesion	Risk of further enhancing and spreading the lesion.
With patients suffering from the following diseases	Risk of exacerbating these pathologies (Cameron et al., 2003; Weisberg et al., 2006):
Active pulmonary tuberculosis	Risk of exacerbation of infection.
Significant kidney, cardiac, and liver diseases	Risk of decreased tolerance of UV radiation.
Hyperthyroidism, diabetes mellitus	Risk of severe itching from interaction of UV light with thyroid medication and insulin.
Acute eczema or dermatitis, systemic lupus rythematosus, porphyrias, pellagra, sarcoidosis, herpes simplex	Risk of exacerbation of these conditions.

TABLE 12-7	RISKS, PRECAUTIONS, AND RECOMMENDATIONS FOR ULTRAVIOLET THERAPY

RISKS	RATIONALE
Over areas recently exposed to other radiation therapies	Increased risk of skin carcinoma (Cameron et al., 2003; Weisberg et al., 2006).
With photosensitive patients (acquired or drug related)	Risk of increased sensitivity to UV radiation results in a decrease in the MED and an increased risk of skin burning if too high a dose is used (Weisberg et al., 2006).
With patients who have a history of skin cancer	Increased risk of skin carcinoma (Weisberg et al., 2006).

PRECAUTION	RATIONALE
With feverish patients	May elevate core temperature (Weisberg et al., 2006).

RECOMMENDATIONS	RATIONALE
Discuss the risk of therapy-induced skin cancer with each patient prior to therapy and obtain written consent	Protection against this risk in case of litigation; record the consent in writing and file it (Ibbotson et al., 2004).
Use of UV day care treatment centers	Facilitate treatment access to outpatients (Warin, 2001).
Plug line-powered device into GFCI receptacles	Prevent the occurrence of macroshocks (see Chapter 27).
Conduct regular maintenance and calibration	Optimize dosimetry and treatment efficacy. Follow the manufacturer's recommendations (Taylor et al., 2002). Change in irradiance can occur as lamp output declines with age. Pairs of internal cabin detectors may be used to automatically adjust treatment time to keep the dose constant (Amatiello et al., 2006). The alternative is to replace lamps as they burn out or otherwise fail.

5. Therapeutic Mode

Select between UVB and UVC therapy. This selection is based on the type of dermatose or dermal wound under treatment.

6. Activating the Device

Follow the manufacturer's instructions about how to power up the UV device and the time needed (warm-up time) before optimal operation.

7. Eye Protection

At all times during treatment both the patient and the phototherapist *must* wear UV-protective goggles. If the facial area is free of lesions and a whole-body device must be used, a UV face shield, instead of simple goggles, may be used to protect the patient's facial area.

8. Lamp Surface Area Perpendicular to Skin Surface

For every treatment session, keep the UV lamp's irradiating surface area perpendicular to the skin surface being treated. This positioning is in accordance with Lambert's cosine law, which stipulates that the greater the radiation incident angle in relation to normal, the lesser the amount of UV energy absorbed by the exposed skin tissue (see Chapter 5). For example, if the UV incident radiating angle is directed perpendicular to the treated skin surface area, or at 0° with reference to the normal (N), then cosinus 0° = 1, which means 100% absorption with 0% reflection. If the incident angle is then directed obliquely at 20° with reference to the N, then cosinus 20° = 0.94, which means 94% absorption and 6% reflection. In other words, the greater the UV incident angle with reference to the normal (N), the lesser the absorption and the greater the reflection of UV rays.

9. Distance Between the Lamp Surface Area and the Skin Surface

For every single treatment session, keep the distance (d) separating the UV lamp's surface from the treated skin surfaces exactly the same. This positioning is in accordance with the inverse square law, which stipulates that the irradiance or dose (if the exposure time is constant) originating from a divergent radiating source declines as the square of the distance from the target surface area increases (see Chapter 5). For example, doubling the distance from the lamp surface area to the exposed skin surface area will reduce to 25% the dose or irradiance per area ($I = 1/d^2$; if d doubles, I will decrease to one-quarter, or 0.25; $1 = 1/1$; $0.25 = 1/2^2 = 1/4$). In contrast, decreasing this distance by 50% will increase irradiance by 400%. Distances of 30 cm (12 in.) and 2.5 cm (1 in.) are recommended for UVB and UVC therapy respectively is often recommended.

10. Dosage

Increase the dosage from one treatment to the next by increasing the exposure time while keeping the UV device's irradiance constant, as shown in **Box 12-1**. This recommendation is in accordance with the reciprocity law, which stipulates that the dose (D) can be increased by augmenting time (T) while keeping irradiance (I) constant. One way to keep irradiance constant is to always use the same UV device or lamp, always keep the lamp surface area the same distance from the skin area being treated, and always position the lamp surface area perpendicular to the skin surface area being treated, as discussed above.

11. Posttreatment Skin Inspection

Always inspect the patient's exposed skin areas after each and every treatment, and record any unusual reaction.

12. Device Maintenance and Calibration

Carefully follow the manufacturer's maintenance and calibration recommendations for the UV device because failure to comply may lead to inaccurate dosimetry. Precise dosimetry is mandatory with UV therapy because the carcinogenic risk increases relative to the cumulative dosage the patient will receive over his or her lifetime.

B. HOME UV PHOTOTHERAPY

UV phototherapy delivered in a clinical setting (hospital or therapeutic UV centers), as discussed in this chapter, is a popular and effective treatment for many patients with skin pathologies. Repeated journeys to these clinical centers for treatments can, however, be time-consuming and expensive for many patients, considering that a given UV treatment session lasts only a few minutes. An alternative is for these patients to treat themselves at home using UV devices found in hospitals. Home-based therapy, therefore, is suitable only if found to be as safe and effective as hospital-based therapy.

1. Consensus

Today's consensus on this subject is that home-based UV therapy should be used with caution and restricted to those patients with overwhelming difficulties in visiting hospitals (Sarkany et al., 1999; Cameron et al., 2002b; Langan et al., 2004; Koek et al., 2006; Yelverton et al., 2006). Moreover, there is strong opinion that home-based UV phototherapy is a suboptimal treatment with greater attendant risks than phototherapy delivered in a hospital environment (Sarkany et al., 1999).

2. Concerns

A key concern with home-based UV therapy relates to legal liability with regard to the safe use of the UV device. There can be no doubt that the safe use of UV therapy is directly related to the carcinogenic risk associated with it (Lee et al., 2005; Man et al., 2005). Dermatologists and phototherapists must be fully aware of this responsibility when prescribing unsupervised home-based UV phototherapy. Before authorizing home-based UV therapy, the treating phototherapist must assure that the patient receives appropriate guidelines, training, and follow-ups (Cameron et al., 2002b; Haykai et al., 2006).

C. DOCUMENTATION

Table 12-8 shows the key parameters to be documented in the patient's file after treatment.

TABLE 12-8	KEY TREATMENT PARAMETERS TO BE DOCUMENTED IN PATIENT'S FILE AFTER UV THERAPY

- UV device type: description
- UV light: description
- Wavelength range: nm
- Treated body area: describe body areas or provide photographs
- Distance between lamp surface and exposed skin surface: cm (in.)
- Patient's skin phototype: from I to IV
- Minimal erythemal dose (MED) or starting dose: mJ/cm^2
- Dose increment regimen: description (see **Box 12-2**)
- Treatment frequency: number of treatments or exposures per week
- Treatment period: number of weeks
- Cumulative dose at the end of the treatment period: J/cm^2

Case Study 12-1 Psoriasis

A 32-year-old active man, diagnosed 4 years ago with severe psoriasis on his trunk, elbows, and knees is referred by his treating dermatologist for UVB therapy. Psoriasis is a non-contagious, common, chronic, and incurable disease that occurs when faulty signals in the immune system causes skin cells to regenerate too quickly. This man has no history of skin cancer. His skin phenotype is II (white, tans minimally; always burns easily). His past treatments included oral drugs, topical creams, as well as five regimens (or therapeutic periods) of oral PUVA. Because of the significant side effects associated with his previous PUVA therapy sessions (nausea, skin phototoxicity), and the growing awareness of his carcinogenic risk, the patient declined further PUVA treatment and asked his dermatologist for an alternative, less carcinogenic, form of UV therapy. His main complaints are pain and restricted elbow, knee, and trunk movements caused by the lesional plaques. He also complains of difficulty with some activities of daily living (ADLs) and with his favorite sport activity, cycling. His goal is to achieve a reasonable, enduring resolution of his plaques, enough to reduce his pain and increase his overall ability to perform most of his daily living and cycling activities. The patient presently suffers from Achilles tendinitis for which he takes the anti-inflammatory and photosensitizing drug Celebrex.

Evidence-Based Steps Toward the Resolution of This Case

1. **List medical diagnosis.**

   Psoriasis

2. **List key impairment(s).**
   - Pain
   - Multiple skin lesional plaques

3. **List key functional limitation(s).**
   - Limited bilateral elbow and knee range of motion (ROM)
   - Limited trunk range of motion (ROM)
   - Difficulty with activity of daily living (ADLs)

4. **List key disabilities.**
   - Difficulty with cycling

5. **Justification of UVB therapy.**

   Is there justification for the use of UVB in this case? This chapter has established that there is *good justification* for the use of UVB for psoriasis, with all studies demonstrating therapeutic benefits (see Section VI). The selection of UVB as the treating EPA is justified on the basis of the following articles: Parrish et al., 1981; Van Weelden et al., 1990, 1990; Bilsland et al., 1997; Green et al., 1988; Coven et al., 1997; Wainwright et al., 1998; Dawe et al., 1998; Dawe et al., 2003; Bandow et al., 2004; Ibbotson et al., 2004; Dogra et al., 2004;

Gambichler et al., 2005. NBUVB is selected over BBUVB because its peak spectral irradiation (313–309 nm) is well within the action spectrum of psoriasis. NBUVB is also selected because it eliminates the nontherapeutic strong erythemogenic response caused by the shorter band (310–290 nm) of BBUVB rays. NBUVB is further justified because it presents no side effects and a lower carcinogenic risk when compared to BBUVB. Because of the broad coverage of his lesions, the patient is treated using a whole-body cubicle device. During therapy the patient's intact skin areas and key organs are protected with a face shield (for facial protection), shorts (for genital protection), gloves, and socks. The repeated erythemal effect of UV light is expected to clear most of the plaques.

6. **Search for contraindications.**

   None is found.

7. **Search for risks and precautions.**

   The use of UVB presents a risk for the patient because he is currently using an anti-inflammatory and photosensitizing drug, Celebrex, for his acute Achilles tendinitis. Caution is advised.

8. **Outline the therapeutic goal(s) you and your patient wish to achieve.**
   - Decrease pain
   - Decrease plaque severity
   - Increase bilateral elbow, knee, and trunk range of motion.
   - Facilitate ADLs
   - Facilitate cycling

9. **List the outcome measurement(s) used to assess treatment effectiveness.**
   - Pain: Visual Analog Scale (VAS)
   - Plaque status: Psoriasis Area Severity Index (PASI)
   - Elbow/knee joint and trunk mobility: goniometry
   - ADL / cycling activity: Personal Specific Function Scale (PSFS)

10. **Instruct the patient about what he/she should experience, do, and not do during the treatment session.**
    - Feel light heating sensation.
    - Refrain from moving

11. **Outline your therapeutic prescription based on the best sources of evidence available.**

    The UV prescription used is based on the following articles: Parrish et al., 1981; Van Weelden et al., 1990, 1990; Bilsland et al., 1997; Green et al., 1988; Coven et al., 1997; Wainwright et al., 1998; Dawe et al., 1998; Dawe et al., 2003; Bandow et al., 2004; Ibbotson et al., 2004; Dogra et al., 2004; Gambichler et al., 2005; Sezer et al., 2007; Kirke et al., 2007.

- **UV device: whole-body cubicle**—NBUVB mounted with 48 fluorescent TL-01 tubes
- **Wavelength range:** 313–309 nm; peak spectra at 311 nm
- **Approximate distance from tube surfaces to treated skin surface:** 45 cm (18 in.)
- **Patient's positioning:** standing
- **Patient's protection:** the aim is to protect normal skin areas from UV light using a faceguard, gloves and socks, and underwear
- **MED or starting dose obtained from phototesting:** 320 mJ/cm^2
- **Treatment frequency:** 3 times weekly (Monday, Wednesday, Friday)
- **Dose incremental regimen:**
  - Week1-MED
  - **2nd to 7th week:** MED increased by 30% over previous dose
- **Total treatment period:** 7 weeks (or until 90% plaque clearance)
- **Total number of treatments:** 21 over 7 consecutive weeks

12. **Collect outcome measurements.**

Pre- and posttreatment comparison:

- Pain: decrease VAS score from 6 to 1
- Plaque lesion status: increase PASI score by 80%
- Joint and trunk mobility: full range of motion
- ADLs/cycling activity: increase PSFS score by 70%

13. **Assess therapeutic effectiveness based on outcome measures.**

The results show that 21 applications of NBUVB therapy, delivered 3 times per week over 7 consecutive weeks, significantly decreased the patient's pain level, which correlates with the significant decrease in his PASI score (less redness, thickness, and scaliness). This UV treatment was also beneficial in restoring full joint and trunk mobility in addition to improving significantly his ability to do his daily living and cycling activities. Overall, this regimen of NBUVB therapy had a beneficial impact on the patient's disablement status created by this dermatosis as illustrated in the **figure below**.

14. **State the prognosis.**

The prognosis is excellent. Considering the unfortunate recurrent nature of this skin disease, it is more than likely that this patient will have to be treated yet again with UVB therapy over the following months and for several years to come. The need for additional UV treatments over this patient's lifetime points to the importance of carefully monitoring his total cumulative doses of UV radiation from one treatment period to the next. Such monitoring will allow the treating phototherapist to assess this patient's overall carcinogenic risk and act accordingly, by modulating the next cumulative doses and treatment periods.

THERAPEUTIC IMPACT on Disablement

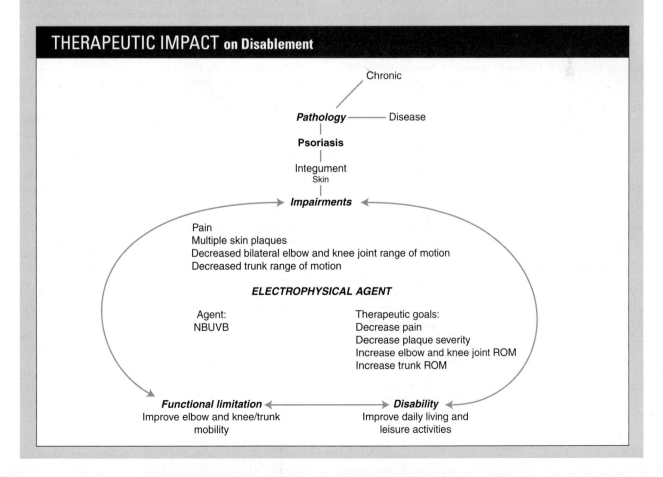

CRITICAL THINKING QUESTIONS

Clarification: What is meant by ultraviolet (UV) therapy?

Assumptions: You have assumed that the carcinogenic risk associated with NBUVB is lower than the one associated with BBUVB? How do you justify making that assumption?

Reasons and evidence: Why do you believe that the use of NBUVB is as effective as and less carcinogenic than PUVA and BBUVB for most dermatoses?

Viewpoints or perspectives: How would you respond to a colleague who says that the use of UVB presents no major advantages over the use of PUVA?

Implications and consequences: What are the implications and consequences of operating a UV device without considering the reciprocity law, Lambert's cosine law, and the inverse square law?

About the question: Why is it so important to do phototesting before UV therapy and monitor cumulative dosages over the patient's lifetime? Why do you think I ask this question?

References

Articles

Ahmad K, Rogers S, McNicholas PD, Collins P (2007) Narrowband UVB and PUVA in the treatment of mycosis fungoides: A retrospective study. Acta Derm Venereol, 87: 413–417

Aydogan K, Karadogan SK, Tunali S, Adim SBG, Ozcelik T (2006) Narrowband UVB phototherapy for small plaque parapsoriasis. J Eur Acad Dermatol Venereol, 20: 573–577

Baldo A, Sammarco E, Monfrecola M (1996) UVB phototherapy for pruritus in polycythaemia vera. J Dermatol Treat, 7: 245–246

Baldo A, Sammarco E, Plaitano R, Martinelli V, Monfrecola A (2002) Narrow (TL-01) ultraviolet B phototherapy for pruritus polycythaemia vera. J Dermatol, 147: 979–981

Berroeta I, Clark C, Ibbotson SH, Ferguson J, Dawe RS (2004) Narrowband (TL-01) ultraviolet B phototherapy for chronic urticaria. Clin Exp Dermatol, 29: 97–99

Bhatnagar A, Kanwar AJ, Parsad D, De D (2007) Comparison of systemic PUVA and NB-UVB in the treatment of vitiligo: An open prospective study. J Eur Acad Dermatol Venereol, 21: 638–642

Bilsland D, George SA, Gibbs NK (1993) A comparison of narrow band phototherapy (TL-01) and phototherapy (PUVA) in the management of polymorphic light eruption. Br J Dermatol, 129: 708–712

Boztepe G, Karaduman A, Sahin S, Hayran M, Koleman F (2006) The effect of maintenance narrow-band ultraviolet B therapy on the duration of remission of psoriasis: A prospective randomized clinical trial. In J Dermatol, 45: 245–250

Brazzelli V, Antoninetti M, Palazzini S, Prestinari F, Berroni G (2007) Narrow-band ultraviolet therapy in early-stage mycosis fungoides: a study on 20 patients. Photodermatol Photoimmunol Photomed, 23: 229–233

Cameron H, Dawe RS, Yule S, Murphy J, Ibbotson SH, Ferguson J (2002a) A randomized observer-blinded trial of twice vs. three times weekly narrowband ultraviolet B phototherapy for chronic plaque psoriasis. Br J Dermatol, 147: 973–978

Cameron H, Yule S, Moseley H, Dawe RS, Ferguson J (2002b) Taking treatment to the patient: Development of a home TL-01 ultraviolet B phototherapy service. Br J Dermatol, 147: 957–965

Clark C, Dawe RS, Evans AT, Lowe G, Ferguson J (2000) Narrowband TL-01 phototherapy for patch-stage mycosis fungoides. Arch Dermatol, 136: 748–752

Clayton TH, Clark, Turner D, Goulden V (2006) The treatment of severe atopic dermatitis in children with narrowband ultraviolet B phototherapy. Clin Exp Dermatol, 32: 28–33

Conner-Kerr TA, Sullivan PK, Gaillard J, Franklin ME, Jones RM (1998) The effect of ultraviolet radiation on antibiotic-resistant bacteria in vitro. Ostomy Wound Manage, 44: 50–56

Coven TR, Burack LH, Gilleaudead R, Keogh M, Ozawa M, Krueger JG (1997) Narrow-band UV-B produces superior clinical and histopathological resolution of moderate-to-severe psoriasis in patients compared with broadband UV-B. Arch Dermatol, 133: 1514–1522

Dawe RS, Cameron H, Yule S, Man I, Wainwright NJ, Ibbotson SH, Ferguson J (2003) A randomized controlled trial of narrowband ultraviolet B vs. bath-psoralen plus ultraviolet A photochemotherapy for psoriasis. Br J Dermatol, 148: 1194–1204

Dawe RS, Wainwright NJ, Cameron H, Ferguson J (1998) Narrow-band (TL-01) ultraviolet B phototherapy for chronic plaque psoriasis: Three times or five times weekly treatment? Br J Dermatol, 139: 833–839

Der-Petrossian M, Seeber A, Honigsmann H, Tanew A (2000) Half-side comparison study on the efficacy of 8-methoxysporalen bath-PUVA versus narrow-band ultraviolet B phototherapy in patients with severe chronic atopic dermatitis. Br J Dermatol, 142: 39–43

Diederen PV, Van Weelden H, Sanders CJ, Toonstra J (2003) Narrowband UVB and psoralen-UVA in the treatment of early-stage mycosis fungoides. A retrospective study. J Am Acad Dermatol, 48: 215–219

Don P, Iuga A, Dacko A, Hardick K (2006) Treatment of vitiligo with broadband ultraviolet B and vitamins. Int J Dermatol, 45: 63–65

Fisher T, Alsins J, Berne B (1984) Ultraviolet action spectrum and evaluation of ultraviolet lamps for psoriasis healing. Int J Dermatol, 23: 633–637

Fitzpatrick TB (1988) The validity and practicality of sun-reactive skin types I through VI. Arch Dermatol, 124: 869–871

Fotiades J, Lim HW, Jiang SB, Soter NA, Sanchez M, Moy J (1995) Efficacy of ultraviolet B phototherapy for psoriasis in patients infected with human immunodeficiency virus. Photodermatol Photoimmunol Photomed, 11: 107–115

Gathers RC, Scherschun L, Malick F, Fivenson DP, Lim HW (2002) Narrowband UVB phototherapy for early-stage mycosis fungoides. J Am Acad Dermatol, 47: 191–197

George SA, Bilsland DJ, Johnson BE, Ferfuson J (1993) Narrowband (TL-01) UVB air-conditioned phototherapy for chronic severe adult atopic dermatitis. Br J Dermatol, 128: 49–56

Gokdemir G, Barutcuoglu B, Sakiz D, Koslu A (2006) narrowband UVB phototherapy for early-stage mycosis fungoides: Evaluation of clinical and histopathological changes. J Eur Acad Dermatol Venereol, 20: 804–809

Gokdemir G, Kivanc-Altunay I, Koslu A (2005) Narrow-band ultraviolet B phototherapy in patients with psoriasis: For which types of psoriasis is it more effective? J Dermatol, 32: 436–441

Gordon PM, Diffey BL, Matthews JN, Farr PM (1999) A randomized comparison of narrow-band TL-01 phototherapy and PUVA photochemotherapy for psoriasis. J Am Acad Dermatol, 41: 728–732

Gordon PM, Saunders PJ, Diffey BL, Farr PM (1998) Phototesting prior to narrow-band (TL-01) ultraviolet B phototherapy. Br J Dermatol, 139: 811–814

Green C, Ferguson J, Lakshmipathi T, Johnson BE (1988) 311 nm UVB phototherapy—An effective treatment for psoriasis. Br J Dermatol, 119: 691–696

Grundmann-Kollmann M, Behrens S, Podda M, Peter RU, Kaufmann R, Kerscher M (1999) Phototherapy for atopic eczema with narrowband UVB. J Am Dermatol, 40: 995–997

Hamzavi I, Jain H, McLean D, Shapiro J, Zeng H, Lui H (2004) Parametric modeling of narrowband UV-B phototherapy for vitiligo using a novel quantitative tool: The vitiligo area scoring index. Arch Dermatol, 140: 677–683

Haykai KA, DesGroseilliers JP (2006) Are narrow-band ultraviolet home units a viable option for continuous or maintenance therapy of photoresponsive diseases? J Cutan Med Surg, 10: 234–240

Hjerppe M, Hasan T, Saksala I, Reunala T (2001) Narrow-band UVB treatment in atopic dermatitis. Acta Derm Venereol, 81: 439–440

Hofer A, Cerroni L, Kerl H, Wolf P (1999) Narrowband (311 nm) UV-B therapy for small plaque parasporiasis and early-stage mucosis fungoides. Arch Dermatol, 135: 1377–1380

Hofer A, Fink-Puches R, Kerl H, Wolf P (1998) Comparison of phototherapy with near vs. far erythemogenic doses of narrow-band ultraviolet B in patients with psoriasis. Br J Dermatol, 138: 96–100

Jekler J (1992) Phototherapy of atopic dermatitis with ultraviolet radiation. Acta Dermatol Venereol, 72: 1–37

Jury CS, McHenry P, Burden AD, Lever R, Bilsland D (2006) Narrowband ultraviolet B (NBUVB) phototherapy in children. Clin Exp Dermatol, 31: 196–199

Kanwar AJ, Dogra S. Parsad D, Kumar B (2005) Narrow-band UVB for the treatment of vitiligo: An emerging effective and well-tolerated therapy. Int J Dermatol, 44: 57–60

Karvonen J, Kokkonen EL, Ruotsalainen E (1989) 311 nmUVB lamps in the treatment of psoriasis with the Ingram regimen. Acta Derm Venereal (Stockh), 69: 82–85

Kaur M, Oliver B, Hu J, Feldman SR (2006) Nonlaser UVB-targeted phototherapy treatment of psoriasis. Cutis, 78: 200–2003

Kirke SM, Lowder S, Lloyd JJ, Diffey BL, Matthews JN, Farr PM (2007) A randomized comparison of selective broadband UVB and narrowband UVB in the treatment of psoriasis. J Invest Dermatol, 127: 1641–1646

Kollner K, Wimmershoff MB, Hintz C, Landthaler M, Hohenleutner U (2005) Comparison of the 308-nm excimer laser and a 308-nm excimer lamp with 311-nm narrow-band ultraviolet B in the treatment of psoriasis. Br J Dermatol, 152: 750–754

Kreuter A, Hyun J, Stiker m, Sommer A, Altmeyer P, Gambichler T (2006) A randomized controlled study of low-dose UVA1, medium dose UVA1, and narrowband UVB phototherapy in the treatment of localized scleroderma. J Am Acad Dermatol, 54: 440–447

Langan SM, Heerey A, Barry M, Barnes L (2004) Cost analysis of narrow-band UVB phototherapy in psoriasis. J Am Acad Dermatol, 50: 623–626

Larko O (1989) Treatment of psoriasis with a new UVB-lamp. Acta Dermatol Venereol (Stockh), 69: 357–359

Leenutaphong V, Nimkulrat P, Sudtim S (2000) Comparison of phototherapy two times and four times a week with low doses of narrowband ultraviolet B in Asian patients with psoriasis. Photodermatol Photoimmunol Photomed, 16: 202–206

Legat FJ, Hofer A, Brabek E, Quehenberger F, Kerl H, Wolf P (2003) Narrowband UV-B vs medium-dose UV-A1 phototherapy in chronic atopic dermatitis. Arch Dermatol, 139: 223–224

Lim C, Brown P (2006) Quality of life in psoriasis improves after standardized administration of narrowband UVB phototherapy. Australas J Dermatol, 47: 37–40

Man I, Crombie OK, Dawe RS, Ibbotson SH, Ferguson J (2005) The photocarcinogenic risk of narrowband UVB (TL-01) phototherapy: Early follow-up data. Br J Dermatol, 152: 755–757

Natta R, Somsak T, Wisuttida T, Laor L (2003) Narrowband ultraviolet B radiation therapy for recalcitrant vitiligo in Asians. J Am Acad Dermatol, 49: 473–476

Njoo MD, Bos JD, Westerhof W (2000) Treatment of generalized vitiligo in children with narrow-band (TL-01) UVB radiation therapy. J Am Acad Dermatol, 42: 245–253

Ortel B, Perl S, Kinaciyan T, Calzavara-Pinton PG, Honigsmann H (1993) Comparison of narrow-band (331 nm) UVB and broad band UVA after oral or bath-water 8-methoxypsoralen in the treatment of psoriasis. J Am Acad Dermatol, 29: 736–740

Otman SG, Edwards C, Gambles B, Anstey AV (2006) Validation of a semiautomated method of minimal etythema dose testing for narrowband ultraviolet B phototherapy. Br J Dermatol, 155: 416–421

Parrish JA, Fitzpatrick TB, Tanenbaum L, Pathak MA (1974) Photochemotherapy of psoriasis with oral methoxsalen and long-wave ultraviolet light. N Engl J Med, 291: 1207–1211

Parrish JA, Jaenicke KF (1981) Action spectrum for phototherapy of psoriasis. J Invest Dermatol, 76: 359–362

Parsad D, Kanwar AJ, Kumar B (2006) Psoralen-ultraviolet A vs. narrowband ultraviolet B phototherapy for the treatment of vertiligo. J Eur Acad Dermatol Venereol, 20: 175–177

Picot E, Meunier I, Picot-Debeze MC (1992) Treatment of psoriasis with a 311-nm UVB lamp. Br J Dermatol, 127: 509–512

Pirkhammer D, Seeber A, Honigsmann H, Tanew A (2000) Narrowband ultraviolet B (TL-01) phototherapy is an effective and safe treatment for patients with seborrhoeic dermatitits. Br J Dermatol, 143: 964–968

Reynolds NJ, Franklin V, Gray JC, Diffey BL, Farr PM (2001) Narrowband ultraviolet B and broad-band ultraviolet A phototherapy in adult atopic eczema: A randomized controlled trial. Lancet, 357: 2012–2016

Saricaoglu H, Karadogan SK, Baskan EB, Tunali S (2003) Narrowband UVB therapy in the treatment of lichen planus. Photodermatol Photoimmunol Photomed, 19: 265–267

Scherschun L, Kim JJ, Lim HW (2001) Narrow-band ultraviolet B is a useful and well-tolerated treatment for vitiligo. J Am Acad Dermatol, 44: 999–1003

Seckin D, Demircay Z, Akin O (2007) Generalized pruritus treated with narrowband UVB. Int J Dermatol, 46: 367–370

Sezer E, Erbil AH, Kurumlu Z, Tastan HB, Etikan I (2007a) Comparison of the efficacy of local narrowband ultraviolet B (NB-UVB) phototherapy versus psoralen plus ultraviolet A (PUVA) paint for palmoplantar psoriasis. J Dermatol, 34: 435–440

Sezer E, Etikan I (2007b) Local narrowband UVB phototherapy vs. local PUVA in the treatment of chronic hand eczema. Photodermatol Photoimmunol Photomed, 23: 10–14

Sjovall P, Christensen O (1987) Local and systemic effect of UV-B irradiation in patients with chronic hand eczema. Acta Dermatol Venereol, 67: 538–541

Stern RS, Armstrong RB, Anderson TF, Bickers DR, Lowe NJ, Harber L, Voorhees J, Parrish J (1986) Effect of continued ultraviolet B phototherapy on the duration of remission of psoriasis: A randomized study. J Am Acad Dermatol, 15: 546–556

Stern RS, Laird N (1994) The carcinogenic risk of treatments for severe psoriasis: photochemotherapy follow-up study. Cancer, 73: 2759–2764

Storbeck K, Holzle F, Schurer N, Lehmann P, Plewig G (1993) Narrowband UVB (311 nm) versus conventional broad-band UVB with and without dithranol in phototherapy for psoriasis. Br J Dermatol, 28: 227–231

Sullivan PK, Conner-Kerr TA, Smith ST (1999) The effects of UVC irradiation on group A streptococcus in vitro. Ostomy Wound Manage, 45: 50–54, 56–58

Tamagawa-Mineoka R, Katoh N, Ueda E, Kishimoto S (2007) Narrowband ultraviolet B phototherapy in patients with recalcitrant nodular prurigo. J Dermatol, 34: 691–695

Tanew A, Radakovic-Fijan S, Schemper M, Honigsmann H (1999) Paired comparison study on narrow-band (TL-01) UVB phototherapy versus photochemotherapy (PUVA) in the treatment of chronic plaque type psoriasis. Arch Dermatol, 135: 519–524

Taneja A, Taylor CR (2002) Narrow-band UVB for lichen planus treatment. Int J Dermatol, 41: 282–283

Tay YK, Morelli JG, Weston WL (1996) Experience with UVB phototherapy in children, Pediatr Dermatol, 13: 406–409

Taylor R (1972) Clinical study of ultraviolet in various skin conditions. Phys Ther, 52: 279–282

Thai TP, Houghton PE, Campbell KE, Woodbury MG (2002) Ultraviolet light C in the treatment of chronic wounds with MRSA: A case study. Ostomy Wound Manage, 48: 52–60

Thai TP, Keast DH, Campbell KE, Woodbury G, Houghton PE (2005) Effect of ultraviolet light C on bacterial colonization in chronic wounds. Ostomy Wound Manage, 51: 32–45

Tjioe M, Gerritsen MJ, Juhlin L, Van Der Kerkof PC (2002) Treatment of vitiligo vulgaris with narrow band UVB (311 nm) for one year and the effect of addition of folic acid and vitamin B12. Acta Derm Venereol, 82: 369–372

Valkova S, Velkova A (2004) UVA/UVB phototherapy for atopic dermatitis revisited. J Dermatolog Treat, 15: 239–244

Van Weelden H, De la Faille B, Young E, Van der Leun JC (1988) A new developement in UVB phototherapy of psoriasis. Br J Dermatol, 119: 11–19

Van Weelden H, De la Faille B, Young E, Van der Leun JC (1990) Comparison of narrowband UV-B phototherapy and PUVA photochemotherapy (PUVA) in the treatment of psoriasis. Acta Derm Venereol, 70: 212–215

Wackernagel A, Legat FJ, Hofer A, Quehenberger F, Kerl H, Wolf P (2007) Psoralen plus UVA vs. UVB-311 nm for the treatment of lichen planus. Photodermatol Photoimmunol Photomed, 23: 15–19

Wainwright NJ, Dawe RS, Ferguson J (1998) Narrowband ultraviolet B (TL-01) phototherapy for psoriasis: Which incremental regimen? Br J Dermatol, 39: 410–414

Weichenthal M, Schwarz T (2005) Phototherapy: How does UV work? Photodermatol Photoimmunol Photomed, 21: 260–266

Westerhof W, Nieuweboer-Krobotova L (1997) Treatment of vitiligo with UV-B radiation vs topical psoralen plus UV-A. Arch Dermatol, 133: 1525–1528

Wills EE, Anderson TW, Beatie LB, Scott A (1983) A randomized placebo controlled trial of ultraviolet in the treatment of superficial pressure sores. J Am Geriatr Soc, 31: 131–133

Wishart J (2001) A new method of phototesting before narrowband UVB therapy. Photodermatol Photoimmunol Photomed, 17: 197–199

Yashar SS, Gielcayk R, Scherschum L, Lim HW (2003) Narrow-band ultraviolet B treatment for vitiligo, pruritis, and inflammatory dermatoses. Photodermatol Photoimmunol Photomed, 19: 164–168

Yelverton CB, Kulkarni AS, Balkrishnan R, Feldman SR (2006) Home ultraviolet B phototherapy: A cost-effective option for severe psoriasis. Manage Care Interface, 19: 33–36, 39

Yones SS, Palmer RA, Garibaldinos TT, Hawk JK (2006) Randomized double-blind trial of the treatment of chronic plaque psoriasis: Efficacy of psoralen-UV-A therapy vs. narrowband UV-B therapy. Arch Dermatol, 142: 836–842

Yones SS, Palmer RA, Garibaldinos TT, Hawk JK (2007) Randomized double-blind of treatment of vitiligo. Efficacy of psoralen-UV-A therapy vs narrowband-UV-B therapy. Arch Dermatol, 143: 578–584

Yones SS, Palmer RA, Kuno Y, Hawk JL (2005) Audit of the use of psoralen photochemotherapy (PUVA) and narrowband UVB phototherapy in the treatment of psoriasis. J Dermatolog Treat, 16: 108–112

Review Articles

Amatiello H, Martin CJ (2006) Ultraviolet phototherapy: Review and options for cabin dosimetry and operation. Phys Med Biol, 51: 299–309

Bandow GD, Koo JY (2004) Narrow-band ultraviolet B radiation: A review of the current literature. Int J Dermatol, 43: 555–561

British Photodermatology Group (1994) Guidelines for PUVA. Br J Dermatol, 130: 246–255

Bilsland D, Dawe R, Diffey BL, Farr P, Ferguson J, George S, Gibbs NK, Green C, McGregor J, Van Weelden H, Wainwright NJ, Young AR (1997) An appraisal of narrowband (TL-01) UVB phototherapy. British Photodermatology Group Workshop Report (April 1996). Br J Dermatol, 137: 327–330

Dawe RS (2003) Ultraviolet A1 phototherapy. Br J Dermatol, 148: 626–637

Dogra S, Kanwar AJ (2004) Narrow band UVB phototherapy in dermatology. Indian J Dermatol Venereal Leprol, 70: 205–209

Gambichler T, Breuckmann F, Booms S, Altmeyer P, Kreuter A (2005) Narrowband UVB phototherapy in skin conditions beyond psoriasis. J Am Acad Dermatol, 52: 660–670

Halpern SM, Anstey AV, Dawe RS, Diffey BL, Farr PM, Ferguson J, Hawk JL, Ibbotson S, McGregor JM, Murphy GM, Thomas SE, Rhodes LE

(2000) Guidelines for topical PUVA: A report of a workshop of the British Photodermatology Group. Br J Dermatol, 142: 22–31

Honigsmann H (2001) Phototherapy for psoriasis. Clin Exp Dermatol, 26: 343–350

Ibbotson SH, Bilsland D, Cox NH, Dawe RS, Diffey B, Edwards C, Farr PM, Ferguson J, Hart G, Hawk J, Loyd J, Martin C, Moseley H, McKenna K, Rhodes LE, Taylor DK (2004) An update and guidance on narrowband ultraviolet B phototherapy: A British Photodermatology Group Workshop Report. Br J Dermatol, 151: 283–297

Karrer S, Eholzer C, Ackermann G (2001) Phototherapy of psoriasis: Comparative experience of different phototherapeutic approaches. Dermatology, 202: 108–115

Kist JM, Van Voorhees AS (2005) Narrowband ultraviolet B therapy for psoriasis and other skin disorders. Adv Dermatol, 21: 235–250

Kitchen S, Partridge C (1991) A review of ultraviolet radiation therapy. Physiotherapy, 77: 423–432

Koek MB, Buskens E, Bruijnzeel-Koomen CA, Sigurdsson V (2006) Home ultraviolet B phototherapy for psoriasis: Discrepancy between literature, guidelines, general opinion and actual use. Results of a literature review, a web search, and a questionnaire among dermatologists. Br J Dermatol, 154: 701–711

Krutmann J (2000) Phototherapy for atopic dermatitis. Clin Exp Dermatol, 25: 552–558

Lebwohl M, Ting PT, Koo JY (2005) Psoriasis treatment: Traditional therapy. Ann Rheum Dis, 64: 83–86

Lee E, Koo J, Berger T (2005) UVB phototherapy and skin cancer risk: A review of the literature. Int J Dermatol, 44: 355–360

Meduri NB, Vandergriff T, Rasmussen H, Jacobe H (2007) Phototherapy in the management of atopic dermatitis: A systematic review. Photodermatol Photoimmunol Photomed, 23: 106–112

Njoo MD, Westerhof W, Bos JD, Bossuyt MM (1999) The development of guidelines for the treatment of vitiligo. Arch Dermatol, 135: 1514–1521

Roelandts R (2002) The history of phototherapy: Something new under the sun? J Am Acad Dermatol, 46: 926–930

Saladi RN, Persaud AN (2005) The causes of skin cancer: A comprehensive review. Drugs Today (Barc), 41: 37–53

Sarkany RP, Anstey A, Diffey BL, Jobling R, Langmack K, McGregor JM, Moseley H, Murphy GM, Rhodes LE, Norris PG (1999). Home phototherapy: Report on a workshop of the British Photodermatology Group., December 1996. Br J Dermatol, 140: 195–199

Stern RS, Laird N (1994) The carcinogenic risk of treatments for severe psoriasis. Cancer, 73: 2793–2764

Su J, Pearce DJ, Feldman SR (2005) The role of commercial tanning beds and ultraviolet A light in the treatment of psoriasis. J Dermatolog Treat, 16: 324–326

Taylor DK, Anstey AV, Coleman AJ, Diffey BL, Farr PM, Ferguson J, Ibbotson S, Langmack K, Lloyd JJ, McCann P, Martin CJ, Menage H, Murphy G, Pye SD, Rhodes LE, Rogers S (2002) Guidelines for dosimetry and calibration in ultraviolet radiation therapy: A report of a British Phototherapy Group Workshop. Br J Dermatol, 146: 755–763

Tuchinda C, Kerr HA, Taylor CR, Jacobe H, Bergamo BM, Elmets C, Rivard J, Lim HW (2006) UVA1 phototherapy for cutaneous diseases: An experience of 92 cases in the United States. Photodermatol Photoimmunol Photomed, 22: 247–253

Van der Leun JC, Forbes PD (2005) Ultraviolet tanning equipment: Six questions. Photodermatol Photoimmunol Photomed, 21: 254–259

Wardin AP (2001) Dermatology day care treatment centres. Clin Exp Dermatol, 26: 351–355

Young AR (1997) Chromophores in human skin. Phys Med Biol, 42: 789–802

Chapters of Textbooks

Cameron MH, Perez D, Otano-Lata S (2003) Electromagnetic radiation. In: Physical Agents in Rehabilitation: From Research to Practice, 2nd Ed. Saunders, New-York, pp 369–413

Conner-Kerr T, Albaugh KW, Woodruff LD, Cameron M, Bill A (2007) Phototherapy in Wound Management. In: Wound Care: A

Collaborative Practice Manual for Health Care Professionnals, 3rd Ed. Sussman C, Bates-Jensen B (Eds). Lippincott Williams & Wilkins, Baltimore, pp 591-611

Davis JM (2002) Ultraviolet therapy. In: Therapeutic Modalities for Physical Therapists, 2nd ed. Prentice WE (Ed). McGraw-Hill, New-York, pp 343–357

Diffey B, Farr P (2002) Ultraviolet therapy. In: Electrotherapy Evidence-Based Practice, 11th ed. Kitchen S (Ed). Churchill Livingstone, London, pp 191–207

Starkey C (2004) Light modalities. In: Therapeutic Modalities, 3rd ed. FA Davis Co., Philadelphia, pp 334—351

Weisberg J, Balogun JA (2006) Ultraviolet radiation. In: Integrating Physical Agents in Rehabilitation, 2nd ed. Hecox B, Mehreteab TA, Weisberg J, Sanko J (Eds). Pearson Prentice Hall, Upper Saddle River, New Jersey, pp 429–446

Textbooks

Morison WL (2005) Phototherapy and Photochemotherapy for Skin Diseases, 3rd Ed. Informa-Healthcare, New York

Zanolli MD, Feldman SR (2005) Phototherapy Treatment Protocols for Psoriasis and other Phototherapy-responsive Dermatoses, 2nd Ed. Informa-Healthcare, New York

Iontophoresis Therapy

Learning Objectives

Knowledge: List the drug ions, with their related proposed physiological and therapeutic effects, most commonly used in iontophoresis in the field of rehabilitation.

Comprehension: Compare the methods of iontophoresis, needle injection, and oral ingestion for the delivery of drugs into the human body.

Application: Carry out the calculation of dosage and the technical steps necessary to deliver an iontophoretic treatment.

Analysis: Differentiate between the process of phoresis and electrolysis related to the practice of drug iontophoresis.

Synthesis: Formulate the strength of scientific evidence related to the practice of iontophoresis in rehabilitation.

Evaluation: Defend the use of iontophoresis over oral ingestion and needle injection for local delivery of drugs into the body.

I. RATIONALE FOR USE

A. DEFINITION AND DESCRIPTION

Iontophoresis is a method of local transfer (*phoresis*), or delivery, of ionized (*ionto*) medicated and nonmedicated substances into the skin and through local microcirculation. Iontophoresis requires the use of electric energy for ion transfer through the skin and is implemented using the traditional wire programmable devices and newer wireless or nonprogrammable patches.

B. IONTOPHORETIC SYSTEMS

Shown in **Figure 13-1** are typical portable (**A**) and cabinet (**B**) wire programmable stimulators presently used for the delivery of iontophoresis therapy. Also available are wireless nonprogrammable patch iontophoretic systems.

1. Wire Programmable Device

Electrical current is generated by a programmable stimulator (**Fig 13-1A**) to which is connected, via wires or cables, a pair of iontophoretic electrodes, positioned over and around the skin overlying the treated area. Each electrode contains a reservoir or gel matrix; one electrode is filled with the medicated solution and the other with tap water.

2. Wireless Nonprogrammable Device

Electrical current is generated by a self-contained battery embedded in a flexible *patch* having positive and negative poles; the patch is positioned also over and around the skin overlying the treated area. One pole is filled with the medicated solution and the other with tap water.

C. IONTOPHORESIS VERSUS OTHER DRUG DELIVERY METHODS

The treatment of soft tissue pathologies very often requires the use of medications such as analgesic drugs to diminish pain and anti-inflammatory drugs to control tissue inflammatory response. Two other basic methods exist, in addition to iontophoresis, to deliver drugs to injured tissues: oral ingestion and needle injection.

1. Oral Ingestion

This method is by far the most utilized for an obvious reason: The only thing the patient needs to do is to swallow the drug tablets. However, drug ingestion involves the

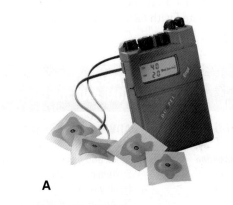

A

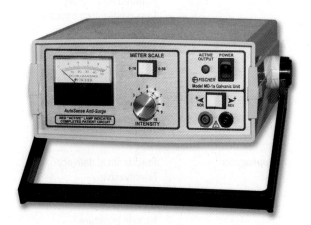

B

FIGURE 13-1 Typical portable (**A**) and cabinet (**B**) iontophoretic devices. (A: Courtesy of Empi; B: Courtesy of RA Fischer.)

gastrointestinal tract in addition to key organs such as the liver, for metabolism, and the kidneys, for elimination.

2. Needle Injection

Needle injection is an invasive technique frequently used by medical specialists. By using a needle to puncture the skin, a given quantity of medication is delivered locally at the site of injury. Just like iontophoresis, and unlike oral ingestion, this method allows the drug to be delivered locally, thus bypassing the systemic route associated with oral ingestion.

D. SYSTEMIC SIDE EFFECTS AND FEAR OF NEEDLES

It is well documented that most orally ingested drugs can induce light, moderate, or severe side effects depending on their nature, dosage, and duration of consumption. Moreover, it is a common clinical observation that many patients are afraid of needles. What, then, are the advantages and disadvantages of using one method of drug delivery over the other?

E. ADVANTAGES AND DISADVANTAGES

Listed in **Table 13-1** are the main advantages and disadvantages associated with each of these three drug delivery methods. The main advantages for using iontophoresis are its less painful and infection-free delivery of the drug, locally, within the vicinity of the tissue lesion, when compared with needle injection, and its bypassing the patient's gastrointestinal tract and liver, when compared with drug ingestion. Its main disadvantage is that drug delivery is limited to the superficial layers of tissues.

F. RATIONALE FOR USE

Using iontophoresis is well justified when oral drug ingestion causes significant problems to the patient's gastrointestinal tract, liver, or kidneys. It is also well justified when the patient's fear of needles plays an important part in the therapeutic plan.

II. HISTORICAL PERSPECTIVE

A. DISCOVERY

According to Licht's (1983) thorough historical account of various electrophysical agents used in the field of rehabilitation, the idea of medications delivered through the skin, via the electromotive force of an electrical current, was first proposed, in 1747, by Pivati and later, in 1833, by Fabre-Palaprat.

TABLE 13-1	ADVANTAGES AND DISADVANTAGES ASSOCIATED WITH ORAL INGESTION, NEEDLE INJECTION, AND IONTOPHORESIS	
METHOD	**ADVANTAGES**	**DISADVANTAGES**
Oral ingestion	Quick and easy Systemic delivery Noninvasive No professional help required for delivery Less costly: drug cost only	Metabolic breakdown by liver Elimination by kidneys Absorption by gastrointestinal tract Potential gastric disorders Amount of drug delivered to the targeted tissue unknown
Needle injection	Precise local delivery Superficial/deep delivery Bypasses gastrointestinal tract Bypasses liver Amount of drug delivered to targeted tissues known	Invasive (skin puncture) Relatively traumatic Relatively painful Potential for infection caused by skin puncture Professional required for delivery More costly than oral ingestion: drug cost plus professional's fee
Iontophoresis	Precise local delivery Noninvasive Bypasses gastrointestinal tract Bypasses liver No skin puncture No risk of infection	Delivery limited to superficial tissues Professional help required for delivery More costly than oral ingestion: drug cost plus professional's fee

B. LE DUC'S EXPERIMENT

There exists a consensus, however, that the experimental work of Le Duc (1900, 1908) on animals, contributed most to the worldwide recognition of what was later to be known as iontophoresis therapy (Licht, 1983; Cummings, 1991; Ciccone, 2008).

1. Physiological Evidence

By using the electromotive force of a continuous direct current (DC) generator after placing a negatively charged potassium cyanide solution (a lethal drug) under the cathode (–) and a positively charged strychnine sulfate solution (a convulsive drug) under the anode (+), with each electrode positioned on a lateral side of two rabbit heads touching one another, Le Duc was able to cause, after turning on the current generator for a few minutes, strong tetanic convulsions in one rabbit and death in the other.

2. Effect Due to Electric Current

To test whether these physiological effects resulted from the driving force generated by the electrical current (iontophoresis) or from the passive diffusion of the two drugs across the skin, Le Duc repeated the experiment, but this time the polarity of the current was reversed. He placed the positively charged strychnine under the cathode (–) and the negatively charged cyanide under the anode (+). After a few minutes of DC flow through the animal heads, Le Duc noticed none of the dramatic and deadly effects that occurred in the earlier experiment.

3. Effect Due to Current Polarity

Le Duc thus concluded that the flow of electric current was responsible for these physiological effects and that iontophoresis can occur only if the ionized medication is placed under the electrode with the same charge, that is, negatively charged ions under the cathode and positively charged ions under the anode. This conclusion, made at the beginning of the 20th century, constitutes the scientific foundation under which the basic biophysical principle related to iontophoresis therapy is established (Le Duc, 1900, 1908; Nair et al., 1999).

C. FIRST CLINICAL USE

According to Chien and Banga's 1983 review, the first clinical use of iontophoresis therapy dates back to 1936, when Ishihashi (1936) noted that excessive sweating of the palms (hyperhidrosis) could be reduced by ion transfer of medicated solutions through iontophoretic techniques. As reported by Stolman (1987), Ishihashi's clinical work went largely unnoticed until 1952, when Bouman et al. (1952) demonstrated the efficacy of tap water–only iontophoresis as an effective therapy for hyperhidrosis.

D. IONTOPHORESIS IN HEALTH CARE

Since the mid-1950s, considerable technical developments, coupled with new clinical applications, have caused iontophoresis to be widely used around the world not only in rehabilitation but also in fields such as medicine and dentistry (see Henley, 1991; Gangarosa et al., 1995; Banga et al., 1998; Grond et al., 2000; Togel et al., 2002; Ting et al., 2004; Eisenach et al., 2005).

E. FOCUS OF CHAPTER

The *focus* of this chapter is on the use of iontophoresis for the management of soft tissue pathologies in the field of rehabilitation. More specifically, the emphasis is on the use of therapeutic ions having analgesic, anti-inflammatory, antiseptic, and sclerolytic effects, including the use of nonmedicated and medicated (anticholinergic) tap water. The use of iontophoresis for medical and dental purposes is *beyond* the scope of this chapter.

F. BODY OF LITERATURE

Over the past two decades, iontophoresis, as an electrophysical agent, has been the subject of several *articles* (see References), many *review articles* (Chien et al., 1989; Lark et al., 1990; Henley, 1991; Costello et al., 1995; Gangarosa et al., 1995; Guy et al., 1996; Kassan et al., 1996; Riviere et al., 1997; Vara Hernando et al., 1997; Banga et al., 1998; Kalia et al., 1998; Stolman, 1998; Zempsky et al., 1998; Nair et al., 1999; Hashmonai et al., 2000; Grond et al., 2000; Togel et al., 2002 Ciccone, 2003; Ting et al., 2004; Eisenach et al., 2005; Fischer, 2005; Hamann et al., 2006; Brown et al., 2006; Dixit et al., 2007; Semalty et al., 2007; Solish et al., 2007; Gurney et al., 2008), and *chapters of textbooks* (Cummings, 1991; Dalzell, 1996; Starkey, 1999; Hayes, 2000; Kahn, 2000; Prentice, 2002; Mehreteab et al., 2006; Ciccone, 2008).

III. BIOPHYSICAL CHARACTERISTICS

A. CONTINUOUS DIRECT CURRENT

The electrophysical agent iontophoresis is described as the use of a continuous, direct electrical current to deliver therapeutically charged ions through the skin into the systemic circulation (Henley, 1991; Banga et al., 1998; Nair et al., 1999; Ciccone, 2008). Shown in **Figure 13-2A** is the typical continuous direct and monophasic current, flowing over time, traditionally generated by wire programmable and lead wireless nonprogrammable iontophoresors.

B. BIOPHYSICAL PRINCIPLE

The biophysical principle underlying therapeutic iontophoresis stipulates that the drug, in its ionic form, be

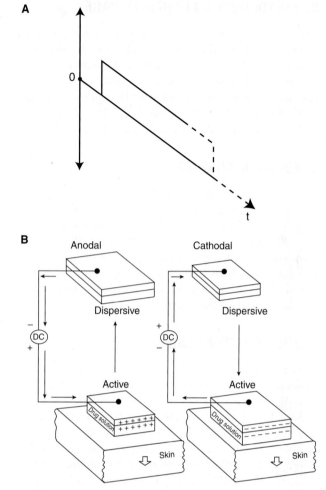

FIGURE 13-2 **A**: Continuous, direct, monophasic electrical current waveform (DC) commonly used to deliver iontophoresis therapy. **B**: Therapeutic charged ions are driven through the skin by the electrical repulsive force created between the electrode and ions with the same polarity. Cathodal and anodal iontophoresis refer to the drug solution placed under the cathode or anode, respectively. The electrode in contact with the drug solution is termed the active electrode. Note that the conductive surface area of the cathode always must be larger than that of the anode, regardless of whether the cathode is used as the active or the dispersive electrode. Cathodal or anodal iontophoresis can be achieved by flicking the device's polarity switch. Changing the polarity creates a reversal of current flow (arrows) between the dispersive and active electrodes without changing the conventional current flow, which still remains from the anode (+) to the cathode (−).

set between the current and drug charges having identical polarity is the driving force behind the iontophoresis phenomenon.

2. Anodal Versus Cathodal

The terms *anodal iontophoresis* and *cathodal iontophoresis* refer to phoresis of a positively and a negatively charged drug solution, respectively (Nair et al., 1999).

C. ELECTRODE LABELING

As shown in **Figure 13-2B**, the electrode under which the therapeutic ions are placed is referred to as the *active*, treatment, or delivery electrode, whereas the other electrode is referred to as the *dispersive*, nontreatment, or return electrode. In this chapter, the terms active and dispersive are used to denote the electrodes. The use of a dispersive electrode is mandatory for iontophoresis because it closes the electrical circuit.

D. SKIN PATHWAY THROUGH PORES

Convincing scientific evidence suggests that the iontophoretic-driven ion process through the skin is *pore* dependent (Banga et al., 1998). It is paramount to understand that the main barrier to transdermal drug intake is the most superficial avascular stratum corneum layer of the epidermis.

1. Hair Follicles and Sweat Glands

Schematically drawn in **Figure 13-3** are *hair follicles* as well as *sweat glands*, which play a crucial role in providing the main pathways, or pores, through which the charged ions can penetrate first the stratum corneum layer and then the remaining layers of the epidermis and dermis (Kalia et al., 1995; Banga et al., 1998).

2. Lower Diffusional Resistance

According to Banga et al. (1998), the diffusional resistance of the skin to permeation of ions is lowest in the hair follicles and sweat gland regions compared with other regions of the epidermis.

E. DRUG PENETRATION DEPTH

Anderson et al. (2003) proposed the following model to explain how drug ions penetrate human tissues during iontophoresis therapy and which key factors may be responsible for such penetration.

1. Penetration Rate

Anderson and colleagues (2003) first proposed that electrical current causes drug penetration through the stratum corneum and the rate of penetration of the drug is proportional to the amplitude of this current.

placed under the electrode bearing the same charge. Another way to state this principle is that *like poles repel* (Kahn, 2000).

1. Repelling Force

The therapeutic ions are driven through the skin, as shown in **Figure 13-2B**, only if a polarity match exists between the charged ions and the electrode under which they are placed, that is, negatively charged ions under the negatively charged electrode (−/−) and positively charged ions under the positively charged electrode (+/+). The *repelling force*

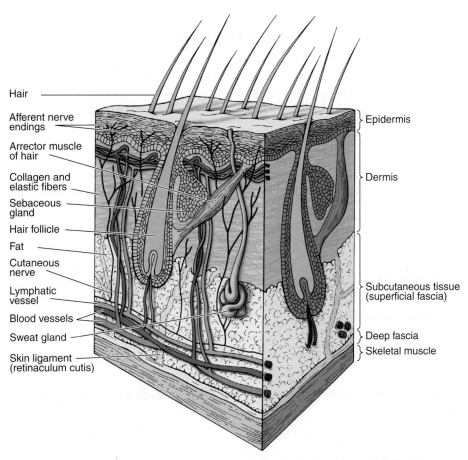

FIGURE 13-3 The skin and its appendages. (Reproduced with permission from Moore KL, Dalley AF (1999), *Clinically Oriented Anatomy,* 4th ed. Lippincott Williams & Wilkins, Philadelphia, p. 13.)

2. Drug Depot Formation

They further hypothesize that these drug ions will collect to form a drug depot, or reservoir, within the avascular epidermal layer just under the active electrode. For this to occur, the authors assume that the ionic current is carried by chloride ions, leaving the drug molecules behind, and that the drug delivery rate exceeds the systemic vascular absorption rate.

3. Penetration Depth

Anderson and colleagues, (2003) final proposal is that drug absorption from the depot and into the dermis of surrounding tissues occurs by diffusion, suggesting that passive diffusion, not the amplitude of current, governs the depth of drug penetration into the tissues.

4. Key Factors to Consider: Time and Local Blood Flow

Anderson and colleagues suggest, on the basis of their model, that for equivalent iontophoretic dosages, it is the factor time (for passive diffusion to occur), not current amplitude, that dictates the ultimate local depth of penetration of the drug. Another key factor to consider, according to these authors, is the state of localized blood flow at the site of injury, indicating that if the local cutaneous capillary

beds under the active electrode are dilated, drug penetration depth will be reduced (due to increased clearance).

5. Summary

From this model it appears that electric current is needed only to induce and regulate the penetration rate of drug ions through the stratum corneum layer of the skin. After that, the process of passive diffusion takes over, thus governing the penetration depth of the drug ions into the tissues during iontophoresis.

IV. PHYSIOLOGICAL AND THERAPEUTIC EFFECTS

A. THERAPEUTIC EFFECTS

Presented in **Figure 13-4** are the proposed physiological and therapeutic effects associated with the use of iontophoresis. These iontophoresis effects are *phoretic, electrolytic,* and *pharmacological* in nature.

1. Phoresis

Drug phoresis (transport) takes place due to the capacity of electrical current to push drug ions through the skin's

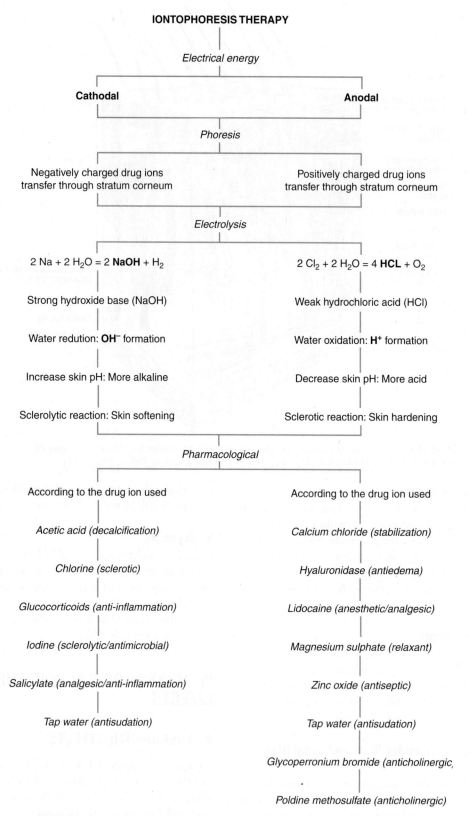

IONTOPHORESIS THERAPY

Electrical energy

Cathodal   **Anodal**

Phoresis

Negatively charged drug ions   Positively charged drug ions
transfer through stratum corneum   transfer through stratum corneum

Electrolysis

$2\ Na + 2\ H_2O = 2\ \textbf{NaOH} + H_2$ $2\ Cl_2 + 2\ H_2O = 4\ \textbf{HCL} + O_2$

Strong hydroxide base (NaOH)   Weak hydrochloric acid (HCl)

Water redution: $\textbf{OH}^-$ formation   Water oxidation: $\textbf{H}^+$ formation

Increase skin pH: More alkaline   Decrease skin pH: More acid

Sclerolytic reaction: Skin softening   Sclerotic reaction: Skin hardening

Pharmacological

According to the drug ion used   According to the drug ion used

Acetic acid (decalcification)   *Calcium chloride (stabilization)*

Chlorine (sclerotic)   *Hyaluronidase (antiedema)*

Glucocorticoids (anti-inflammation)   *Lidocaine (anesthetic/analgesic)*

Iodine (sclerolytic/antimicrobial)   *Magnesium sulphate (relaxant)*

Salicylate (analgesic/anti-inflammation) *Zinc oxide (antiseptic)*

Tap water (antisudation)   *Tap water (antisudation)*

                                           Glycoperronium bromide (anticholinergic,

                                           Poldine methosulfate (anticholinergic)

FIGURE 13-4 Proposed physiological and therapeutic effects of iontophoresis therapy.

first layer (stratum corneum) via the application of one surface electrode (active electrode loaded with medication) directly over the treated area, with the other electrode (dispersive electrode loaded with saline) positioned in the immediate vicinity of the first electrode.

2. Electrolysis

Because iontophoresis involves the passing of a continuous direct current (DC) into water-soluble drug solutions (electrode system) and human tissues over a certain period of time, water electrolysis will occur. *Electrolysis* is the process of decomposition of a compound by passing a direct electrical current through it, leading to the formation of *electrochemical reactions* under both the anode and cathode electrodes.

a. New Compounds

Human tissues are composed of a mixture of approximately 70% sodium chloride (Na^+Cl^-) and water (H_2O); so continuous DC flow through such tissues inevitably leads to electrolysis of this salted water medium at the electrode/skin interface. In turn, over time, during iontophoresis therapy, the continuous DC flow will redistribute the sodium and chlorine ions with water to form *new chemical compounds* at the electrode/skin interface.

b. Weak Hydrochloric Acid

As shown in **Figure 13-4**, the reaction of chlorine with water leads to formation of a *weak hydrochloric acid* ($2\ Cl_2 + 2\ H_2O = 4\ HCl + O_2$) under the anode, because negatively charged chlorine ions migrate toward this positively charged electrode. This weak acidic reaction produced under the anode is *sclerotic* and, over time, tends to *harden* the skin through protein coagulation (Khan, 2000).

c. Strong Sodium Hydroxide Base

The reaction of sodium with water, however, leads to formation of a much *stronger sodium hydroxide base* ($2\ Na + 2\ H_2O = 2\ NaOH + H_2$) under the cathode, because the positively charged sodium ions migrates toward this negatively charged electrode (**Fig 13-4**). This stronger alkaline reaction produced under the cathode is sclerolytic in nature and, over time, tends to soften the skin (due to liquefying of proteins), thus exposing it to potential irritation and burn (Khan, 2000). Such a sclerolytic or caustic reaction is responsible for erythema of the skin and the itching or burning sensation felt under this electrode during therapy (Henley, 1991).

d. Redox

The decomposition of water with electrical current is a *redox* reaction, that is, a reaction that implies the reduction (red-) and the oxidation (-ox) of water. During electrolysis, water present at the electrode/skin interface is reduced ($4\ H_2O + 4\ electrons = 2\ H_2 + 4\ OH^-$) at the cathode and oxidized ($2\ H_2O = O_2 + 4\ H^+ + 4\ electrons$) at the anode. This electrochemical reaction leads, over time, to a net accumulation of *hydrogen ions* (H^+) under the anode and *hydroxyl ions* (OH^-) under the cathode (**Fig 13-4**).

e. Skin pH Shift

This net accumulation of hydrogen and hydroxyl ions creates a pH instability, or shift, at the electrode/skin interface during iontophoresis. The term pH is used to express the hydrogen ion activity of a solution. The average or normal pH value of human skin ranges between 3 and 6, implying that at a physiological pH, the skin is negatively charged (Guffey et al., 1999; Nair et al., 1999). An accumulation of H^+ will induce a *pH drop* (more acid), whereas an accumulation of OH^- will produce a *pH increase* (more alkaline) under the respective electrodes (**Fig 13-4**).

3. Pharmacological

The therapeutic effect of drug iontophoresis is *pharmacological* and relates directly to the specific active ingredient contained in the drug-ionized solution or therapeutic ions.

a. Therapeutic Ions

Table 13-2 lists the *most common* drug ions used in rehabilitation today, including the basic nonmedicated tap water, along with their respective polarities and proposed physiological and therapeutic effects on soft tissues. The type of medication used will depend on the type of pathology and the desired treatment outcomes. Some of these drugs can only be obtained through medical prescription.

b. Nonphysician Practitioners

Because many of the drugs used for the delivery of iontophoresis require a physician's prescription, nonphysician practitioners must first consult the patient's treating physician, first, to inform the person of his or her intention to use iontophoresis and, second, to obtain the drug prescription.

c. Pharmacist

With the prescription on hand, nonphysician practitioners may obtain the desired drug solution, in the form of aqueous solution or ointment, from the pharmacist.

i. Drug concentrations. There is consensus in the literature that the drug ions, listed in **Table 13-2**, should be delivered to soft tissues within the following ranges of aqueous or ointment concentrations: 2–5% aqueous solution; 1–5% ointment (for details see Prentice, 2002; Ciccone, 2008). Medicated ointments are rubbed over the affected area, with the active electrode on top. Medicated aqueous solutions, on the other hand, are injected or impregnated, using a needle, into the electrode reservoir of the active electrode.

ii. Electrode reservoir capacity. Commercial iontophoretic electrodes are sold in various sizes, each having a maximum filling capacity of its reservoir, or fiber matrix, ranging between 1 and 5 cc.

TABLE 13-2	COMMONLY USED THERAPEUTIC IONS IN REHABILITATION	
IONS	**POLARITY**	**PROPOSED PHYSIOLOGICAL AND THERAPEUTIC EFFECTS**
Acetic acid	−	Decalcifying agent. Increases solubility of calcium deposits in tendons and muscles.
Chlorine	−	Sclerolytic agent. Causes a sclerolytic, softening effect on cutaneous tissue.
Glucocorticoid	−	Anti-inflammatory agent. Reduces tissue inflammation by inhibiting biosynthesis of prostaglandins and other pro-inflammatory substances. Includes compounds such as dexamethasone (Decadron), hydrocortisone, prednisone, and other compounds.
Iodine	−	Sclerolytic and antimicrobial agent. Causes a sclerolytic, softening effect on cutaneous tissue in addition to an antimicrobial effect.
Salicylate	−	Analgesic and anti-inflammatory agent. Inhibits the biosynthesis of prostanglandins.
Calcium chloride	+	Membrane-stabilizing agent. Stabilizes excitable cell membranes, thus decreasing excitability threshold in muscle and peripheral nerves.
Hyaluronidase	+	Antiedema agent. Decreases edema by diminishing encapsulation in connective tissues via hydrolization of hyaluronic acid.
Lidocaine	+	Anesthetic and analgesic agent. Decreases local pain through blocking of nerve impulse transmission.
Magnesium sulfate	+	Muscle relaxant agent. Relaxes striated muscles by decreasing the excitability of muscle membrane.
Zinc oxide	+	Antiseptic agent. Enhances tissue healing in addition to acting as a broad antiseptic.
Tap water	+/−	Antisudation/antisweating agent. Suppresses sweating of palms, soles, and armpits by inducing the formation of keratin plugs in the lumen of sweat glands.
Glycoperronium bromide	+	Anticholinergic agent. Suppresses sweating of palms, soles, and armpits through its anticholinergic effect. Mix with tap water.
Poldine methosulfate	+	Anticholinergic agent. Suppresses sweating of palms, soles, and armpits through its anticholinergic effect. Mix with tap water.

iii. To sum up. The practice of iontophoresis thus requires the selection of a drug, the determination of its concentration, and the injection (if aqueous) of this drug solution into the fabric matrix (patch) or electrode reservoir (electrode).

B. UNWANTED SIDE EFFECTS

Water *electrolysis* associated with iontophoresis will cause unwanted electrochemical and electrothermal side effects at the electrode/skin interface if no measures are taken to reduce them. These side effects will manifest themselves in a form of *skin irritation/burn* under the electrodes, particularly under the cathode (see below). This unwanted reaction is caused as follows. First, during the course of iontophoresis, there is an accumulation of extraneous

OH^- ions under the cathode and H^+ ions under the anode (**Box 13-1**). These ions compete with the drug ions of the same charge for the available electrical driving charges, thus reducing drug transfer. Next, this same accumulation of ions, over time, will either raise (at the cathode) or lower (at the anode) skin pH under these electrodes, potentially causing *skin irritation* and, in some cases, when the net deposit is large enough, *a skin burn* (Henley, 1991; Banga et al., 1998; Nair et al., 1999).

C. MINIMIZING SIDE EFFECTS

How can practitioners minimize skin irritation/burn during iontophoresis? As discussed above and illustrated in **Figure 13-4**, the risk of inducing skin irritation, and potentially a skin burn, is related to the accumulation of hydroxyl ions (OH$^-$) under the cathode causing a skin pH increase, which together lead to the formation of a strong alkaline reaction. This alkaline reaction, in turn, causes a strong sclerolytic effect, or softening of the skin, which makes it more susceptible to irritation and burn.

1. Use of Buffered Electrode

One approach to minimize skin irritation/burn is to use buffered electrodes. Such a commercial electrode is characterized by the impregnation of a *buffering agent* into a pad covering the drug reservoir to prevent any pH drift for the duration of the therapeutic application (Henley, 1991; Banga et al., 1998; Guffey et al., 1999; Nair et al., 1999). It is important to know that prior to the use of such commercial buffered electrodes, iontophoresis was delivered using noncommercial/nonbuffered electrodes made of some type of malleable metal such as aluminum, tin, and copper covered by layers of gauze (Ciccone, 2008). The main advantages of using noncommercial/nonbuffered electrodes instead of buffered electrodes are that they are much less expensive, are reusable, and can be used to treat much larger body areas.

a. Buffer

A buffer is any substance that maintains the relative concentrations of hydrogen and hydroxyl ions in a solution by neutralizing (binding) any added acid or alkali. Buffering refers to the process by which the hydrogen ion concentration is maintained at a constant level, thus keeping the pH value stable.

b. Buffered Electrode

Shown in **Figure 13-5** is a cross-sectional view of one such buffered electrode. The buffered layer of the electrode is capable of neutralizing extraneous OH$^-$ and H$^+$ ions, thus stabilizing skin pH in addition to maximizing drug delivery.

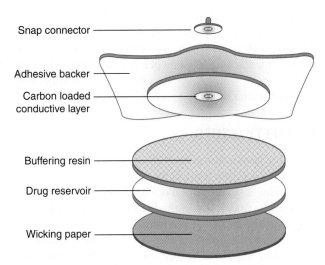

Snap connector

Adhesive backer

Carbon loaded
conductive layer

Buffering resin

Drug reservoir

Wicking paper

FIGURE 13-5 Three-dimensional view of a buffered electrode. (Courtesy of Empi.)

c. Buffering Effect

A study by Guffey et al. (1999) conducted on healthy subjects showed that at dosages of 20 and 40 mA.min (see Section V, Dosimetry) no significant changes in skin pH occurred under the cathode (saturated with saline water), with or without a buffering electrode system (range of mean pH changes, +0.22 to +1.30). Changes in skin pH associated with a dose of 80 mA.min were, however, significantly greater (mean pH change, +3.14) when no buffering system was employed, but were stabilized by each buffering system tested. These results suggest that buffered electrode systems may not be required if therapeutic doses are kept to less than 40 mA.min.

D. CONTROL OVER CURRENT DENSITY

Another approach to minimize this important side effect is to control the current density (CD). Guffey et al. (1999) showed that subjects who received a dose of 80 mA.min with nonbuffered electrodes demonstrated no visible signs of skin irritation despite the skin pH's being increased by an average of three points (mean, +3.14). These results suggest that changes in skin pH after common therapeutic dosages (range, 1–80 mA.min) may not be the prime cause leading to skin irritation/burn and that, perhaps, electrode CD under the electrode may be more to blame. Current density is defined as the magnitude of the applied current (A), measured in milliamperes (mA), divided by the conductive surface area (S) of the electrode, measured in square centimetres (cm^2) (see Section V, Dosimetry, for details). Practitioners should not confuse electrode size with the electrode's conductive surface area, the former being often much larger than the latter. There is a consensus in the literature that in order to minimize skin irritation/burn under the electrodes, the CD of the cathode, if used to deliver the drug, should not exceed 0.5 mA/cm^2 and that of the anode, if used to deliver the drug, should not exceed 1.0 mA/cm^2 (Prentice, 2002; Ciccone, 2008; see below for details).

V. DOSIMETRY

A. DOSIMETRIC PARAMETERS

The dosimetry associated with the practice of iontophoresis depends on four parameters: (1) the drug ions selected for the pathology being treated, (2) the polarity of the aqueous solution or ointment of the drug used, (3) the chemical concentration and volume of the ionic drug solution delivered, and finally (4) the dose used.

1. Drug Selection

Practitioners can choose from a variety, as shown in **Table 13-2**, of drug agents having specific therapeutic properties. The selection is based on the desired therapeutic effects for any given pathology. For example, if the therapeutic goals are to decrease pain or inflammation, analgesic and/or anti-inflammatory drugs will be selected. If the selected drug is under medical control, nonphysician practitioners need to obtain, from the treating physician, the drug prescription and then the prescribed drug solution or ointment, from the pharmacist. Note that nonmedicated and medicated (addition of anticholinergic agents) tap water is selective for the treatment of hand, foot, and armpit hyperhydrosis.

2. Drug Ion Polarity

Knowledge of the drug ion used is *critical* because for phoresis, or transport, to occur at the electrode/skin interface, the negatively charged drug ions *must* be placed under the cathode (negative pole), and the positively charged drug ions, under the anode (positive pole). Because tap water has a double polarity (+/–), it can be placed under the cathode or anode. In such a case, it is recommended to inverse the current polarity midway during treatment to assure an equivalent phoresis of both ions in the skin.

3. Drug Concentration and Volume of Delivery

There is a consensus in the literature that drug concentrations used for iontophoresis usually range within 2–5% aqueous solution or ointment. The drug solution should contain relatively low concentrations of medication, because an increased concentration does not appear to increase the amount of drug delivered (Henley, 1991; Ciccone, 2008). The amount or volume (cc) of drug aqueous solution contained in the electrode reservoir or patch vary according to its filling capacity. The fill volume is indicated, on each electrode, by the manufacturer.

4. Dose

The amount of drug delivered into the tissues, that is, the dose (D), is proportional to the current magnitude used (A) and the total application duration (T). This dose is calculated as D (mA.min) = A (mA) $\times$ T (min).

B. DOSAGE

The literature indicates that the maximum doses used to deliver drug iontophoresis differ significantly from the doses used to deliver tap water iontophoresis.

1. Drug Dose: 1 to 80 mA.min

Doses commonly used to deliver drug ions range between 1 and 80 mA.min, with a maximum available current amplitude of 4 mA. Iontophoresis is commonly delivered using portable wire stimulators and wearable patches.

a. Portable Stimulators

These are constant-current (CC; see Chapter 5) stimulators capable of generating a maximum DC amplitude of 4 mA. Practitioners can program the dose (mA.min) and set the desired current amplitude (A); the application duration (T) may be manually or automatically set and regulated by

the device. For example, to deliver a prescribed dose of 40 mA.min of dexamethasone for treatment of wrist tendonitis, the practitioner may select one of several combinations of current amplitude and application duration, such as 4.0 mA for 10 min, 1.0 mA for 40 min, or 2 mA for 20 min, simply by turning the knobs on the console.

b. Patches

These are *constant-voltage* (CV; see Chapter 5) devices (self-contained battery). These patches are sold at preset dosages (40 mA.min and 80 mA.min). Because current delivery will fluctuate over time due to soft tissue impedance changes, manufacturers recommend an application duration, or wearing time, of 12 hours (720 min) for the 40 mA.min patch and 24 hours (1440 min) for the 80 mA.min. Practitioners have no control over current amplitude settings. The self-contained battery within the patch is activated as soon as the patch is hydrated (i.e., impregnated with the drug solution in one pole of pad and with tap water in the other pad). It will remain activated until the pads are depleted of their solutions.

2. Tap Water Dose: 300 to 500 mA.min

Doses commonly used to deliver tap water iontophoresis for hyperhydrosis, using line-powered devices, are much higher than for drugs, ranging between 300 and 500 mA.min, with maximum current amplitude values ranging between 10 and 20 mA (see Gillick et al., 2004). The need for using a much higher current amplitude is due to the fact that the electrode conductive area (water tray) used is much greater than that used for drug delivery (electrode and patch). In other words, higher current amplitudes can be used safely because current densities under the electrodes are well within the recommended safe values, due to the fact that the electrode conductive areas are much larger.

C. WIRE VERSUS WIRELESS DEVICES

Listed in **Table 13-3** are *key features* related to the use of wire versus wireless iontophoretic devices. A key advantage of wireless devices over wire devices is their wearability, allowing freedom of movement during therapy at home or at work. A key disadvantage of such devices, however, is that the dosage is not programmable.

D. SAFETY ISSUES

There is a limit to the magnitude of current amplitude that can be used within a prescribed dose because of the risk of inducing a skin irritation or burn under the electrodes, particularly under the cathode. The amplitude limit is based on the electrode current denisty (CD), which is the amount of current amplitude (A) applied against the electrode conductive surface area (S). CD is calculated as follows: CD (mA/cm^2) = A (mA)/S (cm^2). It is important to distinguish between electrode *surface area* and

TABLE 13-3	IONTOPHORESORS AND THEIR KEY FEATURES

WIRE PROGRAMMABLE	WIRELESS NONPROGRAMMABLE
Battery-powered electrical stimulator, lead wires and electrodes	Self-contained system (embedded battery with two poles)
Reusable system; only the electrodes are discarded after single application	Disposable system; patch discarded after single application
Constant current (CC) source: current amplitude and delivery kept constant during therapy despite fluctuations of tissue resistance	Constant voltage (CV) source: current amplitude and delivery vary during therapy due to fluctuations of tissue resistance
Drug dose programmable from 1 to 80 mA.min	Drug dose fixed by manufacturer on patch; choice of 40 mA.min or 80 mA.min
Tap water dose (hyperhidrosis) programmable from 300 to 500 mA.min	NA
Current amplitude programmable from 0 to 5 mA for drugs	Current amplitude prefixed at approximately 0.1 mA
Current amplitude programmable from 1 to 20 mA for tap water (hyperhydrosis)	NA
Application duration automatically calculated based on the dosage used	Manufacturers recommend the following continuous wearing time: ■ 12 hours for 40 mA.min patch ■ 24 hours for 80 mA.min patch
No activity allowed during treatment because of electrodes attached to stimulator	Freedom of movement during treatment due to self-contained system

electrode *conductive surface area*, because the latter is always smaller and often unrelated to the former.

1. Safe Limits

The maximum safe CD values recommended for iontophoresis are 0.5 mA/cm^2 for the cathode and 1.0 mA/cm^2 for the anode (Cummings, 1991; Ciccone, 2008). These values correspond to 3.3 mA/in^2 for the cathode and 6.6 mA/in^2 for the anode (1 in^2 = 6.452 cm^2).

2. Calculation of Maximum Current Amplitude

Table 13-4 explains how to determine the maximum current amplitude that can be used in any given application while taking into consideration the recommended safe CD values for each electrode.

3. Electrode Conductive Surface Area

It is strongly recommended that the conductive surface area of the cathode be larger than that of the anode, regardless of whether the cathode is used as the active or dispersive electrode. This is because a skin burn underneath the cathode is more harmful to the skin than one under the anode. The larger the cathodal conductive surface areas, the smaller the CD, and the lower the risk of cathodal skin burn.

E. ELECTRODE PLACEMENT

The recommendation for optimal electrode placement is that the active electrode always be positioned immediately over the treated area, with the dispersive electrode located as far as possible from the active electrode, at a distance longer than the diameter of the smallest electrode (Hayes, 2000; Khan, 2000; Ciccone, 2008).

F. SIMULTANEOUS PHORESIS OF TWO DRUG IONS

The simultaneous iontophoresis of two drug ions with the *same polarity is not recommended*, because both must compete against each other for their share of the delivery force provided by the DC intensity (Ciccone, 2008). If iontophoresis of two drug ions with *different polarity* is performed, a reversal of polarity is required midway during the application to allow an even or balanced delivery of both drugs. Such an application is *not recommended*, because at the end of the application, only a half dose of each drug is delivered to the soft tissues. To sum up, the simultaneous phoresis of two drugs, with or without the same polarity, is *not recommended*.

| TABLE 13-4 | CALCULATING MAXIMUM SAFE CURRENT AMPLITUDE BASED ON ELECTRODE CURRENT DENSITY | |

PARAMETERS	CATHODE	ANODE
Recommended maximum current density (CD)	$CD = 0.5 \text{ mA/cm}^2$	$CD = 1.0 \text{ mA/ cm}^2$
CD = Current amplitude (A)/conductive surface area (S)	If A = 2 mA If S = 6 cm^2	If A = 3 mA If S = 4 cm^2
Is the current density (CD) under each electrode safe?	$CD = 2 \text{ mA} / 6 \text{ cm}^2$ $CD = 0.33 \text{ mA/cm}^2$ Safe	$CD = 3 \text{ mA} / 4 \text{ cm}^2$ $CD = 0.75 \text{ mA/cm}^2$ Safe
What is the maximum safe current amplitude (A) possible under each electrode?	$A = CD \times S$ $A = 0.5 \text{ mA/cm}^2 \times 6 \text{ cm}^2$ $A = 3 \text{ mA}$	$A = CD \times S$ $A = 1.0 \text{ mA/ cm}^2 \times 4 \text{ cm}^2$ $A = 4 \text{ mA}$

VI. EVIDENCE FOR INDICATIONS

A. GUIDED BY THE EVIDENCE

Dictionaries generally define *evidence* as anything that establishes a fact or gives reason to believe something. The aim of this textbook is to present scientific evidence behind therapeutic EPAs. To be guided by the evidence is the process of integrating the evidence from research, however imperfect or scarce this evidence may be, with clinical experience and patients' values. In other words, *evidence-based practice* of EPA requires that practitioners consider evidence from research, in addition to their own clinical experience and the patient's own preference and beliefs about therapy, when the time comes to justify, prescribe, and apply the therapeutic agent. To be guided by evidence is a process, not a search for the absolute truth. Finally, lack of evidence from research in support of any given EPA does not mean that this EPA should never be used. What it means is that no statement can be made about its therapeutic effectiveness and that until more evidence from research is presented its routine use cannot be recommended.

B. EVIDENCE FROM HUMAN RESEARCH

Box 13-1 provides evidence for iontophoresis therapy based on an exhaustive search of published English-language, peer-reviewed studies on humans. The term *indication* is used in reference to a list of pathologies for which iontophoresis is used. Ratings of therapeutic benefit (Yes or No) and grading of the strength of scientific evidence (I, II, or III), including the reference, are included for each pathological condition.

1. Rating Therapeutic Benefit

The rating, expressed as Yes or No, is based on the overall conclusion(s) reached on the issue of therapeutic

effectiveness by the author(s) who conducted the peer-reviewed study.

2. Grading Strength of Evidence

The grading, numerically classified as I, II, and III, is based on the type of research methodology, or experimental design, used by the author(s). All the studies listed are studies on humans published in English-language, peer-reviewed journals. It follows that the strength of evidence in studies graded I is stronger than in those graded II, which itself is stronger than in those graded III.

a. Grade I

Evidence based on *controlled* studies on humans, regardless of their level of randomization and blindness.

b. Grade II

Evidence based on *non-controlled* studies on humans, regardless of their level of randomization and blindness.

c. Grade III

Evidence based on *case* studies of humans, regardless of their level of randomization and blindness.

3. Strength of Evidence Behind the Agent

The strength of evidence in favor of the agent, as presented in the research-based indication box, is arbitrarily assessed in this textbook as *weak, moderate,* or *strong.* For example, the larger the number of studies graded I, regardless of therapeutic benefit, the stronger the scientific evidence behind of the agent.

4. Evidence Justifying Usage of the Agent

The strength of evidence justifying usage of the agent for individual pathologies or groups of pathologies, as listed in the research-based indication box, is arbitrarily assessed in this textbook as *poor, fair, good,* or *conflicting.* For example, where a larger number of grade I studies

Box 13-1	Research-Based Indications for the Use of Iontophoresis Therapy

PATHOLOGY	ION	BENEFIT	GRADE	REFERENCE
Hyperhidrosis	Tap water	Yes	I	Stolman, 1987
		Yes	II	Shrivastava et al., 1977
		Yes	II	Akins et al., 1987
		Yes	II	Midtgaard, 1986
		Yes	II	Levit, 1968
		Yes	II	Levit, 1980
		Yes	II	Holzle et al., 1986
		Yes	II	Holzle et al., 1987
		Yes	II	Bouman et al., 1952
		Yes	II	Goh et al., 1996
		Yes	II	Odia et al., 1996
		Yes	II	Korakoç et al., 2002
		Yes	II	Korakoç et al., 2004
		Yes	II	Dolianitis et al., 2004
		Yes	III	Gillick et al., 2004
		Yes	III	Chan et al., 1999
		Yes	III	Elgart et al., 1987
	Tap water/poldine methosulfate	Yes	II	Grice et al., 1972
		Yes	II	Hill, 1976
	Tap water/glucopyrronium	Yes	II	Abell et al., 1974
Rheumatoid disorders	Dexamethasone/lidocaine	Yes	I	Bertolucci, 1982
		Yes	II	Harris, 1982
		Yes	II	Pellecchia et al., 1994
	Dexamethasone	Yes	II	Akinbo et al., 2007
	Dexamethasone	Yes	III	Hasson et al., 1991
	Dexamethasone	Yes	III	Hasson et al., 1988
	Dexamethasone	No	II	Li et al., 1996
Epicondylitis	Dexamethasone	Yes	I	Nirsch et al., 2003
	Sodium diclofenac/salycilate	Yes	II	Demirtas et al., 1998
	Naproxen	Yes	II	Baskurt et al., 2003
	Lidocaine	Yes	III	Yarrobino et al., 2006
	Cortisone	No	I	Runeson et al., 2002
	Dexamethasone	No	III	Panus et al., 1996
Peyronie's disease	Dexamethasone/lidocaine	Yes	I	Montorsi et al., 2000
	Dexamethasone/lidocaine	Yes	II	Reidl et al., 2000
	Hydrocortisone	Yes	III	Khann, 1982
	Glucocorticoids	Yes	III	Rothfeld et al., 1967
Temporomandibular joint disorders	Dexamethasone/lidocaine	Yes	I	Schiffman et al., 1996
	Dexamethasone	Yes	I	Reid et al., 1994
	Dexamethasone/lidocaine	Yes	III	Braun, 1987
	Hydrocortisone	No	III	Kahn, 1980
Calcifying tendinitis	Acetic acid	Yes	II	Psaki et al., 1955
	Acetic acid	No	I	Perron et al., 1997
	Acetic acid	No	I	Leduc et al., 2003
Plantar faciitis	Dexamethasone	Yes	I	Gudeman et al., 1997
		Yes	II	Chandler, 1998

(Continued)

Box 13-1 Continued

PATHOLOGY	ION	BENEFIT	GRADE	REFERENCE
Plantar warts	Salicylate	Yes	II	Sokoro et al., 2002
	Salicylate	Yes	III	Gordon et al., 1969
Edema	Hyaluronidase	Yes	III	Magistro, 1964
		Yes	III	Boone, 1969
Achilles tendonitis	Dexamethasone	Yes	I	Neeter et al., 2003
Myofascial syndrome	Dexamethasone/lidocaine	Yes	II	Delacerda, 1982
Post–herpetic neuralgia	Prednisone/lidocaine	Yes	II	Ozawa et al., 1999
Myositis ossificans	Acetic acid	Yes	III	Wieder, 1992
Hell pain	Acetic acid	Yes	II	Japour et al., 1999
Postsurgical hip pain	Salicylate	Yes	III	Garzione, 1978
Rheumatoid disorders	Salicylate	Yes	II	Aiyejunusie et al., 2007
Lymphedema	Hyaluronidase	Yes	III	Schwartz, 1955
Scar tissue	Iodine	Yes	III	Tannenbaum, 1980
Tendon adhesion	Iodine	Yes	III	Langley, 1984
Bacterial wounds	Zinc	Yes	III	Balogun et al., 1990
Ischemic skin ulcers	Zinc	Yes	III	Cornwall, 1981
Subdeltoid bursitis	Magnesium sulfate	Yes	II	Weinstein et al., 1958
Carpal tunnel syndrome	Dexamethasone	Yes	II	Banta, 1994
Myopathy	Calcium	Yes	III	Khan, 1975

on an agent show more therapeutic benefit (Yes) than no benefit, for any given pathology, the justification for usage of this agent for that pathology is assessed as *good*. *Conflicting* usage is reported when an equal number of studies with similar grades show therapeutic benefit (Yes) and no benefit (No).

C. STRENGTH OF EVIDENCE AND JUSTIFICATION FOR USAGE

The results accumulated in **Box 13-1** show *weak-to-moderate* strength of evidence behind iontophoresis, with the majority of studies graded II and III. These same results show *good* justification for the use of tap water

iontophoresis for hyperhydrosis disorders and *fair* justification for the treatment of rheumatoid disorders, epicondylitis, Peyronie's disease, and temporomandibular disorders. Finally, the results presented in **Box 13-1** show that iontophoresis therapy has been used to treat a variety of pathologies, using different drugs, but until more evidence from research is provided, the routine use of this EPA *cannot be recommended for the remaining group of pathologies.*

D. THERAPEUTIC IONS MOST INVESTIGATED

Box 13-1 reveals that of all the common therapeutic ions used in iontophoresis therapy, nonmedicated tap water and dexamethasone, either alone or mixed with lidocaine, have been the most investigated.

E. PATHOLOGIES MOST INVESTIGATED

Box 13-1 also reveals that of all the pathologies investigated, *hyperhidrosis* is by far the most studied, followed, in descending order, by rheumatoid disorders, epicondylitis, Peyronie's disease, and temporomandibular joint disorders.

1. Hyperhydrosis

It may come as a surprise to many practitioners that the application of tap water iontophoresis for hyperhydrosis is common and very effective. Hyperhydrosis, a common disorder of excessive sweat, may be generalized (involving the entire body) or focal (involving hands, feet, axillae, and face) (Solish et al., 2007). This painless condition, when moderate to severe in nature, may have significant effects on patients' lives, including difficulty with certain manual employments (e.g., being a carpenter when affected by palmar hyperhydrosis), activities of daily living, interference with intimacy, and social embarrassment (bad body odor). The results presented in this chapter (**Box 13-1**) are in keeping with a recent recommendation made by the Canadian Hyperhydrosis Advisory Committee (Solish et al., 2007) to the effect that tap water iontophoresis should be recognized as a *first-line therapy* for palmar and plantar hyperhydrosis.

2. Other Pathologies

The body of research evidence presented in **Box 13-1** indicate that the main use of iontophoresis has been for the treatment of a variety of painful and inflammatory pathologies using either an anti-inflammatory agent (dexamenthasone) or a mixture of both analgesic and anti-inflammatory drug ions (dexamethasone and lidocaine). It further reveals

the noneffectiveness of acetic acid for calcifying tendons and ligaments. It finally reveals weak evidence of the effectiveness of salicylate for painful disorders, hyaluronidase for edema, and iodine and zinc for cutaneous wound repair.

VII. CONTRAINDICATIONS

Table 13-5 shows the contraindications associated with the practice of therapeutic iontophoresis. It is vital to question the patient about any previous drug sensitivity or allergy before proceeding with iontophoresis therapy.

VIII. RISKS, PRECAUTIONS, AND RECOMMENDATIONS

Iontophoresis is not without risk for the patient. The main risks, along with some precautions and recommendations designed to improve safety and effectiveness, are listed in **Table 13-6**. The risk of skin irritation or, at worst, skin burn, is the factor that most limits the application of drug iontophoresis. Practitioners should pay close attention to assure that the current device (CD) under the active electrode is always kept within the safe limit.

IX. CONSIDERATIONS FOR APPLICATION AND DOCUMENTATION

A. DEVICE TYPES

Presently, drug iontophoresis is commonly delivered, as illustrated in **Figure 13-1**, using reusable wire programmable stimulators followed to a least extent by disposable wireless nonprogrammable patches. Iontophoresis for the treatment of hyperhydrosis using tap water may be

TABLE 13-5	CONTRAINDICATIONS TO IONTOPHORESIS THERAPY
CONTRAINDICATIONS	**RATIONALE**
Over open, damaged, or broken skin	Risk of inducing skin irritation, burn, and severe pain (Ciccone, 2008).
Across the temporal and orbicular regions	Risk of causing transient visual disturbances.
In cases of known sensitivity or allergy to the therapeutic ions	Risk of triggering a life-threatening allergic reaction (Ciccone, 2008).
Over electronic implants (such as cardiac pacemaker)	Risk of interference with normal functioning of the implants if the current flows over the device, cables, or electrodes.

TABLE 13-6	RISKS, PRECAUTIONS, AND RECOMMENDATIONS FOR IONTOPHORESIS

RISKS	RATIONALE

Skin irritation and burn
   Skin irritation will manifest as a transient erythema (redness) under one or both electrodes; should normally disappear within 1 to 3 h after treatment.
   Skin burn is similar to sunburn and may last for a few days. If present, iontophoretic treatment must immediately be discontinued over this area. Periodic application of burn ointments will help to ease the pain, while accelerating healing. For severe burn cases that will not heal by themselves, consult a dermatologist.
	Risk is increased if the dose is too high, nonbuffered electrodes are used, or the current density under the cathode or anode exceeds the recommended safe values.

In the presence of and proximally to flammable sprays or solutions	Risk of igniting the flammable materials, thus posing a risk of explosion.
Over skin area showing severe-to-moderate impaired sensation to heat and pain stimuli	Risk of chemical and/or heat burn under the electrodes due to impaired ability to discriminate sensations of heat or pain.

PRECAUTION	RATIONALE
Ion/electrode polarity match	Failure to ensure polarity match will lead to total ineffectiveness of the iontophoretic treatment because no ion(s) will ever penetrate the skin. The only exception is tap water (+/-), which can be placed under both electrodes irrespective of their polarity.

RECOMMENDATIONS	RATIONALE
Question patients about food and drug allergies prior to first treatment	To prevent complications.
Wash and dry exposed skin areas	Removal of oil and other impurities will facilitate the iontophoretic process.
Shave hair over exposed skin areas	To facilitate the iontophoretic process.
Do not apply iontophoresis over areas where hair has been shaved within the past 24 h.	Will increase skin irritation.
Keep all dosages below 80 mA.min, with the exception of tap water for hyperhydrosis	To minimize the risk of skin irritation and burn.
Use buffered electrode systems	To minimize the risk of skin irritation and burn.
Keep current density under electrode below the recommended safe values (cathode, 0.5 mA/cm2; anode, 1.0 mA/cm2).	To minimize the risk of skin irritation and burn.
Assure even contact between the electrodes and the skin	To assure optimal ion delivery into the treated area.

(Continued)

TABLE 13-6	CONTINUED

RECOMMENDATIONS	RATIONALE
Apply no weight over the electrodes	Increased tissue pressure may lead to relative tissue ischemia, which may interfere with the efficacy of treatment and increase the risk of chemical and/or heat burn under the electrodes.
Use wireless over wired devices	When the patient's time for clinical visit is limited or when he or she prefers to be active while receiving drug therapy, the wireless patch is the selection of choice.
Avoid rearranging electrodes during treatment	Will affect treatment efficacy and create unpleasant sensations for the patient.
Keep adequate distance, or spacing, between the cathode and anode	The distance should be at least equivalent to the diameter of the largest electrode.
Use commercial rather than custom electrodes	Commercial electrodes are to be preferred because of their overall convenience and technical performance.
Work in collaboration with the patient's treating physician and your pharmacist	The adequate prescription and preparation of your drug-ionized solutions depends on the collaboration of these two health professionals; never hesitate to consult them.
Apply soothing skin lotion after treatment	Skin lotions containing aloe vera, lanolin, or other similar substances may alleviate skin irritation posttherapy (Ciccone, 2008).
Discard used commercial electrode systems	Commercial electrode systems are made for single use only.
Plug line-powered devices into GFCI receptacles	Prevent the occurrence of macroshocks (see Chapter 27).
Conduct regular maintenance and calibration	Ensure optimal treatment efficacy. Follow manufacturer's recommendations and scheduling.

delivered using a dedicated line-powered system made of a stimulator, with water tray acting as electrodes. The key features of wired and wireless iontophoresis devices are presented in **Table 13-3**.

B. ELECTRODE TYPES

Iontophoresis is delivered using custom or commercial electrodes. **Figure 13-6** shows samples of such electrodes: custom electrode (**A**) with its clip and metal plate, and wire commercial electrode (**B**). Another type of electrode, wireless patch electrode, is not pictured. **Table 13-7** shows key features that distinguish custom from commercial electrodes. Both types present advantages and disadvantages. The main advantage of commercial electrodes is their buffering system. The main disadvantage is their relatively high cost.

C. ELECTRODE FILLING

Commercial electrodes, used with wire or patch system, are filled with the prescribed drug solution (or tap water when indicated)) using a syringe, with or without a needle. Illustrated in **Figure 13-7** is the filling up of a patch system. The gauzes or cloths used with custom electrodes (see **Fig 13-6A**) are also filled up with drug solution using a syringe.

D. EXAMPLES OF ELECTRODE APPLICATION

Shown in **Figure 13-8** are typical examples of the clinical application of a portable wire electrode system (**A**) and a dedicated line-powered iontophoresor for the treatment of palmar hyperhydrosis (**B**).

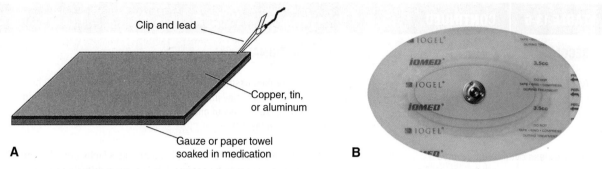

FIGURE 13-6 Iontophoresis electrode types. (**A**) Custom electrode and (**B**) commercial wire electrode (A: From Robinson et al., *Clinical Electrophysiology*, 3rd ed. Lippincott Williams & Wilkins, Philadelphia, 2008, p.361, B: Courtesy of Empi).

E. PROCEDURES

The safe, effective, and optimal application of iontophoresis requires that clinicians perform a systematic set of procedures for every application. Presented below is a list of these procedures.

1. Checklists

Before proceeding with treatment, always check the list of contraindications (**Table 13-5**), as well as the list of risks, precautions, and recommendations (**Table 13-6**).

2. Skin Preparation

Clean the skin area where the active and dispersive electrodes are to be positioned with rubbing alcohol. If necessary, cut and trim excess hair; avoid shaving the hair because of possible skin irritation before treatment. The skin area should be free of open wounds.

3. Device Selection

Select the most appropriate type of iontophoretic device. The wireless type (patch) is the selection of choice for patients who have limited time available for a clinic visit and who want to remain active while receiving drug iontophoresis.

4. Active Versus Dispersive Electrode Preparation

Fill the *active* electrode (gauze or cloth) with the drug solution; *assure a polarity match* (−/−; +/+) between the drug ion and the electrode polarity (cathode −; anode +). Fill the dispersive electrode with tap water (or Ringer solution). The filling capacity (cc) of each electrode is determined by the manufacturer; do not over- or under-fill commercial electrodes. In case of tap water iontophoresis for hyperhydrosis, cover or fill both electrodes with tap water.

TABLE 13-7	CUSTOM VERSUS COMMERCIAL IONTOPHORETIC ELECTRODES
CUSTOM ELECTRODES	**COMMERCIAL ELECTRODES**
Made of malleable metal materials, such as kitchen aluminum foil, under which are applied some layers of absorbent material (gauze or cotton) impregnated with the therapeutic ionic solution (see Khan, 2000).	Made of various materials, such as gel matrix, fiber pad (patch), and plastic reservoir-like material capable of being impregnated with the therapeutic ionic solution (see Ciccone, 2000).
Can be customized to the desired sizes.	Come in predetermined sizes.
No control over skin pH changes during treatment.	Control over skin pH changes due to a buffering agent incorporated within the electrode system (contact plate→drug reservoir→buffering layer). Some commercial electrodes are sold, however, without a buffering system.
Require more preparation time (customizing of electrodes, gauze, or cloth)	Require less preparation time (precut).
Rather messy to use due to leaking of ionic solution from the impregnated gauze or cloth	Cleaner to use, with no leaking of ionic solution from the electrode system.
Require straps, tapes, or elastic bandages to secure electrodes over the skin.	Self-adhesive system.
Relatively inexpensive system.	Relatively more expensive system.

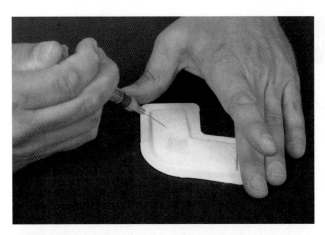

FIGURE 13-7 Patch electrode filled with the drug solution using a syringe (Reprinted with permission from Knight, KL and Draper, DO. *Therapeutic Modalities*. Philadelphia: Lippincott Williams and Wilkins, 2008.)

5. Electrode Placement

Place the active electrode over the soft tissue lesion and the dispersive electrode a few centimeters away. Note that with the patch system the spacing between the two electrodes is fixed.

6. Therapeutic Ions and Dosage

Select the proper therapeutic ions for the condition being treated (see **Table 13-2** and **Box 13-1**). Set the desired dosage (mA.min). For a wired-type device, manually adjust the current amplitude (mA) and the duration of application (min). For a wireless-type device (patch), select the patch that matches your dosage (i.e., 40 or 80 mA.min). For custom or commercial wire electrodes, make sure the CD under the cathode and anode is always kept at less than the recommended values of 0.5 and 1.0 mA/cm^2, respectively.

7. End of Treatment

Carefully remove the electrodes, and immediately inspect the exposed skin areas for any adverse reaction or lesion.

If present, inform the patient, and document these in the patient's file. Discard used commercial wire electrodes, patches, and gauzes (cloths) in biowaste bags. Custom metal plate electrodes may be reused only after thorough cleaning and disinfecting. Apply a lotion over the treated skin areas.

F. DOCUMENTATION

Document the key treatment parameters, as well as any adverse reaction or lesion, in the patient's file. **Table 13-8** shows the key treatment parameters to be documented in the patient's file.

TABLE 13-8	KEY TREATMENT PARAMETERS TO BE DOCUMENTED IN PATIENT'S FILE AFTER IONTOPHORESIS

- *Iontophoresor type or model:* description
- *Drug name and polarity:* description
- *Concentration of ionic drug:* % aqueous solution or % ointment
- *Volume of drug solution impregnated in the reservoir or gel matrix:* cc
- *If patch used:* patch electrode conductive area (cm^2)
- *If electrode system used:* active electrode conductive area (cm^2) and dispersive electrode conductive area: (cm^2)
- *If electrode system used, distance between the active and dispersive electrode:* cm^2
- *Dose:* mA.min—Specify current amplitude (mA) and application duration (min)
- *Application duration: If electrode system:* min *If patch system:* hours per day
- *Electrode placement:* description

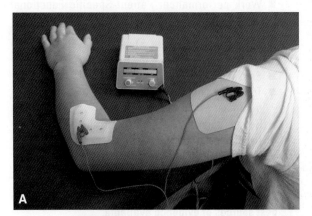

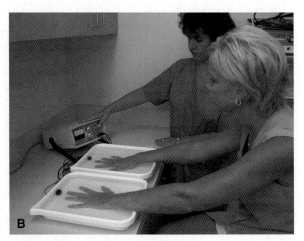

FIGURE 13-8 Typical applications using a portable iontophoresor (**A**) and dedicated cabinet iontophoresor for the treatment of palmar hyperhydrosis (**B**). (A: Reprinted with permission from Knight, KL and Draper, DO. *Therapeutic Modalities*. Philadelphia: Lippincott Williams and Wilkins, 2008; B: Reprinted with permission, © International Hyperhidrosis Society, www.SweatHelp.org).

Case Study 13-1   Epicondylitis

A 49-year-old female worker, working full time for a cleaning company, consults for treatment. She wears a pacemaker, and her present health status is good. She recalls that three weeks ago she sustained a major blow to the lateral side of her right elbow while cleaning a container (the container's cover fell on her elbow). The following day, she was seen by her physician, who diagnosed the presence of a severe traumatic epicondylitis. After three weeks of analgesic and anti-inflammatory oral drug therapy, coupled with rest (absence from work), she reports good improvement. She now experiences no pain at rest and moderate pain during light wrist and hand activities. Physical examination, however, reveals residual signs of inflammation over the lateral epicondyle area; there is moderate swelling, with increasing pain during forceful wrist extension and power grip. She is anxious about prolonging her absenteeism from work. Her goal is to return to work as soon as possible and to stop her oral drug regimen, which is starting to give her some stomach irritation. In other words, she is looking for an alternative treatment to her present oral drug and rest regimen. Finally, she stresses the fact that her physician mentioned that if her condition was to further deteriorate an injection of drugs into the painful area may be needed. She is afraid of needle and wants to avoid this last treatment approach at all costs.

Evidence-Based Steps Toward the Resolution of This Case

1. **List medical diagnosis.**

   Epicondylitis

2. **List key impairment(s).**
   - Pain
   - Decreased grip strength

3. **List key functional limitation(s).**
   - Difficulty to power grip objects and tools

4. **List key disability/disabilities.**
   - Inability to resume full-time work

5. **Justification for dexamethasone iontophoresis therapy.**

   Is there justification for the iontophoresis of an anti-inflammatory agent, such as dexamethasone, in this case? This chapter has established that there is *fair* justification for the use of such a drug agent for the treatment of lateral epicondylitis with the majority of studies demonstrating therapeutic benefits (see Section VI). Local phoresis of this anti-inflammatory agent is expected to reduce the residual inflammation, while promoting the proliferative and maturation phase

of this lesion. It is also expected to reduce pain by decreasing inflammation. The selection of dexamethasone is justified on the basis of the following articles: Demirtas et al., 1998; Baskurt et al., 2003; Nirsch et al., 2003; Hamann et al., 2006. Iontophoresis therapy is further justified by the fact that this patient is afraid of needles and is looking for an alternative to a possible injection of the drug into her elbow. Finally, this treatment, if effective, will eliminate the need for oral drugs, while accelerating her return to full-time work. Note that other glucocorticoid agents could have been used, such as hydrocortisone or prednisone, as well as a nonsteroid agent such as sodium diclofenac (NSAID agent). Because EPAs are rarely used alone, the therapeutic program also includes a progressive regimen of forearm and handgrip strengthening exercises.

6. **Search for contraindications.**

   None is found. The fact that the patient wears a pacemaker *does not* present a contraindication because the delivery of electrical current is far remote, being at the elbow level, from the thoracic area, where the pacemaker unit, cable, and electrodes are located.

7. **Search for dangers and precautions.**

   None is found.

8. **Outline the therapeutic goal(s) you and your patient wish to achieve.**
   - Decrease pain
   - Increase grip strength
   - Resume full working activities

9. **List the outcome measurement(s) used to assess treatment effectiveness.**
   - Pain: Numerical Rating Scale (NRS-101)
   - Grip strength: dynamometry
   - Work performance: Patient-Specific Functional Scale (PSFS)

10. **Instruct the patient about what he/she should experience, do, or not do during the treatment session.**
    - Sensation: light warming/tingling
    - Transient skin redness under the electrode post-treatment
    - Refrain from moving the affected elbow
    - Avoid hand and finger movements
    - If burning sensation is felt, call immediately for assistance

11. **Outline your therapeutic prescription based on the best sources of evidence available.**

    This prescription is based on the following sources of evidence: Demirtas et al., 1998; Baskurt et al., 2003; Nirsch et al., 2003; Hamann et al., 2006; Gurney et al.,

2008. A wire programmable iontophoresis is used with buffered electrodes.

- **Iontophoretic device:** wire programmable iontophoresor
- **Therapeutic ions and polarity:** Dexamethasone (–)
- **Drug concentration:** 4 mg/ml in aqueous solution
- **Dosage:** 40 mA.min, delivered using 2 mA for 20 minutes (see below)
- **Electrodes:** commercial buffered electrodes
- **Active electrode:** Conductive surface area: 4 cm^2
  Fill volume: 2.5 cc
  Electrode fill: 2.5 cc of dexamethasone (4 mg1ml)
  Polarity: negative (cathode) to match drug ion polarity – CD: 0.5 mA/cm^2; safe
- **Dispersive electrode:** Conductive surface area: 6 cm^2
  Fill volume: 3.5 cc
  Electrode fill: 3.5 cc of Ringer solution
- **Active electrode placement:** cathode over the lateral epicondyle area
- **Dispersive electrode placement:** anode over the anterior surface of the forearm
- **Treatment frequency:** once a day for 5 consecutive days
- **Number of treatments:** 10 treatments over 2 consecutive weeks

12. Collect outcome measurements.

Pre- and posttreatment comparison:

- Pain: decrease NRS score from 9 to 2 during forceful wrist extension/power grip
- Grip strength: increase by 25% —within 5% of normal value
- Work performance: PSFS score increased by 80%— resume full work

13. Assess therapeutic effectiveness on the basis of outcome measures.

The results show that 10 applications of dexamethasone iontophoresis therapy, delivered every day for 5 consecutive days over 2 weeks, and coupled with a progressive regimen of forearm and handgrip strengthening regimen, led to a significant decrease in pain during forceful wrist extension movements and power grip. She is now able to resume full work. The patient is more than satisfied with the results of her treatment. She is very pleased with the fact she avoided drug injection in addition to stopping her oral drug therapy regimen. Overall, this regimen of dexamethasone iontophoresis therapy had a beneficial impact on the patient's disablement status created by the pathology, as illustrated in the **figure below**.

14. State the prognosis.

The prognosis is excellent. With a gradual return to those most demanding tasks at work, the probability that this elbow condition worsen is very low. If her condition was to worsen, the possibility of treating by iontophoresis, using a wearable patch system, while remaining at work, should be considered.

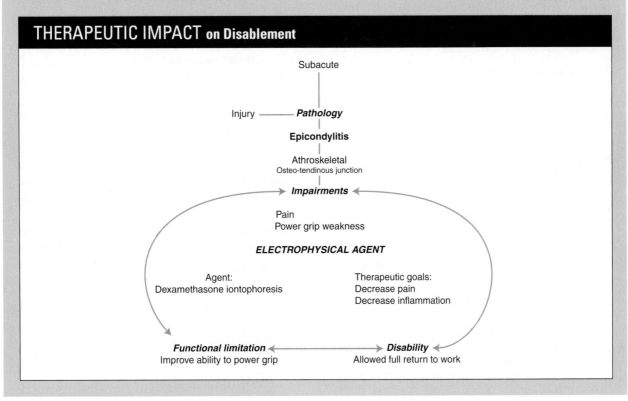

THERAPEUTIC IMPACT on Disablement

Subacute

Injury ———— **Pathology**

Epicondylitis

Athroskeletal
Osteo-tendinous junction

Impairments

Pain
Power grip weakness

ELECTROPHYSICAL AGENT

Agent:
Dexamethasone iontophoresis

Therapeutic goals:
Decrease pain
Decrease inflammation

Functional limitation
Improve ability to power grip

Disability
Allowed full return to work

Case Study 13-2   **Palmar Hyperhidrosis**

A 32-year-old carpenter consults for treatment. His major complaint is excessive sweating of the palmar surface of his hands, which started about a year ago. He explains that his hands are constantly wet and slippery and that the whole thing seems to worsen when he is under pressure at work. He adds that his hand condition led him, over the past 3 months, to improper and unsafe gripping of his hammer and other carpentry tools at work. He indicates that in order to work properly and safely, he has to wear three pairs of cotton gloves a day to absorb the excessive perspiration. He also complains of social embarrassment when he touches his girlfriend and when shaking hands with family members, friends, and coworkers. He reports having consulted a physician two weeks ago for his hand condition. The physician offered to prescribe an oral anticholinergic drug regimen and added that if the medication did not resolve his condition, he would then refer him to a dermatologist for Botulinum toxin injections and, if necessary, for his opinion as to a possible endoscopic thoracic sympathectomy. This young man mentions that before considering any medical or surgical therapeutic interventions his preference is to undertake a more conservative, and much less invasive, type of treatment. A basic Internet search made him aware that tap water iontophoresis may benefit his condition.

Evidence-Based Steps Toward the Resolution of This Case

1. **List medical diagnosis.**
   Idiopathic palmar hyperhidrosis

2. **List key impairment(s).**
   Hand hypersudation (moist)

3. **List key functional limitation(s).**
   Difficulty gripping tools

4. **List key disability/disabilities.**
   - Inability to work safely and effectively
   - Social embarrassment (hand touch)

5. **Justification for tap water iontophoresis therapy.**

   Is there justification for tap water iontophoresis in this case? This chapter has established that there is *good* justification for the use of this EPA with all studies demonstrating therapeutic benefits (see Section VI). This treatment is expected to induce the formation of keratinous plugs in the cutaneous pores, which should decrease sudation for a relatively long period (a few months). The selection of tap water iontophoresis therapy is justified based on the following articles: Shrivastava et al., 1977; Levit, 1968, 1980; Akins et al.,

1987; Stolman, 1987; Korakoç et al., 2002, 2004; Gillick et al., 2004; Solish et al., 2007. It is also justified because it presents no major side effects and, if proven effective, the treatment can later be delivered at home using a dedicated iontophoresor.

6. **Search for contraindications.**
   None is found.

7. **Search for dangers and precautions.**
   None is found.

8. **Outline the therapeutic goal(s) you and your patient wish to achieve.**
   - Increase dryness of both hands
   - Increase grip firmness
   - Decrease social embarrassment
   - Improve safety and effectiveness at work

9. **List the outcome measurement(s) used to assess treatment effectiveness.**
   - Hand dryness: Persprint paper; measurement of hand wetness area in cm^2
   - Grip firmness/safety at work: number of gloves used per day
   - Social embarrassment: personal diary—scale of 0 (none) to 10 (maximum)

10. **Instruct the patient about what he/she should experience, do, and not do during the treatment session.**
    - Sensation: light warming/tingling
    - Transient skin redness following therapy
    - Avoid hand and finger movements
    - Keep a light and constant pressure between the palm and the electrode pad
    - If burning sensation is felt, lift hand off pad and call immediately for assistance

11. **Outline your therapeutic prescription on the basis of the best sources of evidence available.**

    This prescription is based on the following sources of evidence: Shrivastava et al., 1977; Levit, 1968, 1980; Akins et al., 1987; Stolman, 1987; Korakoç et al., 2002, 2004; Gillick et al., 2004; Solish et al., 2007. A dedicated iontophoresis device for hyperhydrosis is used.

    - ***Iontophoretic device:*** any electrical device capable of generating a continuous DC of at least 20 mA amplitude
    - ***Therapeutic ions and polarity:*** tap water (+/−); no anticholinergic agent added
    - ***Dosage:*** 360 mA.min, delivered using 12 mA for 30 minutes
    - ***Water tray:*** two plastic trays, 40 × 25 × 10 cm each, filled with 2 liters of tap water at room temperature (21°C or 70°F)

- **Electrodes:** two custom-made aluminum foil electrodes, 30 × 15 cm each (450 cm²)
  The first electrode is immersed at the bottom of one tray; the other electrode is immersed at the bottom of the other tray
- **Electrode cover:** a piece of cotton cloth covering the entire electrode surface
- **Water level in both trays:** at a level sufficient to cover the palmar surfaces of both hands
- **Connecting cable:** electric wires with alligator clips
- **Upgrading of current amplitude at the beginning of therapy:** gradual increase from 0 to 12 mA during the first 2 minutes, and then maintain 12 mA for 30 minutes
- **Downgrading of current amplitude at the end of therapy:** gradual decrease to 0 mA within 2 minutes, and then maintain 12 mA for 30 minutes
- **Electrode polarity:** reversed after the first 15 minutes of intervention, so that both hands receive anodal and cathodal iontophoresis for an equal amount of time
- **Hand positioning in water tray:** each hand rests inactive; the palmar surface is against each electrode
- **Treatment frequency:** 3 times per week
- **Number of treatments:** 12 treatments over 4 consecutive weeks

12. **Collect outcome measurements.**

Pre- and posttreatment comparison:

- Hand dryness (surface area):
  Right hand: increase of 66%
  Left hand: increased by 55%

- Handgrip firmness/safety at work: cotton gloves required per day decreased from 3 to only 1 pair; improved feeling of safety at work
- Social embarrassment: decreased score from 9 to 2

13. **Assess therapeutic effectiveness on the basis of outcome measures.**

The results show that 12 applications of tap water iontophoresis therapy (without anticholinergic agent added), delivered 3 times per week over 4 consecutive weeks, decreased the patient's right- and left-hand wetness significantly. This improvement led to much improved handgrip firmness and feeling of safety at work. Finally, this noninvasive treatment approach led to a marked decrease in this patient's social embarrassment caused by his condition (dryer touch and handgrip). Overall, this regimen of tap water iontophoresis therapy had a beneficial impact on the patient's disablement status created by the pathology as illustrated in the **figure below**.

14. **State the prognosis.**

The prognosis is good if this patient accepts the need to undergo more treatments after each and every period of remission, unfortunately, for years to come. Now that he is familiar with this treatment, it is recommended that the patient start home therapy, using a commercial line-powered, reusable, and dedicated hyperhydrosis iontophoresor with accessories. To improve treatment effectiveness, the clinician should consider adding an anticholinergic agent to the tap water.

THERAPEUTIC IMPACT on Disablement

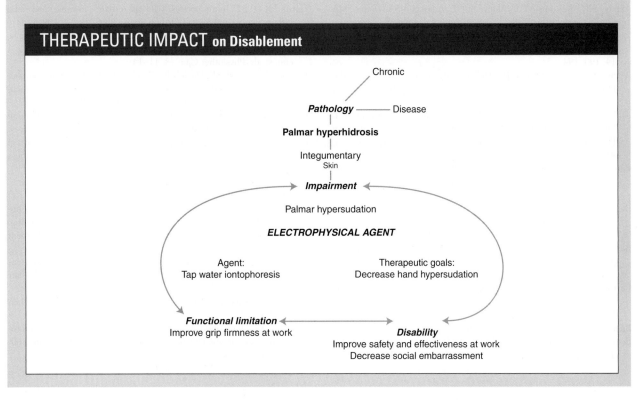

CRITICAL THINKING QUESTIONS

Clarification: How would you describe Le Duc's contribution to the field of iontophoresis?

Assumptions: Can you explain how the phenomenon of water electrolysis causes unwanted electrochemical reactions to the skin during iontophoresis therapy?

Reasons and evidence: Why is a polarity match between the drug ion and the electrode pole under which it is placed critical to the application of iontophoresis?

Viewpoints or perspectives: What is the relationship between skin irritation/burn, skin pH, the use of buffered electrodes, and the concept of electrode current density?

Implications and consequences: What would happen to the depth of penetration of a given drug if the application duration is short, versus long, using the same dose in both situations?

About the question: How would you convince a physician that iontophoresis is an effective and safe method for delivering a drug to a localized region of the body? Why do you think I ask this question?

References

Articles

Abell G, Morgan K (1974) Treatment of idiopathic hyperhidrosis by glycopyrronium bromide and tap water iontophoresis. Br J Dermatol, 91: 87–91

Aiyejusunie CB, Kola-Korolo TA, Ajiboye OA (2007) Comparison of the effects of TENS and sodium salicylate iontophoresis in the management of osteoarthritis of the knee. Nig Q J Hosp Med, 17: 30–34

Akinbo SR, Aiyejunusie CB, Akinyemi OA, Adesegun SA, Danesi MA (2007) Comparison of the therapeutic efficacy of phonophoresis and iontophoresis using Dexamethasone dosium phosphate in the management of patients with knee osteoarthritis. Niger Postgrad Med, 14: 190–194

Akins DL, Meisenheimer JL, Dobson RL (1987) Efficacy of the Drionic unit in the treatment of hyperhidrosis. J Am Acad Dermatol, 16: 828–833

Anderson CR, Morris RL, Boeh SD, Panus PC, Sembrowich WL (2003) Effects of iontophoresis current magnitude and duration on Dexamethasone deposition and localized drug retention. Phys Ther, 83: 161–170

Balogun JA, Abidoye AB, Akala EO (1990) Zinc iontophoresis in the management of bacterial colonized wounds: A case report. Physiother Can, 42: 147–151

Banta CA (1994) A prospective, nonrandomized study of iontophoresis, wrist splinting, and anti-inflammatory medication in the treatment of early mild carpal tunnel syndrome. J Occup Med, 36: 166–168

Baskurt F, Ozcan A, Algun C (2003) Comparison of effects on phonophoresis and iontophoresis of naproxen in the treatment of lateral epicondylitis. Clin Rehab, 17: 96–100

Bertolucci LE (1982) Introduction of anti-inflammatory drugs by iontophoresis: Double-blind study. J Orthop Sports Phys Ther, 4: 103–108

Boone D (1969) Hyaluronidase iontophoresis. Phys Ther, 49: 139–145

Bouman HD, Grunewald Lentzer EM (1952) The treatment of hyperhidrosis of feet with constant current. Am J Phys Med, 31: 158–169

Braun BL (1987) Treatment of an acute anterior disk displacement in the temporomandibular joint: A case report. Phys Ther, 67: 1234–1236

Chan LY, Tang WY, Mok WK, Ly CY, Ip AW (1999) Treatment of palmar hyperhydrosis using tap water iontophoresis: local experience. Hong Kong Med J, 5: 191–194

Chandler TJ (1998) Iontophoresis of 0.4% dexamethasone for plantar fasciitis. Clin J Sport Med, 8: 68

Cornwall MW (1981) Zinc iontophoresis to treat ischemic skin ulcers. Phys Ther, 61: 359–360

Delacerda FG (1982) A comparative study of three methods of treatment for shoulder girdle myofascial syndrome. J Orthop Sports Phys Ther, 4: 51–54

Demirtas RN, Oner C (1998) The treatment of lateral epicondylitis by iontophoresis of sodium salicylate and sodium diclofenac. Clin Rehab, 12: 23–29

Dolianitis C, Scarff CE, Kelly J, Sinclair R (2004) Iontophoresis with glycopyrrolate for the treatment of palmoplantar hyperhydrosis. Australasian J Dermatol, 45: 208–212

Elgart ML, Puchs G (1987) Tapwater iontophoresis in the treatment of hyperhydrosis. Use of the Drionic device. Int J Dermatol, 26: 194–197

Garzione JE (1978) Salicylate iontophoresis as an alternative treatment for persistent thigh pain following hip surgery. Phys Ther, 58: 570–571

Gillick BT, Kloth LC, Starsky A, Cincinelli-Walker L (2004) Management of postsurgical hyperhydrosis with direct current and tap water. Phys Ther, 84: 262–267

Goh CL, Yoyong K (1996) A comparison of tannic acid versus iontophoresis in the medical treatment of palmar hyperhidrosis. Singapore Med J, 37: 466–488

Gordon AH, Weistein MV (1969) Sodium salicylate iontophoresis in the treatment of plantar warts: Case report. Phys Ther, 49: 869–870

Grice K, Sattar H, Baker H (1972) Treatment of idiopathic hyperhidrosis with iontophoresis of tap water and poldine methosulphate. Br J Dermatol, 86:72–78

Gudeman SD, Eisele SA, Heidt RS, Colosimo AJ, Sroupe AL (1997) Treatment of plantar fasciitis by iontophoresis of 0.4% dexamethasone. A randomized, double-blind, placebo-controlled study. Am J Sports Med, 25: 312–316

Guffey JS, Rutherford MJ, Payne W, Phillips C (1999) Skin pH changes associated with iontophoresis. J Orthop Sports Phys Ther, 29: 656–660

Harris PR (1982) Iontophoresis: Clinical research in musculoskeletal inflammatory conditions. J Orthop Sports Phys Ther, 4: 109–112

Hasson SH, Henderson GH, Daniels JC, Schieb DA (1991) Exercise training and dexamethasone iontophoresis in rheumatoid arthritis: A case study. Physiother Can, 43: 11–14

Hasson SM, English SE, Daniels JC, Reich M (1988) Effect of iontophoretically delivered dexamethasone on muscle performance in a rheumatoid arthritic joint: A case study. Arthritis Care Res, 1: 177–182

Hill BH (1976) Poldine iontophoresis in the treatment of palmar and plantar hyperhidrosis. Aust J Dermatol, 17: 92–93

Holzle E, Alberti N (1987) Long-term efficacy and side effects of tap water iontophoresis of palmoplantar hyperhidrosis—The usefulness of home therapy. Dermatologica, 175: 126–135

Holzle E, Ruzicka T (1986) Treatment of hyperhidrosis by a battery-operated iontophoresis device. Dermatologica, 172: 41–47

Ishihashi T (1936) Effects of drugs on the sweat glands by cataphoresis, and an effective method of suppression of local sweating: Observation on the effect of diaphoretics and adiaphoretics. J Orient Med, 25: 101–102

Japour CL, Vohra R, Vohra PK, Garfunkel L, Chin N (1999) Management of heel pain syndrome with acetic acid iontophoresis. J Am Podiatr Med Assoc, 89: 251–257

Kahn J (1975) Calcium iontophoresis in suspected myopathy. Phys Ther, 55: 376–377

Kahn J (1980) Iontophoresis and ultrasound for postsurgical temporomandibular trismus and parasthesia: Case report. Phys Ther, 60: 307–308

Kahn J (1982) Iontophoresis with hydrocortisone for Peyronie's disease. Phys Ther, 62: 975

Kalia YN, Guy RN (1995) The electrical characteristics of human skin in vivo. Pharm Res, 12: 1605–1613

Karakoç Y, Aydemir EH, Kalkan MT (2004) Placebo-controlled evaluation of direct electrical current administration for palmoplantar hyperhidrosis. Int J Dermatol, 43: 503–505

Karakoç Y, Aydemir EH, Kalkan MT, Unal G (2002) Safe control of palmoplantar hyperhidrosis with direct electrical current. Int J Dermatol, 41: 602–605

Langley PL (1984) Iontophoresis to aid in releasing tendon adhesions: Suggestions from the field. Phys Ther, 64: 1395

Le Duc S (1900) Introduction of medicinal substances into depth of tissues by electrical current. Ann Electrobiol, 3: 545–560

Le Duc BE, Caya J, Tremblay S, Bureau NJ, Dumont M (2003) Treatment of calcifying tendonitis of the shoulder by acetic acid Iontophoresis: A double-blind randomized controlled trial. Arch Phys med Rehab, 84: 1523–1527

Levit F (1968) Simple device for the treatment of hyperhidrosis by iontophoresis. Arch Dermatol, 98: 505–507

Levit F (1980) Treatment of hyperhidrosis by tap water iontophoresis. Cutis, 26: 192–194

Li LC, Scudds RA, Heck CS, Harth M (1996) The efficacy of dexamethasone iontophoresis for the treatment of rheumatoid arthritic knees: A pilot study. Arthritis Care Res, 9: 126–132

Magistro CM (1964) Hyaluronidase by iontophoresis in the treatment of edema: A preliminary clinical report. Phys Ther, 44: 169–175

Midtgaard K (1986) A new device for the treatment of hyperhidrosis by iontophoresis. Br J Dermatol, 114: 485–488

Montorsi F, Salonia A, Guazzoni G, Barbieri L, Colombo R, Brausl M, Scattoni V, Rigatti P (2000) Transdermal electromotive multi-drug administration for Peyronie's disease: Preliminary results. J Androl, 21: 85–90

Neeter C, Thomee R, Sillbernagel KG, Thomee P, Karlsson J (2003) Iontophoresis with and without dexamethasone in the treatment of acute Achilles tendon pain. Scand J Med Sci Sports, 13: 376–382

Nirsch RP, Rodin DM, Ochiai DH, Maartmann-Moe C (2003) Iontophoretic administration of dexamethasone sodium phosphate for acute epicondylitis. Am J Sports Med, 31: 189–195

Odia S, Vocks E, Radoski J, Ring J (1996) Successful treatment of dyshidrotic hand eczema using tap water iontophoresis with pulsed direct current. Acta Derm Venereol, 76: 472–474

Ozawa A, Haruki Y, Iwashita K, Sasao Y, Miyahara M, Sugai J, Matsuyama T, Iizuka M, Kawakubo Y, Nakamori M, Ohkido M (1999) Follow-up of clinical efficacy of iontophoresis therapy for postherpetic neuralgia (PHN). J Dermatol, 26: 1–10

Panus PC, Hooper T, Padrones A, Palmer B, Williams D (1996) A case study of exacerbation of lateral epicondylitis by combined use of iontophoresis and phonophoresis. Physiother Can, 48: 27–31

Pellecchia GL, Hamel H, Behnke P (1994) Treatment of infrapatellar tendinitis: A combination of modalities and transverse friction massage versus iontophoresis. J Sports Rehab, 3: 135–145

Perron M, Malouin F (1997) Acetic acid and iontophoresis and ultrasound for the treatment of calcifying tendinitis of the shoulder: A randomized controlled trial. Arch Phys Med Rehab, 78: 379–384

Psaki C, Carol L (1955) Acetic acid ionization: A study to determine the absorptive effects upon calcified tendinitis of the shoulder. Phys Ther, 35: 84–87

Reid KI, Dionne RA, Sicard-Rosenbaum L, Lord D, Dubner RA (1994) Evaluation of iontophoretically applied dexamethasone for painful pathologic temporomandibular joints. Oral Surg Med Pathol, 77: 605–609

Reidl CR, Plas E, Engelhardt P, Daha K, Pfluger H (2000) Iontophoresis for treatment of Peyronie's disease. J Urol, 163: 95–99

Rothfeld SH, Murray W (1967) Treatment of Peyronie's disease by iontophoresis of C21 esterified glucocorticosteroids. J Urol, 97: 874–875

Runeson L, Jaker E (2002) Iontophoresis with cortisone in the treatment of lateral epicondylalgia (tennis elbow)—a double-blind study. Scand J Sci Sports, 12: 136–142

Schiffman EL, Braun BL, Lindgren BR (1996) Temporomandibular joint iontophoresis: A double-blind randomized clinical trial. J Orofac Pain, 10: 157–165

Schwartz MS (1955) The use of hyaluronidase by iontophoresis in the treatment of lymphedema. Arch Intern Med, 95: 662

Shrivastava SN, Sing G (1977) Tap water iontophoresis in palmo-plantar hyperhidrosis. Br J Dermatol, 96: 189–195

Sokoro YT, Repking MC, Clemment JA, Mitchell PL, Berg RL (2002) Treatment of plantar verrucae using 2% sodium salicylate Iontophoresis. Phys Ther, 82: 1184–1191

Stolman LP (1987) Treatment of excess sweating of the palms by iontophoresis. Arch Dermatol, 123: 893–896

Tannenbaum M (1980) Iodine iontophoresis in reduction of scar tissue. Phys Ther, 60: 792

Weinstein MV, Gordon A (1958) The use of magnesium sulfate iontophoresis in the treatment of subdeltoid bursitis. Phys Ther, 38: 96–98

Wieder DL (1992) Treatment of traumatic myositis ossificans with acetic acid iontophoresis. Phys Ther, 72: 133–137

Yarrobino TE, Kalbfleisch JH, Ferslew KE, Panus PC (2006) Lidocaine iontophoresis mediates analgesia in lateral epicondylalgia treatment. Phys Res Int, 11: 152–160

Review Articles

Banga AK, Panus PC (1998) Clinical applications of iontophoretic devices in rehabilitation medicine. Crit Rev Phys Med Rehab, 10: 147–179

Brown M, Marting G, Jones SA, Akomeah FK (2006) Dermal and transdermal drug delivery systems: Current and future prospects. Drug Delivery, 13: 175–187

Chien YW, Banga K (1989) Iontophoretic (transdermal) delivery of drugs: Overview of historical development. J Pharm Sci, 78: 353–354

Ciccone CD (2003) Does acetic acid iontophoresis accelerate the resorption of calcium deposits in calcific tendinitis of the shoulder? Phys Ther, 83: 68–74

Costello CT, Jeske AH (1995) Iontophoresis: Applications in transdermal medication delivery. Phys Ther, 75: 554–563

Dixit N, Bai V, Baboota S, Ahuja A, Ali J (2007) Iontophoresis—an approach for controlled drug delivery: A review. Curr Drug Deliv, 4: 1–10

Eisenach JH, Atkinson JLD, Fealey RD (2005) Hyperhydrosis: Evolving therapies for a well-established phenomenon. Mayo Clin Proc, 80: 657–666

Fischer GA (2005) Iontophoretic drug delivery using IOMED Phoresor system. Expert Opin Drug Deliv, 2: 391–403

Gangarosa LP, Ozawa A, Ohkido M, Shimomura Y, Hill JM (1995) Iontophoresis for enhancing penetration of dermatologic and antiviral drugs. J Dermatol, 11: 865–875

Grond S, Radbrush L, Lehmann KA (2000) Clinical pharmacokinetics of transdermal opioids: Focus on transdermal fentanyl. Clin Pharmacokinet, 38: 59–89

Gurney AB, Washer DC (2008) Absorption of dexamethasone sodium phosphate in human connective tissue using iontophoresis. Am J Sports Med, 36: 753–759

Guy RH (1996) Current status and future prospects of transdermal drug delivery. Pharm Res, 13: 1765–1769

Hamann H, Hodges M, Evans B (2006) Effectiveness of iontophoresis of anti-inflammatory medications in the treatment of common musculoskeletal inflammatory conditions: A systematic review. Phys Ther Rev, 11: 190–194

Hashmonai M, Kopelman D, Assalia A (2000) The treatment of primary palmar hiperhidrosis: A review. Surg Today, 30: 211–218

Henley EJ (1991) Transcutaneous drug delivery: Iontophoresis, phonophoresis. Crit Rev Phys Rehab Med, 2: 139–151

Kalia YN, Merino V, Guy RH (1998) Transdermal drug delivery: Clinical aspects. Dermatol Clin, 16: 289–299

Kassan DG, Lynch AM, Stiller MJ (1996) Physical enhancement of dermatologic drug delivery: Iontophoresis and phonophoresis. J Am Acad Dermatol, 34: 657–666

Lark MR, Gangarosa LP (1990) Iontophoresis: An effective modality for the treatment of inflammatory disorders of the temporomandibular joint and myofascial pain. Cranio, 8: 108–119

Nair V, Pillai O, Poduri R, Panchagnula R (1999) Transermal iontophoresis. Part I: Basic principles and considerations. Methods Find Exp Clin Pharmacol, 21: 139–151

Riviere JE, Heit MC (1997) Electrically assisted transdermal delivery. Pharm Res, 14: 687–697

Semalty A, Semalty M, Singh R, Saraf SK, Saraf S (2007) Iontophoretic drug delivery system: A review. Technol Health Care, 15: 237–245

Solish N, Bertucci V, Dansereau A, Hong HC, Lynde C, Lupin M, Smith KC, Storwick G, Canadian Hyperhidrosis Advisory Committee (2007) A comprehensive approach to the recognition, diagnosis, and severity-based treatment of focal hyperhydrosis: Recommendations of the Canadian Hyperhidrosis Advisory Committee. Dermatol Surg, 33: 908–923

Stolman LP (1998) Treatment of hyperhidrosis. Dermatol Clin, 16: 863–869

Ting WW, Vest CD, Sontheimer RD (2004) Review of traditional and novel modalities of local therapeutics across the stratum corneum. Int J Dermatol, 43: 538–547

Togel B, Greve B, Raulin C (2002) Current therapeutic for hyperhydrosis: A review. Eur J Dermatol, 12 : 219–223

Vara Hernando FJ, Vázquez NG, Ortega JG (1997) The clinical use of iontophoresis. Rehab Int, Fall: 56–58

Zempsky WT, Ashburn MA (1998) Iontophoresis: Noninvasive drug therapy. Am J Anesth, 25: 158–163

Chapters of Textbooks

Ciccone CD (2008) Electrical stimulation for the delivery of medication: Iontophoresis. In: Clinical Electrophysiology, 3rd ed. Robinson AJ, Snyder-Mackler L (Eds). Lippincott Williams & Wilkins, Philadelphia, 2007, pp 351–381

Cummings J (1991) Iontophoresis. In: Clinical Electrotherapy, 2nd ed. Nelson RM, Currier DP (Eds). Appleton & Lange, Norwalk, pp 317–327

Dalzell MA (1996) Tissue healing with electrical stimulation: Wound care and iontophoresis. In: Physical Agents: Theory and Practice for Physical Therapists Assistants. Behrens BJ, Michlovitz SL (Eds). FA Davis, Philadelphia, pp 316–318

Hayes KW (2000) Iontophoresis. Manual of Physical Agents, 5th ed. Prentice-Hall Health, Upper Saddle River, pp 157–163

Kahn J (2000) Iontophoresis. In: Principles and Practice of Electrotherapy, 4th ed. Churchill Livingstone, New York, pp 119–140

Licht S (1983) History of electrotherapy. In: Therapeutic Electricity and Ultraviolet Radiation, 3rd ed. Stillwell GK (Ed). Williams & Wilkins, Baltimore, pp 1–64

Mehreteab TA, Holland (2006) Iontophoresis. In: Integrating Physical Agents in Rehabilitation, 2nd ed. Hecox B, Mehreteab TA, Weisberg, Sanko J (Eds). Appleton & Lange, Norwalk, pp 295–298

Prentice WE (2002) Iontophoresis. In: Therapeutic Modalities for Physical Therapists. McGraw–Hill, New York, pp 133–149

Starkey C (1999) Electrical agents. In: Therapeutic Modalities, 2nd ed. FA Davis, Philadelphia, pp 253–259

Textbook

Le Duc S (1908) Electric Ions and Their Use in Medicine. Rebman, Ltd, Liverpool

Transcutaneous Electrical Nerve Stimulation Therapy

Chapter Outline

Learning Objectives

Knowledge: State and describe the five modes to deliver transcutaneous electrical nerve stimulation (TENS) therapy for pain modulation.

Comprehension: Distinguish between the spinal gate system and the descending endogenous opiate system of pain modulation.

Application: List the considerations for application of TENS therapy.

Analysis: Explain how TENS can close the spinal gate via the spinal gate and descending endogenous opiate system.

Synthesis: Describe how to achieve preferential nerve depolarization of sensory fibers, sensory-motor fibers, and sensory-motor-nociceptive fibers.

Evaluation: Discuss the indication of TENS therapy for the modulation of pain following soft-tissue pathology.

I. RATIONALE FOR USE

A. DEFINITION AND DESCRIPTION

The term *TENS* is the *acronym* for *transcutaneous electrical nerve stimulation*. Literally speaking, this acronym refers to the use of electrical stimulators, capable of delivering pulsed currents, for the purpose of stimulating (depolarizing) nerve fibers through the skin using surface-stimulating electrodes. In this chapter, TENS is *specifically defined* as the application of pulsed electrical current over the skin surface for the purpose of *pain modulation or pain relief*. In other words, TENS is an EPA capable of inducing *electroanalgesia* by means of pulsed electrical current delivered over the skin surface. This definition is consistent with the historic association in the scientific and clinical literature between the terms *TENS* and pain management (see APTA, 2001; and References).

B. PAIN FROM SOFT-TISSUE PATHOLOGY

Because the use of TENS therapy is fundamentally for the management of pain, readers are *urged to review* Chapter 3, which focuses on the topic of pain from soft-tissue pathology, *prior* to considering this chapter. Chapter 3 presents the foundations of pain, its mechanisms of modulation, and its assessment.

C. TENS STIMULATORS

TENS therapy is delivered, as shown in **Figure 14-1**, using portable as well as cabinet-type electrical stimulators. Shown in **14-1A** is a typical *portable* battery-powered TENS stimulator. Such stimulators usually come in a plastic carrying case containing lead wires, reusable electrodes, and electroconductive gel. Shown in **14-1B** is a typical *cabinet-type* line-powered stimulator, also capable of delivering TENS therapy. These cabinet-type stimulators are commonly referred to, in the corporate literature, as *combo* stimulators, meaning that a single stimulator is capable of generating a *combination* (thus the word combo) of different current waveforms simply by pushing a button on the stimulator's console. The combo stimulator may be placed on a plain table or on a therapeutic system *cart*, as show in **14-1B**, which integrates with the stimulator (minimize cord and cable hassles) in addition to providing storage bins and mobility.

D. ELECTRODE TYPES AND COUPLING MEDIUM

TENS therapy is delivered using one or several pairs of surface electrodes, as shown in **Figure 14-2**, made of carbon-impregnated silicon rubber (**A**) or various flexible conductive tissues (**B**). These electrodes, which come in various shapes and sizes, may be reusable or for single use. Sterile

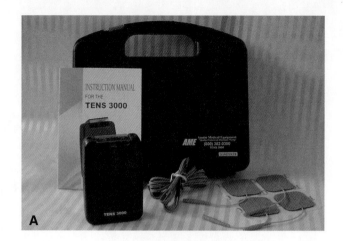

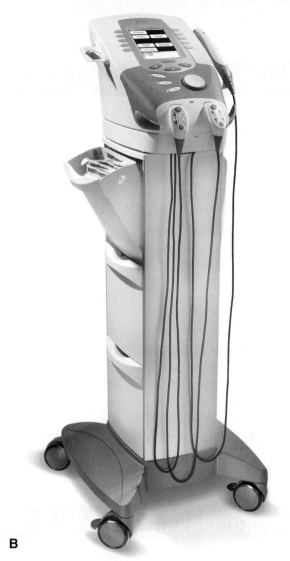

FIGURE 14-1 Typical portable, battery-powered (**A**) and cabinet (**B**), line-powered TENS stimulators (A: Courtesy of Austin Medical; B: Courtesy of Chattanooga Group).

electrodes are also available for postoperative treatment. Silicon-rubber electrodes are covered with an electroconductive gel (**C**) so as to optimize the electrical coupling

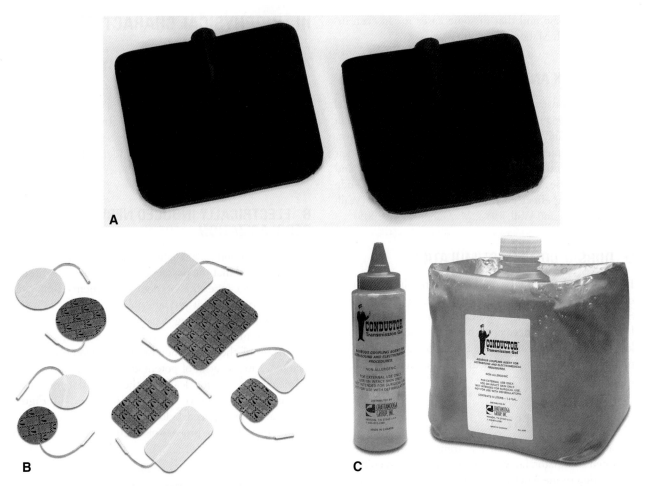

FIGURE 14-2 Typical TENS stimulating electrodes **(A)** made of carbon-impregnated, silicon rubber, and **(B)** of flexible conductive materials, **(C)** electroconductive gel to apply under electrodes (A–C: Courtesy of Chattanooga Group).

at the electrode–skin interface. Note that the use of custom-made metal electrodes is presently on the decline because commercial electrodes are superior and relatively cheap.

E. RATIONALE FOR USE

Pain is by far the dominating symptom that prompts people to consult health-care practitioners. The medical approach to pain therapy is to offer drugs and, if drugs are not successful, to consider surgery. Because these two approaches are invasive and present serious side effects, TENS therapy becomes an attractive therapeutic alternative for managing pain (Berman et al., 2000); it is a noninvasive treatment that has no side effects. The fact that TENS therapy can be administered easily at home and at work makes it even more attractive. Finally, the lower cost, compared with the high cost of drugs and surgery, associated with the delivery of TENS therapy makes this treatment more affordable to patients (Chabal et al., 1998).

II. HISTORICAL PERSPECTIVE

A. ANCIENT TIMES

Use of electrical current for pain relief dates back to the first century, when relief of pain from gout was reported after a torpedo fish, or electric ray, was applied against a patient's skin (McMahon et al., 2005).

B. DESCARTES

The French philosopher and scientist René Descartes can be credited with the first documented attempt to understand pain (DeLeo, 2006). His specificity theory of pain, published in 1664 in his *Treatise of Man* textbook, proposes that a specific pain pathway carries the messages from a pain receptor in the skin to a center in the brain, implying that simply cutting off this pathway should alleviate all pain (DeLeo, 2006). Unfortunately, there is a mountain of evidence in the pain literature to support the view that simply cutting nerve fibers by no means alleviates all pain and that in some cases it can even increase pain (McMahon et al., 2005).

C. MELZACK AND WALL

There is consensus that the discovery of TENS therapy is based on the original work of Ronald Melzack, a Canadian psychologist, and Patrick Wall, a British neuroanatomist. In 1965, they published a landmark paper describing their newly discovered gate control theory of pain (Melzack and Wall, 1965). The authors later revised their theory to include the modulating effect cognition may have on pain (Wall, 1978; Melzack and Wall, 1982; McMahon et al., 2005),

D. DORSAL COLUMN STIMULATION

Immediately after publication of this revolutionary theory, experiments by the American neurosurgeon Norman Shealy and colleagues on humans (Shealy et al., 1967) led to the eventual development of a surgical technique, known as dorsal column stimulation, for pain relief. This technique is based on electrical stimulation of dorsal column nerve fibers.

E. TENS DISCOVERY

Shealy and colleagues used a transcutaneous battery-operated stimulator, known as *Electreat*, as a screening device to determine whether patients were good candidates for dorsal column stimulation (Walsh, 1997). Unexpectedly, their preliminary work revealed that some responded better to this simple, noninvasive TENS therapy than to the more technically complicated invasive dorsal column stimulation (Shealy, 1974). This remarkable observation, combined with the work of Melzack and Wall, led to the discovery of TENS therapy.

F. BODY OF LITERATURE

The use of TENS for pain management, also called electroanalgesia, has been the subject, over the past quarter of a century, of numerous *articles* (see References), *review articles* (Belanger, 1985; Gersh et al., 1985; Roche et al., 1990; Richardson, 1994; Oosterwijk et al., 1994; Lundeberg, 1995; APTA, 1996a,b; Carroll et al., 1996; Reeve et al., 1996; Robinson, 1996; Walsh et al., 1996; Carroll et al., 1997; Kaplan et al., 1997; Johnson, 2000, 2001; Dickenson, 2002; Bjordal et al., 2003; Sluka et al., 2003; Brosseau et al., 2004; Khadilkar et al., 2005; Miller et al., 2005; Allen, 2006; Johnson et al., 2007; Ying et al., 2007), *chapters of textbooks* (Woolf et al., 1994; Mayer et al., 1995; Snyder-Mackler, 1995; Behrens et al., 1996; Frampton, 1996; Barr, 1999; Foley, 2000; Khan, 2000; Johnson, 2002; Behrens, 2006; Weisberg et al., 2006; Manal et al., 2008), and of a few *textbooks* (Mannheimer et al., 1984; Ottoson et al., 1988; Walsh, 1997).

III. BIOPHYSICAL CHARACTERISTICS

A. TRANSCUTANEOUS DELIVERY

The biophysical principle underlying the use of TENS is the delivery of pulsed electrical currents through the skin, using single or multiple pairs of electrodes, for the purpose of *activating, that is, stimulating, exciting, or depolarizing* groups of nerve fibers that underlie the process of pain perception and modulation.

B. ELECTRICALLY INDUCED NERVE DEPOLARIZATION

Research has long established that nerves are excitable structures and that the passage of pulsed currents through such nerves can excite or depolarize them (Robinson, 2008). Nerve fibers at rest are polarized, with the inside of their membranes being negatively charged. To *depolarize* a nerve means to reverse this polarized state, causing the inside of the nerve membrane to become positively charged. This reversal of potential across the nerve semipermeable membrane leads to the formation of an action potential, or nerve impulse. Illustrated in **Figure 14-3**, and summarized below, are the key physiological events related to the process of electrically induced nerve depolarization.

1. Resting Membrane Potential

At rest (stimulator OFF), excitable nerve membranes are readily permeable to potassium (K^+) ions, slightly permeable to sodium (Na^+) and chloride (Cl^-) ions, and impermeable to a number of large, negatively (−) charged proteins and phosphates named anions (A^-). Research has shown that the flow or gating of Na^+ and K^+ ions in and out of the membrane is regulated by voltage-sensitive channels (Robinson, 2008; see below). Because anions (A^-) are trapped within the intracellular space, the inside of the nerve membrane remains negatively charged. A resting membrane potential (RMP) is thus established and measure, in humans, at approximately −70 mV (**Fig 14-3**).

2. Electrical Stimulation Threshold

What will happen to the nerve RMP if a pulsed electrical current of gradually increasing amplitudes, as is the case with TENS, is applied over the nerve membrane? The gradual increase of current amplitude will decrease the RMP, passing from approximately −70 to −30 mV (**Fig 14-3A–B**). When the nerve membrane potential finally reaches a critical voltage level (**B**), a cascade of events (**B–E**) leads to the process of nerve depolarization (**B–C**), which leads to the formation of an action potential or nerve impulse (**B–E**). This critical voltage level corresponds to the nerve membrane *threshold* of activation (**B**).

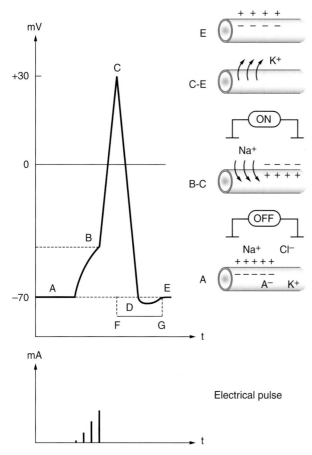

FIGURE 14-3 Electrically induced nerve depolarization. Schematized are the key events (**A–E**) leading to the production of an action potential or nerve impulse. (**A**) Stimulator OFF—resting membrane potential. (**B**) Stimulator ON—nerve threshold of activation achieved following the application of an electrical pulse. (**B** and **C**) depolarization phase. (**C** and **E**) repolarization and hyperpolarization (**D**) phases. (**F** and **G**) nerve refractory period.

3. Depolarization

This process (**B–C**) is caused by the rapid and massive opening of voltage-gated Na^+ channels, resulting in the reversal of potential inside the nerve membrane. In other words, the massive influx of positively charged sodium ions makes the inside of the nerve membrane more positive. This depolarization phase coincides with the beginning of the action potential (**B–C**).

4. Repolarization/Hyperpolarization

After being depolarized, the nerve membrane quickly repolarizes itself (**C–D**). This process begins with the complete closure of the voltage-gated Na^+ channels (**C**) and manifests itself by the rapid and massive opening of the voltage-gated potassium (K^+) channels. In other words, the massive efflux of positively charged potassium ions makes the inside of the nerve membranes more negative until its RMP is once again restored (from **C** to **D**). During this repolarization phase, the nerve membrane is slightly *hyperpolarized* (**D–E**) for a very short period of time because the potassium channels stay open a bit too

long in the process. The RMP is quickly restored by the Na^+—K^+ ATPase pumps.

5. Chain Reaction

The process of depolarization–repolarization is self-perpetuating, triggering a chain reaction of action potential along the nerve fiber. The influx of Na^+ depolarizes the axon and the outflow of K^+ repolarizes it (**Fig 14-3**).

6. Action Potential/Nerve Impulse Propagation

As shown in **Figure 14-3**, the passage of a pulse current through a nerve membrane results in the creation of an action potential (**B–D**), also called nerve impulse. Such nerve impulses propagate, or travel, along the nerves carrying neural information from organs to the central nervous system (CNS) or from the CNS to the organs.

a. All-Or-None Principle

When the threshold for stimulation (**B**) is achieved, an action potential of a fixed size will always be generated. In other words, there is no big- or small-amplitude action potential—all action potentials, for a given nerve, are of the same size. We have, therefore, two possibilities—either the nerve threshold for depolarization is not achieved (no action potential generated—*none*) or the threshold is achieved (full action potential generated—*all*). This is the all-or-none situation that underlies the all-or-none principle. In other words, there is no such thing as a fraction of action potential generated—the potential is either full or none. This also means that increasing the electrical pulse amplitude (subthreshold to supramaximal levels) will not induce larger-size action potentials.

b. Nerve Refractory Period

Nerve fibers require a certain period of time to recover before they can be depolarized again. In other words, there is a short period of time, as shown in **Figure 14-3F** and **G**, during which the nerve fiber will be refractory to the delivery (incapable of being depolarized) of another subthreshold electrical pulse. Within the refractory period, which lasts less than 1 ms, there is an *absolute* period, during which it is impossible to depolarize the nerve, and a *relative* period, during which an action potential can be generated if one applies an electrical pulse having a greater amplitude. The refractory period limits the pulse frequency that practitioners can choose to depolarize peripheral nerve fibers. For example, if the absolute refractory period is of 1 ms, then the maximum pulse frequency (or burst frequency) one can use to depolarize nerve fibers will be 1000 pps (1000 = 1 / 0.001).

C. KEY PARAMETERS

The pulsed currents used to deliver TENS therapy are characterized, as described below, by waveform, pulse/burst duration, pulse/burst frequency, and current amplitude. To further facilitate learning, readers are requested to *review* Chapter 5, which contains an illustrated glossary of EPA terminology of key concepts, definitions, and formulas related to electrical terminology.

1. Waveform

The basic current waveform generated by most modern TENS stimulators, as illustrated in **Figure 14-4**, is biphasic, either symmetrical or asymmetrical, and balanced. The delivery of balanced waveforms (those with an equal number of electrical charges in each phase, which is equivalent to having a zero net DC component) is critical because the duration of electrical stimulation for pain control is often prolonged, that is, more than 1 hour per application, with more than one application per day, for many consecutive days, weeks, and sometimes months (Johnson et al., 1991). To put it differently, using nonbalanced waveforms could lead to an adverse net accumulation of charges under the electrode, thus increasing the risk of skin irritation and burn under the electrodes, especially if the duration of application is relatively long (a few hours).

2. Pulses Versus Bursts of Pulses

Modern TENS units may be programmed, as illustrated in **Figure 14-5**, to deliver single pulses (**A**) or bursts of pulses (**B**).

a. Pulse/Interpulse Duration

Pulse duration (PD) is defined as the elapsed time between the beginning and end of all phases within a single pulse (**Fig 14-5A**). PD usually varies between 50 and 400 μs. The interpulse duration (IPD) is the elapsed time between each pulse. Its value varies according to the set pulse frequency and pulse duration.

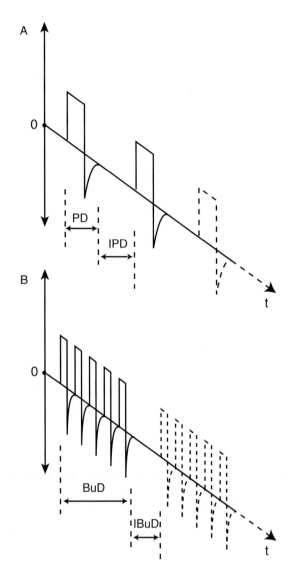

FIGURE 14-5 Determination of (**A**) pulse duration (PD) and interpulse duration (IPD) measurements from the delivery of single pulses. Determination of (**B**) burst duration (BuD) and interburst duration (IBuD) measurements with regard to the burst mode of TENS.

b. Pulse Frequency

Pulse frequency is defined as the number of pulses delivered per second (pps) and is commonly expressed in hertz (Hz). The frequency (f) is calculated using the following formula: $f = 1/P$, where P is the period. The period of a pulsed current is the summation of PD plus IPD. Consider the following example: A PD of 200 μs coupled with an IPD of 9800 μs yields a pulse frequency of 100 Hz (100 Hz = 1 / (0.0002 s + 0.00980 s), or 100 Hz = 1,000,000 / (200 μs + 9800 μs). Pulse frequency in most TENS devices ranges between 1 and 200 Hz.

c. Burst of Pulses

Among the five classic modes of delivering TENS therapy, one is known as *burst TENS*. In this mode, electrical pulses are delivered in bursts (Bu) of pulses, as illustrated in **Figure 14-5B**, as opposed to the repeated delivery

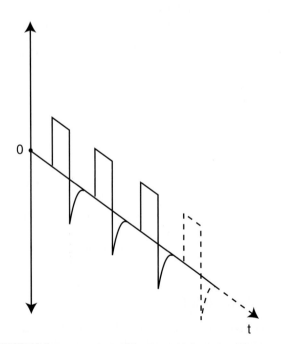

FIGURE 14-4 Typical pulsed, biphasic, and balanced current waveforms delivered from modern TENS devices. Note that the waveforms are not drawn to scale to show balance.

of single pulses over time, as discussed and illustrated in **Figure 14-5A**.

d. Number of Pulses Per Burst
The number of pulses per burst varies from one TENS unit to the next. For example, shown in **Figure 14-5B** is a burst made of five pulses.

e. Burst/Interburst Duration
Burst duration (BuD) is the time elapsed from the beginning to the termination of one burst, whereas the interburst duration (IBuD) is the duration between two bursts (**Fig 14-5B**).

f. Burst Frequency
Burst frequency (f), expressed in bursts per second (bups), is calculated on the basis of the following formula: f = 1/ (BuD + IBuD). Let us consider the following example: A BuD of 50 ms coupled with an IBuD of 150 ms yields a burst frequency of 5 bups. Burst frequency in most TENS units is low, ranging between 1 and 10 bups, and the number of pulses per burst often ranges between 5 and 10 pulses.

3. Current Amplitude
Current amplitude refers to the magnitude of current delivered by the TENS unit and is measured in milliamps (mA). In most TENS stimulators, current amplitude varies between 0 and 120 mA. Such a range of current amplitude is more than necessary to depolarize all peripheral nerve fibers within and through the skin.

D. CONSTANT CURRENT STIMULATOR

TENS devices are constant current-type (CC-type) stimulators, meaning that the set current amplitude (say, 80 mA read on the digital meter) remains constant (hence the term constant current) during treatment, regardless of changes in tissue impedance over time (see Chapter 5). The main advantage of CC-type stimulators is that they deliver predictable levels of electrical stimulation, making therapy more comfortable for the patient (no surge of current).

IV. PHYSIOLOGICAL AND THERAPEUTIC EFFECTS

A. PAIN MODULATION

There is a substantial body of evidence to suggest that the selective, or preferential, depolarization of specific groups of afferent nerve fibers, as illustrated in **Figure 14-6**, affects two key pain modulation systems, known as the *gate* and *opiate* systems (Lundeberg, 1995; Mayer et al., 1995; Walsh, 1997; Barr, 1999; McMahon et al., 2005). The physiological and therapeutic effect of TENS therapy, as

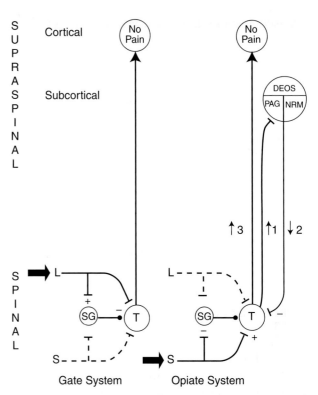

FIGURE 14-6 Schematic representation of both the gate and the opiate system of pain modulation in relation to TENS therapy (see text). DEOS, descending endogenous opiate system; L, large fibers; NRM, nucleus raphe magnus; PAG, periaquaductal gray matter; S, small fibers; SG, substantia gelatinosa; T, pain-transmitting cells; 1, excitatory synapse; 2, inhibitory synapse; arrow L, preferential electrical stimulation of large-diameter sensory fibers (A beta); arrow S, preferential electrical stimulation of small-diameter sensory fibers (A delta and C); arrows 1 and 2, negative feedback loop; arrow 3, pathway to the brain.

shown in **Figure 14-7**, is for the management of pain. Prior to considering the following material, readers are *strongly* advised to review Chapter 3, which deals with the topics of pain modulation and pain assessment and scoring.

1. Pain-Afferent Nerve Fibers
Research has shown that three peripheral afferent nerve fibers, or axons, namely, the larger-diameter *A-beta* and smaller-diameter *A-delta* and C fibers, play a major role in the process of pain modulation (McMahon et al., 2005; see Chapter 3).

a. Large A-Beta Fibers
These large-diameter nerve fibers are mechanosensitive in nature, carrying information from mechanoreceptors responsible for touch and vibration to the brain (McMahon et al., 2005).

b. Small C and A-Delta Fibers
These two smaller-diameter nerve fibers are nociceptive in nature, carrying information from nociceptors (nerve-free endings) buried in soft tissues to the brain (McMahon et al., 2005; DeLeo, 2006).

TRANSCUTANEOUS ELECTRICAL NERVE STIMULATION THERAPY

Electrical energy

Peripheral nerve depolarization

Sensory nerve   Motor nerve   Nociceptive nerve

Gate system   **Opiate system**

Gate closing

Pain modulation

Pain management

FIGURE 14-7 The proposed physiological and therapeutic effects of TENS therapy.

2. Dorsal Horn

Neurophysiologic studies have demonstrated that these peripheral afferent nerve fibers travel toward the dorsal horn of the spinal cord (**Fig 14-6**) to make synaptic contacts with key neurons and interneurons known to play an important role in pain modulation (Melzack et al., 1965; Sluka et al., 2003; McMahon et al., 2005).

B. GATE SYSTEM

The gate control system, proposed by Melzack and Wall in 1965, states that peripheral neural inputs from A-beta, A-delta, and C fibers into the dorsal horn will decrease or increase the flow of impulses to higher processing centers in the brain. In other words, this system implies,

as illustrated in **Figure 14-6**, the action of a spinal gating system, where the gate may be closed (decreased input) or open (increased input), depending on the net neural input coming from the peripheral A-beta, A-delta, and C fibers. When the gate is closed it means that no nociceptive inputs can reach the brain, resulting in pain relief. How can TENS close this gate?

1. Gate Closing

Research (see McMahon et al., 2005) has shown that gate closing is associated with the preferential evoked activity or depolarization (*indicated by the large bolded arrow*) of the peripheral large-diameter A-beta fiber (*designated by the letter L for large*) over the smaller-diameter A-delta and C fibers (*designated by the letter S for small*) (**Fig 14-6**), According to the gate control theory of pain, preferential activity in these large (L) fibers is presumed to activate inhibitory interneurons located in the substantia gelatinosa (SG) of the dorsal horn of the spinal cord. Activation of these inhibitory interneurons results in the inhibition of pain-transmitting cells, called T (transmission) cells, located in the dorsal horn of the spinal cord. Inhibition of T cells causes the gate to close, thus preventing nociceptive inputs to reach the supraspinal level (subcortical and cortical). The end result is no perceived pain.

2. Preferential Nerve Fiber Depolarization

Research has shown that selective, or preferential, depolarization of sensory, motor, and nociceptive nerve fibers using TENS may be achieved through appropriate settings of the following two key electrical parameters: current amplitude and pulse duration (see McMahon et al., 2005). The interaction between these two stimulation parameters is illustrated in the classical nerve strength/duration curve (S/D curve) presented in **Figure 14-8**. The term *strength* (S) is synonymous with current amplitude, measured in

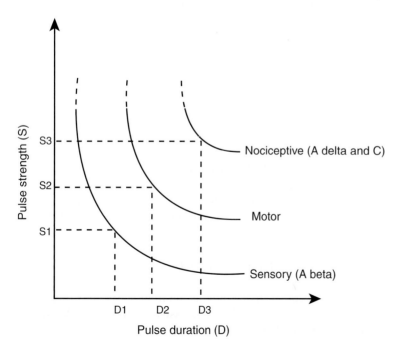

FIGURE 14-8 The classical strength/duration (S/D) curve on which the preferential, electrically evoked depolarization of one group of nerve fibers is made possible during TENS therapy. By selecting a given combination of pulse current amplitude or strength (S) and pulse duration (D), such as seen with S1-D1, S2-D2, and S3-D3 combinations, the preferential depolarization of sensory-only, sensory-motor-only, and sensory-motor-nociceptive nerve fibers can be achieved.

mA, and the term *duration* (D) corresponds to pulse duration, measured in microseconds.

a. Sensory-Level Stimulation

With a combination of low current amplitude (S) and short pulse duration (D), as illustrated by the S1–D1 combination in **Figure 14-8**, preferential depolarization of large-diameter sensory fibers, such as A-beta fibers, is theoretically possible. Preferential sensory stimulation (S1–D1) is clinically confirmed when the patient reports sensations of pins and needles and tingling, with no sensation of muscle contraction under the stimulating electrode, and no pain. This sensory stimulation, below the motor and nociceptive threshold, is perceived as comfortable. Sensory threshold stimulation causes the depolarization of large-diameter A-delta fibers.

b. Motor-Level Stimulation

Combinations of higher current amplitudes (S) and longer pulse durations (D), as illustrated by the S2–D2 combination, leads to the concomitant preferential depolarization of large-diameter afferent sensory (A-beta), and large-diameter efferent motor nerve fibers (alpha), causing muscle contraction (**Fig 14-8**). Preferential stimulation of these two types of fibers (S2–D2) can be clinically confirmed when the patient feels a mixed sensation of tingling combined with muscle contraction, without pain. Practitioners can confirm the patient's motor sensation by visualizing or palpating the evoked muscle contraction during stimulation.

c. Noxious-Level Stimulation

Combinations of still higher current amplitudes (S) and longer pulse durations (D), as illustrated by the S3–D3 combination, will lead to the concomitant depolarization of all three nerve fibers, namely, sensory (A-beta), motor (alpha), and nociceptive (A-delta and C fibers) (**Fig 14-8**). This level of stimulation can be clinically confirmed when the patient experiences a strong and mixed sensation of muscle contraction and pain during stimulation. In other words, this level of stimulation is present when a muscle contraction is clearly apparent and when the patient describes the electrically evoked sensation as being just below the threshold of being intolerable, or too painful.

3. Gate Opening

As stated previously, TENS may either close or open the gate. For a patient to perceive pain, on the basis of Melzack and Wall's gate control theory, the spinal gate must be open, that is, T cells must be depolarized or activated, so that nociceptive inputs reach the brain (cortical level), where pain is decoded. How can TENS decrease pain while opening the gate further? Can TENS open the gate and by what mechanism is pain modulation achieved? The gate control theory stipulates that TENS opens the gate, as illustrated in **Figure 14-6**, through the preferential depolarization (*indicated by the large bolded arrow*) of the peripheral afferent smaller-diameter A-delta and C fibers (*designated by the letter S for small*) over the larger-diameter (*designated by the letter L for large*) A-beta fibers. This opening of the gate, as shown in **Figure 14-6**, allows T-cells to depolarize, sending nociceptive inputs to key subcortical neural structures, which activate another pain-modulating system, commonly called the opiate system.

C. OPIATE SYSTEM

There is a substantial body of evidence (McMahon et al., 2005) to suggest that the human body possesses its own pain-modulation system, known as the descending endogenous opiate system (DEOS). This system, schematized in **Figure 14-6**, operates at the supraspinal level and involves neurohumonal activity from particular subcortical areas, such as the periaqueductal gray matter (PAG) and the nucleus raphe magnus (NRM).

1. Descending Endogenous Opiate System

The term *descending* indicates that this system operates in a descending fashion, from the supraspinal to the spinal levels. The term *endogenous opiate* indicates that pain modulation occurs through the release of opiate-like substances secreted by the body itself. These endogenous opiate substances are known by the generic term endorphins.

2. Preferential A-Delta and C Fiber Depolarization

As shown in **Figure 14-6**, the preferential depolarization of the nociceptive smaller-diameter (see bold arrow pointing to S) A-delta and C fibers *opens* the spinal gate by inducing a powerful inhibitory effect on the inhibitory neurons contained in the SG. The resulting T-cell depolarization triggers a negative feedback loop within the DEOS that will lead to pain modulation or relief.

3. Negative Feedback Loop

This feedback loop, represented by arrows (1, 2, and 3) in **Figure 14-6**, is said to be negative because it begins with T-cell depolarization (arrow 1) and ends with T-cell inhibition (arrow 2) and pain relief (arrow 3) as more and more endogenous opiate substances are secreted within the suffering patient's blood plasma and cerebrospinal fluid (Mayer et al., 1995).

4. Naloxone Test

That pain is modulated through an endogenous opiate system in humans was demonstrated by numerous studies on the use of naloxone, a potent antagonist to exogenous and endogenous opiates (Mannheimer et al., 1984; McMahon et al., 2005). Theoretically speaking, pain modulation is mediated through the opiate system when TENS-induced analgesia is reversed after injection of naloxone. If TENS-induced analgesia is not reversed by naloxone, then pain modulation is presumed to occur through other pain-modulating mechanisms, most likely through the spinal gate system described earlier.

D. RECAP

TENS-induced analgesia can occur through the spinal gate system or the DEOS. Modulation of pain via the spinal gate system implies the closing of the gate by the preferential electrical activation of large-diameter afferent A-beta fibers. Modulation of pain via the opiate system, on the other hand, implies the opening of the spinal gate by the preferential electrical activation of small-diameter A-delta and C fibers. This gate opening triggers the opiate system, which, via its negative loop, closes the gate by releasing more endorphins in the body.

V. DOSIMETRY

A. TENS MODES

The dosimetry of TENS therapy is primarily based on the selection of one of the following five modes of delivery: conventional, acupuncture-like, brief-intense, burst, and modulation (Walsh, 1997; Barr, 1999; Foley, 2000). Each mode, as illustrated in **Table 14-1**, may be characterized on the basis of three stimulation parameters (pulse/burst duration, pulse/burst frequency, and current amplitude) and four physiological and therapeutic correlates (preferential fiber depolarization, preferential mechanism

behind pain relief, onset of analgesia, and duration of analgesia).

1. Conventional TENS

This mode involves delivery of electrical pulses with relatively short durations, high frequencies, and with current amplitudes corresponding to sensory-level stimulation (**Table 14-1**). It is called *conventional* because, by convention or clinical experience, clinicians usually select this mode to begin TENS therapy as it is perceived by most patients as the most comfortable of all modes. This mode implies the preferential depolarization of large-diameter A-beta fibers using current amplitudes and pulse durations within the sensory-level range (see **Figure 14-7**). Electrical stimulation is perceived as comfortable (pins and needles; tingling; no muscle contraction), and pain modulation occurs through the gate system. The onset of analgesia is relatively rapid, and analgesia itself is relatively brief.

2. Acupuncture-like TENS

This mode refers to the delivery of electrical pulses with relatively long durations, low frequencies, and with current amplitudes capable of sensory- and motor-level stimulation (**Table 14-1**). It is described as *acupuncture-like* because the pulse frequency is low, resembling traditional needle acupuncture therapy, in which the practitioner

TABLE 14-1	BIOPHYSICAL AND PHYSIOLOGICAL ASPECTS OF CLASSIC MODES OF TRANSCUTANEOUS ELECTRICAL NERVE STIMULATION THERAPY				
	CONVENTIONAL	**ACUPUNCTURE-LIKE**	**BRIEF-INTENSE**	**BURST**	**MODULATION**
Pulse duration	Short (<150 ms)	Long (>150 ms)	Long (>150 ms)	N/A	Variable
Frequency	High (>80 Hz)	Low (<10 Hz)	High (>80 Hz)	Low (<10 bups)	Variable
Current amplitude	Comfortable / Sensory level	Comfortable/ tolerable / Sensory / motor level	Tolerable / Noxious level	Comfortable / Sensory / motor level	Variable
Nerve fibers preferentially depolarized	A-beta	A-delta and C	A-delta and C	A-delta and C	Variable
Preferential mechanism for pain modulation	Gate	Opiate	Opiate	Opiate	Variable
Onset of analgesia	Rapid (within minutes)	Slow (within hours)	Rapid (within minutes)	Slow (within hours)	Variable
Duration of analgesia	Brief (<few hours)	Long (>few hours)	Long (>few hours)	Long (>few hours)	Variable

slowly rotates the needle in the patient's skin. This mode implies the preferential and concomitant depolarization of afferent large-diameter A-beta and efferent alpha motor fibers innervating skeletal muscles. Electrical stimulation is perceived as tolerable as well as a mixed sensation of tingling and muscle contraction. Pain is presumed to occur via the opiate system. Onset of analgesia is relatively slow, and analgesia is sustained for a relatively long period.

3. Brief-Intense TENS

This mode involves the delivery of electrical pulses with relatively long durations, high frequencies, and with current amplitudes capable of noxious stimulation (**Table 14-1**). It is described as *brief-intense* because durations of application are briefer and current amplitudes much higher, or more intense, than in the other modes, triggering a somewhat brief yet intense, and sometimes painful, stimulation during therapy. This mode implies the preferential depolarization of all nerve fibers (A-beta, A-delta, and C fibers), causing a mixed sensation of strong muscle contraction and maximum tolerable pain. Pain modulation occurs through the opiate system. The onset of analgesia is relatively rapid, and analgesia is sustained for a relatively long period.

4. Burst TENS

This mode refers to the delivery of bursts of pulses (not individual pulses as in the first three modes) of relatively low burst frequencies, with current amplitudes capable of sensory and motor stimulation (**Table 14-1**). It is described as *burst* to emphasize the use of bursts of pulses rather than individual pulses. This mode implies the preferential depolarization of sensory A-delta and motor alpha fibers. Electrical stimulation is felt as a mixed sensation of tingling and moderate motor contraction. Pain modulation occurs through the opiate system. The onset of analgesia is relatively slow, and analgesia is sustained for a relatively long period.

5. Modulation TENS

This mode calls upon the random electronic modulation (cycles of increasing and decreasing values) of pulse duration, pulse frequency, and current amplitude (**Table 14-1**). It is called *modulation* because one, or two, or all three stimulation parameters are electronically and randomly modulated at the same time during therapy (for details see current modulation, Chapter 5.) This mode is presumed to decrease brain (sensation) and nerve (depolarization) *habituation* to electrical input. Because there is a variable modulation (cycles of increasing and decreasing values), variability is expected to occur with regard to the types of fibers preferentially depolarized and the pain modulation present, as well as the onset and duration of analgesia.

B. WHICH MODE IS BEST?

The current body of evidence does not support the view that one mode of TENS delivery is better than any other for any painful pathological conditions. Evidence obtained from long-term users of TENS therapy reveals no correlation between patient, site, and cause of pain versus TENS mode selection (Johnson et al., 1991). The selection of one mode in preference to the other, therefore, is still based on trial and error and the patient's comfort during therapy (Johnson et al., 1991). This explains why the general recommendation is to begin therapy with the conventional mode, because it is perceived as being more comfortable than the other four modes of TENS. Review articles by Bjordal et al. (2003) and Johnson et al. (2007) suggest that TENS therapy, regardless of mode of delivery, can provide significant pain relief and, as a result, presents as a viable alternative to drug and surgical therapy.

VI. EVIDENCE FOR INDICATIONS

A. GUIDED BY EVIDENCE

Dictionaries generally define *evidence* as anything that establishes a fact or gives reason to believe something. The aim of this textbook is to present *scientific* evidence on therapeutic EPAs. To be guided by the evidence is the process of integrating evidence from research, however imperfect or scarce this evidence may be, with clinical experience and patients' values. In other words, the *evidence-based practice* of EPA requires that practitioners consider the evidence from research, in addition to their own clinical experience and patients' own preference and beliefs about a given EPA, when the time comes to justify, prescribe, and apply the therapeutic agent. To be guided by evidence is a process, not a search for the absolute truth. Finally, a lack of evidence from research in support of any given EPA does not mean that this EPA should never be used. What it means is that no statement can be made about its therapeutic effectiveness and that until more evidence from research is presented, its routine use cannot be recommended.

B. EVIDENCE FROM HUMAN RESEARCH

Box 14-1 provides evidence for TENS therapy based on an exhaustive search of published English-language, peer-reviewed studies on humans. The term *indication* is used in reference to a list of pathologies for which TENS therapy is employed. Ratings of clinical benefit (Yes or No) and grading of strength of scientific evidence (I, II, or III), including the reference, are included for each pathological condition.

1. Rating Therapeutic Benefit

The rating, expressed as Yes or No, is based on the overall conclusion(s) reached on the issue of therapeutic effectiveness by the author(s) who conducted the peer-reviewed study.

Box 14-1	**Research-Based Indications for the Use of Transcutaneous Electrical Nerve Stimulation**

PATHOLOGY	BENEFIT	GRADE	REFERENCE
Postoperative abdominal pain	Yes	I	Cooperman et al., 1977
	Yes	I	Vander Ark et al., 1975
	Yes	I	Smith et al., 1986
	Yes	I	Hargreaves et al., 1989
	Yes	I	Hollinger, 1986
	Yes	I	Chen et al., 1998
	Yes	I	Sims, 1991
	Yes	I	Rosenberg et al., 1978
	Yes	I	Solomon et al., 1980
	Yes	I	Hamza et al., 1999
	Yes	II	Torres et al., 1992
	Yes	II	Hymes et al., 1974
	Yes	II	Caterine et al., 1988
	Yes	II	Ali et al., 1981
	Yes	II	Bussey et al., 1981
	Yes	II	Merril, 1987
	Yes	II	Merril, 1988
	Yes	II	Merril, 1989
	Yes	II	Schomburg et al., 1983
	No	I	Galloway et al., 1984
	No	I	Cuschieri et al., 1985
	No	I	Conn et al., 1986
	No	I	Reynolds et al., 1987
	No	I	Rawatt et al., 1991
	No	I	Taylor et al., 1983
	No	I	Laitinen et al., 1991
	No	I	Reuss et al., 1988
	No	I	Smedley et al., 1988
	No	I	Gilbert et al., 1986
Low-back pain	Yes	I	Melzack et al., 1983
	Yes	I	Cheing et al., 1999
	Yes	I	Gemignani et al., 1991
	Yes	I	Bertalanffy et al., 2005
	Yes	II	Bates et al., 1980
	Yes	II	Magora et al., 1983
	Yes	II	Woolf et al., 1978
	Yes	II	Fried et al., 1984
	Yes	II	Brill et al., 1985
	Yes	II	Fox et al., 1976
	Yes	II	Ersek et al., 1976
	Yes	II	Laitinen, 1976
	Yes	II	Rutkowski et al., 1977
	Yes	II	Ersek, 1977
	Yes	II	Loeser et al., 1975
	Yes	II	Ebersold et al., 1975
	No	I	Lehmann et al., 1986
	No	I	Deyo et al., 1990
	No	I	Melzack et al., 1980
	No	I	Marchand et al., 1993
	No	I	Herman et al., 1994
	No	I	Warke et al., 2006
	No	II	Indeck et al., 1975
	No	II	Pope et al., 1994

(Continued)

| Box 14-1 | Continued |

PATHOLOGY	BENEFIT	GRADE	REFERENCE
Labor and postlabor pain	Yes	I	Harrison et al., 1987
	Yes	I	Mannheimer et al., 1985
	Yes	I	Grim et al., 1985
	Yes	I	Chao et al., 2007
	Yes	II	Bundsen et al., 1981
	Yes	II	Bundsen et al., 1982
	Yes	II	Augustinsson et al., 1977
	Yes	II	Kaplan et al., 1998
	Yes	II	Bortoluzzi, 1989
	Yes	II	Olsen et al., 2007
	Yes	III	Keenan et al., 1985
	No	I	Harrison et al., 1986
	No	I	Lee et al., 1990
	No	I	Vander Ploeg et al., 1996
	No	I	Thomas et al., 1988
	No	I	Erkkola et al., 1980
	No	I	Chia et al., 1990
	No	I	Nesheim, 1981
Postoperative thoracic pain	Yes	I	Bayindir et al., 1991
	Yes	I	Navarathnam et al., 1984
	Yes	I	Warfield et al., 1985
	Yes	I	Benedetti et al., 1997
	Yes	I	Rooney et al., 1983
	Yes	I	Erdogan et al., 2005
	Yes	II	Ho et al., 1987
	Yes	II	Neary, 1981
	Yes	II	Klin et al., 1984
	Yes	III	Carrol et al., 2001
	No	I	Foster et al., 1994
	No	I	Stubbing et al., 1988
	No	I	Lim et al., 1983
Chronic pain syndromes	Yes	II	Bates et al., 1980
	Yes	II	Fishbain et al., 1996
	Yes	II	Abram et al., 1981
	Yes	II	Tulgar et al., 1991
	Yes	II	Guieu et al., 1991
	Yes	II	Chabal et al., 1998
	Yes	II	Long, 1974
	Yes	II	Meyler et al., 1994
	Yes	II	Eriksson et al., 1979
	Yes	II	Loeser et al., 1975
	Yes	II	Koke et al., 2004
	No	I	Oosterhof et al., 2006
Osteoarthritis pain	Yes	I	Taylor et al., 1981
	Yes	I	Fargas-Babjak et al., 1989
	Yes	I	Smith, Lewith, et al., 1983
	Yes	I	Grimmer, 1992
	Yes	I	Lewis et al., 1984
	Yes	I	Zizic et al., 1995
	Yes	I	Cheing et al., 2003

(Continued)

Box 14-1   **Continued**

PATHOLOGY	BENEFIT	GRADE	REFERENCE
	Yes	II	Yurtkuran et al., 1999
	Yes	II	Paker et al., 2006
	No	I	Lewis et al., 1994
	No	I	Law et al., 2004
	No	I	Cheing et al., 2002
	No	II	Fargas-Babjak et al., 1992
	No	II	Jensen et al., 1991
Dysmenorrheal pain	Yes	I	Lundeberg et al., 1985
	Yes	I	Dawood et al., 1990
	Yes	I	Mannheimer et al., 1985
	Yes	I	Milsom et al., 1994
	Yes	I	Neighbors et al., 1987
	Yes	I	Lewers et al., 1989
	Yes	II	Smith et al., 1991
	Yes	II	Kaplan et al., 1994
	Yes	II	Kaplan et al., 1997
	Yes	II	Schietz et al., 2007
Rheumatoid arthritis pain	Yes	I	Abelson et al., 1983
	Yes	II	Mannheimer et al., 1979
	Yes	II	Mannheimer et al., 1978
	Yes	II	Bruce et al., 1988
	Yes	II	Kumar et al., 1982
	No	I	Langley et al., 1984
	No	I	Moystad et al., 1990
Postoperative orthopedic pain	Yes	I	Arvidsson et al., 1986
	Yes	I	Jensen et al., 1985
	Yes	I	Cornell et al., 1984
	Yes	I	Finsen et al., 1988
	Yes	II	Harvie, 1979
	Yes	II	Smith, Hutchins, et al., 1983
	Yes	III	Gyori et al., 1977
Orofacial pain	Yes	I	Hansson et al., 1983
	Yes	II	Hansson et al., 1986
	Yes	II	Pike, 1978
	Yes	II	Stabile et al., 1978
	Yes	II	Eriksson et al., 1984
	Yes	III	Murphy, 1990
Postoperative spinal pain	Yes	I	Solomon et al., 1980
	Yes	II	Schuster et al., 1980
	Yes	II	Issenman et al., 1985
	No	II	McCallum et al., 1988
Painful spasticity	Yes	I	Levin et al., 1992
	Yes	I	Potisk et al., 1995
	Yes	II	Bajd et al., 1985
	No	I	Miller et al., 2007

(Continued)

Box 14-1 Continued

PATHOLOGY	BENEFIT	GRADE	REFERENCE
Total joint replacement pain	No	I	Walker et al., 1991
	No	I	Angulo et al., 1990
	No	I	Breit et al., 2004
Phantom pain	Yes	II	Katz et al., 1991
	Yes	II	Carabelli et al., 1985
	Yes	II	Miles et al., 1978
Painful peripheral neuropathies	Yes	I	Thorsteinsson et al., 1977
	Yes	II	Bohm, 1978
	Yes	III	Somers et al., 1999
Dental pain	Yes	I	Harvey et al., 1995
	Yes	I	Meechan et al., 1998
	No	II	Oztas et al., 1997
Migraine/headache	Yes	I	Solomon et al., 1980
	Yes	II	Jay et al., 1989
Trigeminal neuralgia	Yes	I	Taylor et al., 1993
	Yes	III	Thorsen et al., 1997
Painful stroke arm dysfunction	Yes	I	Sonde et al., 1998
	Yes	II	Tekeoglu et al., 1998
Painful reflex sympathetic dystrophy	Yes	II	Robaina et al., 1989
	Yes	III	Ashwal et al., 1988
Myofascial pain	Yes	I	Graff-Radford et al., 1989
	No	I	Kruger et al., 1998
Detrusor muscle pain	Yes	II	Okada et al., 1998
	Yes	II	Hasan et al., 1996
Acute posttraumatic pain	Yes	I	Ordog, 1987
	Yes	II	Sloan et al., 1986
Painful Sudeck's atrophy	Yes	III	Bodenheim et al., 1983
Central pain	No	II	Leijon et al., 1989
Whiplash dystonic pain	Yes	III	Foley-Nolan et al., 1990
Hemorrhoidectomy pain	Yes	I	Chiu et al., 1999
Painful open perineal lesions	Yes	III	Merkel et al., 1999
Neck pain	Yes	I	Nordemar et al., 1981
Painful shoulder	Yes	I	Leandri et al., 1990
Brachial plexus pain	Yes	III	Frampton, 1996
Postherpetic neuralgia	Yes	II	Nathan et al., 1974

(Continued)

Box 14-1 Continued

PATHOLOGY	BENEFIT	GRADE	REFERENCE
Paraplegic pain	Yes	II	Richardson et al., 1980
Unstable angina pectoris pain	Yes	I	Borjesson et al., 1997
Chronic intractable angina	Yes	II	Nitz et al., 1993
Temporomandibular pain	No	II	Linde et al., 1995
Renal colic pain	Yes	I	Mora et al., 2006
Posttraumatic hip pain	Yes	I	Lang et al., 2007
Diabetic neuropathy	Yes	III	Somers et al., 1999

2. Grading Strength of Evidence

The grading, numerically classified as I, II and III, is based on the type of research methodology, or experimental design used by the author(s). All those listed are studies on humans published in English-language, peer-reviewed journals. It follows that the evidence in studies graded I is stronger than in those graded II and the evidence in studies graded II are stronger than in those graded III.

a. Grade I

Evidence based on *controlled* studies on humans, regardless of their level of randomization and blindness.

b. Grade II

Evidence based on *non-controlled* studies on humans, regardless of their level of randomization and blindness.

c. Grade III

Evidence based on *case* studies on humans, regardless of their level of randomization and blindness.

3. Strength of Evidence Behind the Agent

The strength of evidence behind the agent, as presented in the research-based indication box, is arbitrarily assessed in this textbook as *weak, moderate,* or *strong*. For example, the larger the number of studies graded I, regardless of therapeutic benefit, the stronger the scientific evidence in support of the agent.

4. Evidence Justifying Usage of Agent

The strength of evidence justifying the usage of an agent for an individual pathology or groups of pathologies, as listed in the research-based indication box, is arbitrarily assessed in this textbook as *poor, fair, good,* or *conflicting*. For example, where a larger number of grade I studies show therapeutic benefit (Yes) than no benefit, for a given pathology, the justification for the usage of this agent for that pathology is assessed as *good*. A *conflicting* usage is reported when an equal number of studies with similar grades show therapeutic benefit (Yes) and no benefit (No).

C. STRENGTH OF EVIDENCE AND JUSTIFICATION FOR USAGE

The results presented in **Box 14-1** show *moderate-to-strong* strength of evidence for TENS therapy, with practically all studies graded as I and II. These results also show *conflicting* evidence for the use of this EPA for postoperative abdominal pain, low-back pain, and labor and postlabor pain, with a relatively equal number of studies showing therapeutic benefit and no benefit. They also show *good* evidence in support of the use of TENS therapy for the management of postoperative thoracic pain, chronic pain syndromes, osteoarthritis pain, dysmenorrheal pain, postoperative orthopedic pain, and orofacial pain. **Box 14-1** also reveals *poor-to-fair* evidence for the use of this EPA for the remaining pathologies listed. Until more evidence from research is provided with regard to those remaining pathologies listed, or any other pathology, the routine use of TENS therapy for such pathologies *cannot be recommended*.

VII. CONTRAINDICATIONS

A. HEART ELECTRONIC IMPLANTS

Table 14-2 shows the contraindications associated with the practice of TENS therapy. The issue related to the application of TENS on people wearing implanted *pacemakers* and *implanted cardioverter defibrillators* (ICDs) deserves particular attention because of the continued controversy about this subject (Eriksson et al., 1978; Kimberley et al., 1987; Hauptman et al., 1992; Sliwa et al., 1996; Weitz et al., 1997; Glotzer et al., 1998; Philbin et al., 1998; Curwin et al., 1999; Broadley, 2000).

TABLE 14-2	CONTRAINDICATIONS TO TRANSCUTANEOUS ELECTRICAL NERVE STIMULATION THERAPY
CONTRAINDICATIONS	**RATIONALE**
Over the anterior cervical area	Risk of stimulating key organs, such as the vagus nerve, phrenic nerve, and carotid sinuses, resulting in adverse effects such as hypotensive reaction and laryngeal spasm.
Over the thoracic region	Risk of affecting normal heart function. Stimulation over intercostal muscles led to a respiratory failure in one cardiac patient (Mann, 1996).
Over the cranial area	Risk of affecting normal brain function.
With patients wearing rate-responsive pacemakers	Risk of interference with normal functioning of the device (Eriksson et al., 1978; Rasmussen et al., 1988; Marples, 2000). *Important note*: TENS may be used with these patients *only* after cardiac monitoring during TENS, by means of an ECG, reveals no interference (Chen et al., 1990). If no such cardiac monitoring is available in your working facility, *obtain authorization from the patient's treating cardiologist before using TENS.*
With patients wearing cardioverter defibrillators (ICDs)	Risk of interference with normal functioning of the device (Glotzer et al., 1998; Philbin et al., 1998; Pyatt et al., 2003; Siu et al., 2005; Occheta et al., 2006; Holmgren et al., 2008). *Important note*: TENS may be used with these patients *only* if the ICU unit is *turned off* during therapy (Glotzer, 1999).
Over the abdominal, pelvic, or lumbar areas of pregnant women in their first trimester	Risk of inducing labor.
Over metal implants	Risk of causing unnecessary pain due to electrical current-induced overheating of implants.
With epileptic patients	Risk of causing an epileptic episode (Scherder et al., 1999).
Over hemorrhagic area	Risk of enhanced bleeding due to increased blood flow in the treated area.
Over a malignant area	Risk of increasing and spreading the tumor due to increased blood flow in the treated area.
Over damaged skin	Risk of causing unnecessary and severe pain.

1. Pacemakers

These electronic devices are prescribed for people of all ages who have an abnormal heart rate (e.g., slower or faster than average, or irregular beating patterns). Their purpose is to assure a normal heart rate, or to pace the heart. There are several models of pacemakers on the market today. For example, *Medtronic Inc.*, one of the leading manufacturers of pacemakers in the world, offers six different categories of pacemakers that cardiologists and heart surgeons can choose from to treat their cardiac patients. There are presently two basic *types* of pacemakers commonly implanted in cardiac patients: fixed and rate responsive.

a. Fixed Type

Early pacemakers were of the fixed type, also known as asynchronous type, in that they continuously paced the heart at a set fixed rate. These pacemakers have been shown to be *unaffected* by TENS application (Jones, 1976; Eriksson et al., 1978; Shade, 1985; Rasmussen et al., 1988; Chen et al., 1990). The use of TENS, therefore, is not contraindicated for patients with implanted fixed-type pacemakers.

b. Rate-Responsive Type

Newer pacemakers are of the rate-responsive type, also known as synchronous or demand type (see www.medtronic.com). This type of pacemaker is needed when a heart cannot appropriately increase its rate according to a person's needs. This pacemaker varies the pacing rate depending upon a person's level of activity, respiration, or other factors. Most pacemakers implanted today are rate responsive because they respond to the body's needs, similar to how a healthy heart works. The pacemaker automatically adjusts the pacing rate to match the level of activity, including periods of time during which the patient is at rest or sleeping. Rate-responsive pacemakers, unfortunately, *can be affected* by TENS (Jones, 1976; Eriksson et al., 1978; Chen et al., 1990). Medtronic Inc., on their Web site, lists the use of TENS under precaution, meaning that there could be electronic interference in the pacemaker due to the electrical field generated by the TENS unit (www.medtronic.com). This interference means that no pacing beat, or extra pacing beats, may be generated by the pacemaker, thus seriously affecting heart function. Considering that the patient's safety always come first, this textbook states that the use of TENS on patients wearing rate-responsive pacemakers is *contraindicated, unless* a screening heart monitoring test, using ECG, reveals no interference during TENS application (see **Table 14-2**). Although testing heart and pacemaker functions by monitoring ECG during TENS application must be done as a screening test, research has shown that TENS may cause ECG artifacts that may be *wrongly* interpreted as pacemaker dysfunction (Kimberley et al., 1987; Hauptman et al., 1992; Sliwa et al., 1996; Weitz et al., 1997; Marples, 2000). This finding only reinforces the need to have the treating cardiologist's authorization before considering TENS therapy in these patients.

2. Cardioverter Defibrillators

These devices are prescribed for people who have a faster-than-normal heart rate, or tachycardia, as well as for patients suffering from ventricular fibrillation. For example, when tachycardia occurs, the implanted ICD device immediately delivers a mild shock to the heart, redirecting its rhythm to a normal beating pattern. Interference between TENS and ICDs has been reported in numerous case reports (Glotzer et al., 1998; Philbin et al., 1998; Pyatt et al., 2003; Siu et al., 2005; Occheta et al., 2006; Holmgren et al., 2008). Consequently, the use of TENS in patients with ICDs is *contraindicated, unless* the unit is *turned off* during the application (see **Table 14-2**).

B. MANUFACTURER'S SAFETY RECOMMENDATIONS

To ensure maximal safety during TENS therapy with patients wearing pacemakers or ICDs, practitioners should always refer to the manufacturers' lists of contraindications, precautions, and warnings regarding the use of this therapeutic agent with such devices.

VIII. RISKS, PRECAUTIONS, AND RECOMMENDATIONS

The practice of TENS therapy is not without risks for the patient. The main risks associated with this electrophysical agent, including some precautions and recommendations designed to improve safety and effectiveness, are listed in **Table 14-3**.

IX. CONSIDERATIONS FOR APPLICATION AND DOCUMENTATION

A. CONSIDERATIONS AND PROCEDURES

The safe, effective, and optimal application of this electrophysiological agent requires that clinicians go through a systematic set of considerations and procedures for each and every application. Presented below is a list of such considerations and procedures.

1. Checklists

Before going ahead with treatment, always go through the list of contraindications (**Table 14-2**) and the list of risks, precautions, and recommendations (**Table 14-3**).

2. Skin Preparation

Before each application, cleanse the skin surface in the area of the stimulating electrode with rubbing alcohol to remove impurities and reduce skin impedance.

TABLE 14-3	**RISKS, PRECAUTIONS, AND RECOMMENDATIONS FOR TRANSCUTANEOUS ELECTRICAL NERVE STIMULATION**
RISKS	**RATIONALE**
Prolonged use of electrode, electroconductive gel, and adhesive tape over the same skin areas	Risk of causing contact dermatitis from the materials the electrode, gel, and adhesive tape are made of (Fisher, 1978; Zugerman, 1982; Bolton, 1983, 1999; Castelain et al., 1986; Marren et al., 1991; Dwyer et al., 1994; Meuleman et al., 1996; Corazza et al., 1999).
Usage near functioning shortwave diathermy (SWD) device	Risk of causing electronic interference. A patient reporting a sudden and variable surge of current output when an SWD unit is functioning in the neighborhood may be indicative of such electronic interference.

(Continued)

TABLE 14-3	CONTINUED

PRECAUTIONS	RATIONALE
With confused and unreliable patients	May result in unreliable information, which may have a negative impact on treatment effectiveness.
Home TENS therapy	Instruct patients to keep the portable TENS unit out of the reach of children at all time.

RECOMMENDATIONS	RATIONALE
Clean and dry exposed skin surface areas before each treatment	To reduce skin impedance significantly as well as to remove impurities, and thus allow an optimal electrical coupling at the skin–electrode interface.
Clip hair over exposed skin areas	To ensure optimal electrode–skin coupling.
Wash and dry reusable electrodes after each treatment	To ensure optimal performance; follow the manufacturer's instructions.
Check electrode impedance monthly	To ensure appropriate electrode impedance for optimal conduction, because electrodes will deteriorate with use and time. Use an ohm-meter to check impedance.
Monitor the patient's medication	To allow practitioners to determine if the observed analgesic effect is more attributable to TENS or to medication. Discuss with the treating physician if patients should continue or discontinue intake of painkiller drugs during the course of TENS therapy.
Monitor patient's caffeine intake	Caffeine may decrease the pain-relieving effect of TENS (Marchand et al., 1995).
Keep all TENS units at least 3 m (10 feet) away from any functioning shortwave diathermy (SWD) device	To minimize the risk of electronic interference.
Plug line-powered stimulators into GFCI receptacles	Prevent the risk of electrocution (see Chapter 27).
Conduct regular maintenance and calibration	To ensure optimal treatment efficacy. Follow the manufacturer's recommendations and schedule.

3. Modes of Delivery

Select one among the five common modes described in **Table 14-1**. The *conventional mode* is often selected to begin therapy because the sensation of electrical stimulation is felt as comfortable. If this mode fails to decrease pain after a few treatments, select another mode. Note that there is no evidence to suggest that one mode of delivery is better than the other one for the treatment of any given pathology.

4. Electrode Type

TENS devices are operated with commercially made reusable or disposable surface electrodes of various shapes and sizes, as shown in **Figure 14-2**, that best suit the condition, localization, and size of the treated area (see Walsh, 1997; Barr 1999; Behrens, 2006).

a. Common Electrodes

The most commonly used electrodes are of the reusable, nonsterile type, which can be made from a variety of materials. Carbonized rubber electrodes and siliconized carbon rubber electrodes are among the most commonly used.

b. Specialized Electrodes

Sterile, disposable electrodes of various sizes and shapes are available for postoperative conditions in which infection of the surgical wound is likely.

c. Electrode Maintenance

Routine use of common electrodes requires that clinicians adopt a strict maintenance program, including frequent visual inspection and periodic measurement of electrode impedance. With time and use, electrode material will become less flexible, will show signs of degradation (e.g., breaks, cracks), and will show higher electrical impedance (i.e., more drain on the battery), leading to less-than-optimal applications (Behrens, 2006).

5. Electrode Preparation

Ensure that a thin and evenly distributed coating of electroconductive gel is applied to each electrode to optimize conduction at the electrode–skin interface. Note that sterile electrodes are pre-gelled.

6. Electrode Placement

Much has been written about TENS optimal electrode placements (Mannheimer et al., 1984; Ottoson et al., 1988). To sum up, three basic *electrode placements* are described in the literature. These placements are (1) over and around the painful area, (2) along the dermatome(s) corresponding to the painful site, and (3) over specific body points.

a. Over and Around the Painful Area

This is the most common electrode placement observed in the literature. The rationale for this placement is that the electrical field within the electrodes will depolarize nerve fibers anatomically associated with the site of injury, or with the injured soft tissues. In other words, this placement allows for the stimulation of nerve fibers that enter the same spinal segment as the nerue fibers associated with the origin of the pain.

b. Along the Dermatome(s) Corresponding to the Painful Site

The rationale of this electrode placement is that the electrical field within the electrodes will depolarize nociceptive fibers belonging to the dermatome(s) associated with the site of injury or with the injured soft tissues. Such a placement also allows for the stimulation of nociceptive fibers that enter the same spinal dermatome segment as the nociceptive fibers associated with the origin of the pain.

c. Over Specific Body Points

The third electrode placement is characterized by applications over specific points identified as acupuncture and trigger points. This placement may or may not allow the stimulation of nociceptive fibers that enter the same spinal segment as the nociceptive fibers associated with the origin of the pain. Various charts of acupuncture and trigger points are available (e.g., Mannheimer et al., 1984; Ottoson et al., 1988).

d. Which Electrode Placement Is Best?

Considering the limited body of evidence one can find on this subject (Woolf et al., 1981; Wheeler et al., 1984), *no* *conclusion* can be drawn as to which electrode placement is best for TENS therapy. Until more evidence is provided, practitioners must continue to rely on trial and error when considering the best electrode placement for use with their patients (Walsh, 1997).

7. Electrode Attachment

Electrodes are mechanically attached to the skin using basic surgical tapes (which are cheaper) or precut self-adhesive patches (which are more expensive).

8. Electrode Connection

The electrodes are connected to the stimulator circuit output using regular or bifurcarted lead wires of various lengths.

9. End of Treatment

Carefully remove the electrodes and immediately inspect the exposed skin areas for any adverse reaction or lesion. If present, inform the patient, and document these in the patient's file. Wash (with warm water) and hang dry the reusable electrodes. Dispose of single-use electrodes in a biowaste bag.

B. DOCUMENTATION

Document the key treatment parameters, as well as any adverse reaction or lesion, in the patient's file. **Table 14-4** shows the key parameters to be documented in the patient's file.

TABLE 14-4	KEY TREATMENT PARAMETERS TO BE DOCUMENTED IN PATIENT'S FILE AFTER TRANSCUTANEOUS ELECTRICAL NERVE STIMULATION

- *Stimulator type:* portable; cabinet
- *TENS mode:* conventional; acupuncture-like; brief-intense; burst; modulation
- *Stimulation parameters for each mode:* pulse duration (µs); current amplitude (mA); pulse frequency (burst frequency) Hz; bups
- *Electrode type:* nonsterile reusable; sterile disposable
- *Electrode number and size:* number of pairs and size description
- *Electrode placement:* over and around the painful area; along the dermatome(s) associated with the painful area; over specific body points
- *Application duration:* min
- *Treatment sessions per day:* number
- *Analgesic drug intake during therapy (when applicable):* type and number of tablets

Case Study 14-1 Postoperative Abdominal Pain

A 58-year-old man, wearing an implanted cardioverter defibrillator (ICD), is resting in his hospital room following an open cholecystectomy (gallbladder removal), performed a few hours ago. Postoperative pain management is done using a patient-controlled analgesia device. The device is programmed to deliver set boluses of morphine at different lockout intervals. The surgeon is aware that this patient has a history of experiencing opiate-related side effects, such as nausea, vomiting, dizziness, and depressed respiration. His goal is to provide the patient with adequate postoperative abdominal pain relief, while minimizing the opiate-related side effects. The patient is instructed to request the prescribed narcotics when needed. The surgeon consults you to see if an additional nonpharmacological pain therapy, with no side effects, can be used to manage the patient's postoperative abdominal pain. You propose using TENS therapy until the patient is discharged from the hospital. Your main goal is to decrease postoperative opiate analgesic requirements and opiate-related side effects, while providing adequate pain relief. Your secondary goal is to increase the patient's alertness level, in addition to increasing his body mobility. The patient's first goal is to minimize pain, while taking a minimum amount of drugs. His second goal is to return to work as soon as possible.

Evidence-Based Steps Toward the Resolution of This Case

1. **List medical diagnosis.**

   Cholecystitis—treated by open cholecystectomy.

2. **List key impairment(s).**
   - Severe postoperative abdominal pain over and around the area of incision
   - Surgical cutaneous wound

3. **List key functional limitation(s).**
   - Decreased trunk mobility
   - Difficulty moving in bed
   - Difficulty sitting
   - Difficulty walking

4. **List key disability/disabilities.**
   - Unable to work

5. **Justification for TENS therapy.**

   Is there justification to use TENS therapy in this case? This chapter has established that there is *moderate-to-strong* strength of evidence and *conflicting* justification for the use of TENS therapy for pain, particularly for postoperative abdominal pain (see Section VI). This textbook recommends the use of this EPA for the following reasons. First, the patient's condition is acute and the postoperative pain is severe. Second, there is a need to modulate pain using minimum amount of narcotic because the patient has a past history of severe side effects with such medication. Third, there is evidence that TENS therapy is justi-

fied based on specific clinical studies (Hymes et al., 1974; Vander Ark et al., 1975; Cooperman et al., 1977; Rosenberg et al., 1978; Solomon et al., 1980; Ali et al., 1981; Bussey et al., 1981; Schomburg et al., 1983; Hollinger, 1986; Smith et al., 1986; Caterine et al., 1988; Merrill, 1987, 1988, 1989; Hargreaves et al., 1989; Sims, 1991; Torres et al., 1992; Chen et al., 1998; Hamza et al., 1999) and meta-analysis (Bjordal et al., 2003). Because EPAs should never be used in isolation or as a sole intervention, TENS therapy is used here *concomitantly* with a regimen of drugs, where the aim is to eventually decrease and eliminate them for pain management.

6. **Search for contraindications.**

   The patient wears an ICD. In the present case, TENS is not contraindicated because the treating cardiologist has authorized the *deactivation* of the ICD during each treatment session.

7. **Search for risks and precautions.**

   None is found.

8. **Outline the therapeutic goal(s) you and your patient wish to achieve**
   - Decrease postoperative pain
   - Decrease opiate analgesic requirements during hospitalization
   - Increase bed mobility
   - Increase ability to sit and walk
   - Accelerate return to work

9. **List outcome measurement(s) used to assess treatment effectiveness.**
   - Pain: Short-Form McGill Pain Questionnaire (SF-MPQ)
   - Narcotic intake: daily tablets count
   - Opiate-related side effects: daily number of episodes of nausea and vomiting
   - Overall pain disability: Pain Disability Index (PDI)

10. **Instruct patient about what he/she should experience, do, and not do during the treatment session.**
    - Should feel sensation of pins and needles, and tingling
    - Do not touch electrodes, cables, and TENS unit

11. **Outline your therapeutic prescription based on the best sources of evidence available.**

    This prescription is based on several articles (Hymes et al., 1974; Vander Ark et al., 1975; Cooperman et al., 1977; Rosenberg et al., 1978; Solomon et al., 1980; Ali et al., 1981; Bussey et al., 1981; Schomburg et al., 1983; Hollinger, 1986; Smith et al., 1986; Caterine et al., 1988; Merrill, 1987, 1988, 1989; Hargreaves et al., 1989; Sims, 1991; Torres et al., 1992; Chen et al., 1998; Hamza et al., 1999) and a meta-analysis study (Bjordal et al., 2003). The *conventional mode* (sensory-level stimulation) is chosen because the other modes are likely to evoke

(Continued)

Case Study 14-1   Continued

abdominal muscle contraction (motor- and nociceptive-level stimulation), which may interfere with the healing of the incision wound, in addition to unduly enhanced pain. This mode of TENS delivery is expected to induce a rapid analgesia, which may last a few hours (see **Table 14-1**). Sterile disposable electrodes are used in order to minimize wound infection. Electrodes are kept in place during the whole period, separating wound bandaging, and are replaced with each bandaging session.

- ■ ***TENS device:*** portable
- ■ ***TENS mode:*** burst
- ■ ***Current amplitude:*** just below the maximum comfortable level
- ■ ***Pulse frequency:*** 8 bups
- ■ ***Pulse duration:*** 100 μs
- ■ ***Patient position:*** supine in bed
- ■ ***Electrode type:*** sterile, disposable, pre-gelled, auto-adhesive
- ■ ***Electrode size:*** 3 cm × 10 cm
- ■ ***Electrode number:*** 2 (1 pair)
- ■ ***Electrode placement:*** para-incisional (above and below the surgical incision)
- ■ ***Application duration:*** 60 minutes
- ■ ***Frequency of treatments:*** every 4 hours
- ■ ***Treatment sessions per day:*** 6
- ■ ***Total number of treatments:*** 24 treatments spread over the 4-day hospitalization period.

12. **Collect outcome measurements.**

Pre- and posttreatment comparison:

- ■ Pain: decrease SF-MPQ score by 70%

- ■ Narcotic intake: decrease count by 70%
- ■ Narcotic-related side effects: decrease number of episodes by 80%
- ■ Overall pain disability: decrease PDI score by 90%

13. **Assess therapeutic effectiveness based on outcome measures.**

The results show that 24 applications of TENS therapy, every 4 hours for 4 consecutive days, used in conjunction with narcotic drug therapy for postsurgical abdominal pain, significantly decreased the patient's pain level, narcotic analgesic requirements, and narcotic-related side effects. By providing adequate pain relief with less narcotic intake, this patient improved his alertness level, while improving his overall pain disability level. The patient, now more mobile, was discharged from the hospital after 4 days. The patient plans to return to work within the few days. Overall, the use of TENS therapy had a beneficial impact on the patient's disablement status caused by the pathology, as illustrated in the **figure below**.

14. **State the prognosis.**

The prognosis is excellent if no postsurgical complication occurs and if the patient continues, at home, the care of his abdominal wound and takes the prescribed oral drug analgesics as needed. Pain is expected to disappear over the next few days, and he should enjoy full recovery in addition to full return to work within the next few days.

THERAPEUTIC IMPACT on Disablement

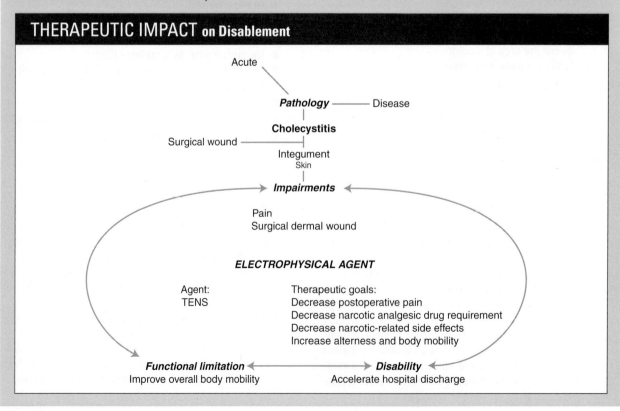

CRITICAL THINKING QUESTIONS

Clarification: What is meant by transcutaneous electrical nerve stimulation (TENS) therapy?

Assumptions: You have assumed that TENS stimulators can be programmed such that it will trigger the spinal gate system without simultaneously triggering the DEOS. How do you justify making that assumption?

Reasons and evidence: What led you to believe that TENS therapy could decrease pain without any side effects?

Viewpoints or perspectives: How would you respond to a colleague who says that there is no way to scientifically determine whether the analgesic effect caused by TENS therapy is modulated or not via the release of endorphins in the body?

Implications and consequences: What are the implications and consequences of using TENS therapy in (1) a patient implanted with a rate-responsive-type pacemaker and (2) in a patient with an implanted cardioverter defibrillator (ICD)?

About the question: Why is it that the electrical waveforms generated by TENS units can be delivered daily, for a few hours at a time, and for several weeks, with a minimal risk of causing contact dermatitis? Why do you think I ask this question?

References

Articles

Abelson K, Langley GB, Sheppeard H, Vlieg M, Wigley RD (1983) Transcutaneous electrical nerve stimulation in rheumatoid arthritis. N Z Med J, 96: 156–158

Abram SE, Reynolds AC, Cusick JF (1981) Failure of naloxone to reverse analgesia from transcutaneous electrical stimulation in patients with chronic pain. Anesth Analg, 60: 81–84

Ali J, Yaffe CS, Serrette C (1981) The effect of transcutaneous electric nerve stimulation on postoperative pain and pulmonary function. Surgery, 89: 507–512

Angulo DL, Colwell CW (1990) Use of postoperative TENS and continuous passive motion following total knee replacement. J Orthop Sports Phys Ther, 11: 599–604

Arvidsson J, Eriksson E (1986) Postoperative TENS pain relief after knee surgery: Objective evaluation. Orthopedics, 9: 1346–1351

Ashwal S, Tomasi L, Neumann M, Schneider S (1988) Reflex sympathetic dystrophy syndrome in children. Pediatr Neurol, 4: 38–42

Augustinsson LE, Bohlin P, Bundsen P, Carlsson CA, Forssman L, Sjöberg P, Tyreman NO (1977) Pain relief during delivery by transcutaneous electrical nerve stimulation. Pain, 4: 59–65

Bajd T, Gregoric M, Vodovnik L, Benko H (1985) Electrical stimulation in treating spasticity resulting from spinal cord injury. Arch Phys Med Rehab, 66: 515–517

Bates JAV, Nathan PW (1980) Transcutaneous electrical nerve stimulation for chronic pain. Anaesthesia, 35: 817–822

Bayindir O, Paker, T, Akpinar B, Erenturk S, Askin D, Aytac A (1991) Use of transcutaneous electrical nerve stimulation in the control of postoperative chest pain after cardiac surgery. J Cardiothorac Vasc Anesth, 5: 589–591

Benedetti F, Amanzio M, Casadio C, Cavallo A, Gianci R, Giobbe R, Mancusso M, Ruffini E, Maggi C (1997) Control of postoperative pain by transcutaneous electrical nerve stimulation after thoracic operations. Ann Thorac Surg, 63: 773–776

Berman BM, Bausell RB (2000) The use of non-pharmacological therapies by pain specialists. Pain, 85: 313–315

Bertalanffy A, Kober A, Bertalanffy P, Gustroff B, Gore O, Adel S, Hoerauf K (2005) Transcutaneous electrical nerve stimulation reduces acute low back pain during emergency transport. Acad Emerg Med, 12: 607–611

Bodenheim R, Bennett JH (1983) Reversal of a Sudeck's atrophy by the adjunctive use of transcutaneous electrical nerve stimulation. A case report. Phys Ther, 63: 1287–1288

Bohm E (1978) Transcutaneous electrical nerve stimulation in chronic pain after peripheral nerve injury. Acta Neurochir (Wien), 40: 277–283

Bolton L (1983) TENS electrode irritation. J Am Acad Dermatol, 8: 134–135

Borjesson M, Eriksson P, Dellborg M, Eliason T, Mannkeimer C (1997) Transcutaneous electrical nerve stimulation in unstable angina pectoris. Coronary Artery Dis, 8: 543–550

Bortoluzzi G (1989) Transcutaneous electrical nerve stimulation in labour: Practicality and effectiveness in a public hospital ward. Austr J Physiother, 35: 81–87

Breit R, Van der Wall H (2004) Transcutaneous electrical stimulation for postoperative pain relief after total knee arthroplasty. J Arthroplasty, 19: 45–48

Brill MM, Whiffen JR (1985) Application of 24-hour burst TENS in a back school. Phys Ther, 65: 1355–1357

Broadley AJ (2000) The diagnostic dilemma of "pseudopacemaker spikes." Pacing Clin Electrophysiol, 23: 286–288

Bruce JR, Riggin CS, Parker JC (1988) Pain management in rheumatoid arthritis: Cognitive behavior modification and transcutaneous neural stimulation. Arthritis Care Res, 32: 1178–1184

Bundsen P, Ericson K, Peterson LE, Thiringer K (1982) Pain relief in labor by transcutaneous electrical nerve stimulation. Acta Obstet Gynaecol Scand, 61: 129–136

Bundsen P, Peterson LE, Selstam U (1981) Pain relief in labor by transcutaneous electrical nerve stimulation. Acta Obstet Gynaecol Scand, 60: 459–468

Bussey JG, Jackson A (1981) TENS for postsurgical analgesia. Contemp Surg, 18: 35–41

Carabelli RA, Kellerman WC (1985) Phantom limb pain: Relief by application of TENS to contralateral extremity. Arch Phys Med Rehab, 66: 466–467

Carrol EN, Badura AS (2001) Focal intense brief transcutaneous electric nerve stimulation for treatment of radicular and postthoracotomy pain. Arch Phys Med Rehabil, 82: 262–264

Castelain PY, Chabeau G (1986) Contact dermatitis after transcutaneous electric analgesia. Contact Dermatitis, 15: 32–35

Caterine JM, Smith DC, Olivencia J (1988) TENS for postsurgical analgesia following gastroplasty. Iowa Med, 78: 369–371

Chabal C, Fishbain DA, Weaver M, Heine LW (1998) Long-term transcutaneous electrical nerve stimulation (TENS) use: Impact on medication and physical therapy costs. Clin J Pain, 14: 66–73

Chao AS, Chao A, Wang TH, Chang YC, Peng HH, Chang SD, Chao A, Chang CJ, Lai CH, Wong AM (2007) Pain relief by applying transcutaneous electrical nerve stimulation (TENS) on acupuncture points during the first stage of labor: A randomized double-blind placebo-controlled trial. Pain, 127: 214–220

Cheing GL, Tsui AY, Lo SK, Hui-Chan CW (2003) Optimal stimulation duration of TENS in the management of osteoarthritis knee pain. J Rehabil Med, 35: 62–68

Cheing GL, Hui-Chan CW (1999) Transcutaneous electrical nerve stimulation: Non paralleled antinociceptive effects on chronic pain and acute experimental pain. Arch Phys Med Rehab, 80: 305–312

Cheing GL, Hui-Chan CW, Chan KM (2002) Does four weeks of TENS and/or isometric exercice produce cumulative reduction of osteoarthritis knee pain? Clin Rehabil, 16: 749–760

Chen D, Philip M, Philip PA, Monga TN (1990) Cardiac pacemaker inhibition by transcutaneous electrical nerve stimulation. Arch Phys Med Rehab, 71: 27–30

Chen L, Tang J, White PF, Sloninsky A, Wender RH, Naruse R, Kariger R (1998) The effect of location on transcutaneous electrical nerve stimulation on postoperative opioid analgesic requirement: Acupoint versus nonacupoint stimulation. Anaesth Analg, 87: 1129–1234

Chia YT, Arulkumaran S, Chua S, Ratnam SS (1990) Effectiveness of transcutaneous electric nerve stimulator for pain relief in labour. Asia Oceania J Obstet Gynecol, 16: 145–151

Chiu JH, Chen WS, Chen CH, Jiang JK, Tang GJ, Lui WY, Lin JK (1999) Effect of transcutaneous electrical nerve stimulation for pain relief on patients undergoing hemorrhoidectomy: Prospective, randomized, controlled trial. Dis Colon Rectum, 42: 180–185

Conn IG, Marshall AH, Yadav SN, Daly JC, Jaffer M (1986) Transcutaneous electrical nerve stimulation following appendicectomy: The placebo effect. Ann R Coll Surg Engl, 68: 191–192

Cooperman AM, Hall B, Mikalacki K, Hardy R, Sardar E (1977) Use of transcutaneous electrical stimulation in the control of postoperative pain: Results of a prospective, randomized, controlled study. Am J Surg, 133: 185–187

Corazza M, Maranini C, Bacilieri S, Virgili A (1999) Accelerated allergic contact dermatitis to a transcutaenous electric nerve stimulation device. Dermatology, 199: 281

Cornell PE, Lopez AL, Malofsky H (1984) Pain reduction with transcutaneous electrical nerve stimulation after foot surgery. J Foot Surg, 23: 326–333

Curwin JH, Coyne RF, Winters SL (1999) Inappropriate defibrillator (ICD) shocks caused by transcutaneous electronic nerve stimulation (TENS) units. Pacing Clin Electrophysiol, 22: 692–693

Cuschieri RJ, Morran CG, McArdle CS (1985) Transcutaneous electrical stimulation for postoperative pain. Ann R Coll Surg Engl, 67: 127–129

Dawood MY, Ramos J (1990) Transcutaneous electrical nerve stimulation (TENS) for the treatment of primary dysmenorrhea: A randomized crossover comparison with placebo TENS and ibuprofen. Obstet Gynecol, 75: 656–660

Deyo RA, Walsh NE, Martin DC, Schoenfeld LS, Ramamurthy S (1990) A controlled trial of transcutaneous electrical nerve stimulation (TENS) and exercise for chronic low back pain. N Engl J Med, 322: 1627–1634

Dwyer CM, Chapman RS, Forsyth A (1994) Allergic contact dermatitis from TENS gel. Contact Dermatitis, 30: 305

Ebersold MJ, Laws EK, Stonnington H, Stillwell GK (1975) Transcutaneous electrical stimulation for treatment of chronic pain: A preliminary report. Surg Neurol, 4: 96–99

Erdogan M, Erdogan A, Erbil N, Karakaya HK, Demircan A (2005) Prospective, randomized, placebo-controlled study of the effect of TENS on postthoracotomy pain and pulmonary function. World J Surg, 29: 1563–1570

Eriksson M, Schuller H, Sjolund B (1978) Hazard from transcutaneous nerve stimulation in patients with pacemakers. Lancet, i: 1319 (Letter)

Eriksson MB, Sjölund B, Nielzen S (1979) Long term results of peripheral conditioning stimulation as an analgesic measure in chronic pain. Pain, 6: 335–347

Eriksson MB, Sjölund BH, Sundbärg G (1984) Pain relief from peripheral conditioning stimulation in patients with chronic facial pain. J Neurosurg, 61: 149–155

Erkkola R, Pikkola P, Kanto J (1980) Transcutaneous nerve stimulation for pain relief during labour: A controlled study. Ann Chir Gynaecol, 69: 273–277

Ersek RA (1976) Low back pain: Prompt relief with transcutaneous neuro-stimulation—A report of 35 consecutive patients. Orthop Rev, 5: 27–31

Ersek RA (1977) Transcutaneous electrical neurostimulation: A new therapeutic modality for controlling pain. Clin Orthop, 128: 314–323

Fargas-Babjak A, Pomeranz B, Rooney PJ (1992) Acupuncture-like stimulation with Codetron for rehabilitation of patients with chronic pain syndrome and osteoarthritis. Acupunct Electrother Res, 17: 99–105

Fargas-Babjak A, Rooney P, Gerecz E (1989) Randomized trial of Codetron for pain control in osteoarthritis of the hip/knee. Clin J Pain, 5: 137–141

Finsen V, Persen L, Lovlien M, Veslegaard EK, Simensen M, Gasvann AK, Benum P (1988) Transcutaneous electrical nerve stimulation after major amputation. J Bone Joint Surg, 70B: 109–112

Fishbain DA, Chabal C, Abbot A, Heine LW, Cutler R (1996) Transcutaneous electrical nerve stimulation (TENS) treatment outcome in long-term users. Clin J Pain, 12: 201–214

Fisher AA (1978) Dermatitis associated with transcutaneous electrical stimulation current. Cutis, 21: 24–47

Foley-Nolan D, Kinirons M, Coughlan RJ, O'Connor P (1990) Post-whiplash dystonia well controlled by transcutaneous electrical nerve stimulation (TENS): Case report. J Trauma, 30: 909–910

Forster EL, Kramer JF, Lucy SD, Scudds RA, Novick RJ (1994) Effect of TENS on pain, medications, and pulmonary function following coronary artery bypass graft surgery. Chest, 106: 1343–1348

Fox EJ, Melzack R (1976) Transcutaneous electrical stimulation and acupuncture: Comparison of treatment for low back pain. Pain, 2: 141–148

Frampton V (1996) Management of pain in brachial plexus lesions. J Hand Ther, 9: 339–343

Fried T, Johnson R, McCracken W (1984) Transcutaneous electrical nerve stimulation: Its role in the control of chronic pain. Arch Phys Med Rehab, 65: 228–231

Galloway DJ, Boyle P, Burns HJ, Davidson PM, George WD (1984) A clinical assessment of electroanalgesia following abdominal operations. Surg Gynecol Obstet, 159: 453–456

Gemignani G, Olivieri L, Ruju G, Pasero G (1991) Transcutaneous electrical nerve stimulation in ankylosing spondylitis: A double-blind study. Arthritis Rheum, 34: 788–789

Gilbert JM, Gledhill T, Law N, George C (1986) Controlled trial of transcutaneous electrical nerve stimulation (TENS) for postoperative pain relief following inguinal herniorrhaphy. Br J Surg, 73: 749–751

Glotzer TV, Gordon M, Sparta M, Radoslovich G, Zimmerman J (1998) Electromagnetic interference from a muscle stimulation device causing discharge of an implantable cardioverter defibrillator: Epicardial bipolar and endocardial bipolar sensing circuits are compared. Pacing Clin Electrophysiol, 21: 1996–1998

Graff-Radford SB, Reeves JL, Baker RL, Chiu D (1989) Effects of transcutaneous electrical nerve stimulation on myofascial pain and trigger point sensitivity. Pain, 37: 1–5

Grim LC, Morey SH (1985) Transcutaneous electrical nerve stimulation for relief of parturition pain: A clinical report. Phys Ther, 65: 337–340

Grimmer K (1992) A controlled double-blind study comparing the effects of strong burst mode TENS and high rate TENS on painful osteoarthritic knees. Austr J Physiother, 38: 49–56

Guieu R, Tardy-Gervet MF, Roll JP (1991) Analgesic effects of vibration and transcutaneous electrical nerve stimulation applied separately and simultaneously to patients with chronic pain. Can J Neurol Sci, 18: 115–119

Györy AN, Caine DC (1977) Electrical pain control (EPC) of a painful forearm amputation stump. Med J Austr, 2: 156–158

Hamza MA, White PF, Ahmed HE, Ghoname EA (1999) Effect of the frequency of transcutaneous electrical nerve stimulation on the postoperative opioid analgesic requirement and recovery profile. Anesthesiology, 91: 1232–1238

Hansson P, Ekblom A (1983) Transcutaneous electrical nerve stimulation (TENS) as compared to placebo TENS for the relief of acute oro-facial pain. Pain, 15: 157–165

Hansson P, Ekblom A, Thomsson M, Fjellner B (1986) Influence of naloxone on relief of acute oro-facial pain by transcutaneous electrical nerve stimulation (TENS) or vibration. Pain, 24: 323–329

Hargreaves A, Lander J (1989) Use of transcutaneous electrical nerve stimulation for postoperative pain. Nurs Res, 38: 159–161

Harrison RF, Shore M, Woods T, Mathews G, Gardiner J, Unwin A (1987) A comparative study of transcutaneous electrical nerve stimulation (TENS), entonox, pethidine plus promazine and lumbar epidural for pain relief in labor. Acta Obstet Gynaecol Scand, 66: 9–14

Harrison RF, Woods T, Shore M, Mathews G, Unwin A (1986) Pain relief in labour using transcutaneous electrical nerve stimulation (TENS): A TENS/TENS placebo controlled study in two parity groups. Br J Obstet Gynaecol, 93: 739–746

Harvey M, Elliott M (1995) Transcutaneous electrical nerve stimulation (TENS) for pain management during cavity preparations in pediatric patients. J Dent Child, Jan–Feb: 49–51

Harvie KW (1979) A major advance in the control of postoperative knee pain. Orthopedics, 2: 26–27

Hasan ST, Robson WA, Pridie AK, Neal DE (1996) Transcutaneous electrical nerve stimulation and temporary S3 neuromodulation of idiopathic detrusor instability. J Urol, 155: 2005–2011

Hauptman PJ, Raza M (1992) Electrocardiographic artifact with a transcutaneous electrical nerve stimulation unit. Int J Cardiol, 34: 110–112

Herman E, Williams R, Stratford P, Fargas-Babjak A, Trott M (1994) A randomized controlled trial of transcutaneous electrical nerve stimulation (CODETRON) to determine its benefits in a rehabilitation program for acute occupational low back pain. Spine, 19: 561–568

Ho A, Hui PW, Cheung J, Cheung C (1987) Effectiveness of transcutaneous electrical nerve stimulation in relieving pain following thoracotomy. Physiotherapy, 73: 33–35

Hollinger JL (1986) Transcutaneous electrical nerve stimulation after cesarean birth. Phys Ther, 66: 36–38

Holmgren C, Carlsson T, Mannheimer C, Edvardsson N (2008) Risk of interference from transcutaneous electrical nerve stimulation on the sensing function of implantable defibrillators. PACE, 31: 151–158

Hymes AC, Raab DE, Yonehiro EG, Nelson GD, Printy AL (1974). Electrical surface stimulation for control of acute postoperative pain and prevention of ileus. Surg Forum, 24: 447–449

Indeck W, Printy A (1975) Skin application of electrical impulses for relief of pain in chronic orthopedic conditions. Minn Med, 58: 305–309

Issenman J, Nolan MF, Rowley J, Hobby R (1985) Transcutaneous electrical nerve stimulation for pain control after spinal fusion with Harrington rods. Phys Ther, 65: 1517–1520

Jay GW, Brunson J, Bronson SJ (1989) The effectiveness of physical therapy in the treatment of chronic daily headaches. Headache, 29: 156–162

Jensen JE, Conn RR, Hazelrigg G, Hewett JE (1985) The use of transcutaneous neural stimulation and isokinetic testing in arthroscopic knee surgery. Am J Sports Med, 13: 27–33

Jensen H, Zesler R, Christensen T (1991) Transcutaneous electrical nerve stimulation (TENS) for painful osteoarthritis of the knee. Int J Rehab Res, 14: 356–358

Johnson MI, Asthon CH, Thompson JW (1991) An in-depth study of long term users of transcutaneous electrical nerve stimulation (TENS). Implications for clinical users of TENS. Pain, 44: 221–229

Jones SL (1976) Electromagnetic field interference and cardiac pacemakers. Phys Ther, 56: 1013–1018

Kaplan B, Peled Y, Pardo J, Rabinerson D, Hirsh M, Ovadia J, Neri A (1994) Transcutaneous electrical nerve stimulation (TENS) as a relief for dysmenorrhea. Clin Exp Obstet Gynecol, 21: 87–90

Kaplan B, Rabinerson D, Lurie S, Bar J, Krieser UR, Neri A (1998) Transcutaneous electrical nerve stimulation (TENS) for adjuvant pain-relief during labor and delivery. Int J Gynaecol Obstet, 60: 251–255

Kaplan B, Rabinerson D, Lurie S, Peled Y, Royburt M, Neri A (1997) Clinical evaluation of a new model of a transcutaneous electrical nerve stimulation device for the management of primary dysmenorrhea. Gynecol Obstet Invest, 44: 255–259

Katz J, Melzack R (1991) Auricular transcutaneous electrical nerve stimulation (TENS) reduces phantom limb pain. J Pain Symptom Manage, 6: 73–83

Keenan DL, Simonsen L, McCrann DJ (1985) Transcutaneous electrical nerve stimulation for pain control during labor and delivery: A case report. Phys Ther, 65: 1363–1364

Kimberley AP, Soni N, Williams TR (1987) Transcutaneous nerve stimulation and the electrocardiograph. Anaesth Intens Care, 15: 358–359

Klin B, Uretzky G, Magora F (1984) Transcutaneous electrical nerve stimulation (TENS) after open heart surgery. J Cardiovasc Surg (Torino), 25: 445–448

Koke AJ, Schouten JS, Lamerichs-Geelen MJ, Lipsch JS, Waltje EM, van Kleef M, Pa J (2004) Pain reducing effects of three types of transcutanenous electrical nerve stimulation in patients with chronic pain: A randomized crossover trial. Pain, 108: 36-42

Kruger LR, van der Linden WJ, Cleaton-Jones PE (1998) Transcutaneous electrical nerve stimulation in the treatment of myofascial pain dysfunction. S Afr J Surg, 36: 35–38

Kumar VN, Redford JB (1982) Transcutaneous electrical nerve stimulation in rheumatoid arthritis. Arch Phys Med Rehab, 63: 595–596

Laitinen J (1976) Acupuncture and transcutaneous electrical stimulation in the treatment of chronic sacrolumbalgia and ischialgia. Am J Chin Med, 4: 169–175

Laitinen J, Nuutinen L (1991) Failure of transcutaneous electrical nerve stimulation and indomethacin to reduce opiate requirement following cholecystectomy. Acta Anaesthesiol Scand, 35: 700–705

Lang T, Barker R, Steinlechner B, Gustorff B, Puskas T, Gore O, Kober A (2007) TENS relieves acute posttraumatic hip pain during emergency transport. J Trauma, 62: 184–188

Langley GB, Sheppeard H, Johnson M, Wigley RD (1984) The analgesic effects of transcutaneous electrical nerve stimulation and placebo in chronic pain patients: A double-blind non-crossover comparison. Rheumatol Int, 4: 119–123

Law PP, Cheing, Tsui AY GL (2004) Does transcutaneous electrical nerve stimulation improve the physical performance of people with knee osteoarthritis? J Clin Rheumatol, 10: 295–299

Leandri M, Parodi CI, Corrieri N, Rigardo S (1990) Comparison of TENS treatments in hemiplegic shoulder pain. Scand J Rehab Med, 22: 69–72

Lee EW, Chung IW, Lee JY, Lam PW, Chin RK (1990) The role of transcutaneous electrical nerve stimulation in management of labour in obstetric patients. Asia Oceania J Obstet Gynaecol, 16: 247–254

Lehmann TR, Russell DW, Spratt KF, Colby H, King Liu Y, Fairchild ML, Christensen S (1986) Efficacy of electroacupuncture and TENS in the rehabilitation of chronic low back pain patients. Pain, 26: 277–290

Leijon G, Boivie J (1989) Central post-stroke pain—The effect of high and low frequency TENS. Pain, 38: 187–191

Levin MF, Hui-Chan CW (1992) Relief of hemiparetic spasticity by TENS is associated with improvement in reflex and voluntary motor functions. Electroencephalogr Clin Neurophysiol, 85: 131–142

Lewers D, Clelland JA, Jackson JR, Varner RE, Bergman J (1989) Transcutaneous electrical nerve stimulation in the relief of primary dysmenorrhea. Phys Ther, 69: 277–290

Lewis B, Lewis D, Cumming G (1994) The comparative analgesic efficacy of transcutaneous electrical nerve stimulation and non-steroidal anti-inflammatory drug for painful osteoarthritis Br J Rheumatol, 33: 455–460

Lewis D, Lewis B, Sturrock R (1984) Transcutaneous electrical nerve stimulation in osteoarthritis: A therapeutic alternative? Ann Rheum Dis, 43: 47–49

Lim AT, Edis G, Kranz H, Mendelson G, Selwood T, Scott DF (1983) Postoperative pain control: Contribution of psychological factors and transcutaneous electrical stimulation. Pain, 17: 179–188

Linde C, Isacsson G, Jonsson BG (1995) Outcome of 6-week treatment with transcutaneous electrical nerve stimulation compared with splint on symptomatic temporomandibular joint disk displacement without reduction. Acta Odontol Scand, 53: 92–98

Loeser JD, Black RG, Christman RA (1975) Relief of pain by transcutaneous stimulation. J Neurosurg, 42: 308–314

Long DM (1974) External electrical stimulation as a treatment of chronic pain. Minn Med, 5: 195–198

Lundeberg T, Bondesson L, Lundström V (1985) Relief of primary dysmenorrhea by transcutaneous electrical nerve stimulation. Acta Obstet Gynaecol Scand, 64: 491–497

Magora F, Aladjemoff L, Tannenbaum J, Magora A (1978) Treatment of pain by transcutaneous electrical stimulation. Acta Anaesthesiol Scand, 22: 589–592

Mann JC (1996) Respiratory compromise. A rare complication of transcutaneous electrical stimulation for angina pectoris. J Accid Emerg Med, 13: 68

Mannheimer C, Carlsson CA (1979) The analgesic effect of transcutaneous electrical nerve stimulation (TENS) in patients with rheumatoid arthritis. A comparative study of different pulse patterns. Pain, 6: 329–334

Mannheimer C, Lund S, Carlsson CA (1978) The effect of transcutaneous electrical nerve stimulation (TNS) on joint pain in patients with rheumatoid arthritis. Scand J Rheumatol, 7: 13–16

Mannheimer JS, Whalen EC (1985) The efficacy of transcutaneous electrical nerve stimulation in dysmenorrhea. Clin J Pain, 1: 75–83

Marchand S, Charest J, Li J, Chenard JR, Lavignolle B, Laurencelle L (1993) Is TENS purely a placebo effect ? A controlled study on chronic low back pain. Pain, 54: 99–106

Marchand S, Li J, Charest J (1995) Letter to the Editor. Effects of caffeine on analgesia from transcutaneous electrical nerve stimulation. N Engl J Med, 333: 325

Marples IL (2000) Transcutanenous electrical nerve stimulation (TENS): An unusual source of electrocardiogram artifact. Anaesthesia, 55: 719– 720

Marren P, DeBerker D, Powell S (1991) Methacrylate sensitivity and transcutaneous electrical nerve stimulation (TENS). Contact Dermatitis, 25: 190–191

McCallum MI, Glynn CJ, Moore RA, Lammer P, Phillips AM (1988) Transcutaneous electrical nerve stimulation in the management of acute postoperative pain. Br J Anaesth, 61: 308–312

Meechan JG, Gowans AJ, Welbury RR (1998) The use of patient-controlled electronic nerve stimulation (TENS) to decrease the discomfort of regional anaesthesia in dentistry: A randomized controlled clinical trial. J Dent, 26: 417–420

Melzack R, Jeans ME, Stratford JG, Monks RC (1980) Ice massage and transcutaneous electrical stimulation: Comparison of treatment for low-back pain. Pain, 9: 209–217

Melzack R, Vetere P, Finch L (1983) Transcutaneous electrical nerve stimulation for low back pain: A comparison of TENS and massage for pain and range of motion. Phys Ther, 63: 489–493

Melzack R, Wall PD (1965) Pain mechanisms: A new theory. Science, 150: 971–979

Merkel SI, Gutstein HB, Malviya S (1999) Use of transcutaneous electrical nerve stimulation in a young child with pain from open perineal lesions. J Pain Symptom Manage, 18: 376–381

Merrill DC (1987) Electroanalgesia in urologic surgery. Urology, 29: 494–497

Merril DC (1988) FasTENS—A disposable transcutaneous electrical nerve stimulator designed specifically for use in postoperative pain. Urology, 31: 78–79

Merrill DC (1989) Clinical evaluation of FasTENS, an inexpensive, disposable transcutaneous electrical nerve stimulator designed specifically for postoperative electroanalgesia. Urology, 33: 27–30

Meuleman V, Busschots AM, Dooms-Goossens A (1996) Contact allergy to a device for transcutaneous electrical neural stimulation (TENS). Contact Dermatitis. 35: 52–54

Meyler WJ, de Jongste MJ, Rolf CA (1994) Clinical evaluation of pain treatment with electrostimulation: A study on TENS in patients with different pain syndromes. Clin J Pain, 10: 22–27

Miles J, Lipton S (1978) Phantom limb pain treated by electrical stimulation. Pain, 5: 373–382

Milsom I, Hedner N, Mannheimer C (1994) A comparative study of the effect of high-intensity transcutaneous nerve stimulation and oral naproxen on intrauterine pressure and menstrual pain in patients with primary dysmenorrhea. Am J Obstet Gynecol, 170: 123–129

Miller L, Mattison P, Paul L, Wood L (2007) The effects of transcutaneous electrical nerve stimulation (TENS) on spasticity in multiple sclerosis. Mult Sler, 13: 527–533

Mora B, Giorni E, Dobrovits M, Barker R, Lang T, Gore C, Kober A (2006) Transcutaneous electrical nerve stimulation: An effective treatment for pain caused by renal colic in emergency care. J Urol, 175: 1737–1741

Moystad A, Krogstard BS, Larheim TA (1990) Transcutaneous electrical nerve stimulation in a group of patients with rheumatic disease involving the temporomandibular joint. J Prosthet Dent, 64: 596–600

Murphy GJ (1990) Utilization of transcutaneous electrical nerve stimulation in managing craniofacial pain. Clin J Pain, 6: 64–69

Nathan PW, Wall PD (1974) Treatment for post-herpetic neuralgia by prolonged electrical stimulation. Br Med J, 3: 645–647

Navarathnam RG, Wang IY, Thomas D, Klineberg PL (1984) Evaluation of the transcutaneous electrical nerve stimulator for postoperative analgesia following cardiac surgery. Anaesth Intensive Care, 12: 345–350

Neary JM (1981) Transcutaneous electrical nerve stimulation for the relief of post-incisional pain. Am Assoc Nurs J, 49: 151–155

Neighbors LE, Clelland J, Jackson JR, Begman J, Orr J (1987) Transcutaneous electrical nerve stimulation for pain relief in primary dysmenorrhea. Clin J Pain, 3: 17–22

Nesheim BI (1981) The use of transcutaneous nerve stimulation for pain relief during labor. A controlled clinical study. Acta Obstet Gynaecol Scand, 60: 13–16

Nitz J, Cheras F (1993) Transcutaneous electrical nerve stimulation and chronic intractable angina pectoris. Austr J Physiother, 39: 109–113

Nordemar R, Thörner C (1981) Treatment of acute cervical pain—A comparative group study. Pain, 10: 93–101

Occhetta E, Bortnik M, Magnami A, Francalacci G, Marino P (2006) Inappropriate implantable cardioverter-defibrillator discharges unrelated to supraventricular tachyarrythmias. Europace, 8: 863–869

Okada N, Igawa Y, Ogawa A, Nishizawa O (1998) Transcutaneous electrical stimulation of thigh muscles in the treatment of detrusor overactivity. Br J Urol, 81: 560–564

Olsen MF, Elden H, Janson ED, Lilja H, Stener-Victorin E (2007) A comparison of high- versus low-intensity, high –frequency transcutaneous electric nerve stimulation for painful postpartum uterine contractions. Acta Obstet Gynecol Scand, 86: 310–314

Oosterhof J, De Boo TM, Oostendorp BA, Wilder-Smith OG, Crul BJ (2006) Outcome of transcutaneous electrical nerve stimulation in chronic pain: Short-term results of a double-blind, randomized, placebo-controlled trial. J Headeache Pain, 7: 196–205

Ordog GJ (1987) Transcutaneous electrical nerve stimulation versus oral analgesic: A randomized double-blind controlled study in acute traumatic pain. Am J Emerg Med, 5: 6–10

Oztas N, Olmez A, Yel B (1997) Clinical evaluation of transcutaneous electrical nerve stimulation for pain control during tooth preparation. Quintessence Int, 28: 603–608

Paker N, Tekdos D, Kesiktas N, Soy D (2006) Comparison of the therapeutic efficacy of TENS versus intra-articular hyaluronic acid injection in patients with knee osteoarthritis: A prospective randomized study. Adv Ther, 23: 342–353

Philbin DM, Marieb MA, Aithal KH, Schoenfeld MH (1998) Inappropriate shocks delivered by an ICD as a result of sensed potentials from a transcutaneous electronic nerve stimulation unit. Pacing Clin Electrophysiol, 21: 2010–2011

Pike PM (1978) Transcutaneous electrical stimulation: Its use in the management of postoperative pain. Anaesthesia, 33: 165–171

Pope MH, Philips RB, Haugh LD (1994) A prospective randomized three-week trial of spinal manipulation, transcutaneous muscle stimulation, massage and corset in the treatment of subacute low-back pain. Spine, 19: 2571–2577

Potisk KP, Gregoric M, Vodovnik L (1995) Effects of transcutaneous electrical stimulation (TENS) on spasticity in patients with hemiplegia. Scand J Rehab Med, 27: 168–174

Pyatt JR, Trenbath D, Chester M, Connelly DT (2003) The simultaneous use of a biventricular implantable defibrillator (ICD) and transcutaenous electrical nerve stimulation (TENS) unit: Implication for device interaction. Europace, 5: 91–103

Rasmussen MJ, Hayes DL, Vlietstra RE, Thorsteinsson G (1988) Can transcutaneous electrical nerve stimulation be safely used in patients with permanent cardiac pacemakers? Mayo Clin Proc, 63: 443–445

Rawat B, Genz A, Fache JS, Ong M, Coldman AJ, Burhenne HJ (1991) Effectiveness of transcutaneous electrical nerve stimulation (TENS) for analgesia during biliary lithotripsy. Invest Radiat, 26: 866–869

Reuss R, Cronen P, Abplanalp L (1988) Transcutaneous electrical nerve stimulation for pain control after cholecystectomy: Lack of expected benefits. South Med J, 81: 1361–1363

Reynolds RA, Gladstone N, Ansari AH (1987) Transcutaneous electrical nerve stimulation for reducing narcotic use after cesarean section. J Reprod Med, 32: 843–846

Richardson RR, Meyer PR, Cerullo LJ (1980) Neurostimulation in the modulation of intractable paraplegic and traumatic neuroma pains. Pain, 8: 75–84

Robaina FJ, Rodriguez JL, de Vera JA, Martin MA (1989) Transcutaneous electrical nerve stimulation and spinal cord stimulation for pain relief in reflex sympathetic dystrophy. Stereotact Funct Neurosurg, 52: 53–62

Rooney SM, Jain S, Goldiner PL (1983) Effect of transcutaneous nerve stimulation on postoperative pain after thoracotomy. Anesth Analg, 62: 1010–1012

Rosenberg M, Curtis L, Bourke DL (1978) Transcutaneous electrical nerve stimulation for the relief of postoperative pain. Pain, 5: 129–133

Rutkowski B, Niedzialkowska J (1977) Electrical stimulation in low-back pain. Br J Anaesth, 49: 629–632

Scherder E, Van Someren E, Swaab D (1999) Epilepsy: A possible contraindication for transcutaenous electrical nerve stimulation. J Pain Sympt Manag, 17: 151–153

Schietz HA, Jettestad M, Al-Heeti D (2007) Treatment of dysmenorrhoea with a new TENS device (OVA). J Obstet Gynaecol, 27: 726–728

Schomburg FL, Carter-Baker SA (1983) Transcutaneous electrical nerve stimulation for postlaparotomy pain. Phys Ther, 63: 188–193

Schuster GD, Infante MC (1980) Pain relief after low back surgery: The efficacy of transcutaneous electrical nerve stimulation. Pain, 8: 299–302

Shade SK (1985) Use of transcutaneous electrical nerve stimulation for a patient with a cardiac pacemaker. A case report. Phys Ther, 65: 206–208

Shealy CN (1974) Six years' experience with electrical stimulation for control of pain. Adv Neurol, 4: 775–782

Shealy CN, Mortimer JT, Reswick JB (1967) Electrical inhibition of pain by stimulation of the dorsal column: Preliminary clinical report. Anesth Analg, 46: 489–491

Sims DT (1991) Effectiveness of transcutaneous electrical nerve stimulation following cholecystectomy. Physiotherapy, 77: 715–722

Siu CW, Tse HF, Lau CP (2005) Inappropriate implantable defibrillator shock from a transcutaneous muscle stimulation device therapy. J Interv Card Electrophysiol, 13: 73–75

Sliwa JA, Marinko MS (1996) Transcutaneous electrical nerve stimulation-induced electrocardiogram artifact. A brief report. Am J Phys Med Rehab, 75: 307–309

Sloan JP, Muwanga CL, Waters EA, Dove AF, Dave SH (1986) Multiple rib fractures: Transcutaneous nerve stimulation versus conventional analgesia. J Trauma, 26: 1120–1122

Smedley F, Taube M, Wastell C (1988) Transcutaneous electrical nerve stimulation for pain relief following inguinal hernia repair: A controlled trial. Eur Surg Res, 20: 233–237

Smith CR, Lewith GT, Machin D (1983) TENS and osteoarthritis: Preliminary study to establish a controlled method of assessing transcutaneous electrical nerve stimulation as a treatment for pain caused by osteoarthritis. Physiotherapy, 69: 266–268

Smith CM, Guralnick MS, Gelfand MM, Jeans ME (1986) The effects of transcutaneous electrical nerve stimulation on post-cesarean pain. Pain, 27: 181–193

Smith MJ, Hutchins RC, Hehenberger D (1983) Transcutaneous electrical nerve stimulation in postoperative knee rehabilitation. Am J Sports Med, 11: 75–81

Smith RP, Heltzel JA (1991) Interrelation of analgesia and uterine activity in women with primary dysmenorrhea. A preliminary report. J Reprod Med, 36: 260–264

Solomon RA, Viernstein MC, Long DM (1980) Reduction of postoperative pain and narcotic use by transcutaneous electrical nerve stimulation. Surgery, 87: 142–146

Somers DL, Somers MF (1999) Treatment of neuropathic pain in a patient with diabetic neuropathy using transcutaneous electrical nerve stimulation applied to the skin of the lumbar region. Phys Ther, 79: 767–777

Sonde L, Gip C, Fernaeus SE, Nilsson CG, Viitanen M (1998) Stimulation with low frequency (1.7 Hz) transcutaneous electric nerve stimulation (low-TENS) increases motor function of the post-stroke paretic arm. Scand J Rehab Med, 30: 95–99

Stabile ML, Mallory TH (1978) The management of postoperative pain in total joint replacement. Orthop Rev, 7: 121–123

Stubbing JF, Jellicoe JA (1988) Transcutaneous electrical nerve stimulation after thoracotomy. Pain relief and peak expiratory flow rate: A trial of transcutaneous electrical nerve stimulation. Anaesthesia, 43: 296–298

Taylor AG, West BA, Simon B, Sketon J, Rowlingson JC (1983) How effective is TENS for acute pain? Am J Nurs, 83: 1171–1174

Taylor DN, Katims JJ, Ng LK (1993) Sine-wave auricular TENS produces frequency-dependent hypoesthesia in the trigeminal nerve. Clin J Pain, 9: 216–219

Taylor P, Hallett M, Flaherty L (1981) Treatment of osteoarthritis of the knee with transcutaneous electrical nerve stimulation. Pain, 11: 233–240

Tekeoglu Y, Adak B, Goksoy T (1998) Effect of transcutaneous electrical nerve stimulation (TENS) in Barthel Activities of Daily Living (ADL) index score following stroke. Clin Rehab, 12: 277–280

Thomas IL, Tyle V, Webster J, Neilson A (1988) An evaluation of transcutaneous electrical nerve stimulation for pain relief in labour. Aust N Z J Obstet Gynaecol, 28: 182–189

Thorsen SW, Lumsden SG (1997) Trigiminal neuralgia: Sudden and long-term remission with transcutaneous electrical nerve stimulation. J Manipulative Physiol Ther, 20: 415–419

Thorsteinsson G, Stonnington HH, Stillwell GK, Elveback LR (1977) Transcutaneous electrical stimulation: A double-blind trial of its efficacy for pain. Arch Phys Med Rehab, 58: 8–13

Torres WE, Fraser NP, Baumgartner BR, Nelson RC, Evans GR, Jones V, Peterson J (1992) The use of transcutaneous electrical nerve stimulation during the biliary lithotripsy procedure. J Stone Dis, 4: 41–45

Tulgar M, McGlone F, Bowsher D, Miles J (1991) Comparative effectiveness of different stimulation modes in relieving pain. Part II: A double blind controlled long-term clinical trial. Pain, 47: 157–162

Vander Ark GD, McGrath KA (1975) Transcutaneous electrical stimulation in treatment of postoperative pain. Am J Surg, 130: 338–340

Vander Ploeg JM, Vervest HA, Liem AL, Schagen van Leewen JH (1996) Electrical nerve stimulation (TENS) during the first stage of labour: A randomized clinical trial. Pain, 68: 75–78

Walker RH, Morris BA, Angulo DL, Schneider J, Colwell CW (1991) Postoperative use of continuous passive motion, transcutaneous electrical nerve stimulation, and continuous cooling pad following total knee arthroplasty. J Arthroplasty, 6: 151–156

Wall PD (1978) The gate control theory of pain modulation. An examination and restatement. Brain, 101: 1–18

Warfield CA, Stein JM, Frank HA (1985) The effect of transcutaneous electrical nerve stimulation on pain after thoracotomy. Ann Thorac Surg, 39: 462–465

Warke K, Al-Smadi J, Baxter D, Walsh DM, Lowe-Strong AS (2006) Efficacy of transcutaneous electrical nerve stimulation (TENS) for chronic low-back pain in multiple sclerosis population: A randomized, placebo-controlled clinical trial. Clin J Pain, 22: 812–819

Weitz SH, Tunick PA, McElhinney L, Mitchell T, Kronzon I (1997) Pseudoatrial flutter: Artifact simulating atrial flutter coursed by a transcutaneous electrical nerve stimulation (TENS). Pacing Clin Electrophysiol, 20: 3010–3011

Wheeler JB, Doleys DM, , Harden RS, Clelland JA (1984) Conventional TENS electrode placement and pain threshold. Phys Ther, 64: 745

Woolf SL, Gersh MR, Rao VR (1981) Examination of electrode placements and stimulating parameters in treating chronic pain with conventional transcutaneous electrical nerve stimulation (TENS). Pain, 11: 37–47

Woolf CJ, Mitchell D, Myers RA, Barrett GD (1978) Failure of naloxone to reverse peripheral transcutaneous electro-analgesia in patients suffering from acute trauma. S Afr Med J, 53, 179–180

Yurtkuran M, Kocagil T (1999) TENS, electroacupuncture and ice massage: Comparison of treatment for osteoarthritis of the knee. Am J Acupunct, 27: 133–140

Zizic TM, Hoffman KC, Holt PA, Hungerford DS, Odell JR, Jacobs MA, Lewis CG, Deal CL, Caldwell JR, Cholewczuski JG, Free SM (1995) The treatment of osteoarthritis of the knee with pulsed electrical stimulation. J Rheumatol, 22: 1757–1761

Zugerman C (1982) Dermatitis from transcutaneous electrical nerve stimulation. J Am Acad Dermatol, 6: 936–939

Review Articles

Allen RJ (2006) Physical agents used in the management of chronic pain by physical therapists. Phys Med Rehabil Clin N Am, 17: 315–345

APTA (1996a) Management of the individual with pain. Part 1—Physiology and evaluation. PT Magazine, November: 54–63

APTA (1996b) Management of the individual with pain. Part 2—Treatment. PT Magazine, December: 58–65

Belanger AY (1985) Physiological evidence for an endogenous opiate-related pain-modulating system and its relevance to TENS: A review. Physiother Can, 37: 163–168

Bjordal JM, Johnson MI, Ljunggreen AE (2003) Transcutaneous electrical nerve stimulation (TENS) can reduce postoperative analgesics consumption. A meta-analysis with assessment of optimal treatment parameters for postoperative pain. Eur J Pain, 7: 181–188

Brosseau L, Yonge K, Marchand S, Robinson V, Osiri M, Wells G, Tugwell P (2004) Efficacy of transcutanenous electrical nerve stimulation for osteoarthritis of the lower extremities: A meta-analysis. Phys Ther Rev, 9: 213–233

Carroll D, Tramer M, McQuay H, Nye B, Moore A (1996) Randomization is important in studies with pain outcomes: Systematic review of transcutaneous electrical nerve stimulation in acute postoperative pain. Br J Anaesth, 77: 798–803

Carroll D, Tramer M, McQuay H, Nye B, Moore A (1997) Transcutaneous electrical nerve stimulation in labour pain: A systematic review. Br J Obstet Gynaecol, 104: 169–175

DeLeo JA (2006) Basic science of pain. J Bone Joint Surg (A), 88: 58–62

Dickenson AH (2002) Gate control theory of pain stands the test of time. Br J Anaesth, 88: 755–757

Gersh MR, Wolf SL (1985) Applications of transcutaneous electrical nerve stimulation in the management of patients with pain: State-of-the-art update. Phys Ther, 65: 314–336

Johnson MI (2000) The clinical effectiveness of TENS in pain management. Crit Rev Phys Med Rehab, 12: 131–149

Johnson MI (2001) Transcutaneous electrical nerve stimulation (TENS) and TENS-like devices: Do they provide pain relief? Pain Rev, 8: 121–158

Johnson M, Martinson M (2007) Efficacy of electrical nerve stimulation for chronic musculoskeletal pain: A meta-analysis of randomized controlled trials. Pain, 130: 157–165

Kaplan B, Rabinerson D, Pardo J, Krieser RV, Neri A (1997) Transcutaneous electrical nerve stimulation (TENS) as a pain-relief device in obstetrics and gynecology. Clin Exp Obstet Gynecol, 24: 123–126

Khadilkar A, Milne S, Brosseau L, Wells G, Tugwell P, Robinson V, Shea B, Saginur M (2005) Transcutaneous electrical nerve stimulation for the treatment of chronic low back pain: A systematic review. Spine, 30: 2657–2666

Lundeberg T (1995) Pain physiology and principles of treatment. Scand J Rehab Med (Suppl), 32: 13–42

Miller L, Mattison P, Paul L, Wood L (2005) The effects of transcutaneous electrical nerve stimulation on spasticity. Phys Ther Rev, 10: 201–208

Oosterwijk RF, Meyler WJ, Henley EJ, Scheer SS, Tannenbaum J (1994). Pain control with TENS and Team nerve stimulators: A review. Crit Rev Phys Med Rehab, 6: 219–258

Reeve J, Menon D, Corabian P (1996) Transcutaneous electrical nerve stimulation (TENS): A technology assessment. Int J Technol Assess Health Care, 12: 299–324

Richardson PH (1994) Placebo effects in pain management. Pain Rev, 1: 15–32

Robinson AJ (1996) Transcutaneous electrical nerve stimulation for the control of pain in musculoskeletal disorders. J Orthop Sports Phys Ther, 24: 208–226

Roche PA, Wright A (1990) An investigation into the value of transcutaneous electrical nerve stimulation (TENS) for arthritic pain. Physiother Theory Pract, 6: 25–33

Sluka KA, Walsh D (2003) Transcutaneous electrical nerve stimulation: Basic science mechanisms and clinical effectiveness. J Pain, 4: 109–121

Walsh DM, Baxter, GD (1996) Transcutaneous electrical nerve stimulation (TENS): A review of experimental studies. Eur J Phys Med Rehab, 6: 42–51

Ying KN, While A (2007) Pain relief in osteoarthritis and rheumatoid arthritis. Br J Community Nurs, 12: 364–371

Chapters of Textbooks

Barr JO (1999) Transcutaneous electrical nerve stimulation for pain management. In: Clinical Electrotherapy, 3rd ed. Nelson RM, Hayes KW, Currier DP (Eds). Appleton & Lange, Stamford, pp 291–354

Behrens BJ (2006) Electrodes: Material and care. In: Physical Agents—Theory and Practice, 2nd ed. Behrens BJ, Miclovitz SL (Eds). F.A Davis Co, Philadelphia, pp 163–173

Behrens BJ, Michlovitz SL (1996) Appendix: Optimal stimulation sites for TENS-electrodes. In: Physical Agents: Theory and Practice for the Physical Therapist Assistant. Behrens BJ, Michlovitz SL (Eds.) FA Davis Co., Philadelphia, pp 390–406

Foley RA (2000) Transcutaneous electrical nerve stimulation. In: Manual for Physical Agents, 5th ed. Hayes KW (Ed). Prentice-Hall Health, Upper Saddle River, pp 121–147

Frampton V (1996) Transcutaneous electrical nerve stimulation (TENS). In: Clayton's Electrotherapy, 10th ed. Kitchen S, Bazin S (Eds). WB Saunders, London, pp 287–305

Johnson M (2002) Transcutaneous electrical nerve stimulation (TENS). In: Electrotherapy Evidence-Based Practice. 11th ed. Kitchen S, (Ed). Churchill-Livingstone, Edinburg, pp 259–286

Kahn J (2000) Transcutaneous electrical nerve stimulation. In: Principles and Practice of Electrotherapy, 4th ed. Churchill Livingstone, New York, pp 101–117

Manal TJ, Snyder-Mackler L (2008) Electrical stimulation for pain. In: Clinical Electrophysiology—Electrotherapy and Electrophysiologic Testing, 3rd ed. Robinson AW, Snyder-Mackler L (Eds). Lippincott Williams & Wilkins, Philadelphia, pp151–196

Mayer DJ, Price DD (1995) Neural mechanisms of pain. In: Clinical Electrophysiology: Electrotherapy and Electrophysiologic Testing, 2nd ed. Robinson AW, Snyder-Mackler L (Eds). Williams & Wilkins, Baltimore, pp 211–278

Robinson AJ (2008) Physiology of muscle and nerve. In: Clinical Electrophysiology—Electrotherapy and Electrophysiologic Testing,

3rd ed. Robinson AW, Snyder-Mackler L (Eds). Lippincott Williams & Wilkins, Philadelphia, pp 71–105

Snyder-Mackler L (1995) Electrical stimulation for pain modulation. In: Clinical Electrophysiology: Electrotherapy and Electrophysiologic Testing, 2nd ed. Robinson AW, Snyder-Mackler L (Eds). Williams & Wilkins, Baltimore, pp 279–310

Weisberg J, Troiano R (2006) Transcutaneous Electrical Nerve Stimulation (TENS). In: Integrated Physical Agents in Rehabilitation, 2nd ed. Hecox B, Mehreteab TA, Weisberg J, Sanko J (Eds). Pearson Prentice Hall, Upper Saddle River, pp 295–306

Woolf CJ, Thompson JW (1994) Stimulation-induced analgesia: Transcutaneous electrical nerve stimulation (TENS) and vibration. In: Textbook of Pain, 3rd ed. Wall PD, Melzack R (Eds). Churchill Livingstone, Edinburgh, pp 1191–1208

Textbooks

Mannheimer JS, Lampe GN (1984) Clinical Transcutaneous Electrical Stimulation. FA Davis Co., Philadelphia

McMahon S, Koltzenburg M (2005) Wall and Melzack's Textbook of Pain. Churchill Livingstone, London

Melzack R, Wall PD (1982) The Challenge of Pain. Penguin Books Ltd., New York

Ottoson D, Lundeberg T (1988) Pain Treatment by Transcutaneous Electrical Nerve Stimulation: A Practical Manual. Springer-Verlag, New York

Walsh DM (1997) TENS: Clinical Applications and Related Theory. Churchill Livingstone, Edinburgh

Monograph

American Physical Therapy Association (2001) Electrotherapeutic Terminology in Physical Therapy. APTA Publications, Alexandria, p 36

Microcurrent Therapy

Chapter Outline

Learning Objectives

Knowledge: State the physiological rationale for the use of microcurrent therapy for the management of dermal wounds.

Comprehension: Distinguish between the concept of skin battery and current of injury.

Application: Show the placement of the active versus the dispersive electrode in relation to the wound site.

Analysis: Explain the galvanotaxis and anti-inflammatory effects attributed to microcurrent therapy.

Synthesis: Explain how microcurrent therapy can enhance wound healing.

Evaluation: Discuss the place microcurrent therapy should have, in relation to the other therapeutic electrophysical agents (EPAs) available, in the management of slow-to-heal dermal wounds.

I. RATIONALE FOR USE

A. DEFINITION AND DESCRIPTION

The term *microcurrent electrical stimulation*, designated by the acronym *MES*, is defined as the transcutaneous delivery of continuous and pulsed electrical current waveforms of amplitudes within the microamperage range, that is, from 1 to 999 μA, or less than 1 mA (APTA, 2001). Microcurrent therapy falls under the field of *electrical stimulation for tissue healing and repair*, designated under the acronym ESTHR. More specifically, MES is used to promote and accelerate the healing process of slow-to-heal cutaneous wounds (APTA, 2001; Robinson, 2008). The use of ESTHR was approved, in 2002, in the United States, for the treatment of various lower-extremity ulcers caused by pressure, vascular insufficiency and diabetes (Centers for Medicare and Medicaid Services, 2004).

B. MICROCURRENT STIMULATOR

Shown in **Figure 15-1** is a typical cabinet-type, line-powered, stimulator also capable of delivering continuous or pulsed microcurrent therapy, limiting the current amplitude below 1 mA. These cabinet-type stimulators are commonly referred to, in the corporate literature, as *combo* stimulators, meaning that a single stimulator, or unit, is capable of generating a *combination* (thus the word combo) of current waveforms simply by pushing a button on the stimulator's console.

C. ELECTRODE TYPES

Microcurrent therapy is commonly delivered, as shown in **Figure 15-2**, using reusable carbon-impregnated silicon rubber (**A**); fiber electrodes (**B**); and disposable homemade aluminum foil electrodes (**C**). Unlike commercial carbon electrodes, aluminum foil electrodes are very cost-effective and time efficient for treatment of open wounds (Sussman, 2007). They are very good conductors of electricity, are nontoxic, and are easily molded to fit the wound size and configuration.

D. RATIONALE FOR USE

The treatment of slow-to-heal chronic cutaneous wounds remains a significant health problem especially in the aging population (Kloth, 2002, 2005; Sussman et al., 2007a,b). Various therapeutic interventions are available to treat wounds, including topical and systemic antibiotics, topical antiseptics and dressings, hydrotherapy (Chapter 9), and surgical skin grafting (Kloth, 2005a). Unfortunately, many wounds worsen or do not heal despite the use of such therapies. Research for alternative therapies led to the discovery and application of microcurrent therapy, which is based on the fact that the human body has an endog-

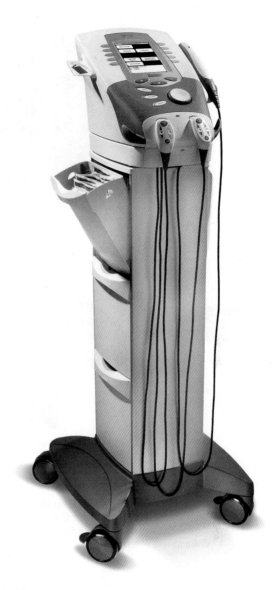

FIGURE 15-1 Typical cabinet and combo-type microcurrent stimulator. (Courtesy of Chattanooga Group.)

enous bioelectric system that enhances soft-tissue wound healing. When the patient's endogenous bioelectric system fails to contribute to the wound-healing process, therapeutic electrical stimulation dosages, within the microamperage range, are delivered externally to the wound to boost the weak endogenous healing system, thus enhancing and accelerating the wound-healing process.

II. HISTORICAL PERSPECTIVE

A. ROOTS

The delivery of electrical current into refractory wounds for the purpose of enhancing tissue healing is not new. Several reports dating from the seventeenth century describe the use of electrostatically charged gold leaf to treat various skin lesions (Kloth, 2005a,b; Sussman et al., 2007).

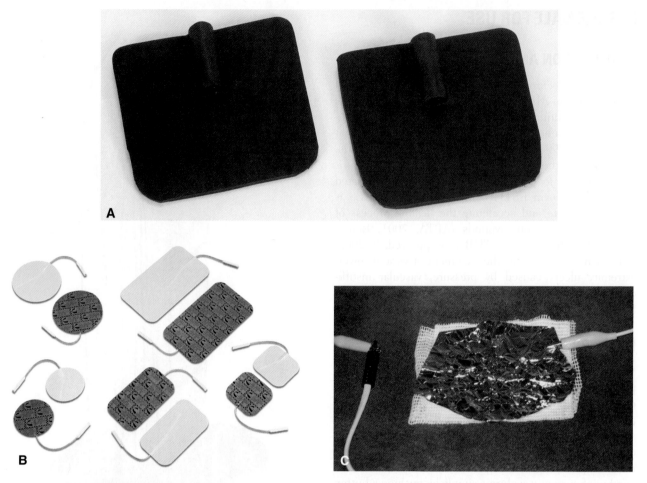

FIGURE 15-2 Typical carbon rubber (**A**), carbon fiber (**B**) and custom aluminum foil (**C**) electrodes. (A–B: Courtesy of Chattanooga Group; C: Reprinted with permission from Sussman C, Bates-Jensen B. *Wound Care: A Collaborative Practice Manual for Health Professionals*, 3rd ed. Baltimore, Maryland: Lippincott Williams and Wilkins, 2007.)

B. CONCEPTS

The development of microcurrent electrical therapy (MES) rests on the concept of *current of injury*, driven by *skin batteries*, originally proposed by Robert O. Becker, during the late 1960s, following research on animal soft-tissue healing and limb regeneration mechanisms.

1. Current of Injury

On the basis of both his original publication regarding cell dedifferentiation produced by very small electrical currents (Becker et al., 1967) and his well-publicized textbook (Becker et al., 1987), Becker theorized that a so-called *current of injury*, in the microampere range, is present in human tissues after trauma and diseases, and that such an endogenous current may be important in soft-tissue repair.

2. Skin Battery

Becker's hypothesis was also based on experimental discoveries, made during the 1970s and 1980s, of natural or endogenous direct currents in the vicinity of regenerating amphibian and mammalian stumps that are driven by so-called *skin batteries* (Borgens et al., 1977, 1984).

C. HUMAN SKIN BATTERIES

Inspired by findings in animals, similar studies were conducted on humans during the early 1980s to identify and measure such skin-battery voltages and currents of injury. Illingsworth et al. (1980) reported endogenous electrical currents at the stump surface of fingers, the tips of which had been accidentally amputated in children. Two years later, Barker et al. (1982) reported microcurrents leaving a wound in human skin immersed in saline. Then Foulds et al. (1983) set up an experiment to determine whether normal, or noninjured, human skin possessed battery potentials similar to those demonstrated in amphibians. Their results, obtained in 17 healthy subjects, revealed that there are skin batteries in healthy human cutaneous tissue with voltages comparable to those of animal skin batteries (see Section III, Biophysical Characteristics).

D. THERAPEUTIC ANALOGY

Based on the results of animal and human studies, injured cells originating from tissues such as skin, muscle, and nerve are believed to possess their own injury currents, and these endogenous electrical currents may play a major role in tissue repair. It logically follows that, if human tissue repair is mediated, at least in part, by electrical signals, then an exogenous electrical current delivered at the site of wounds may enhance the healing process.

E. FIRST CLINICAL STUDIES

The first two published reports of microcurrent therapy for wound healing in humans were those of Assimacopoulos (1968) for venous ulcers and Wolcott et al. (1969) for diabetic ulcers.

F. BODY OF LITERATURE

Microcurrent (MES) therapy has been the subject of several *articles* (see References), *review articles* (Picker, 1988a,b; Dayton et al., 1989; Gersh, 1989; Weiss et al., 1990; Gentzkow et al., 1991; Wieder, 1991; Gentzkow, 1993; Kloth, 1995; Makiov, 1995; Kloth et al., 1996; Mercola et al., 1995; Lampe, 1998; Gardner et al., 1999; Houghton, 1999; Houghton et al., 1999; Bogie et al., 2000; Kloth, 2005a; Keast et al., 2007) and *chapters of textbooks* (Byl, 1999; Sussman et al., 1999; Kloth, 2002; Watson, 2002; Kloth, 2005; Sussman, 2007; Robinson, 2008). *Brief coverage* of microcurrent therapy can also be found in *textbooks* focused on wound care (Kloth et al., 2002; Shai et al., 2005; Falabella et al., 2005; Sussman et al., 2007).

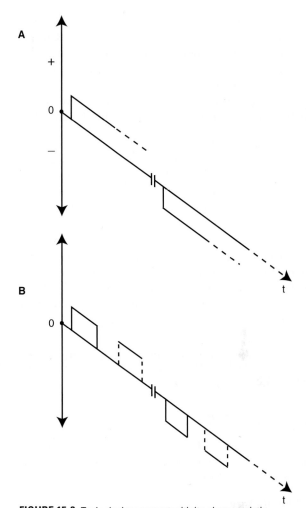

FIGURE 15-3 Typical microcurrent with its characteristic continuous (**A**) or pulsed (**B**) monophasic waveform, and optional polarity reversal.

III. BIOPHYSICAL CHARACTERISTICS

A. CURRENT WAVEFORM

Microcurrent therapy is delivered using constant or pulsed direct current with maximum current amplitude never exceeding 1 mA or 1000 μA. The current waveform shown in **Figure 15-3A** corresponds to a continuous monophasic waveform with optional polarity reversal, whereas that shown in **Figure 15-3B** refers to a pulsed monophasic rectangular waveform, with a similar optional polarity reversal.

B. CONFUSING TERMINOLOGY

The biophysical terminology used in microcurrent therapy is confusing in many aspects, and clarifications are needed.

1. MENS Versus MES

Microcurrent therapy was originally referred to in the literature as microcurrent electrical nerve stimulation, or MENS. The term *nerve* was quickly abandoned because current amplitudes within the microamperage range (less than 1 mA) are too weak to stimulate or depolarize nerve fibers. This led to the correct designation of microcurrent electrical stimulation, or MES.

2. MES Versus LIDC

The APTA booklet on Electrophysiological Terminology (APTA, 2001) defines low-intensity direct current, or LIDC, as the use of *direct* (or continuous) current of less than 1 mA. It also defines MES as the delivery of a *pulsed* current at maximum amplitude of less than 1 mA. In this textbook, therefore, microcurrent therapy is defined as the use of both direct and pulsed current waveforms of amplitudes less than 1 mA.

3. Microamperage Versus Milliamperage Stimulation

Because MES refers to the use of electrical currents in the microamperage range, as opposed to the milliamperage range, the designation *microamperage stimulation* (MS) was also introduced in reference to MES. For example, the electrical currents used to deliver iontophoresis therapy (Chapter 13), TENS therapy (Chapter 14), Russian current therapy (Chapter 17), interferential current therapy (Chapter 18), and diadynamic current therapy (Chapter 19), all belong to the field of *milliamperage stimulation* because their waveforms have current amplitudes greater than 1 mA, often within 1–120 mA.

4. Crediting Benefits

It is important to distinguish microamperage from milliamperage stimulation or therapy because one can *erroneously credit* to the field of microcurrent therapy the therapeutic outcomes obtained using milliamperage therapy. For example, one *cannot* credit to the field of microcurrent therapy, as mentioned in some textbooks and scientific articles, the therapeutic benefits on human wound repair reported by Kaada (1983), Mulder (1991), Gentzkow et al. (1991), Feedar et al. (1991), and Baker et al. (1996) because the current amplitudes used in these studies were greater than 1 mA.

IV. PHYSIOLOGICAL AND THERAPEUTIC EFFECTS

A. FOUNDATIONS

Presented in **Figure 15-4** are schematic illustrations of the principle or foundation underlying the physiological and therapeutic effects of MES on wound repair.

1. Skin Battery

Figure 15-4A shows a typical skin battery, located at the interface between the stratum corneum and the dermis, demonstrated experimentally by Foulds et al. (1983) in normal human skin tissue. Becker hypothesized that a direct current bioelectrical system is present in the human body and that this system is responsible for maintaining tissue health (Becker et al., 1987).

2. Currents of Injury

Figure 15-4B illustrates the currents of injury driven by those skin batteries located at the wound site after trauma or disease. Becker further hypothesized that when the body is injured a disturbance within the body's electrical system causes a shift in the current flow at the site of injury, which he labeled the current of injury (Becker et al., 1987).

3. Mimic and Amplification

Figure 15-4C shows Becker's fundamental proposition that an exogenous source of electrical current applied over an injured tissue, such as MES applied over a dermal wound, enhances the healing process. In the present case, MES *mimics* and *amplifies* those endogenous, weak human skin batteries at the wound site to enhance and maintain, with repeated applications over time, the skin's healing process.

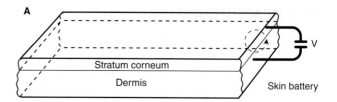

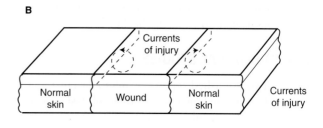

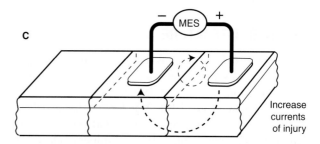

FIGURE 15-4 Schematic representation of a human skin battery (**A**), currents of injury flow after a wound to the skin (**B**), and increased current of injury amplitude by application of MES (**C**). Continuous flow of endogenous current (circling arrow), which is driven by the skin battery, is presumed to sustain the normal repair process of skin tissue in the absence of injury (**A**). Injury to the skin (wound) causes the flow of this endogenous current, now called currents of injury, to flow at the interface between the damaged and the normal skin tissue (**B**). Delivery of MES at the wound site mimics and augments the amplitude of those weak currents of injury to enhance tissue healing.

B. ENHANCED CURRENTS OF INJURY

The rationale behind this therapeutic approach is the fact that animals as a whole, and amphibians in particular, have a much greater capacity for tissue self-healing than humans do. This concept suggests that, through the evolutionary process, human currents of injury have become less efficient; hence the need to mimic and amplify those weak skin batteries to obtain stronger, more efficient currents of injury to enhance soft-tissue repair. In other words, by providing an external current to the wound, MES mimics and augments those weak, natural bioelectric currents to enhance wound repair. To facilitate learning of the material to follow, readers are *strongly advised to review* Chapter 2, which describes the healing process underlying soft tissue pathology.

C. GALVANOTAXIS AND GERMICIDAL EFFECTS

Presented in **Figure 15-5** are the proposed physiological and therapeutic events and effects underlying MES therapy (Kloth, 2005a,b; Robinson, 2008). The application of MES is presumed to enhance the currents of injury generated by the skin battery. These stronger currents of injury are then presumed to induce *galvanotaxis* and *bacterial growth inhibition* effects on dermal wounds.

1. Galvanotaxis Effect

Because many key cells involved in the process of wound healing carry a negative or a positive charge, Kloth et al., (1996, Kloth, 2005a,b) hypothesized that the monophasic nature of MES facilitates the *galvanotaxic* attraction of these cells into the wound via application of a cathode or anode over or around the wound, thereby promoting the different phases of wound healing (**Fig 15-5**). The term galvanotaxis stems for the word *galvano*—for electrical galvanic cell producing direct current having monophasic waveforms—and the word *taxis*—for orderly arrangement of motile organisms in response to a stimulus either toward the cathode (positively charged cells) or the anode (negatively charged cells).

a. Inflammatory Phase

There is experimental evidence to suggest that negatively charged cells, such as macrophages (−) and neutrophils (−), will migrate toward the anode (+), thus promoting the inflammatory phase (phagocytosis and autolysis) of wound healing (Kloth, 1995, 2005; Robinson, 2008). This makes anodal stimulation the treatment option of choice for the management inflamed wounds (**Fig 15-5**).

b. Proliferative Phase

There is also experimental evidence to suggest that positively charged cells, such as fibroblasts (+), will migrate toward the cathode (−) during MES therapy, thus promoting the proliferative (collagen formation) phase of wound healing (Kloth, 1995, 2005a,b; Robinson, 2008). Cathodal stimulation may therefore be the treatment option of choice for the management of wounds in their proliferative phase (**Fig 15-5**).

c. Remodeling/Maturation Phase

There is experimental evidence to also suggest that positively charged cells, such as keratinocytes (+) and epidermal (+) cells, will migrate toward the cathode (−), thus promoting the remodeling/maturation phase of wound healing. Once again, cathodal stimulation may be the preferred treatment option for the management of wounds in this phase of repair (**Fig 15-5**).

2. Germicidal Effect

There is limited experimental evidence to suggest that passing a monophasic electrical current, such as the case with

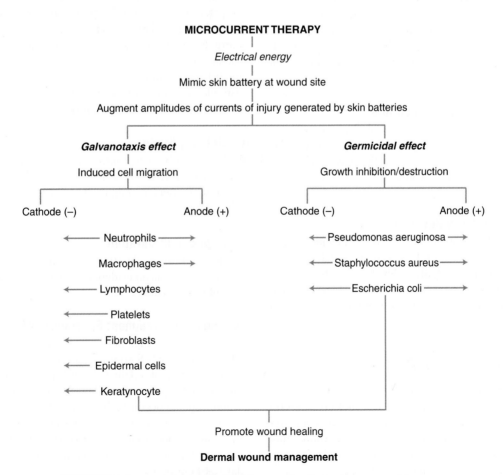

FIGURE 15-5 Proposed physiological and therapeutic effects of microcurrent therapy.

MES therapy, into a wound may have a *germicidal effect* on germs, as shown in **Figure 15-5**, that commonly colonize or infect human wounds, such as *E-coli*, *Pseudomonas aeruginosa*, and *Staphylococcus aureus* (Watson, 2002; Kloth, 2005a,b; Sussman et al., 2007; Robinson, 2008). There is slightly better evidence to suggest that the passage of such monophasic current waveforms may have, instead, a *growth inhibition* effect on bacteria (Merriman et al., 2004; Kloth, 2005a,b; Robinson, 2008).

D. ELECTRODE POLARITY

As stated earlier and based on **Figure 15-5**, which electrode polarity should best facilitate the proposed galvanotaxis and germicidal effects following microcurrent therapy?

1. Anodal Stimulation

This stimulation mode should be used in cases where wound *inflammation* is present because the migration (galvanotaxis) of key cells such as macrophages and neutrophils to the wound site will stimulate the inflammatory response, thus improving tissue repair.

2. Cathodal Stimulation

After the inflammatory phase has subsided, cathodal stimulation of the wound should be used in order to facilitate the *proliferative/remodeling/maturation* phases of healing through the migration of key cells such as fibroblasts, keratynocytes, and epidermal cells to the wound site.

3. Anodal or Cathodal Stimulation

Practitioners may use either cathodal or anodal stimulation first over the *infected* wound as the evidence seems to suggest that both electrode polarities may induce germ growth inhibition at the wound site (Merriman et al., 2004).

4. Electrode Polarity Reversal

Because the different phases of wound healing overlap over time (see Chapter 2), it is recommended that electrode polarity *be reversed* after a few treatments to ensure migration of both negatively (anti-inflammatory) and positively (repair) charged cells at the wound site during the entire course of therapy.

E. MOIST ENVIRONMENT

Research has shown that currents of injury are sustained in a moist wound environment but will shut off when the wound dries out (Kloth, 2005a,b). The clinical implication of this finding is that, to facilitate healing, the wound must be covered by occlusive, moisture-retentive dressings at all times (Kloth, 2005a,b; Sussman et al., 2007).

V. DOSIMETRY

A. PARAMETERS

Dosimetry for MES consists in setting the following parameters: current amplitude, electrode polarity, delivery mode, application duration, number of treatment sessions per day, and number of treatment days per week.

1. Current Amplitude

As the topic of this chapter implies, current amplitude must be within the microamperage range, that is, between 1 and 999 μA. This setting is largely determined by the patient's ability to tolerate the set current amplitude at the wound site for a relatively long period of time.

2. Electrode Polarity

Selection is based on the healing phase the practitioner wants to facilitate (see **Fig 15-5**). Anodal stimulation is recommended during the inflammatory phase of wound healing. Cathodal stimulation, on the other hand, is recommended to facilitate the proliferative, remodeling/maturation phases of wound healing. Cathodal or anodal stimulation may be used to manage germ wound infection, when present. Because the phases of wound healing overlap over time, it is recommended that the stimulator be programmed for a periodic reversal of the current polarity during the entire treatment session. This automatic current polarity reversal leads to an equal period of cathodal and anodal stimulation of the wound site per treatment session. Another suggestion is to alternate between cathodal and anodal stimulation at the wound site every 3 days for the duration of treatment.

3. Delivery Mode

Delivery can be with *continuous* or *pulsed* mode, with or without polarity reversal (**Fig 15-3**). Pulsed mode is applied at frequencies ranging from 0.1 to 200 pulses per second (pps).

4. Application Duration

Single application duration may range from 30 to 120 minutes. There is no evidence on which to base the selection of this parameter.

5. Number of Treatment Sessions per Day

Treatments can range between 1 and 4 sessions per day. Most portable MES stimulators feature a switch that allows presetting of a daily ON:OFF time stimulation regimen. For example, setting a daily ON:OFF time regimen of 1 hour:5 hours over a 12-hour period automatically yields two treatment sessions per day. This feature is practical, in that it allows practitioners to program all the parameters at one time for half the day, as just mentioned, or for the full day (24-hour period).

6. Number of Treatment Days per Week

Treatment days can range from 5 to 7 days per week. There is no evidence on which to base the selection of this parameter.

VI. EVIDENCE FOR INDICATIONS

A. GUIDED BY EVIDENCE

Dictionaries generally define *evidence* as anything that establishes a fact or gives reason to believe something. The aim of this textbook is to present *scientific* evidence behind therapeutic electrophysical agents (EPAs). To be guided by evidence is the process of integrating the evidence from research, however imperfect or scarce this evidence may be, with clinical experience and patients' values. In other words, the *evidence-based practice* of EPA requires that practitioners consider the evidence from research, in addition to their own clinical experience and patients' own preferences and beliefs about a given EPA, when the time comes to justify, prescribe, and apply the therapeutic agent. To be guided by evidence is a process, not a search for the absolute truth. Finally, a lack of evidence from research to support any given EPA does not mean that this

EPA should never be used. What it means is that no statement can be made about its therapeutic effectiveness and that until more evidence from research is presented, its routine use cannot be recommended.

B. EVIDENCE FROM HUMAN RESEARCH

Box 15-1 provides evidence for MES therapy based on an exhaustive search of published English-language, peer-reviewed studies on humans. The term *indication* is used in reference to a list of pathologies for which microcurrent therapy is used. Ratings of therapeutic benefit (Yes or No) and a grading of the strength of scientific evidence (I, II, or III), including the reference, are included for each pathological condition.

1. Rating Therapeutic Benefit

The rating, expressed as Yes or No, is based on the overall conclusion(s) reached on the issue of therapeutic effectiveness by the author(s) who conducted the peer-reviewed study.

2. Grading Strength of Evidence

The grading, numerically classified as I, II, and III, is based on the type of research methodology, or experimental

---

Box 15-1	Research-Based Indications for the Use of Microcurrent Therapy		
PATHOLOGY	**BENEFIT**	**GRADE**	**REFERENCE**
Dermal wounds	Yes	I	Wood et al., 1993
	Yes	I	Gault et al., 1976
	Yes	I	Carley et al., 1985
	Yes	II	Wolcott et al., 1969
	Yes	II	Assimacopoulos, 1968
	Yes	III	Barron et al., 1985
	Yes	III	Weiss et al., 1989
Delayed-onset muscle soreness	No	I	Allen et al., 1999
	No	I	Weber et al., 1994
	No	I	Bonacci et al., 1997
	No	II	Denegar et al., 1992
Resistant myofascial trigger points	Yes	II	McMakin, 1998
Epicondylitis	Yes	I	Johannsen et al., 1993
Myocontracture	Yes	III	Maenpaa et al., 2004
Shoulder peritendinitis	Yes	I	Hatten et al., 1990
Low-back disorders	Yes	I	Lerner et al., 1981
Temporomandibular joint disorders	Yes	I	Bertolucci et al., 1995

design used by the author(s). All the studies listed are on humans, published in English-language, peer-reviewed journals. It follows that the evidence in studies graded I is stronger than in those graded II, where the evidence is stronger than in studies graded III.

a. Grade I

Evidence based on *controlled* studies on humans, regardless of their level of randomization and blindness.

b. Grade II

Evidence based on *noncontrolled* studies on humans, regardless of their level of randomization and blindness.

c. Grade III

Evidence based on *case* studies on humans, regardless of their level of randomization and blindness.

3. Strength of Evidence Behind the Agent

The strength of evidence behind the agent, as presented in the research-based indication box, is arbitrarily assessed in this textbook as *weak*, *moderate*, or *strong*. For example, the larger the number of studies graded I, regardless of therapeutic benefit, the stronger the scientific evidence behind the agent.

4. Strength for Justifying Usage of Agent

The strength of evidence justifying the usage of an agent for an individual pathology or groups of pathologies, as listed in the research-based indication box, is arbitrarily assessed in this textbook as *poor*, *fair*, *good*, or *conflicting*. For example, where a larger number of grade I studies show therapeutic benefit (Yes) than no benefit, for a given pathology the justification for usage of this agent for that pathology is assessed as *good*. *Conflicting* usage is reported when an equal number of studies with similar grades show therapeutic benefit (Yes) and no benefit (No).

C. STRENGTH OF EVIDENCE AND JUSTIFICATION FOR USAGE

The results presented in **Box 15-1** show *moderate* strength of evidence behind the use of MES therapy for dermal wounds, with the majority of studies, all showing benefit, graded I and II. These results also show that the justification for usage of MES therapy is *fair to good* for dermal wounds. This finding is consistent with the recent FDA approval (2002) of the use of electrical stimulation, such as microcurrent therapy, for tissue healing and repair (ESTHR). Results presented in **Box 15-1** also show *no justification* for the use of this EPA for management of delayed-onset muscle soreness. Until more evidence from research is provided with regard to those remaining pathologies listed, or any other pathology, the routine use of MES therapy for such pathologies *cannot be recommended*.

VII. CONTRAINDICATIONS

Table 15-1 lists the contraindications associated with microcurrent therapy. Note that the use of this EPA over the anterior cervical area is contraindicated, although the risk of nerve stimulation is minimal, considering the very low current amplitude (less than mA) used to deliver microcurrent therapy.

VIII. RISKS, PRECAUTIONS, AND RECOMMENDATIONS

The practice of MES therapy is not without risks for the patient. The main risks associated with this EPA, as well as some precautions and recommendations designed to improve safety and effectiveness, are listed in **Table 15-2**.

TABLE 15-1	CONTRAINDICATIONS TO MICROCURRENT THERAPY
CONTRAINDICATIONS	**RATIONALE**
Over osteomyelitis[a] area	Risk of blinding the site of observation (wound penetration to the bone) because tissue growth after MES therapy may superficially cover the osteomyelitis area (Sussman et al., 1999).
Over cancerous areas	Risk of further enhancing and spreading the tumor due to increased blood flow into the treated area.
Over electronic implants	Risk of interference with normal functioning of these devices.
Over anterior cervical area (pulsed mode)	Risk of stimulating key organs such as the vagus nerve, phrenic nerve, and carotid sinuses (Picker, 1988b). The risk is *minimal* because the maximum current amplitude is very low (less than 1 mA), which makes depolarization of such nerves practically impossible.

[a]Osteomyelitis is the inflammation of bone marrow, adjacent bone, and epiphysial cartilage.

TABLE 15-2	RISKS, PRECAUTIONS, AND RECOMMENDATIONS FOR MICROCURRENT THERAPY

RISK	RATIONALE
Over a hemorrhagic area	Risk of promoting further bleeding due to increased blood circulation into the treated area.

PRECAUTIONS	RATIONALE
Auto- and cross-contamination with open wound	May induce auto- and cross-contamination if adequate measures are not taken (see Recommendations).
Coupling media temperature	Cool media may chill the wound, increasing the possibility of slowing down mitotic activity, thus delaying or slowing down wound healing (Sussman et al., 1999, see Recommendations).

RECOMMENDATIONS	RATIONALE
Wear protective gown, gloves, mask, and goggles	To assure adequate protection against cross-contamination and/or infection of the wound.
Clean, irrigate, and debride the wound before treatment	Removal of necrotic material, foreign material, heavy metals, and previous topical medication, including petroleum gel or paste, from the wound will prevent penetration, caused by current flow, of foreign materials and medication that may hinder or adversely affect wound healing (Kloth et al., 1996; Sussman et al., 1999).
Use disposable rather than reusable electrodes	Prevent the risk of auto- and cross-contamination of the wound.
Ensure that the coupling media temperature is warmer than the wound surface, but no hotter than 38°C (100°F), before applying over the wound.	This measure will prevent chilling of the wound, which may slow healing. Use portable infrared thermometer to record temperature (see Chapter 26).
Plug line-powered stimulater into GFCI receptacle	Prevent the risk of electrocution (see Chapter 27).
Discard coupling media and disposable electrodes in biowaste bucket	Prevent the risk of auto- and cross-contamination.
Conduct regular maintenance and calibration	Ensure optimal treatment efficacy. Follow the manufacturer's recommendations and schedules.

IX. CONSIDERATIONS FOR APPLICATION AND DOCUMENTATION

A. CONSIDERATIONS AND PROCEDURES

The safe, effective, and optimal application of this EPA requires that practitioners go through a systematic set of considerations and procedures for each and every application. Presented here is a list of such considerations and procedures.

1. Checklists

Before proceeding with treatment, always go through the list of contraindications (**Table 15-1**) and list of risks, precautions, and recommendations (**Table 15-2**).

2. Wound Preparation

Before each application, the wound should be washed, cleansed, and debrided using mechanical or hydrotherapeutic interventions. To prevent contamination, practitioners *must* adopt protective measures, that is, wearing

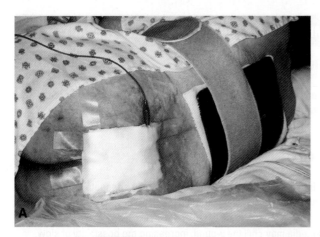
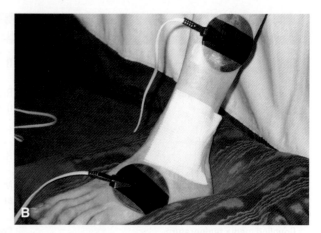

FIGURE 15-6 Electrode placement over (**A**) and around (**B**) the wound. (Reprinted with permission from Sussman C, Bates-Jensen B. *Wound Care: A Collaborative Practice Manual for Health Professionals,* 3rd ed. Baltimore, Maryland: Lippincott Williams and Wilkins, 2007.)

of masks, gloves, goggles, and gowns during wound preparation and treatment.

3. Electrode Placements

Illustrated in **Figure 15-6** are the two common electrode placements used by practitioners to deliver microcurrent therapy for dermal wound management. These placements can be described as *over the wound* (**A**) and *around the wound* (**B**).

a. Over the Wound

This first electrode placement is as follows: one electrode is positioned directly *over the wound,* and the other a few centimeters away (**Fig 15-6A**). The electrode over the wound is called the *active* electrode, and the other the *dispersive* electrode.

b. Around the Wound

This second electrode placement is as follows: both electrodes are positioned around the wound, over healthy tissues adjacent to the wound margins (**Fig 15-6B**).

4. Electrode Preparation

Over the wound placement: Wrap the active electrode with layers of sterile gauze pads, saturate the pads with Ringer solution or normal saline solution, and position the electrode/pad arrangement over the wound (**Fig 15-6A**). The pads must be warmer than the wound before application, but not warmer than 38°C (100°F). Cover the dispersive electrode with electroconductive gel. *Around the wound:* Cover both electrodes with electroconductive gel and secure to the skin using hypoallergic tape (**Fig 15-6B**).

5. Electrode Polarity

Select electrode polarity according to the wound healing phase. Kloth (2002, 2005a,b; Robinson, 2008) proposes the following polarity settings: *Anodal* stimulation should be used to manage the inflammatory phase of healing. *Cathodal* stimulation, on the other hand, should be used to facilitate the proliferative, remodeling, and maturation phases of wound healing. Both anodal and cathodal stimulation can be used to manage infected wounds.

6. Polarity Reversal

It is recommended that electrode polarity be reversed periodically over the course of therapy (i.e., every 3–4 treatments). This will ensure a balanced migration of positively and negatively charged cells at the wound site.

7. Current Amplitude

Set the current amplitude between 1 and 999 μA; there is no precise guideline on this subject. Setting of this parameter must be guided by the patient's sensation at the wound site during stimulation.

8. Delivery Mode

Set continuous or pulsed mode. There is no evidence to suggest that one mode is better than the other.

9. Treatment Schedule

Determine the application duration and the number of treatment sessions per day by setting the ON:OFF time ratio on the stimulator. The wound may be treated for 30–60 minutes, 2 or 3 times a day. Treatments may be delivered between 5 and 7 days a week.

10. End of Treatment

Inspect the wound and question the patient on the sensation perceived during treatment. Any unusual sensation felt during treatment should be documented in the patient's file. To optimize treatment effectiveness, *do not remove* the sterile gauze pad covering the wound after treatment. Keep this coupling medium moist and in place until the next treatment. Proceed with wound dressing. Discard used material in a biowaste bag. If the active electrode is reusable, make sure that it is properly washed and disinfected before using again. Disposable electrodes are highly recommended in preference to reusable electrodes, especially if the over-the-wound method of application is used.

11. Treatment Discontinuation

Treatment is stopped when the wound shows a 100% epithelialized wound bed, or when the wound is closed (Kloth, 2002, 2005a,b).

B. DOCUMENTATION

Table 15-3 shows the key parameters to be documented in the patient's file when using microcurrent therapy.

TABLE 15-3	KEY TREATMENT PARAMETERS TO BE DOCUMENTED IN PATIENT'S FILE AFTER MICROCURRENT THERAPY

- *MES stimulator type:* portable or cabinet
- *Delivery mode:* pulsed or continuous
- *If pulsed mode:* waveform duration (μs)
  pulse frequency (Hz)
- *Current amplitude:* μA
- *Electrode type and size:* description
- *Coupling medium:* sterile cotton gauze, electroconductive gel, hydrogel pad
- *Active electrode polarity:* cathode (−) or anode (+)
- *Electrode placement:* over the wound; around wound margins
- *Dispersive electrode positioning:* cm away from active electrode
- *Application duration:* min
- *Number of treatment sessions per day:* number

Case Study 15-1   Infected Ischial Pressure Ulcer

A well-oriented and underweight 76-year-old woman, showing evidence of poor hygiene and malnutrition, is admitted to the hospital with an infected pressure ulcer over the right ischial tuberosity. This woman lives alone and presents with difficulty walking. She reports spending long hours sitting on her hard wooden chair playing cards with friends, knitting, and watching television. These long and repeated sitting hours have caused significant pressure on the buttock soft tissues leading to the development of her ischial pressure ulcer. Physical examination reveals the presence of a painful stage II pressure ischial ulcer approximately 2 cm in diameter. Laboratory results confirm that the ulcer is colonized, or infected, with the bacteria *Pseudomonas aeruginosa*. She states that the ulcer began approximately 6 months ago. Over the past few weeks, she recalls that the ulcer has enlarged, become more painful, enabling her to sit for only a brief amount of time and forcing her to consult at the hospital. The treating physician at the hospital is aware that electrical stimulation may benefit the healing and repair of this ulcer. He refers his patient for ESTHR. Your goals, and those of the treating physician, are to eliminate infection and promote wound healing until complete closure. The patient's goals are to be able to sit with a minimum of pain, to see complete healing of her ulcer, and to resume playing cards with her friends at home. One of her friends is a former nurse who is more than willing to assist her (i.e., wound preparation and electrode setup) with her home MES treatment. The therapeutic plan is to begin therapy on an inpatient basis and, after

hospital discharge, to continue on an outpatient basis at home. During her hospital stay, the patient will also receive nursing care (optimize hygiene) and nutritional (weight control) counseling.

Evidence-Based Steps Toward the Resolution of This Case

1. **Establish medical diagnosis.**

   Stage II pressure ischial ulcer with bacterial infection

2. **List key impairment(s).**
   - Right ischial pain
   - Open ischial wound
   - Bacterial infection

3. **List key functional limitation(s).**
   - Difficulty with sitting
   - Difficulty with walking

4. **List key disabilities.**
   - Difficulty with prolonged sitting while playing cards

5. **Justification for MES therapy.**

   Is there justification to use MES therapy in this case? This chapter has established that there is *moderate* strength of evidence and *fair-to-good* justification for the use of microcurrent therapy for dermal ulcers (see Section VI.). This textbook recommends the use of this EPA for the following reasons. First, MES is expected to promote wound healing through its galvanotaxis

(Continued)

Case Study 15-1   Continued

and germicidal effects. Second, MES can be easily delivered on an outpatient basis at home. Third, there is evidence that MES therapy is justified based on the following articles: Wolcott et al., 1969; Gault et al., 1976, Carley et al., 1985; Wood et al., 1993; Gardner et al., 1999; Kloth, 2002; Kloth, 2005a,b. Because EPAs should never be used in isolation or as a sole intervention, a regimen MES of hydrotherapy, which consists of cleansing, irrigating, and debriding the wound before each daily therapeutic session, and wound dressing, applied between treatment sessions, is also used.

6. Search for contraindications.

None is found.

7. Search for risks and precautions.

None is found.

8. Outline the therapeutic goal(s) you and your patient wish to achieve.

- Decrease pain
- Eliminate wound infection
- Close the wound
- Resume normal sitting and walking
- Facilitate leisure (playing cards)

9. List outcome measurement(s) used to assess treatment effectiveness.

- Pain: 101-point Numerical Rating Scale (NRS-101)
- Wound infection status: bacterial culture counts
- Wound healing status: Pressure Sore Status Tool (PSST)
- Sitting/walking performance: Patient-Specific Function Scale (PSFS)

10. Instruct patient about what he/she should experience, do, and not do during the treatment session.

- Should feel very light tingling under electrodes
- Do not touch stimulator, electrodes, and wires during treatment

11. Outline your therapeutic prescription based on the best sources of evidence available.

The following MES prescription is based on the following literature: Wolcott et al., 1969; Gault et al., 1976; Carley et al., 1985; Wood et al., 1993; Kloth, 2005a,b.

- *MES stimulator type:* portable
- *Waveform type:* monophasic
- *Delivery mode:* pulsed, 10 Hz
- *Waveform duration:* 600 μs
- *Current amplitude:* 800 μA
- *Electrode placement:* over the wound
- *Active electrode type and size:* aluminum foil cut to wound size and shape

- *Dispersive electrode type and size:* carbon rubber—4 $\times$ 8 cm^2 (2 $\times$ 3 in)
- *Coupling media:* under active electrode; sterile saline-soaked gauze packed into the wound under dispersive electrode: hydrogel pad
- *Electrode polarity reversal:* every 5 treatments
- *Dispersive electrode positioning:* 15 cm away from left gluteal area
- *Body positioning:* lying on left side
- *Application duration:* 90 min
- *Number of treatment sessions per day:* 2
- *Treatment frequency:* daily
- *Total treatment duration:* 4 weeks
- *Inpatient / outpatient schedule:* Inpatient—3 days (6 treatments); outpatient—25 days (50 treatments)

12. Collect outcome measurements.

Pre- and posttreatment comparison:

- Pain: decrease NRS-101 score from 70 to 25
- Wound infection status: test culture negative after 12 treatments
- Wound healing status: PSST score improved by 100%
- Sitting/walking performance: PSFS score improved by 100%

13. Assess therapeutic effectiveness based on outcome measures.

The results show that microcurrent therapy (MES), combined with nursing and nutritional counseling while hospitalized and regular hydrotherapy, delivered twice a day on an inpatient and outpatient basis for four consecutive weeks, led to complete healing of the wound. This elderly patient is now able to sit normally and comfortably at home enjoying her favorite leisure activity, playing cards with her friends. This treatment approach had a beneficial impact on the patient's disablement status created by the pathology, as illustrated in the **figure** shown on the next page.

14. State the prognosis.

The prognosis is excellent in that such an ulcer is unlikely to recur if the patient put into practice the nursing (better skin hygiene) and nutritional (increase weight gain through healthy nutrition) advices she received while at the hospital. She is advised to always put cushions on her chairs and limit prolonged sitting to no more than 30 minutes at a time (walk for a few minutes in between sitting sessions). She is also advised to massage her gluteal region and to regularly monitor this region, using a mirror, for any sign of irritation or ulceration.

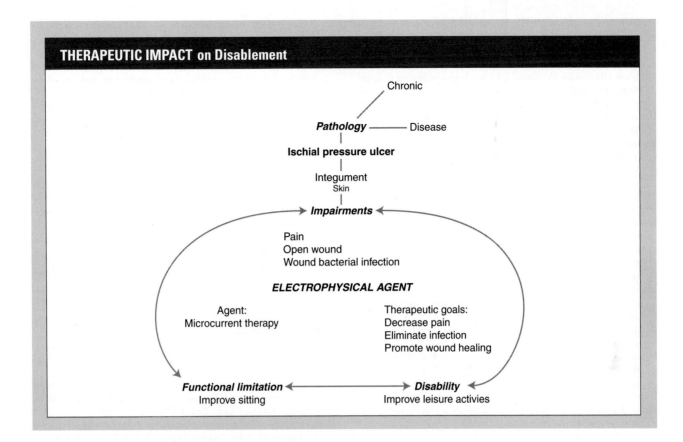

THERAPEUTIC IMPACT on Disablement

Chronic

Pathology ——— Disease

Ischial pressure ulcer

Integument
Skin

Impairments

Pain
Open wound
Wound bacterial infection

ELECTROPHYSICAL AGENT

Agent:
Microcurrent therapy

Therapeutic goals:
Decrease pain
Eliminate infection
Promote wound healing

Functional limitation
Improve sitting

Disability
Improve leisure activies

CRITICAL THINKING QUESTIONS

Clarification: What is meant by microcurrent electrical therapy (MES)?

Assumptions: You have assumed that the human body possesses an endogenous bioelectrical system that plays an important role in the process of dermal tissue healing. How do you justify making that assumption?

Reasons and evidence: What led you to believe that delivering an external source of monophasic electrical current to the wound site can enhance tissue repair?

Viewpoints or perspectives: How would you respond to a colleague who says that only microamperage electric current can enhance wound repair?

Implications and consequences: What are the implications or consequences of not maintaining a moist environment for the wound in between treatment, and of alternating electrode polarity during the course of treatment?

About the question: Is it true that MES therapy is only indicated for noninfected wounds? Why do you think I ask this question?

References

Articles

Allen JD, Mattacola CG, Perrin DH (1999) Effect of microcurrent stimulation on delayed-onset muscle soreness: A double-blind comparison. J Athl Train, 34: 334–337

Assimacopoulos D (1968) Low-intensity negative electric current in the treatment of ulcers of the leg due to chronic venous insufficiency: Preliminary reports of three cases. Am J Surg, 115: 683–687

Baker LL, Rubayi S, Villar F, DeMuth SK (1996) Effect of electrical stimulation waveform on healing of ulcers in human beings with spinal cord injury. Wound Repair Regen, 4: 21–28

Barker AT, Jaffe LF, Vanable JW (1982) The glabrous epidermis of cavies contain a powerful battery. Am J Physiol, 242: 358–366

Barron JJ, Jacobson WE, Tidd G (1985) Treatment of decubitus ulcers: A new approach. Minn Med, 68: 103–106

Becker RO, Murray DG (1967) Method of producing cellular dedifferentiation by means of very small electrical current. Trans N Y Acad Sci, 29: 606–615

Bertolucci LE, Grey T (1995) Clinical comparative study of microcurrent electrical stimulation to mid-laser and placebo treatment in degenerative joint disease of the temporomandibular joint. Cranio, 13: 116–120

Bonacci JA, Higbie EJ (1997) Effects of microcurrent treatment on perceived pain and muscle strength following eccentric exercises. J Athl Train, 32: 119–123

Borgens RB, McGinnis ME, Vanable JW, Miles ES (1984) Stump currents in regenerating salamanders and newts. J Exp Zool, 23: 249–256

Borgens RB, Vanable JW, Jaffe LF (1977) Bioelectricity and regeneration: Large currents leaves the stumps of regenerating newt limbs. Proc Natl Acad Sci USA, 74: 4528–4532

Carley PJ, Wainapel SF (1985) Electrotherapy for acceleration of wound healing: Low-intensity direct current. Arch Phys Med Rehab, 66: 443–446

Denegar CR, Yoho AP, Borowicz AJ, Bifulco N (1992) The effects of low-volt microamperage stimulation on delayed onset muscle soreness. J Sport Rehabil, 1: 95–102

Feedar JA, Kloth LC, Gentzkow CD (1991) Chronic dermal ulcer healing enhanced with monophasic pulsed electrical stimulation. Phys Ther, 71: 639–649

Foulds IS, Barker AT (1983) Human skin battery potentials and their possible role in wound healing. Br J Dermatol, 109: 512–522

Gault WR, Gatens PF (1976) Use of low-intensity direct current in management of ischemic skin ulcers. Phys Ther, 56: 265–269

Gentzkow GD, Pollack SV, Kloth LC (1991) Improved healing of ulcers using Dermapulse, a new electrical stimulation device. Wounds, 3: 158–160

Hatten E, Hervik JB, Kalheim T, Sundvor T (1990) Pain treatment with Rebox. Fysiotherapeuten, 11: 8–13

Illingsworth CM, Barker AT (1980) Measurement of electrical currents emerging during the regeneration of amputated finger tips in children. Clin Phys Physiol Meas, 1: 87–89

Johannsen F, Gam A, Haudschild B, Mathiesen B, Jensen L (1993) Rebox: An adjunct in physical medicine? Arch Phys Med Rehab, 74: 438–440

Kaada B (1983) Promoted healing of chronic ulceration by transcutaneous nerve stimulation (TNS). Vasa, 12: 262–269

Lerner FN, Kirsh DL (1981) A double blind comparative study of microstimulation and placebo effect in short term treatment of the chronic back pain patient. J Chiropract, 15: 101–106

Maenpaa H, Jaakkola R, Sandstrom M, Von Wendt L (2004) Does microcurrent stimulation increase the range of movement of ankle dorsiflexion in children with cerebral palsy? Disabil Rehabil, 26: 669–677

McMakin C (1998) Microcurrent treatment of myofascial pain in the hand, neck and face. Top Clin Chiropract, 5: 29–35, 73–75

Merriman HL, Heygi CA, Albright-Overton, Carlos J, Putnam RW, Mulcare JA (2004) A comparison of four electrical stimulation types on *Staphylococcus aureus* growth in vitro. J Rehab Res Dev, 41: 139–146

Mulder GD (1991) Treatment of open skin wounds with electric stimulation. Arch Phys Med Rehab, 72: 375–377

Weber MD, Servedio FJ, Woodall WR (1994) The effect of three modalities on delayed-onset muscle soreness. J Orthop Phys Ther, 20: 236–242

Weiss DS, Eagstein WH, Falanga V (1989) Exogenous electric current can reduce the formation of hypertrophic scars. J Dermatol Surg Oncol, 15: 1272–1275

Wolcott LE, Wheeler PC, Hardwicke HM, Rowley BA (1969) Accelerated healing of skin ulcer by electrotherapy: Preliminary clinical results. South Med J, 62: 795–801

Wood JM, Evans PE, Shallreuter KU, Jacobson WE, Sufit R, Newman J, White C, Jacobson M (1993) A multicenter study on the used of pulsed low intensity direct current for healing chronic stage II and III decubitus ulcers. Arch Dermatol, 129: 999–1009

Review Articles

Bogie KM, Reger SI, Levine SP (2000) Electrical stimulation for pressure sore prevention and wound healing. Assist Technol, 12: 50–66

Dayton PD, Palladino SJ (1989) Electrical stimulation of cutaneous ulcerations: A literature review. J Am Podiatr Med Assoc, 79: 318–321

Gardner SE, Frantz RA, Schmidt FL (1999) Effects of electrical stimulation on chronic wound healing: A meta-analysis. Wound Rep Regul, 7: 495–503

Gentzkow GD (1993) Electrical stimulation to heal dermal wounds. J Dermatol Surg Oncol, 19: 753–758

Gentzkow GD, Miller KH (1991) Electrical stimulation for dermal wound healing. Clin Podiatr Med Surg, 4: 827–841

Gersh MR (1989) Microcurrent electrical stimulation: Putting it in perspective. Clin Manage, 9: 51–54

Houghton PE (1999) Effects of therapeutic modalities on wound healing: A conservative approach to the management of chronic wounds. Phys Ther Rev, 4: 167–182

Houghton PE, Campbell KE (1999) Choosing adjunctive therapy for the treatment of chronic wound. Ostomy Wound Manag, 45: 43–53

Keast DH, Parslow N, Houghton PE, Norton L, Fraser C (2007) Best practice recommendations for the prevention and treatment of pressure ulcers: Update 2006. Adv Skin Wound Care, 20: 447–460

Kloth LC (1995) Physical modalities in wound management: UVC, therapeutic heating and electrical stimulation. Ostomy Wound Manage, 41: 18–20, 22–24, 26–27

Kloth LC (2005a) Electrical stimulation for wound healing: A review of evidence from in vitro studies, animal experiments, and clinical trials. Int J Low Extrem Wounds, 4: 23–44

Kloth LC, McCulloch JM (1996) Promotion of wound healing with electrical stimulation. Adv Wound Healing, 9: 42–45

Lampe KE (1998) Electrotherapy in tissue repair. J Hand Ther, 11(2): 131–139

Mercola JM, Kirch DL (1995) The basis for microcurrent electrical therapy in conventional medical practice. J Adv Med, 8: 107–120

Makiov MS (1995) Electrical current and electromagnetic field effects on soft tissue: Implications for wound healing. Wounds, 7: 94–110

Picker RI (1988a) Current trends: Low-volt pulsed microamp stimulation. Part I. Clin Manage, 9: 10–14

Picker RI (1988b) Current trends: Low-volt pulsed microamp stimulation. Part II. Clin Manage, 9: 28–33

Weiss DS, Krisner R, Eaglstein WH (1990) Electrical stimulation and wound healing. Arch Dermatol, 126: 222–225

Wieder DL (1991) Microcurrent therapy: Wave of the future? Rehab Manage, 4(2): 34–35

Chapters of Textbooks

Byl NN (1999) Electrical stimulation for tissue repair: Basic information. In: Clinical Electrotherapy, 3rd ed. Nelson RM, Hayes, KW, Currier DP (Eds). Appleton & Lange, Stamford, pp 183–227

Kloth LC (2002) Electrical stimulation in tissue repair. In: Wound Healing: Alternatives in Management, 3rd ed. Kloth LC, McCulloch JM (Eds). FA Davis Corp, Philadelphia, pp 271–315

Kloth LC (2005b) Electrical stimulation. In: Wound Healing. Falabella AF, Kirsner RS (Eds). Taylor & Francis, New York, pp 439–479

Robinson AJ (2008) Electrical stimulation to augment healing of chronic wounds. In: Clinical Electrophysiology: Electrotherapy and Electrophysical Testing, 3rd ed. Robinson AJ, Snyder-Mackler L (Eds). Lippincott Williams & Wilkins, Philadelphia, pp 275–299

Sussman C, Byl NN (1999) Externally applied electric current for tissue repair. In: Clinical Electrotherapy, 3rd ed. Nelson RM, Hayes, KW, Currier DP (Eds). Appleton & Lange, Stamford, pp 229–290

Sussman C (2007) Electrical stimulation for wound healing. In: Wound Care: A Collaborative Manual for Health Professionals, 3rd ed. Sussman C, Bates-Jensen B (Eds). Lippincott Williams & Wilkins, Philadelphia, pp 505–553

Watson T (2002) Electrical stimulation for wound healing: A review of current knowledge. In: Electrotherapy Evidence Based Practice, 11th ed. Kitchen S (Ed). Churchill Livingstone, London, pp 313–334

Textbooks

Becker RO, Selden G (1987) The Body Electric. Electromagnetism and the Foundation of Life. William Morrow Co., New York

Falabella AF, Kirsner RS (2005) Wound Healing. Taylor & Francis, New York, pp 1–723

Kloth LC, McCulloch JM (2002) Wound Healing: Alternatives in Management, 3rd ed. FA Davis Corp., Philadelphia, pp 1–568

Shai A, Maibach HI (2005) Wound Healing and Ulcers of the Skin. Springer, Berlin, pp 1–270

Sussman C, Bates-Jensen B (2007) Wound Care: A Collaborative Manual for Health Professionals, 3rd ed. Lippincott Williams & Wilkins, Philadelphia, pp 1–768

Monographs and Documents

American Physical Therapy Association (APTA) (2001) Electrotherapeutic Terminology in Physical Therapy. APTA Publications, Alexandria, p 38

Centers for Medicare and Medicaid Services (2004) National Coverage: Determination for Electrical Stimulation and Electromagnetic Therapy for the Treatment of Wounds. NCD 270.1. Washington DC

CHAPTER 16

High-Voltage Pulsed Current Therapy

Chapter Outline

Learning Objectives

Knowledge: Describe the waveform that characterizes the delivery of high-voltage pulsed current (HVPC) therapy.

Comprehension: Discuss why the delivery of HVPC waveforms requires a high-voltage source.

Application: Demonstrate the application of HVPC therapy for wound management.

Analysis: Explain how HVPC therapy may be beneficial for wound management, soft-tissue edema, and muscle spasm.

Synthesis: Formulate the physiological rationale behind electrode polarity for wound management using HVPC.

Evaluation: Discuss the body and strength of the English-language-based scientific evidence supporting the use of HVPC therapy.

I. RATIONALE FOR USE

A. DEFINITION AND DESCRIPTION

The term *high-voltage pulsed current*, designated under the acronym HVPC, is defined as the percutaneous delivery of pulsed, twin-peak, monophasic pulses, each pulse having a very short phase duration of less than 200 μs, which employs a high-driving peak voltage, usually higher than 150 volts and up to 500 volts (APTA, 2001). As was the case with *microcurrent therapy (MES)* covered in the previous chapter (Chapter 15), HVPC is used primarily in the field of electrical stimulation for tissue healing and repair (ESTHR). More specifically, HVPC therapy is used to promote and accelerate the healing process of slow-to-heal cutaneous wounds (APTA, 2001; Sussman, 2007; Robinson, 2008). The use of ESTHR was approved in 2002 in the United States for the treatment of various lower-extremity ulcers caused by pressure, vascular insufficiency, and diabetes (Centers for Medicare and Medicaid Services, 2004).

B. HVPC STIMULATORS

High-voltage pulsed current therapy is delivered using portable as well as cabinet-type electrical stimulators. Shown in **Figure 16-1A** is a typical *cabinet-type*, line-powered stimulator also capable of delivering HVPC therapy. These cabinet-type stimulators are commonly referred to, in the corporate literature, as *combo* stimulators, meaning that a single stimulator, or unit, is capable of generating a *combination* (thus the word combo) of current waveforms simply by pushing a button on the stimulator's console. Shown in **Figure 16-1B** is a typical *portable*, battery-powered HVPC stimulator. Such stimulators usually come in a plastic carrying case containing wires or cables, reusable electrodes, and electroconductive gel.

C. ELECTRODE TYPES

HVPC therapy is delivered, as illustrated in **Figure 16-2**, using a variety of commercial reusable surface carbon rubber (**A**), home-made aluminum foil (**B**), and intravaginal (**C**) and intrarectal (**D**) electrodes. The former two types of electrodes (**A**, **B**) are used for the management of dermal wounds and posttraumatic edema, and the latter two (**C**, **D**) for the management of pelvic floor muscle spasm.

D. RATIONALE FOR USE

It remains a challenge for practitioners to electrically stimulate deep excitable soft tissues without causing pain. The challenge is to be able to depolarize these sensory and motor nerve fibers without depolarizing pain or nociceptive fibers. To meet this challenge, the electrical waveform duration must be very short, and its amplitude very high, according to the classic relationship between current strength (S) and pulse duration (D) known as the SD curve (for details, see Chapter 14). HVPC stimulation, characterized

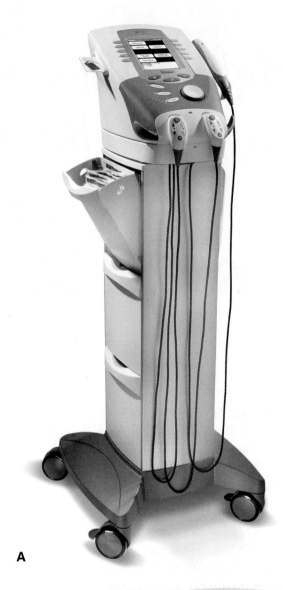

A

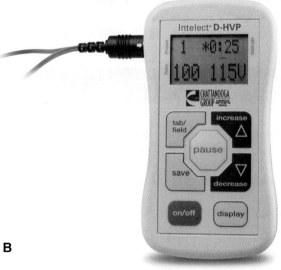

B

FIGURE 16-1 Typical (**A**) cabinet-type and (**B**) portable stimulators. (Courtesy of Chattanooga Group.)

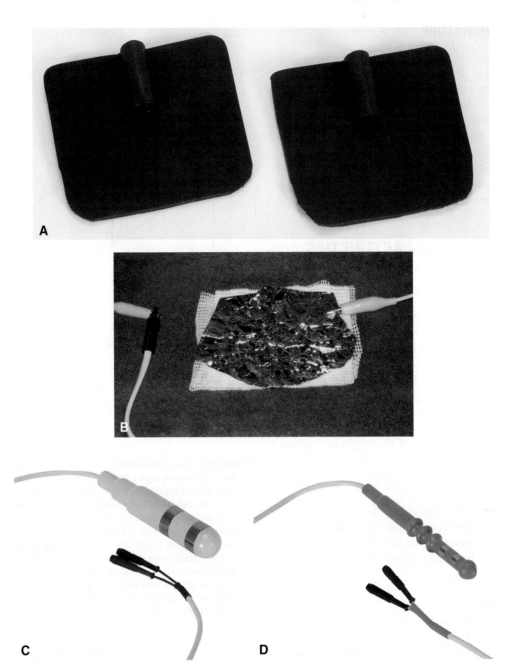

FIGURE 16-2 Typical reusable (**A**, **B**) surface electrodes, (**C**) intravaginal, and (**D**) intrarectal electrodes (A, C, D: Courtesy of Enraf-Nonius; B: Reprinted with permission from Sussman C, Bartes-Jenson B. Wound Care; *A Collaborative Practice Manual for Health Professionals*. Philadelphia: Lippincott Williams and Wilkins, 2007).

by its ultrashort phase duration and very high-driving voltage, meets these two electrophysiological requirements. HVPC therapy is used today primarily for the management of dermal wounds and secondarily for the management of pelvic floor muscle spasm and edema.

II. HISTORICAL PERSPECTIVES

A. ROOTS

The first HVPC electrical stimulator, marketed under the name DynaWave Neuromuscular Stimulator, was devel-

oped in the 1940s by American scientists at Bell Laboratories (Newton, 1991).

B. EARLY STUDIES

The first published article on the application of HVPC was by Young, who in 1966 reported that this current effectively decreased limb edema and prevented gangrene in dogs that had their hind limb circulation compromised for 12 hours via a tourniquet (Young, 1966). Five years later, Thurman et al. (1971) published what appears to be the first study on the therapeutic use of HVPC on humans, reporting benefit for the treatment of a purulent septic diabetic abscess in a single patient.

C. BODY OF LITERATURE

HVPC therapy has been the topic of several *articles* (see Reference), *review articles* (Lampe, 1998; Ovington, 1999; Taradaj, 2003; Kloth, 2005), *chapters of textbooks* (Newton, 1991; Snyder-Mackler, 1995; Sussman et al., 1999; Hayes, 2000; Kloth, 2002; Watson, 2002; Kloth, 2005; Sussman, 2007; Robinson, 2008), in addition to *brief coverage* in some *textbooks* dedicated to wound healing (Falabella et al., 2005; Shai et al., 2005). The overall management of wounds is presented in the following two textbooks: Kloth et al., 2002 and Sussman et al., 2007.

III. BIOPHYSICAL CHARACTERISTICS

A. FOUNDATIONS

The biophysics of HVPC therapy lies in the production, as shown in **Figure 16-3**, of a twin-peak, monophasic pulsed electrical current driven by a high electromotive force, or voltage, that always exceeds 150 V to reach a maximum of 500 V. Voltage stimulators having an output of less than 150 V are labeled as low-voltage stimulators. Before considering the following material, readers are *urged to review* Chapter 5, which presents an illustrated glossary of terms and concepts related to the use of electrophysical agents capable of delivering electric energy to soft tissues.

1. Waveform

Figure 16-3 shows the typical twin-peak, monophasic pulses generated by current commercial HVPC stimulators. Each pulse is made of a pair of spike-like waveforms that have an almost instantaneous rise, followed by an exponential decline.

2. Pulse Duration

A pulse duration (PD) corresponds to the phase duration of both spikes plus, if applicable, the interspike duration. HVPC pulse durations are characteristically very short, ranging from 100 to 200 μs, and are usually fixed by the manufacturers. The interspike duration may vary between HVPC stimulators and may be fixed, or programmable, by the operator.

3. Interpulse Duration

An interpulse duration (IPD) corresponds to the duration between two pulses.

B. PULSE FREQUENCY

HVPC stimulators generate pairs of monophasic, spike-like pulses at frequencies ranging from 1 to 200 pulses per second (pps) through automatic adjustment of interpulse duration (**Fig 16-3**). For example, manually selecting a pulse frequency (f) of 100 pps, with a fixed pulse duration (PD) of 200 μs, yields an automatic interpulse duration (IPD)

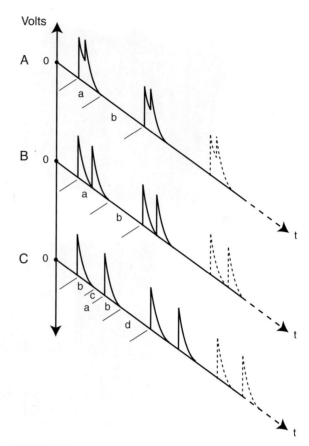

FIGURE 16-3 Typical monophasic, twin-peak pulse patterns generated by a commercial high-voltage pulsed current (HVPC) stimulator. Some stimulators include a control switch that allows the operator to set the time between the first spike waveform and the beginning of the second waveform. **A:** The time between the two spikes is set so that the two waveforms overlap: (a) pulse duration; (b) interpulse duration. **B:** The time is adjusted so that the second spike waveform begins immediately after the end of the first waveform: (a) pulse duration; (b) interpulse duration. **C:** The time is adjusted so that an interpulse duration occurs between each twin-peak pulse. Note that pulse duration (a) is made of the summation of both spike duration (b) and interspike duration (c); interpulse duration (d).

of 9800 μs (f = 1 / (PD = IPD); 100 pps = 1,000,000 μs / 200 μs + 9800 μs).

C. PULSE VERSUS PEAK

Do not confuse the terms pulse and peak when discussing HVPC. The term *pulse* refers to the waveform, not to the number of peaks within the waveform. For example, the display of an HVPC having a 60-pps frequency on the oscilloscope screen will show 60 monophasic pulses and 120 peaks, because each pulse has twin peaks.

D. HIGH-VOLTAGE SOURCE

The need for a high-voltage source, as the name of this electrophysical agent (EPA) implies, is based on the fact that to depolarize excitable tissues using ultrashort pulse duration, a large peak current must be generated.

According to Ohm's law (V = RI), the higher the voltage (V), for a given resistance (R), the higher the current amplitude (I) delivered. The term *high voltage* refers to the use of voltage amplitudes of 150 to 500 V (APTA, 2001).

E. CONFUSING TERMINOLOGY

High-voltage pulsed current stimulators were originally marketed in the mid-1970s under the name high-voltage electro galvanic stimulator (Newton, 1991). To label a pulsed current stimulator as a galvanic stimulator is technically incorrect because a current cannot be pulsed *and* galvanic, meaning direct or continuous, at the same time. The term high-voltage electro galvanic stimulator was thus eliminated and replaced by the correct term, *high-voltage pulse current stimulator*.

IV. PHYSIOLOGICAL AND THERAPEUTIC EFFECTS

A. GENERAL EFFECTS

Figure 16-4 summarizes the proposed physiological and therapeutic effects associated with HVPC therapy (Taradaj, 2003; Kloth, 2005; Sussman, 2007; Robinson, 2008). The evidence gathered from the peer-reviewed literature (see Section VI) reveals that this EPA has been used primarily for the management of dermal wounds, soft-tissue edema, and pelvic floor muscle spasm.

1. Dermal Wounds

The physiological and therapeutic effects of HVPC on dermal wounds are identical to those proposed for microcurrent therapy (Chapter 15). Delivery of HVPC at the wound site is believed to mimic and augment the weak endogenous skin battery voltages, which in turn increase the amplitude of those currents of injury, thus promoting wound healing (**Fig 16-4**). As was the case with microcurrent therapy, HVPC therapy is proposed to promote wound healing through its galvanotaxis and germicidal effects.

a. Galvanotaxis Effect

As discussed in Chapter 15, the galvanotaxis effect involves the migration of polarized cells toward the cathode or anode. The migration of neutrophils, macrophages, lymphocytes, and platelets enhances the inflammatory phase of healing. Migration of fibroblasts enhances the proliferative phase. Finally, migration of epidermal cells and keratynocytes facilitates the final phase of healing, namely, the remodeling/maturation phase. For details on the process of galvanotaxis and cell migration, consult Kloth (2005), Sussman (2007), and Robinson (2008).

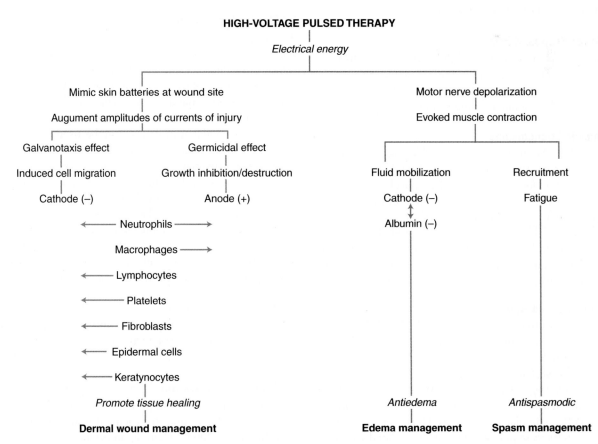

FIGURE 16-4 The proposed physiological and therapeutic effects of high-voltage pulsed current therapy.

b. Germicidal Effect

As was the case with microcurrent therapy (Chapter 15), HVPC therapy is presumed to inhibit the growth of and destroy germs at the wound site. This effect is presumed to occur under both electrodes (**Fig 16-4**). Maximal germicidal effects were found using HVPC in vitro, with a voltage of 250 V at the cathode, for a period of 2 hours (Kincaid et al., 1989; Weiss et al., 1989). Guffey et al. (1989) found that an application of at least 30 minutes was necessary to produce a germicidal effect in vitro using HVPC.

2. Antiedema Effect

The antiedema effect attributed to HVPC is presumed to be caused by the repulsion, under the cathode, of negatively charged albumin proteins found in the blood, causing a fluid shift and thus reducing edema at the electrode site (Sussman, 2007), as shown in **Figure 16-4**.

3. Antispasmodic Effect

The antispasmodic effect attributed to HVPC is presumed to be caused by induced muscle fatigue (prolonged motor unit recruitment) leading to muscle exhaustion (**Fig 16-4**). The use of HVPC for the management of levator ani syndrome (chronic anal spasm) rests on the capacity of HVPC stimulators to depolarize motor nerves, thus inducing evoked muscle contractions. Prolonged evoked contraction of the levator ani muscle is believed to induce fatigue, which in turn promotes its relaxation (no contraction—no spasm) by breaking the muscle spasm–pain cycle.

4. Other Proposed Effects

Some authors have suggested that HVPC may also be used for muscle strengthening and for increasing muscle blood flow. As discussed below, *no evidence* can be found to support such therapeutic applications.

a. Muscle Strengthening

Alon (1985), Mohr et al. (1985), and Wong (1986) have shown the capacity of HVPC to evoke relatively strong muscle contractions that may lead to muscle strengthening over time. Only one article was found in the English-language, peer-reviewed literature on the muscle-strengthening effect of HVPC. The controlled study by Mohr et al. (1985) found HVPC stimulation to be *ineffective* for increasing quadriceps muscle force compared with a voluntary isometric muscle contraction regimen.

b. Muscle Blood Flow

HVPC is presumed to increase muscle blood flow after bouts of evoked muscle contractions. Only two peer-reviewed articles, involving healthy subjects, were found in the English-language literature. These two studies report *conflicting* results. Carlson-Walker et al. (1988) found *no increase* of blood flow in the popliteal artery after HVPC stimulation, whereas Heath et al. (1992) did find an *increase* in blood flow that correlated with the voltage amplitude used to contract the calf muscle.

B. UNWANTED ELECTROCHEMICAL CHANGES

The delivery of monophasic current waveform, such as seen with HVPC therapy, may lead to electrochemical changes, such as skin irritation and burn under the electrodes, especially when applied continuously over the skin for a relatively long period of time. Newton et al. (1983) revealed no chemical buildup under the electrodes, as measured by skin pH, when HVPC was delivered continuously for 30 minutes. There is a consensus that a monophasic HVPC pulse, because of its ultrashort pulse duration, when applied over a relatively short period of time (15–45 minutes), induces no significant unwanted electrochemical effects under the electrodes during treatment (Sussman, 2007).

V. DOSIMETRY

A. PARAMETERS

Dosimetry for HVPC therapy requires specific parameters to be set according to the desired therapeutic effects: voltage amplitude, electrode polarity, pulse frequency, application duration, and treatment schedule.

1. Voltage Amplitude

The voltage may be set between 150 and 500 V.

2. Electrode Polarity

As was the case with MES therapy (Chapter 15), polarity selection is based on the healing phase the practitioner wants to facilitate. Cathodal stimulation is used during the inflammatory phase of wound healing. Anodal stimulation, on the other hand, is used to facilitate the proliferative, remodeling, and maturation phases of wound healing. Cathodal or anodal stimulation may be used to manage wound infection, when present. Because the phases of wound healing overlap one another over time, it is recommended to program the stimulator for a periodic reversal of the current polarity during the entire treatment session. This automatic current polarity reversal leads to equal periods of cathodal and anodal stimulation of the wound site per treatment session. Another suggestion is to alternate between cathodal and anodal stimulation at the wound site every 3 days for the duration of treatment.

3. Pulse Frequency

The frequency range is from 0.1 to 200 pulses per second (pps). Frequencies between 30 and 50 pps are used to evoke muscle contraction.

4. Application Duration

The duration may range from 30 to 90 minutes. Application durations for wound management often last 60 minutes (Sussman, 2007). There is no evidence on which to base the selection of this parameter.

5. Treatment Schedule

For wound management, treatments are usually given daily or at a rate of 5–7 times a week (Sussman, 2007). Treatment schedules for the management of edema and muscle spasm will vary according to the pathology under consideration. Treatments may be delivered daily or 3 times per week.

B. WOUND MANAGEMENT

The voltage amplitude used is relatively low (150–250 V) because the purpose here is to jump-start the skin batteries. As was the case for microcurrent therapy (Chapter 15), the cathode or anode may be placed directly over the wound or around its margins. There is no evidence to suggest that one polarity is better than the other or that the continuous delivery mode is better than the pulsed mode for wound therapy. Reusable carbon rubber-type or aluminum foil-type electrodes are used.

C. EDEMA AND MUSCLE SPASM MANAGEMENT

The voltage amplitude used is higher, ranging between 250 and 500 V, because moderate-to-strong electrically evoked muscle contractions are needed. Reusable carbon rubber electrodes are used for both conditions; when pelvic muscle spasm is present, intravaginal or intrarectal electrodes are used.

VI. EVIDENCE FOR INDICATIONS

A. GUIDED BY EVIDENCE

Dictionaries generally define *evidence* as anything that establishes a fact or gives reason to believe something.

The aim of this textbook is to present scientific evidence on therapeutic EPAs. To be guided by evidence is the process of integrating the evidence from research, however imperfect or scarce this evidence may be, with clinical experience and patients' values. In other words, the *evidence-based practice* of EPA requires that practitioners consider the evidence from research, in addition to their own clinical experience, and patients' own preference and beliefs about a given EPA, when the time comes to justify, prescribe, and apply the therapeutic agent. To be guided by evidence is a process, not a search for the absolute truth. Finally, a lack of evidence from research in support of any given EPA does not mean that this EPA should never be used. What it means is that no statement can be made about its therapeutic effectiveness and that until more evidence from research is presented, its routine use cannot be recommended.

B. EVIDENCE FROM HUMAN RESEARCH

Box 16-1 provides evidence for HVPC therapy based on an exhaustive search of published English-language, peer-reviewed studies on humans. The term *indication* is used in reference to a list of pathologies for which HVPC therapy is employed. Ratings of therapeutic benefit (Yes or No) and grading of strength of scientific evidence (I, II, or III), including the reference, are included for each pathological condition.

1. Rating Therapeutic Benefit

The rating, expressed as Yes or No, is based on the overall conclusion(s) reached on the issue of therapeutic effectiveness by the author(s) who conducted the peer-reviewed study.

Box 16-1	Research-Based Indications for the Use of High-Voltage Pulsed Current Therapy		
PATHOLOGY	**BENEFIT**	**GRADE**	**REFERENCE**
Dermal wounds	Yes	I	Houghton et al., 2003
	Yes	I	Peters et al., 2001
	Yes	I	Unger, 1985
	Yes	I	Kloth et al., 1988
	Yes	I	Goldman et al., 2004
	Yes	II	Gilcreast et al., 1998
	Yes	II	Griffin et al., 1991
	Yes	II	Akers et al., 1984
	Yes	II	Franek et al., 2000
	Yes	II	Goldman et al., 2003
	Yes	III	Mawson et al., 1993
	Yes	III	Goldman et al., 2002
	Yes	III	Thurman et al., 1971
	Yes	III	Fitzgerald et al., 1993

(Continued)

Box 16-1   Continued

PATHOLOGY	BENEFIT	GRADE	REFERENCE
Levator ani syndrome	Yes	II	Morris et al., 1987
	Yes	II	Nicosia et al., 1985
	Yes	II	Oliver et al., 1985
	Yes	II	Sohn et al., 1982
	Yes	II	Billingham et al., 1987
	Yes	II	Hull et al., 1993
	Yes	II	Park et al., 2005
Posttraumatic edema	Yes	II	Lamboni et al., 1983
	Yes	II	Voight, 1984
	Yes	II	Ross et al., 1981
	No	I	Griffin et al., 1990
	No	II	Michlovitz et al., 1988
Delayed-onset muscle soreness	No	I	Butterfield et al., 1997
	No	I	Tourville et al., 2006
Chronic low-back pain	Yes	III	Quirion de Girardi et al., 1984
Hand/wrist pain	Yes	I	Stralka et al., 1998
Bell's palsy	Yes	III	Shrode, 1993

2. Grading Strength of Evidence

The grading, numerically classified as I, II and III, is based on the type of research methodology or research design used by the author(s). All those listed are studies on humans published in English-language, peer-reviewed journals. It follows that the evidence in studies graded I is stronger than in those graded II and the evidence in studies graded II is stronger than in those graded III.

a. Grade I

Evidence based on *controlled* studies on humans, regardless of their level of randomization and blindness.

b. Grade II

Evidence based on *non-controlled* studies on humans, regardless of their level of randomization and blindness.

c. Grade III

Evidence based on *case* studies on humans, regardless of their level of randomization and blindness.

3. Strength of Evidence Behind the Agent

The strength of evidence in support of the agent, as presented in the research-based indication box, is arbitrarily assessed in this textbook as *weak*, *moderate*, or *strong*. For example, the larger the number of studies graded I,

regardless of therapeutic benefit, the stronger the scientific evidence in support of the agent.

4. Evidence Justifying Usage of Agent

The strength of evidence justifying the usage of an agent for an individual pathology or groups of pathologies, as listed in the research-based indication box, is arbitrarily assessed in this textbook as *poor*, *fair*, *good*, or *conflicting*. For example, where the number of grade I studies showing therapeutic benefit (Yes) for any given pathology is larger than that of similar studies showing no benefit, the justification for the of usage of this agent for that pathology is assessed as *good*. A *conflicting* usage is reported when an equal number of studies with similar grades show therapeutic benefit (Yes) and no benefit (No).

C. STRENGTH OF EVIDENCE AND JUSTIFICATION FOR USAGE

The results presented in **Box 16-1** show *weak-to-moderate strength* of evidence for the use of HVPC therapy, with a relatively balanced number of studies graded I, II, and III, the majority showing therapeutic benefit. These results suggest that the *justification for usage* of HVPC therapy is *fair to good* for dermal wounds. This finding is in keeping with the recent FDA approval (2002) of the use of electrical stimulation, such as HVPC therapy, for

TABLE 16-1	CONTRAINDICATIONS TO HIGH-VOLTAGE PULSED CURRENT THERAPY
CONTRAINDICATIONS	**RATIONALE**
Over osteomyelitis[a] area	Risk of blinding the site of observation (wound penetration to the bone) because tissue growth after HVPC therapy may superficially cover the osteomyelitis area (Sussman, 2007).
Over malignant area	Risk of further enhancing and spreading the tumor due to increased blood flow into the treated area.
Over electronic implants	Risk of interference with normal functioning of these devices (see Chapter 14 for details).
Over anterior cervical area	Risk of stimulating key organs such as the vagus nerve, phrenic nerve, and carotid sinuses.
Over the thoracic region	Risk of affecting normal heart function.
Over the cranial area	Risk of affecting normal brain function.
Over metallic implants	Risk of causing unnecessary pain due to electrical current–induced overheating of implants.
Over the abdominal pelvic and lumbar areas of pregnant women in their first trimester	Risk of inducing labor.
Over heavy scarring and thick adipose tissues	Risk of impeding current flow from crossing these skin areas because of their high electrical resistance, thus minimizing treatment effectiveness.
Over hemorrhagic area	Risk of promoting further bleeding due to increased blood circulation into the treated area.

[a]Osteomyelitis is the inflammation of bone marrow, adjacent bone, and epiphysial cartilage.

tissue healing and repair (ESTHR). Results also show *fair justification* for the use of this EPA for management of pelvic floor muscle spasm. Until more evidence from research is provided with regard to the remaining listed pathologies or any other pathology, the routine use of HVPC therapy for such pathologies *cannot be recommended*.

VII. CONTRAINDICATIONS

Table 16-1 describes the contraindications associated with HVPC therapy. Because this EPA is capable of nerve deplorization, its contraindications are similar to those listed for TENS therapy (Chapter 14). Always ensure that the electrode placements used never allow the current field between the electrodes to cross the transcranial, transthoracic, and anterior cervical areas of the body.

VIII. RISKS, PRECAUTIONS, AND RECOMMENDATIONS

The practice of HVPC therapy is not without risks for the patient. The main risks associated with this EPA, as well as some precautions and recommendations de-

signed to improve safety and effectiveness, are listed in **Table 16-2**.

IX. CONSIDERATIONS FOR APPLICATION AND DOCUMENTATION

A. CONSIDERATIONS AND PROCEDURES

The safe, effective, and optimal application of this electrophysical agent requires that practitioners go through a systematic set of considerations and procedures for each and every application. Presented here is a list of these considerations and procedures.

1. Checklists
Before proceeding with treatment, always go through the list of contraindications (**Table 16-1**) and the list of risks, precautions, and recommendations (**Table 16-2**).

2. Wound Management
The considerations and procedures are similar to those described for the use of microcurrent therapy. To avoid duplication, readers should review Chapter 15, Sections IX, A, 2–11.

TABLE 16-2	RISKS, PRECAUTIONS, AND RECOMMENDATIONS FOR HIGH-VOLTAGE PULSED CURRENT THERAPY

RISK	RATIONALE
Usage near functioning shortwave (SWD) device	Risk of causing electronic interference.

PRECAUTIONS	RATIONALE
Auto- and cross-contamination—wound and pelvic floor muscle spasm management	May induce auto and cross-contamination if adequate measures are not taken (see Recommendations).
Coupling media temperature—wound management	Cool media may chill the wound, thus slowing down mitotic activity, which in turn delays wound healing (Sussman et al., 1999). Ensure that the coupling media (saline-soaked cotton gauze/hydrogel pad) is *warmer* than the wound surface, but not hotter than 38°C (100°F), before applying it over the wound. This measure will prevent chilling of the wound, which may slow down mitotic activity.

RECOMMENDATIONS	RATIONALE
Wear protective gown, gloves, mask, and goggles	To ensure adequate protection against cross-contamination and/or infection of the wound.
Clean, irrigate, and debride the wound before treatment	Removal of necrotic material, foreign material, heavy metals, and previous topical medication, including petroleum gel or paste, from the wound will prevent penetration, caused by current flow, of foreign materials and medication that may hinder or adversely affect wound healing.
Use disposable electrodes—wound management	To prevent the risk of auto- and cross-contamination of the wound. If reusable electrodes are used, wash, disinfect, and dry them after each usage.
Use reusable intrarectal or intravaginal electrodes	Use intrarectal electrode for the management of levator ani syndrome. Use intravaginal electrode for the management of urinary incontinence (not covered in this text). Wash, disinfect, and dry electrodes after each usage.
Discard coupling media (gauze) and disposable electrodes (aluminum foil) in biowaste bucket	To prevent the risk of auto- and cross-contamination.
Plug line-powered stimulation into GFCI receptacle	Prevent the risk of electrocution (see Chapter 27 for details).
Conduct regular maintenance and calibration	To ensure optimal treatment efficacy. Follow the manufacturer's recommendations and schedules.

3. Pelvic Floor Muscle Spasm

Use intrarectal or intravaginal electrodes. Lubricate them with sterile gel prior to insertion. Set current amplitude and current frequency such that sustained and comfortable muscle contractions are felt by the patient. Wash, disinfect, and dry the electrodes after each usage.

4. Edema Management

Use surface electrodes. Cover them with electroconductive gel. Apply the electrodes directly over the edematous area. Set current amplitude and current frequency such that sustained and comfortable muscle contractions are felt by the patient. Wash, disinfect, and dry the electrodes after each usage.

B. DOCUMENTATION

Table 16-3 shows the key parameters to be documented in the patient's file.

TABLE 16-3	KEY TREATMENT PARAMETERS TO BE DOCUMENTED IN PATIENT'S FILE AFTER HIGH-VOLTAGE PULSED CURRENT THERAPY

- *HVPC stimulator type:* portable or cabinet
- *Pulse duration:* μs
- *Pulse frequency:* Hz
- *Voltage amplitude:* V
- *Electrode type and size:* description
- *Active electrode polarity:* + or −
- *Coupling media:* description
- *Treatment session duration:* minutes to hours
- *Treatment frequency:* description

Case Study 16-1   Levator Ani Syndrome

Note: This chapter shows that the main indication of HVPC therapy, based on the assessment for strength of evidence and justification for usage, is for the management of dermal wounds (**Box 16-1**). This textbook, which focuses on the evidence behind practice, should therefore present a case study related to wound management. Because the rationale and methods of application of HVPC therapy are identical to that discussed and described for microcurrent therapy (see Chapter 15), another case related to the use of HVPC for wound management in this chapter would be redundant. Therefore, in order to avoid duplication or redundancy, a case study related to the management of muscle spasm (levator ani syndrome) is presented.

A 56-year-old woman, with a history of pelvic surgery, complains of rectal pain associated with symptoms of pressure and spasm. She has a feeling of rectal fullness and incomplete evacuation. She reports that her symptoms, which have now lasted for approximately 6 months, are aggravated by sitting for prolonged periods, especially when driving her car for leisure and going to work. She adds that the frequency of symptoms is increasing. She consulted her physician, who diagnosed, after a complete physical and anal palpation, a levator ani syndrome, also known as *proctalgia fugax.* The levator ani muscle is a major component of the pelvic floor musculature. Symptoms associated with this syndrome are believed to be referred from inter-mittent spasm of this muscle, lasting seconds to several hours. Her physician prescribed nonnarcotic analgesic and muscle relaxant drugs. After 2 months of drug therapy, she consulted her physician again, reporting minor improvements. The physician stopped the medication and referred her for a conservative treatment. The patient's goals are to decrease pain/spasm, decrease sensation of rectal fullness, improve ability to prolong sitting, and improve ability to drive her car for relatively long periods of time without stopping. You propose HVPC therapy. It is important to note that HVPC therapy is generally not employed to treat patients while they are experiencing symptoms, since the attacks usually last only for seconds to minutes. HVPC therapy is thus employed, in the present case, as a prophylactic treatment, which aim is to reduce the incidence of attacks.

Evidence-Based Steps Toward the Resolution of This Case

1. **Establish medical diagnosis.**

   Levator ani syndrome

2. **List key impairment(s).**

   - Rectal pain
   - Anal pressure
   - Anal spasm

(Continued)

Case Study 16-1 Continued

3. List key functional limitation(s).

Difficulty with prolonged sitting

4. List key disability/disabilities

Difficulty driving her car at will

5. Justification for HVPC therapy

Is there justification to use HVPC therapy in this case? This chapter has established that there is *weak-to-moderate* strength of evidence and *fair* justification for the use of HVPC therapy for levator ani syndrome (see Section VI). This textbook recommends the use of this EPA for the following reasons. First, the drug approach, used over a 2-month period, has yielded only minor improvement. Second, there is enough evidence (Sohn et al., 1982; Nicosia et al., 1985; Oliver et al., 1985; Billingham et al., 1987; Morris et al., 1987; Hull et al., 1993; Park et al., 2005) to suggest that HVPC therapy may significantly decrease the anal muscle spasm by inducing repeated levator ani muscle contractions and thus creating a fatigue state, or muscle exhaustion, to such a degree that the muscle cannot contract anymore. This effect is presumed to break the spasm–pain cycle (antispasmodic), bringing relief. Another effect of HVPC therapy is to reduce the frequency of these painful muscle spasms, acting, therefore, as a prophylactic measure. This EPA is used concomitantly with a self-regimen of anal massage.

6. Search for contraindications.

None is found.

7. Search for risks and precautions.

None is found.

8. Outline the therapeutic goal(s) you and your patient wish to achieve.

- Decrease pain/spasm cycle
- Decrease frequency of spasm episodes
- Increase ability to prolong sitting at home
- Increase ability to drive a car at will

9. List outcome measurement(s) used to assess treatment effectiveness.

- Pain: Verbal Rating Scale (VRS-5)
- Frequency of episodes: daily recording in log book
- Ability to prolong sitting at home/car: Pain-Specific Function Scale (PSFS)

10. Instruct patient about what he/she should experience, do, and not do during the treatment session.

Sensation of mild discomfort during electrode placement and electrical stimulation

Do not move during treatment

11. Outline your therapeutic prescription based on the best sources of evidence available.

This prescription is based on the following clinical studies: Sohn et al., 1982; Nicosia et al., 1985; Oliver et al., 1985; Billingham et al., 1987; Morris et al., 1987; Hull et al., 1993; and Park et al., 2005.

- **HVPC stimulator type:** portable
- **Waveform type:** monophasic twin peak
- **Pulse duration:** 100 microseconds
- **Pulse frequency:** 80 pps
- **Interspike interval:** 0 s
- **Voltage amplitude:** between 250 and 500 V, depending upon patient tolerance
- **Patient's position:** left lateral decubitus
- **Active electrode:** intrarectal
- **Coupling medium—active electrode:** surgilube—sterile and bacteriostatic surgical lubricant placed around the anal opening
- **Active electrode polarity:** negative
- **Active electrode placement:** inserted into the anus
- **Dispersive electrode:** Carbon rubber (15 × 15 cm) (6 × 6 in)
- **Coupling medium—dispersive electrode:** electroconductive gel
- **Dispersive electrode placement:** 30 cm away over right hip
- **Application duration:** 60 min
- **Treatment frequency:** every 3 days
- **Total number of treatment:** 6
- **Protective measures—practitioner:** gown, glove, and mask

12. Collect outcome measurements.

Pre- and posttreatment comparison

- Pain: decreased VRS-5 score from 4 to 1
- Frequency of spasmodic episode: reduced by 70% over past 12 months
- Ability to prolong sitting at home and in car: PSFS score improved by 100%

13. Assess therapeutic effectiveness based on outcome measures.

The results show that HVPC therapy, used as a prophylactic measure and combined with a self-regimen of anal massage, delivered every 3 days for 2 weeks, led to a significant decrease in the number of spasmodic episodes when measured over the next 12 months. The episodes, when present, are much less painful. The sensation of rectal fullness during spasm has disappeared. She can now sit and drive her car at will. Overall, this treatment approach had a beneficial effect on the impairments, functional limitations, and disabilities created by the pathology, as illustrated in the **figure below**.

14. State the prognosis.

The prognosis is excellent. If the number of episodes increases, the patient may consider using HVPC therapy again as a treatment and prophylactic measure.

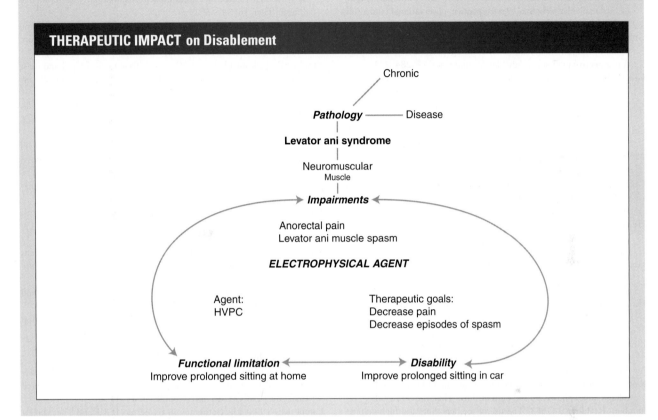

THERAPEUTIC IMPACT on Disablement

Chronic

Pathology ——— Disease

Levator ani syndrome

Neuromuscular
Muscle

Impairments

Anorectal pain
Levator ani muscle spasm

ELECTROPHYSICAL AGENT

Agent:
HVPC

Therapeutic goals:
Decrease pain
Decrease episodes of spasm

Functional limitation
Improve prolonged sitting at home

Disability
Improve prolonged sitting in car

CRITICAL THINKING QUESTIONS

Clarification: What is meant by high-voltage pulsed current (HVPC) therapy?

Assumptions: Many of your colleagues assume that the use of HVPC is strictly for tissue repair. How can you disprove this assumption?

Reasons and evidence: What led you to believe that delivering an ultrashort, very high-voltage pulse, such as these HVPC pulses, is likely to depolarize sensory and motor nerves but unlikely to depolarize nociceptive nerve fibers?

Viewpoints or perspectives: How would you respond to a colleague who says that, on the basis of scientific evidence available, HVPC therapy is more effective for wound management than microcurrent therapy?

Implications and consequences: What are the potential implications and consequences of using intravaginal or intrarectal electrodes as opposed to surface reusable electrodes for HVPC therapy?

About the question: Why is the passage of an HVPC presumed to trigger a galvanotaxis response under the electrodes? Why do you think I ask this question?

References

Articles

Akers TK, Gabrielson AL (1984) The effect of high-voltage galvanic stimulation on the rate of healing of decubitus ulcers. Biomed Sci Instrum, 20: 99–100

Alon G (1985) High-voltage stimulation: Effects of electrode size on basic excitatory responses. Phys Ther, 65: 890–895

Billingham RP, Isler JT, Firend WG, Hostetier J (1987) Treatment of levator syndrome using high-voltage electrogalvanic stimulation. Dis Colon Rectum, 30: 584–587

Butterfield DL, Draper DO, Richard MD (1997) The effects of high-volt pulsed current electrical stimulation on delayed-onset muscle soreness. J Athl Train, 32: 15–20

Carlson-Walker D, Currier DP, Threlkeld AJ (1988) Effects of high-voltage pulsed electrical stimulation on blood flow. Phys Ther, 68: 481–485

Fitzgerald GK, Newsome D (1993) Treatment of a large infected thoracic spine wound using high-voltage pulsed monophasic current. Phys Ther, 73: 355–360

Franek A, Polak A, Kucharzewski M (2000) Modern application of high voltage stimulation for enhanced healing of venous crural ulceration. Med Eng Phys, 22: 647–655

Gilcreast DM, Stotts NA, Froelicher ES, Baker LL, Moss KM (1998) Effect of electrical stimulation on foot skin perfusion in persons with or at risk for diabetic foot ulcers. Wounds Repair Regen, 6: 434–441

Goldman RJ, Brewley BI, Golden MA (2002) Electrotherapy reoxygenates inframalleolar ischemic wounds on diabetic patients: A case series. Adv Skin Wound Care, 15: 112–120

Goldman R, Brewley B, Zhou L, Golden M (2003) Electrotherapy reverses inframalleolar ischemia: A retrospective, observational study. Adv Skin Wound Care, 16: 79–89

Goldman R, Rosen M, Brewley B, Golden M (2004) Electrotherapy promotes healing and microcirculation of infrapopliteal ischemic wounds: A prospective pilot study. Adv Skin Wound Care, 17: 284–294

Griffin JW, Newsome LS, Stralka SW, Wright PE (1990) Reduction of chronic posttraumatic hand edema: A comparison of high-voltage pulsed current, intermittent pneumatic compression and placebo treatments. Phys Ther, 70: 279–286

Griffin JW, Tooms RE, Mendius RA, Clifft JK, Vander Swaag R, El-Zeky F (1991) Efficacy of high-voltage pulsed current for healing of pressure ulcers in patients with spinal cord injury. Phys Ther, 71: 433–442; discussion 442–444

Guffey JS, Asmussen MD (1989) In vitro bactericidal effects of high voltage pulsed current versus direct current against Staphylococcus aureus. Clin Electrophysiol, 1: 5–9

Heath ME, Gibbs SB (1992) High-voltage pulsed galvanic stimulation: Effects of frequency of current on blood flow in the human calf muscle. Clin Sci (Lond), 82: 607–613

Houghton PE, Kincaid CB, Lovell M, Campbell KE, Keast DH, Woodbury MG, Harris KA (2003) Effect of electrical stimulation on chronic leg ulcer size and appearance. Phys Ther, 83: 17–28

Hull Tl, Milsom JW, Church J, Oakley J, Lavery I, Fazio V (1993) Electrogalvanic stimulation for levator syndrome: How effective is it in the long term? Dis Colon Rectum, 36: 731–733

Kincaid CB, Lavoie KH (1989) Inhibition of bacterial growth in vitro following stimulation with high-voltage, monophasic, pulsed current. Phys Ther, 69: 651–655

Kloth LC, Feedar JA (1988) Acceleration of wound healing with high-voltage, monophasic, pulsed current. Phys Ther, 68: 503–508

Lamboni P, Harris B (1983) The use of ice, airsplint, and high-voltage galvanic stimulation in effusion reduction. Athl Train, 118: 23–27

Mawson AR, Siddiqui FH, Connelly BJ, Sharp CJ, Stewart GW, Summer WR, Biundo JJ (1993) Effect of high-voltage pulsed galvanic stimulation on sacral transcutaneous oxygen tension levels in the spinal cord injured. Paraplegia, 31: 311–319

Michlovitz S, Smith W, Watkins M (1988) Ice and high-voltage stimulation in treatment of acute lateral ankle sprains. J Orthop Sports Phys Ther, 9: 301–304

Mohr T, Carlson B, Sulentic C, Landry R (1985) Comparison of isometric exercise and high-volt galvanic stimulation on quadriceps femoris muscle strength. Phys Ther, 65: 606–609

Morris L, Newton RA (1987) Use of high-voltage pulsed galvanic stimulation for patients with levator ani syndrome. Phys Ther, 67: 1522–1525

Newton RA, Karselis TC (1983) Skin pH following high-voltage pulsed galvanic stimulation. Phys Ther, 63: 1593–1596

Nicosia JF, Abcarian H (1985) Levator syndrome: A treatment that works. Dis Col Rectum, 28: 406–408

Oliver GC, Robin RJ, Salvati EP, Eisenat E (1985) Electrogalvanic stimulation in the treatment of levator syndrome. Dis Col Rectum, 28: 662–663

Park DH, Yoon SG, Kim KU, Hwang DY, Kim HS, Lee JK, Kim KY (2005) Comparison study between electrogalvanic stimulation and local injection therapy in levator ani syndrome. In J Colorectal Dis, 20: 272–276.

Peters EJ, Lavery LA, Armstrong DG, Fleischli JG (2001) Electric stimulation as an adjunct to heal diabetic foot ulcers. A randomized clinical trial. Arch Phys Med Rehab, 82: 721–725

Quirion de Girardi CQ, Seaborne D, Savard-Goulet F, Nieto MW, Lambert J (1984) The analgesic effect of high-voltage galvanic stimulation combined with ultrasound in the treatment of low back pain: A one-group pre-test/post-test study. Physiother Can, 36: 327–333

Ross CR, Segal D (1981) High-voltage galvanic stimulation: An aid to postoperative healing. Curr Podiatry, 30: 19–25

Shrode LW (1993) Treatment of facial muscles affected by Bell's palsy with high-voltage electrical muscle stimulation. J Manipulative Physiol Ther, 16: 347–352

Sohn N, Weinstein MA, Robbins RD (1982) The levator syndrome and its treatment with high-voltage electrogalvanic stimulation. Am J Surg, 44: 580–582

Stralka SW, Jackson JA, Lewis AR (1998) Treatment of hand and wrist pain. A randomized clinical trial of high-voltage, pulsed, direct current built into a wrist splint. AAOHN J, 46: 233–236

Thurman BF, Christian EL (1971) Response of a serious circulatory lesion to electrical stimulation. A case report. Phys Ther, 51: 1107–1110

Tourville TW, Connelly DA, Reed BV (2006) Effects of sensory-level high-volt pulsed electrical current on delayed-onset muscle soreness. J Sports Sci, 24: 941–949

Unger PG (1985) Wound healing using high-voltage galvanic stimulation. Stimulus, 10: 8–10

Voight ML (1984) Reduction of posttraumatic ankle edema with high-voltage pulsed galvanic stimulation. Athl Train, 19: 278–279, 311

Weiss DS, Eaglstein WH, Falanga V (1989) Exogenous electric current can reduce the formation of hypertrophic scars. J Dermatol Surg Oncol, 15: 1272–1275

Wong RT (1986) Force of induced muscle contraction and perceived discomfort in healthy subjects. Phys Ther, 66: 1209–1214

Young HG (1966) Electrical impulse therapy aids wound healing. Mod Vet Pract (Anim), 47: 60–62.

Review Articles

Kloth LC (2005) Electrical stimulation for wound healing: A review of evidence from in vitro studies, animal experiments, and clinical trials. Int J Lower Extremity Wounds, 4: 23–44

Lampe KE (1998) Electrotherapy in tissue repair. J Hand Ther, 11(2): 131–139

Ovington LG (1999) Dressings and adjuvant therapies: AHCPR guidelines revisited. Ostomy Wound Manage, 45 (1A Suppl): 94S–106S

Taradaj J (2003) High-voltage stimulation (HVS) for enhanced healing of wounds. Phys Ther Rev, 8: 131–134

Chapters of Textbooks

Hayes KW (2000) High-voltage pulsed current. In Manual for Physical Agents, 5th ed., Prentice Hall Health, Upper Saddle River, pp 165–171

Kloth LC (2002) Electrical stimulation in tissue repair. In Wound Healing: Alternatives in Management, 3rd ed., Kloth LC, McCulloch JM (Eds). FA Davis Corp, Philadelphia, pp 271–315

Kloth LC (2005) Electrical stimulation. In Wound Healing. Falabella AF, Kirsner RS (Eds). Taylor & Francis, New York, pp 439–479

Newton R (1991) High-voltage pulsed current theoretical bases and clinical applications. In Clinical Electrotherapy, 2nd ed., Nelson RM, Currier DP (Eds). Appleton & Lange, Norwalk, pp 201–220

Robinson AJ (2008) Electrical stimulation to augment healing of chronic wounds. In Clinical Electrophysiology: Electrotherapy and Electrophysical Testing, 3rd ed., Robinson AJ, Snyder-Mackler L (Eds). Lippincott Williams & Wilkins, Philadelphia, pp 275–299

Snyder-Mackler L (1995) Electrical stimulation for tissue repair. In Clinical Electrophysiology: Electrotherapy and Electrophysiologic Testing, 2nd ed., Robinson AJ, Snyder Mackler L (Eds). Williams & Wilkins, Baltimore, pp 311–332

Sussman C (2007) Electrical stimulation for wound healing. In Wound Care: A Collaborative Practice Manual for health Professionals, 3rd ed., Sussman C, Bates-Jensen B (Eds). Lippincott Williams & Wilkins, Philadelphia, pp 505–554

Sussman C, Byl NN (1999) Externally applied electric current for tissue repair. In Clinical Electrotherapy, 3rd ed., Nelson RM, Hayes KW, Currier DP (Eds). Appleton & Lange, Stamford, pp 229–289

Watson T (2002) Electrical stimulation for wound healing: A review of current knowledge. In Electrotherapy Evidence-Based Practice, 11th ed., Kitchen S (Ed). Churchill Livingstone, London, pp 313–334

Textbooks

Falabella AF, Kirsner RS (2005) Wound Healing. Taylor & Francis, New York, pp 1–723

Kloth LC, McCulloch JM (2002) Wound Healing: Alternatives in Management, 3rd ed., FA Davis Corp, Philadelphia, pp 1–568

Shai A, Maibach HI (2005) Wound Healing and Ulcers of the Skin. Springer, Berlin, pp 1–270

Sussman C, Bates-Jensen B (2007) Wound Care: A Collaborative Manual for Health Professionals, 3rd ed., Lippincott Williams & Wilkins, Philadelphia, pp 1–768

Monographs and Documents

American Physical Therapy Association (APTA) (2001) Electrotherapeutic Terminology in Physical Therapy. APTA Publications, Alexandria, p 38

Centers for Medicare and Medicaid Services (2004) National Coverage: Determination for Electrical Stimulation and Electromagnetic Therapy for the Treatment of Wounds. NCD 270.1. Washington, DC.

Russian Current Therapy

Chapter Outline

Learning Objectives

Knowledge: Describe the electrical current modulation that characterizes the delivery of Russian current therapy.

Comprehension: Compare the muscle-strengthening mechanisms of volitional contractions with those of electrically evoked contractions.

Application: Demonstrate the four electrode placements related to the usage of Russian current therapy for muscle strengthening.

Analysis: Explain how the current modulation produced in Russian stimulators differs from that produced in other neuromuscular stimulators.

Synthesis: Explain the three stimulating modes (synchronous, reciprocal, and overlap) used to deliver neuromuscular electrical stimulation.

Evaluation: Discuss the strength behind, and justification for, the use of Russian current therapy for muscle strengthening.

I. RATIONALE FOR USE

A. DEFINITION AND DESCRIPTION

The term *Russian current* stems from the work conducted in the mid-1970s by Russian (thus the word Russian) physiologist Yakov Kots (1971, 1977) in the field of neuromuscular electrical stimulation, known under the acronym *NMES*. This current is defined as the time modulation, in the form of bursts of electrical pulses (or cycles), of a continuous alternating sine-wave current with a carrier frequency of 2500 cycles per second (cps).

B. NEUROMUSCULAR ELECTRICAL STIMULATION (NMES)

The practice of NMES focuses on *improving muscle performance*, in both healthy individuals and patients, using transcutaneous electrical stimulators that generate various pulsed electrical currents and waveforms. Improving muscle performance by the use of NMES, delivered using Russian current or any other pulsed currents, means enhancing muscle *strength*, muscle *endurance* as well as enhancing *control of movement and posture*.

1. Muscle Strengthening

The body of literature presented in this chapter indicates that the *primary usage* of NMES is to enhance muscle strengthening by replacing *maximal voluntary* muscle contractions by maximal *electrically evoked* contractions. The objective is to improve motor unit (MU) recruitment, while inducing muscle hypertrophy, through a series or bouts of *short duration* maximal electrically evoked muscle contractions done against resistance or load.

2. Muscle Endurance

The *secondary* usage of NMES is for enhancing muscle endurance by replacing *submaximal* voluntary muscle contraction by *submaximal* electrically evoked muscle contractions. The objective is to improve the ability to recruit fatigue-resistant muscle fibers through series of bouts of longer duration submaximal electrically evoked contractions.

3. Control of Movement and Posture

The use of NMES for the purpose of enhancing the control of movement and posture falls under the field of *functional electrical stimulation*, known by the acronym FES. More specifically, this therapeutic field focuses on the enhancement of impaired motor functions, such as hand grasping, locomotion, respiration, and incontinence, using complex transcutaneous and percutaneous electrical muscle stimulation systems (Peckham et al., 2005; Glinsky et al., 2007; Stackhouse, 2008). The main purpose of using FES therapy is thus to enable motor function by replacing, or assisting, a patient's voluntary ability to execute or control the impaired functions.

C. SCOPE OF CHAPTER

The focus of this chapter is on the use of Russian current for the delivery of NMES, the purpose of which is to *enhance muscle strengthening* in healthy individuals and patients suffering from soft-tissue pathologies. The coverage of NMES for the purpose of enhancing muscle endurance and the control of movement and posture is thus *beyond* the scope of this chapter. Readers interested in an overview of the use of NMES for enhancing muscle endurance, and for the control of movement and posture, may refer to the following chapters in these recent textbooks: on endurance—Farquhar et al., 2008; on control of movement and posture—Stackhouse, 2008.

D. RUSSIAN VERSUS OTHER NEUROMUSCULAR STIMULATORS

It is important for the reader to recognize that Russian current is not the only electrical current capable of motor nerve depolarization inducing evoked muscle contractions in humans. The body of literature presented in this chapter indicates that many other pulsed, *biphasic* current waveforms, such as the one used for TENS therapy (Chapter 15) and interferential therapy (Chapter 18), as well as pulsed *monophasic* waveforms such as the one used for HVPC therapy (Chapter 16) and diadynamic therapy (Chapter 19) are capable of evoking muscle contractions in healthy individuals and patients.

E. RUSSIAN STIMULATORS

Figure 17-1 shows typical portable, battery-powered (**A**) and cabinet, line-powered-type (**B**) Russian current stimulators. Most portable stimulators have two independent stimulating channels and are sold in a carrying case containing pairs of cables and surface electrodes. Are portable battery-operated stimulators capable of producing output

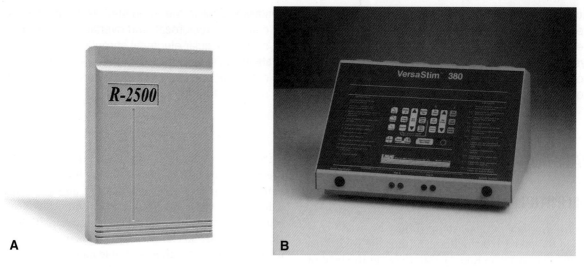

FIGURE 17-1 Typical portable (**A**) and cabinet-type (**B**) Russian current stimulators. (A: Courtesy of Heliohealth; B: Courtesy of Electro-Med Health.)

of similar torque/force/generating power as cabinet line-powered stimulators? There is evidence to suggest that battery-powered stimulators are as effective as line-powered stimulators in producing current amplitudes necessary to generate the training muscle force/torque outputs required for therapy (Laufer et al., 2001; Lyons et al., 2005).

F. ELECTRODES AND COUPLING GEL

The practice of NMES using Russian stimulators, as shown in **Figure 17-2**, is done using reusable surface electrodes made of various materials and having various shapes. The most common types of electrodes are reusable and made

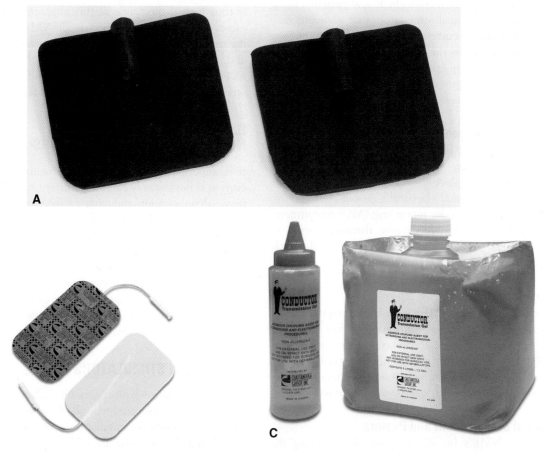

FIGURE 17-2 Typical surface carbon rubber (**A**) and pliable stainless steel knit fabric (**B**) electrodes used to deliver Russian current therapy with electroconductive gel (**C**). (A–C: Courtesy of Chattanooga Group.)

of carbon rubber material (**A**) and pliable stainless steel knit fabrics (**B**). The electroconductive coupling at the electrode–skin interface is assured with the use of electroconductive gel (**C**). Non–pre-gelled electrodes require the application of a thin film of gel.

G. RATIONALE FOR USE

There is strong evidence in the scientific literature on muscle strengthening to show that the best method practitioners can use to enhance muscle strength is to subject their patients to regimens of maximum voluntary contractions (MVCs) (exercises), done under isometric, isotonic, or isokinetic conditions. But which muscle-strengthening method should be used when the patient is unable to generate MVCs, and thus maximum force or torque, following physical deconditioning or pathologies leading to moderate-to-severe muscle weakness and atrophy? Use of NMES provides practitioners with an alternative muscle-strengthening method that *mimics* volitional training methods. By using NMES alone, or by superimposing it during voluntary muscle contractions as described later in this chapter, practitioners can enhance muscle strengthening by improving motor unit (MU) activation while inducing muscle hypertrophy.

II. HISTORICAL PERSPECTIVE

A. MINIMIZING MUSCLE WEAKNESS

Before the 1970s, NMES was used primarily to retard muscle atrophy, or minimize muscle weakness, in patients suffering from various disorders of the nervous and arthroskeletal systems. For example, NMES was used to minimize muscle atrophy from disuse after prolonged peripheral denervation or postfracture immobilization. The goal was to minimize muscle weakness while patients regained their ability to perform MVCs or recovered full strength, on their own.

B. MAXIMIZING MUSCLE STRENGTH

The introduction, by Kots, of Russian current in the mid-1970s shocked the field of NMES by forcing practitioners and researchers to rethink its foundation and use. His work opened the door to the practice of NMES, alone or in combination with voluntary muscle contraction, to promote muscle strengthening in patients suffering from a wide variety of soft-tissue pathologies, and in healthy people who want to increase their muscle strength without doing regimens of voluntary muscle exercises (Delitto, 2002; Ward et al., 2002). Kots is recognized as the father of Russian current.

C. COMMERCIAL RUSSIAN STIMULATORS

In response to the scientific and public interest in this newly discovered current, commercial production of Russian current stimulators began in Canada and the United States. The first generation of these stimulators, sold under the name *Electro-Stim 180*, became clinically available in 1980.

D. BODY OF LITERATURE

Since its first introduction in the late 1970s, Russian current therapy has been the topic of several *articles* (see References), *review articles* (Kramer et al., 1982; Kramer, 1989; Selkowitz, 1989; Belanger, 1991; Lake, 1992; Ward et al., 2002; Quinn et al., 2003; Bax et al., 2005; Paillard et al., 2005; Glinsky et al., 2007), and *chapters of textbooks* (Greathouse et al., 1992; Alon, 1999; Baker, 1999; Gerleman et al., 1999; Selkowitz, 1999; Speilholz, 1999; Van Swearingen, 1999; Hayes, 2000; Hooker, 2002; McDonough et al., 2002; Shapiro, 2003; Starkey, 2004; Johnson, 2005; Cohn et al., 2006; Farquhar et al., 2008; Stackhouse, 2008).

III. BIOPHYSICAL CHARACTERISTICS

A. ORIGINAL RUSSIAN CURRENT

Figure 17-3 illustrates the biophysical characteristics associated with the *original* Russian current. There is a

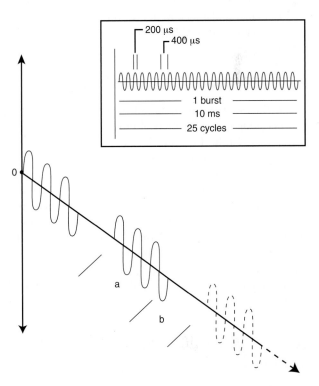

FIGURE 17-3 Typical Russian current, with its sine-wave carrier frequency of 2500 cps delivered in bursts of 10 ms (a) followed by 10-ms interburst duration (b), leading to a burst frequency of 50 bups (not drawn to scale). The inset shows the 25 cycles contained in each 10-ms burst, with each half-cycle and cycle in the burst lasting 200 and 400 ms, respectively.

consensus in the literature (Kramer et al., 1982, 1989; Alon, 1999) that the *original* Russian current stems from time modulation of a continuous alternating sine-wave current (AC) having a carrier frequency of 2500 cycles per second (cps).

1. Burst Modulation

This continuous sine-wave current, as shown in **Figure 17-3**, is modulated in bursts of cycles, each burst (Bu) having a fixed duration (BuD) of 10 ms, followed by a fixed interburst duration (IBuD) of 10 ms, resulting in a pulsed AC current with a fixed-burst frequency of 50 bursts per second [f = 1 / (BuD + IBuD); 50 bups = 1000 / (10 ms + 10 ms)].

2. Burst Characteristics

The inset in **Figure 17-3**, shows a typical Russian burst of current, lasting 10 ms and consisting of 25 continuous biphasic symmetrical sinusoidal cycles. With a carrier frequency of 2500 cps, the duration of each sine-wave cycle within a burst is 400 μs (2500 cps = 1,000,000 / 400 μs), with each half-cycle having a duration of 200 μs. A 10 ms burst thus consists of 25 cycles, each cycle lasting 400 μs (25 cycles = 10,000 μs / 400 μs).

3. Modern Russian Current

As described, the original Russian current is generated on the basis of a biphasic sinusoidal waveform. Modern neuromuscular stimulators now deliver Russian current based not only on a sinusoidal but also on square or rectangular waveforms.

B. OTHER STIMULATING CURRENTS

Before the Russian current was introduced, NMES therapy was performed using a variety of pulsed current types and waveforms. **Table 17-1** provides a comparison between the biophysical characteristics of Russian current versus other NMES current waveforms found in older and newer neuromuscular electrical stimulators. Russian current *differs* from the other stimulating currents in delivering bursts of pulses (sinusoidal waveform) as opposed to single pulses (rectangular or square waveform). It also differs in having fixed burst duration (10 ms), interburst duration (10 ms), and burst frequency (50 bups), as opposed to variable pulse duration, pulse interval, and pulse frequency for all the other currents.

IV. PHYSIOLOGICAL AND THERAPEUTIC EFFECTS

A. MOTOR NERVE DEPOLARIZATION

Figure 17-4 shows the proposed physiological and therapeutic effects of Russian current therapy. The key physiological effect is the electrically evoked depolarization of

TABLE 17-1	RUSSIAN VERSUS OTHER STIMULATING CURRENTS	
PARAMETERS	**RUSSIAN**	**OTHERS**
Modulation	Burst of pulses	Single pulse
Carrier frequency	Fixed—2500 Hz	Variable
Waveform	Sinusoidal	Square/ Rectangular
	Biphasic Symmetrical	Biphasic Symmetrical/ asymmetrical
	Balanced	Balanced
Burst duration	Fixed—10 ms	NA
Burst interval	Fixed—10 ms	NA
Burst frequency	Fixed—50 bups	NA
Pulse duration	NA	Variable
Pulse interval	NA	Variable
Pulse frequency	NA	Variable
Brand name (sample)	Electro-Stim	Respond II
	Versa-Stim 180 R-2500	Respond Select Empi 300PV

motor nerve leading to induced MU activation. Readers are *advised to review* Chapter 14, which deals with TENS therapy, for details on the process of evoking nerve *depolarization* using pulsed electrical currents.

1. Motor Unit

An MU is made of a motoneurone along with its axon and all the muscle fibers it innervates. A motor nerve is made of several large-diameter myelinated axons. It is well established that skeletal muscles are made of several MUs and that for muscle force to be generated, these MUs must be activated.

2. Motor Unit/Muscle Fiber Type

Research has established that a skeletal muscle is made of a mosaic of three types of MUs. The first type is the fast-twitch/fatigable (FF) units made of fast-twitch glycolytic (FG) muscle fibers. The second type is the fast-twitch/fatigue-resistant (FR) units made of fast-twitch, oxidative-glycolytique (FOG) muscle fibers. The third and final type of MU is the slow-twitch (S) unit made of slow-twitch, oxidative (SO) fibers, which are very resistant to fatigue. FG and FOG muscle fibers contract faster and generate more force than SO fibers. SO units are also

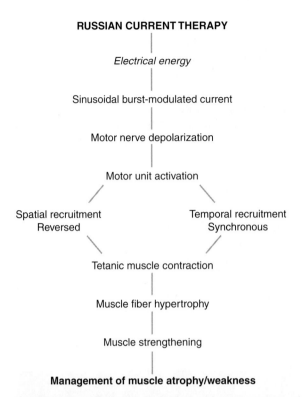

RUSSIAN CURRENT THERAPY

Electrical energy

Sinusoidal burst-modulated current

Motor nerve depolarization

Motor unit activation

Spatial recruitment
Reversed

Temporal recruitment
Synchronous

Tetanic muscle contraction

Muscle fiber hypertrophy

Muscle strengthening

Management of muscle atrophy/weakness

FIGURE 17-4 Proposed physiological and therapeutic effects of Russian current therapy.

classified as type I units, whereas FF and FR units are classified as type IIB and type IIA units, respectively.

B. TETANIC CONTRACTION

All electrical currents used to evoke muscle contractions *must be pulsed* (periodically interrupted over time) for the electrically produced muscle twitches to fuse together (**Table 17-1**). Pulsating current leads to repeated delivery of electrical bursts of pulses (Russian current) or individual pulses (other currents) that will cause repeated motor nerve depolarization, triggering a series of muscle twitches that will combine—if the frequency at which they are generated is high enough—to form an evoked smooth fused tetanic muscle contraction similar to that of maximal voluntary contraction.

C. OPTIMAL FUSION FREQUENCY

Neuromuscular research has shown that full tetanic muscle contraction of human skeletal muscles occurs at a fusion frequency of about 50 Hz (i.e., 50 pps; 50 cps or 50 bups). Some muscles may fuse at a higher frequency (i.e., 60–80 Hz) if their MU content is primarily made of FF and FR units, and some at lower frequency (i.e., 30–40 Hz) if their MU content is primarily made of S motor units.

D. BURST OF PULSES VERSUS PULSES

The motor nerve depolarization that results from the delivery of Russian bursts of electrical pulses is independ-

ent of the intrinsic number of pulses contained in each burst. The total number of bursts delivered per second (i.e., burst frequency), not the total number of pulses *within* each burst (i.e., 25 pulses), along with the current amplitude used, determines the magnitude or force of the evoked tetanic muscle contraction. It is important to remember that at the nerve/muscle membrane level, each burst of pulses is perceived as a single pulse. This explains why the delivery of single pulses (other stimulating pulsed currents), as opposed to burst of pulses (Russian current), is as effective as depolarizing motor nerves.

E. REVOLUTIONARY CLAIMS

Kots made three revolutionary claims, never before heard in the field of NMES, when he introduced the Russian current to the clinical and research communities (Kots, 1971, 1977; Belanger 1991; Ward et al., 2002).

1. Painless Current

Kots's *first* claim was that his Russian current, unlike all the other known neuromuscular stimulating currents (**Table 17-1**), is painless; it produces no sensory discomfort during maximal evoked muscle tetanic contraction. Because it is painless, Kots postulated that higher current amplitude can be delivered to soft tissues so that the deeper motor nerve fibers, which are associated with those larger high-force, fast-twitch motor units (FF; FR), can be depolarized, thus increasing the magnitude of the electrically evoked tetanic contraction.

2. Greater Force

Kots's *second* claim was that his Russian current, delivered at a higher current amplitude than all the other stimulating currents, could generate up to 30% more force than that generated during the course of a maximum voluntary effort or contraction. He postulated that during an MVC, a percentage of those large FF motor units (FG muscle fibers) are not recruited. There is a substantial body of scientific evidence to support this theory (Belanger et al., 1981; Rutherford et al., 1986; Dowling et al., 1994; Behm et al., 1996). Kots theorized further that applying his painless and deeply penetrating current would compensate for this lack of voluntary motor unit activation by activating, or depolarizing, those inactive large motor units, and thus generating more muscle force.

3. Lasting Force Gains

Kots's *third* and final claim was that a few weeks of muscle training using his Russian current could produce lasting gains in muscle strength in healthy people.

F. CLAIMS TESTED

Deeply intrigued by Kots's revolutionary claims, several neuromuscular physiologists spent more than a decade conducting studies on patients and healthy subjects using

Russian current stimulation. Their goal was to gather human scientific evidence to either support or refute each and every one of Kots's claims.

G. EVIDENCE BEHIND CLAIMS

Table 17-2 lists the body of English-language, peer-reviewed literature on human research that either supports or refutes Kots's claims about the unique properties of his Russian current.

1. Painless Current: Refuted

No evidence can be found to substantiate Kots's claim that his Russian current yields no sensory discomfort during high-level muscle tetanic contraction. In fact, all subjects enrolled in the studies listed in **Table 17-2** have reported various levels of sensory discomfort and pain when subjected to Russian current stimulation. There is evidence to support the view that pain experienced during electrically evoked tetanic muscle contraction, using Russian as well

as other stimulating currents, results from the depolarization of sensory nerve fibers originating not only from skin nociceptors but also from muscle nociceptors (Belanger et al., 1992). This claim is thus refuted.

2. Greater Force: Refuted

Only one study (Selkowitz, 1985) supports Kots's claim that Russian current-evoked muscular contractions lead to greater muscular force than those obtained after MVCs (**Table 17-2**). Unless more evidence is presented, this claim must also be refuted.

3. Lasting Force Gains: Supported

There is a substantial body of evidence to support Kots's claim that sole application of electrically evoked muscular training, using not only Russian current but also other types of pulsed current waveforms, leads to lasting gains in strength in healthy people (**Table 17-2**). This claim is thus supported.

TABLE 17-2	EVIDENCE TO SUPPORT OR REFUTE KOTS'S CLAIMS	
CLAIMS	**SUPPORT**	**REFUTE**
Painless contraction	No studies found	Owens et al., 1983
		Hartsell et al., 1992
		Laughman et al., 1983
		Ferguson et al., 1989
		Selkowitz, 1985
		Rooney et al., 1992
		Grimby et al., 1989
		Noel et al., 1987
		Delitto et al., 1986a,b
		Brooks et al., 1990
		Balogun, 1986
		Boutelle et al., 1985
		Kubiak et al., 1987
		Delitto et al., 1992
		Franklin et al., 1991
		Underwood et al., 1990
		Curwin et al., 1980
		Currier et al., 1984
		Snyder-Mackler et al., 1989
		Laufer et al., 2001
Maximum electrically evoked muscle force greater than maximum voluntary muscle force	Selkowitz, 1985	Owens et al., 1983
		Hartsell et al., 1992
		Snyder-Mackler et al., 1989
		Noel et al., 1987
		Laufer et al., 2001
Lasting strength gain	Laughman et al., 1983	St-Pierre et al., 1986
	Selkowitz, 1985	
	Soo et al., 1988	
	Kubiak et al., 1987	
	Currier et al., 1983	

H. WHICH CURRENT TYPE IS SUPERIOR?

The body of scientific evidence presented in this chapter reveals that none of the current types (pulsed AC or DC) and waveforms (sinusoidal, rectangular, or square) described in **Table 17-1** is superior to the others for enhancing muscle strength in patients and healthy populations. This explains why commercial pulsed DC stimulators such as the *Respond II* and *Respond Select* are still used today with commercial Russian stimulators such as the *R-2500* and *Versa-Stim* for muscle strengthening purposes in clinical settings.

I. NEUROPHYSIOLOGIC MECHANISMS

There are *fundamental differences*, as shown in **Table 17-3**, between the neurophysiologic mechanisms at work during a voluntary versus electrically evoked muscle contraction. Research has shown that MUs vary in *size* from small (few muscle fibers) to large (several muscle fibers). It has also been shown that smaller MUs produce less force than larger MUs because the former contain fewer muscle fibers or contractile elements (i.e., actin and myosin). Motor unit activation or recruitment is based on two interrelated neurophysiological processes: spatial and temporal recruitment.

1. Spatial MU Recruitment

This process refers to the number and to the order of MUs that are recruited or activated during the process of muscle contraction. The number of MUs refers to the amount, or percentage, of MUs activated within a given muscle or muscle group. The order of MU activation refers to the sequence of activation based on the size of each MU, that is, from the smaller to the larger or vice versa.

2. Temporal MU Recruitment

This process refers to the rate of discharge, or frequency, with which MUs are recruited during the process of muscle contraction. Temporal recruitment is also referred to in the literature as rate coding.

3. Voluntary Contraction

During a voluntary effort, the command for muscle contraction originates in the upper motoneurones (volition) which is then transmitted down to the spinal motoneurones. MUs are activated (spatial recruitment) according to their *size*, that is, from the smaller (S) to the larger (FG, FR) units. This is known as the *size principle* of MU activation (Henneman et al., 1965). MUs are also recruited (temporal recruitment) *asynchronously*, which means that a given MU may be activated several times per second (rate coding) while another MU may be activated only a few times per second, or not at all, during a particular voluntary muscle contraction. In other words, asynchronous recruitment means that MUs are activated randomly over time.

4. Electrically Evoked Contraction

During an electrically evoked muscle contraction, the command for muscle contraction is given by the electrical stimulator, which generates electrical pulses of given amplitudes and frequencies. In such a case, the motoneurone pool is bypassed, meaning that muscle contraction results from the local depolarization of motor nerves buried in soft tissues as opposed to the impulses generated by motoneurones. In contrast to the voluntary contraction process described above, research has shown that MUs are activated (spatial recruitment) in the reversed size order, that is, from the larger (FF; FG) to the smaller (S) motor units (Kramer, 1989; Delitto et al., 1990; Sinacore et al., 1990; Trimble et al., 1991). Also demonstrated is the fact that MUs are now activated (temporal recruitment) *synchronously*, that is, at a fixed frequency that is dictated by the frequency setting on the electrical stimulator.

5. Recap

During electrically evoked muscle contraction, as shown in **Figure 17-4**, current passes through soft tissues and depolarizes motor nerve fibers causing nerve impulses to reach neuromuscular junctions initiating muscle contractions. Spatial motor unit activation occurs in a reverse size order (from the larger to the smaller units) and temporal recruitment is synchronous (fixed frequency) in nature.

TABLE 17-3	ELECTRICALLY EVOKED VERSUS VOLUNTARY MUSCLE CONTRACTION	
MECHANISM	**ELECTRICALLY EVOKED**	**VOLUNTARY**
Spatial MU recruitment	Large to small	Small to large
Temporal MU recruitment	Synchronous	Asynchronous
Muscle loading	Against resistance	Against resistance
Strengthening	Increased MU recruitment Increased muscle hypertrophy	Increased MU recruitment Increased muscle hypertrophy

J. TROPHIC MECHANISM

Research has shown that repeated muscle contractions, whether voluntarily or electrically evoked, against an external load leads to muscle hypertrophy. In strenuous strength-training regimens using Russian current, skeletal muscles get larger and stronger from the hypertrophy, or enlargement, of their muscle fibers, not from the addition of new muscle fibers (hyperplasia).

K. MUSCLE-STRENGTHENING MECHANISM

As shown in **Figure 17-4** and described in **Table 17-3**, muscle strengthening following Russian current therapy results from the interaction between a *neural* (improved MU recruitment and firing) and a *trophic* (hypertrophy) mechanism. The patient's or subject's ability to improve MU activation and to enlarge muscle fibers through voluntary or electrically evoked training will determine the extent of muscle strengthening achieved.

V. DOSIMETRY

A. PARAMETERS

The dosimetry of Russian current therapy requires setting specific parameters to achieve the desired level of evoked muscular contraction. These key parameters are current amplitude, burst frequency, ON:OFF time ratio and duty cycle, ramp-up and ramp-down times, training method, and training protocol. Remember that Russian current, regardless of whether the waveform is sinusoidal, square, or rectangular, always delivers biphasic pulses at a carrier frequency of 2500 cps, modulated to produce 50 bups, each burst lasting 10 ms (2500 cps/50bups/10ms). Readers are *urged to review* Chapter 5 which presents an illustrated glossary of terms related to the practice of NMES and discussed in the following paragraphs.

B. CURRENT AMPLITUDE

To set the level of evoked muscle contraction used for therapy, adjust the stimulator's current amplitude. The body of research indicates that training levels between 40% and 60% of that of MVC are necessary to achieve lasting strength gains. Note that the Russian current stimulator may be calibrated as peak (A_{pk}, for square or rectangular waveform) or as root-mean-square (A_{rms}, for sinusoidal waveform) amperage. As discussed in Chapter 5, A_{rms} is equivalent to 70.7% of amplitude peak value (Gerleman et al., 1999). For example, setting the current amplitude at 80 A_{pk} is equivalent to setting it at 56 A_{rms}. Take note that the order of motor unit recruitment is *reversed*, meaning that the larger, more superficial motor units (FF and FR) will be activated first, with the smaller motor units (S) recruited last as more and deeper motor nerve fibers are depolarized.

C. BURST FREQUENCY

This parameter is commonly set at 50 bups because fused tetanic muscle contraction is achieved in most human muscles at this frequency. Recall that temporal MU recruitment is *synchronous* because all the activated MUs are firing at the same frequency, that is, that which is set on the stimulator.

D. ON:OFF TIME RATIO AND DUTY CYCLE

Setting this ratio corresponds to setting the contraction (ON) and the rest (OFF) time in between two evoked muscle contractions. This ratio is defined as the time during which the muscle is electrically activated (ON time, muscle contraction) to the time during which it is not (OFF time, no contraction). For example, a 10-second ON time followed by a 40-second OFF time yields a 10s:40s ratio.

1. Russian 10s:50s Ratio

The recommended ON:OFF ratio for optimal muscle strengthening is 10s:50s (Kots, 1971, 1977). It is important to set an adequate period of muscle inactivation or relaxation (OFF time) between successive evoked contractions (ON time) to prevent muscle fatigue. Practitioners may vary this ratio during the course of a strength training program to accommodate muscle fatigability. The more fatigable the muscle is, the shorter the ON time and/or the longer the OFF time.

2. Duty Cycle

Setting the ON:OFF time ratio automatically sets up the duty cycle, which is clinically defined as the proportion of ON time to the combined total of the ON and OFF times, expressed as a percentage: duty cycle = [ON / (ON + OFF)] × 100. For example, an ON:OFF ratio of 10s:50s sets up a duty cycle of 16.7% (16.7% = [10 s / (10 s + 50s)] × 100).

3. ON:OFF Time Ratio Versus Duty Cycle

To document or chart only the duty cycle value *without* the corresponding ON:OFF time ratio is *misleading* because, for example, ON:OFF time ratios of 5s:20s and 10s:40s yield exactly the same 20% duty cycle value but different ON and OFF times. Both the duty cycle and its corresponding ON:OFF time ratio must be charted in the patient's file.

4. Practical Meaning

An ON:OFF time ratio of 10s:50s means that the resting time between two successive evoked contractions is five times that of contraction time. The duty cycle, calculated to be 16.7% in the example above, means that muscle contraction occurs during an amount of time (10 seconds) that is 16.7% of the total period of time (60 seconds) between two successive electrically evoked muscle contractions.

E. RAMP-UP AND RAMP-DOWN TIMES

Setting a ramp-up and ramp-down time within the ON time will favor the evoked contraction to *mimic* as closely as possible the gradual build-up and relaxation phases seen at the beginning and the end of a voluntary muscle contraction. Technically, and contrary to the view expressed in some textbooks, both the ramp-up time and the ramp-down time *are part of the total ON time*, along with the plateau time, because during the ramp-up and ramp-down times the process of muscle contraction is occurring (see Chapter 5 for details). Ramp-up and ramp-down times usually last 1–2 seconds.

F. TRAINING METHODS

Practitioners can choose between two electrically evoked muscle training methods: electrical stimulation alone or electrical stimulation plus volition.

1. Electrical Stimulation Alone

In this method, electrical current is applied to a *noncontracting* muscle or muscle group. The evoked muscle contraction thus results solely from the electrical energy delivered to the target muscle. No volitional muscle contraction is required during therapy.

2. Electrical Stimulation Plus Volition

In this method, electrical current is applied to a *voluntarily contracting* muscle or muscle group. In other words, this method consists of *superimposing* the electrical current on the patient's voluntary muscle contraction. The resulting muscle contraction reflects the combined effect of both the electrical energy delivered to the muscle and the volitional energy generated by the brain.

3. Which Training Method is Best?

The body of evidence presented in this chapter reveals that neither method is better than the other in enhancing muscle strength. The choice of one method over the other is a matter of preference.

G. TRAINING PROTOCOL—10c/10s/50s

Of all dosimetric parameters related to the practice of Russian current therapy, the training protocol originally described by Kots (1971, 1977) has received most attention in the literature. This protocol is known as the *10c/10s/50s protocol*. This protocol stands for 10 electrically evoked contractions (c) per training session, with each contraction lasting 10 seconds, and separated by a rest period of 50 seconds. In other words, this protocol calls for a series of 10 contractions with an ON:OFF time ratio of 10s:50s. On the basis of his series of experiments on Russian athletes, Kots reported (1971, 1977) that this 10c/10s/50s protocol was the best protocol for achieving maximum strength gain without inducing significant muscle fa-

tigue during training. Most investigators have faithfully applied this Russian protocol in their studies to either support or refute Kots's claims (**Table 17-2**), and to determine the therapeutic effectiveness of Russian current therapy (**Box 17-1**).

VI. EVIDENCE FOR INDICATIONS

A. GUIDED BY EVIDENCE

Dictionaries generally define *evidence* as anything that establishes a fact or gives reason to believe something. The aim of this textbook is to present *scientific* evidence behind therapeutic EPAs. To be guided by the evidence is the process of integrating the evidence from research, however imperfect or scarce this evidence may be, with clinical experience and patient's preferences. In other words, the *evidence-based practice* of EPA requires that practitioners consider the evidence from research, in addition to their own clinical experience and patient's own preference and beliefs about a given EPA, when the time comes to justify, prescribe, and apply the therapeutic agent. To be guided by the evidence is a process, not a search for the absolute truth. Finally, a lack of evidence from research in support of any given EPA does not mean that this EPA should never be used. What it means is that no statement can be made about its therapeutic effectiveness and that until more evidence from research is presented, its routine use cannot be recommended.

B. EVIDENCE FROM HUMAN RESEARCH

Box 17-1 provides evidence for Russian current therapy, and other NMES currents, based on an exhaustive search of published English-language, peer-reviewed studies on humans. The term *indication* is used in reference to a list of pathologies for which Russian current therapy is employed. Ratings of therapeutic benefit (Yes or No) and grading of strength of scientific evidence (I, II, or III), including the reference, are included for each pathological condition.

1. Rating Therapeutic Benefit

The rating, expressed as Yes or No, is based on the overall conclusion(s) reached on the issue of therapeutic effectiveness by the author(s) who conducted the peer-reviewed study.

2. Grading Strength of Evidence

The grading, numerically classified as I, II, and III, is based on the type of research methodology or experimental design used by the author(s). All those listed are studies on humans published in English-language, peer-reviewed journals. It follows that the evidence in studies graded I is stronger than in those graded II and the evidence in studies graded II is stronger than in those graded III.

Box 17-1	**Research-Based Indications for the Use of Russian Current and Other Neuromuscular-Stimulating Current Therapy**

PATHOLOGY	BENEFIT	GRADE	REFERENCE
Muscle weakness	Yes	I	Laughman et al., 1983
	Yes	I	Parker et al., 2003
	Yes	I	Nuhr et al., 2004
	Yes	I	Quittan et al., 2001
	Yes	II	Dobsak et al., 2006
	Yes	II	Harris et al., 2003
	Yes	II	Caggiano et al., 1994
	Yes	II	Romero et al., 1982
	Yes	II	Currier et al., 1983
	Yes	II	Fahey et al., 1985
	Yes	II	McMiken et al., 1983
	Yes	II	Parker et al., 2005
	Yes	II	Laufer et al., 2001
	Yes	II	Hortobagyi et al., 1992
	Yes	II	Pfeifer et al., 1997
	Yes	II	Selkowitz, 1985
	Yes	II	Soo et al., 1988
	Yes	II	Underwood et al., 1990
Muscle weakness, post–anterior cruciate ligament (ACL) reconstruction	Yes	II	Fitzgerald et al., 2003
	Yes	II	Lieber et al., 1996
	Yes	II	Wigerstad-Lossing et al., 1988
	Yes	II	Delitto et al, 1988b
	Yes	II	Anderson et al., 1989
	Yes	II	Draper et al., 1991
	Yes	II	Snyder-Mackler et al., 1995
	Yes	II	Snyder-Mackler et al., 1994
	Yes	II	Snyder-Mackler et al., 1991
	Yes	III	Delitto et al., 1988a
	Yes	III	Eriksson et al., 1979
	No	II	Sisk et al., 1987
	No	II	Paternostro-Sluga et al., 1999
Muscle weakness—total knee arthroplasty	Yes	II	Williams et al., 1986
	Yes	II	Curwin et al., 1980
	Yes	III	Petterson et al., 2006
	Yes	III	Stevens et al., 2004
	Yes	III	Lewek et al., 2001
	Yes	III	Mintken et al., 2007
Muscle weakness—Bell's palsy	Yes	II	Farragher et al., 1987
	Yes	III	Targan et al., 2000
	Yes	III	Weiss, 1976
	Yes	III	Paniora, 1994
Muscle weakness—cerebral palsy	Yes	III	Daichman et al., 2003
	No	I	Kerr et al., 2006
Knee osteoarthritis	No	II	Gaines et al., 2004
Patellofemoral syndrome	Yes	II	Callaghan et al., 2001
Post–knee sprain muscle atrophy	Yes	III	Nitz et al., 1987
Post–ankle sprain edema	No	I	Man et al., 2007

a. Grade I
Evidence based on *controlled* studies on humans, regardless of their level of randomization and blindness.

b. Grade II
Evidence based on *noncontrolled* studies on humans, regardless of their level of randomization and blindness.

c. Grade III
Evidence based on *case* studies on humans, regardless of their level of randomization and blindness.

3. Strength of Evidence Behind the Agent
The strength of evidence behind the agent, as presented in the research-based indication box, is arbitrarily assessed in this textbook as *weak*, *moderate*, or *strong*. For example, the larger the number of studies graded I, regardless of therapeutic benefit, the stronger the scientific evidence behind the agent.

4. Strength for Justifying Usage of the Agent
The strength of evidence to justify the usage of an agent for an individual pathology or groups of pathologies, as listed in the research-based indication box, is arbitrarily assessed in this textbook as *poor*, *fair*, *good*, or *conflicting*. For example, where a larger number of grade I studies show therapeutic benefit (Yes) than no benefit, for any given pathology, the justification for usage of this agent for that pathology is assessed as *good*. *Conflicting* usage is reported when an approximately equal number of studies with similar grades show therapeutic benefit (Yes) and no benefit (No).

C. STRENGTH OF EVIDENCE AND JUSTIFICATION FOR USAGE
The results presented in **Box 17-1** shows *moderate-to-strong* strength of evidence for the use of Russian current for the management of quadriceps muscle atrophy in healthy (de-conditioning) individuals and patients who have undergone knee surgical interventions (partial and total knee reconstruction), with the majority of studies graded II showing benefit. These results also show that the justification for usage of Russian therapy is *good* for quadriceps muscle strength enhancement in such healthy individuals and patients. Until more evidence from research is provided with regard to those remaining pathologies listed, or any other pathology, the *routine use* of Russian current therapy for such pathologies *cannot be recommended*.

VII. CONTRAINDICATIONS
Table 17-4 describes the contraindications for using therapeutic Russian current stimulation. Because this EPA is capable of nerve depolarization, its contraindications are similar to those listed for TENS therapy (Chapter 14). Always ensure that electrode placement never allows the current field between the electrodes to cross the transcranial, transthoracic, and anterior cervical areas of the body.

TABLE 17-4	CONTRAINDICATIONS TO RUSSIAN CURRENT THERAPY
CONTRAINDICATIONS	**RATIONALE**
Over the anterior cervical area	Risk of stimulating key organs, such as the vagus nerve, phrenic nerve, and carotid sinuses, resulting in adverse effects such as hypotensive reaction and laryngeal spasm.
Over the thoracic region	Risk of affecting normal heart function. Stimulation over intercostal muscles led to a respiratory failure in one cardiac patient.
Over the cranial area	Risk of affecting normal brain function.
With patients wearing rate-responsive pacemakers or implanted cardioverter defibrillators (ICDs)	Risk of electronic interference with units (Crevenna et al., 2003, 2004—for more details, see Chapter 14). *Important note:* NMES may be used with these patients *only* if the ICU unit is *turned OFF* during therapy.
Over the abdominal, pelvic, or lumbar areas with pregnant women in their first trimester	Risk of inducing labor.
Over metal implants	Risk of causing unnecessary pain due to electrical current-induced overheating of implants.
With epileptic patients	Risk of causing an epileptic episode (Scherder et al., 1999).

(Continued)

TABLE 17-4	CONTINUED

CONTRAINDICATIONS	RATIONALE
Over a hemorrhagic area	Risk of enhanced bleeding due to increased blood flow in the treated area.
Over a malignant area	Risk of increasing and spreading the tumor due to increased blood flow in the treated area.
Over damaged skin	Risk of causing unnecessary and severe pain.

VIII. RISKS, PRECAUTIONS, AND RECOMMENDATIONS

The practice of Russian current therapy is not without risk for the patient. The major risks associated with this electrophysical agent, as well as some precautions and recommendations designed to improve safety and effectiveness, are listed in **Table 17-5**.

IX. CONSIDERATIONS FOR APPLICATION AND DOCUMENTATION

A. CONSIDERATIONS AND PROCEDURES

Safe, effective, and optimal application of Russian current therapy requires that clinicians run through a systematic set of considerations and procedures for every single application. Presented here is a list of such considerations and procedures.

1. Checklists
Before proceeding with treatment, practitioners should always go through the list of contraindications (**Table 17-4**) and list of risks, precautions, and recommendations (**Table 17-5**).

2. Skin Preparation
Before each application, cleanse the skin on the stimulating area with rubbing alcohol to remove impurities and reduce skin impedance.

3. Stimulator Type
There is evidence to suggest that portable battery-powered stimulators are as good as cabinet line-powered stimulators to deliver therapeutic NMES. The selection is a matter of preference.

TABLE 17-5	RISKS, PRECAUTIONS, AND RECOMMENDATIONS FOR RUSSIAN CURRENT THERAPY

RISKS	RATIONALE
Prolonged use of electrode, electroconductive gel, and adhesive tape over the same skin areas	Risk of causing contact dermatitis related to the materials with which the electrode, gel, or adhesive tape are made (for details, see Chapter 14).
Usage near functioning shortwave diathermy (SWD) device	Risk of causing electronic interference. A patient reporting a sudden and variable surge of current output when a SWD unit is functioning in the neighborhood may be indicative of such electronic interference.

PRECAUTIONS	RATIONALE
With confused and unreliable patients	May result in unreliable information, which may have a negative impact on treatment effectiveness.
Home NMES therapy	Instruct patients to keep the portable NMES unit out of the reach of children at all times.

(Continued)

TABLE 17-5	CONTINUED

RECOMMENDATIONS	RATIONALE
Clean and dry exposed skin surface areas before each treatment	Wiping the skin surface with alcohol will reduce its impedance significantly in addition to removing impurities, thus allowing an optimal electrical coupling at the skin–electrode interface.
Clip hair over exposed skin areas	To ensure optimal electrode–skin coupling.
Wash and dry reusable electrodes after each treatment	To ensure optimal performance; follow the manufacturer's instructions.
Check cables and electrodes regularly for visible wear and tear	To ensure optimal efficacy; to prevent macroshock if line-powered stimulators are used.
Check electrode impedance monthly	To ensure appropriate electrode impedance for optimal conduction because electrodes will deteriorate with use and time. Use an ohmmeter to check impedance.
Keep all NMES units at least 3 m (10 ft) away from any functioning SWD device.	To minimize the risk of electronic interference.
Discard all electrodes after 6 months of usage.	Material deterioration will increase electrode impedance thus reducing treatment efficacy.
Plug line-powered stimulation into GFCI receptacle	Prevent the risk of electrocution (see Chapter 27 for details).
Conduct regular maintenance and calibration	To ensure optimal treatment efficacy. Follow the manufacturer's recommendations and schedule.

4. Stimulator Output Channel

Portable Russian stimulators, as is the case with most therapeutic electrical stimulators, offer two stimulating channels (bi-channels) while cabinet stimulators may offer more than two channels (multichannels). The majority of applications of Russian current therapy for muscle strengthening are done using either one or two channels. A pair of electrodes is usually connected, using a bipolar cable, to each stimulating channel. Multiple electrodes can be connected to a single channel using bifurcated cables. The rationale for using bifurcated cables, thus the number of electrodes per channel, is to enlarge the stimulation area per channel.

3. Electrode Type

Practitioners can choose from a variety of commercial reusable electrodes made of carbon-impregnated rubber and flexible mesh metals, available in different sizes and shapes (**Fig 17-2**).

4. Electrode Preparation

Make sure that a thin and evenly distributed coating of electroconductive gel is applied to each electrode to optimize conduction at the electrode–skin interface. Note that some electrodes may be pre-gelled.

5. Electrode Current Density

Current density is the ratio of maximum current amplitude to electrode stimulating surface area, and is usually expressed as milliamperes per square centimeter (mA/cm^2). Research shows that the higher the current density under the electrode, the more discomfort or pain the patient feels beneath that electrode. Because the current density under a given electrode often dictates whether the application is more or less comfortable, using a larger electrode size is recommended, especially when the current amplitude used to evoke the muscle contraction is relatively high.

6. Electrode Spacing and Penetration Depth

The spacing between a pair of electrodes influences current dispersion within the tissues, which in turn affects the current's penetration depth. The wider the spacing between electrodes is, the deeper the current penetration into the tissue. In contrast, the closer the two electrodes, the more superficial the stimulating effect.

7. Electrode Orientation

Each pair of electrodes should be placed parallel, not perpendicular, to the direction of muscle fibers (Brooks et al., 1990). A rule of thumb is to orient each pair of electrodes parallel to the estimated line of pull of the muscle or the muscle group.

8. Electrode Attachment

Most surface electrodes are mechanically attached to the skin with hypoallergic tape. Some electrodes are self-adhesive. Good skin surface attachment is necessary to ensure that the entire electrode stimulating surface area is in contact with the skin surface to avoid unintentional variations of current density in one region of the skin during the application.

9. Electrode Placement Methods

Three methods of electrode placement are routinely mentioned in the NMES literature: *monopolar*, *bipolar*, and *quadripolar*. This textbook introduces a fourth method, called *multipolar*. These methods, each illustrated in **Figure 17-5**, are based on clinical situations in which only one stimulator, with two or three channels, is used. Recall that each electrode has a pole; hence the term polar.

a. Monopolar

One (mono-) electrode is placed *over* the targeted muscle contractile area with the other positioned at some distance away from the targeted muscle or muscle group. In the example shown in **Figure 17-5A**, one electrode, within the pair connected to a single channel, is placed over the targeted quadriceps area with the other positioned away from the targeted area, over the upper lateral hip area.

b. Bipolar

Two (bi-) electrodes are placed *over* the targeted muscle area. **Figure 17-5B** shows a pair of electrodes positioned over the targeted quadriceps muscle area.

c. Quadripolar

Four (quadri-) electrodes are placed *over* the targeted muscle area. **Figure 17-5C** shows two pairs of electrodes positioned over the targeted quadriceps muscle area. Note that this method can also be applied via one channel only if a bifurcated cable is used.

d. Multipolar

More than four (multi-) electrodes are placed over the targeted muscle contractile area. In **Figure 17-5D**, six electrodes are positioned over the quadriceps contractile area using a multichannel stimulator, to which is connected three pairs of electrodes using three pairs of bipolar cables. Note that this electrode placement method can also be applied using a bi-channel stimulator to which is connected two pairs of three electrodes, each pair connected to the stimulator using a bifurcated cable.

e. Electrode Over Motor Point

When placing an electrode over the target muscle, practitioners should consider placing it over the muscle's motor points. A *motor point* is clinically defined as a specific skin area where the targeted muscle is best stimulated with the smallest amount of current amplitude and the shortest pulse duration. Anatomically speaking, this

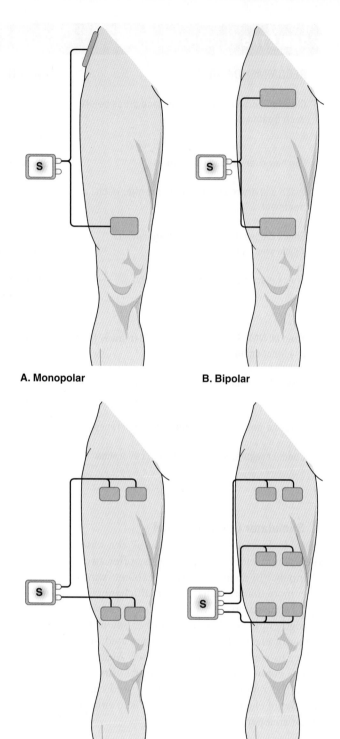

A. Monopolar   **B. Bipolar**

C. Quadripolar   **D. Multipolar**

FIGURE 17-5 Monopolar (**A**), bipolar (**B**), quadripolar (**C**), and multipolar (**D**) electrode placement methods.

same motor point is defined as the surface entry point of a bundle of motor nerve fibers into a fascicle of muscle fibers. Some muscles may have more than one motor point. Various charts of human motor points are available to facilitate localization on the body (see Prentice, 1998; Starkey, 2004).

10. Stimulation Modes

As stated earlier, all modern neuromuscular electrical stimulators, such as Russian current stimulators, feature at least two independent channels and a *time-delay switch*, allowing both channels to be triggered or activated independently. When such a stimulator is used, manually setting the time delay between channel 1 and channel 2, as illustrated in **Figure 17-6**, allows practitioners to chose between three stimulation modes: synchronous, reciprocal, and overlapping.

a. Synchronous

The synchronous mode, illustrated in **Figure 17-6A**, is achieved by setting the time delay switch (D for delay) of channel 2 at 0 seconds, with the ON time and OFF time of channel 1 equal to the ON and OFF times of channel 2; for example: D = 0 s; channel 1: ON = 5 s; OFF= 15 s; channel 2: ON = 5 s; OFF =15 s). In such a setting, both channels are *synchronously* activated (ON) and deactivated (OFF) for the full duration of the treatment session. This

mode allows synchronous stimulation of two different muscle groups or two muscle parts within a muscle group.

b. Reciprocal

The reciprocal mode, shown in **Figure 17-6B**, is achieved by setting the time delay (D) value of channel 2 equivalent to the ON time of channel 1 while setting the ON time of channel 1 equal to the OFF time of channel 2; for example: D = 5 s; channel 1: ON = 5 s; OFF = 15 s; channel 2: ON = 15 s; OFF = 5 s. This setting results in a *reciprocal* activation of both channels for the full duration of the treatment session. This mode allows reciprocal, or alternating, stimulation of two different muscles or muscle groups, such as the agonist versus the antagonist.

c. Overlap

The overlap mode, shown in **Figure 17-6C**, is achieved by setting the time delay (D) switch of channel 2 greater than 0 second but less than the ON time of channel 1,

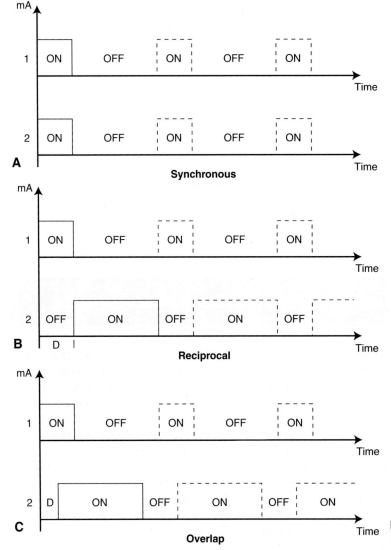

FIGURE 17-6 Synchronous (**A**), reciprocal (**B**), and overlapping (**C**) stimulation modes.

while keeping the ON time and OFF time of both channels identical; for example: D = 3 s; channel 1: ON = 5 s; OFF =15 s; channel 2: ON = 5 s; OFF =15 s. Setting this time delay value implies that both channels now *overlap*, as channel 2 is activated 3 seconds after channel 1, for the full duration of the treatment session. This mode allows overlapping stimulation or contraction of two different muscles or muscle groups.

11. Dosimetry

Set the dosimetric parameters, which include current amplitude, burst duration, interburst duration, burst frequency, ramp-up and ramp-down times, ON and OFF times with duty cycle, and number of contractions per training bout. Recall that Russian current therapy for muscle strengthening is commonly delivered using the so-called Russian protocol—10c/10s/50s—meaning 10 electrically evoked contractions per training bout, each lasting 10 seconds and separated by 50 seconds.

12. Stimulation Training Method

Practitioners can choose between two methods: *electrical stimulation alone* and *electrical stimulation plus volition*. The second method differs from the first in that electrical stimulation is superimposed on a given level of voluntary or volitional muscle contraction. In other words, electrical stimulation is delivered concomitantly with voluntary muscle contraction.

13. Number of Bouts per Training Session

Determine the number of training bouts per training session. For example, 3 bouts of 10 contractions, each bout separated by a 5-minute rest period.

14. End of Treatment

Inspect the skin under each stimulating electrode. Document any unusual sensation the patient felt during treatment in the patient's file. Wipe off electroconductive gel.

Wash dry reusable electrode. Discard disposable electrode in biowaste bags.

15. Cable and Reusable Electrode Maintenance

Check cables and electrodes regularly for visible wear and tear. Check electrode impedance regularly with ohmmeter because their impedance may increase with usage and over time. Discard all electrodes after 6 months of usage.

B. DOCUMENTATION

Table 17-6 shows the key parameters to be documented in the patient's file with regard to the application of Russian current therapy.

TABLE 17-6	KEY TREATMENT PARAMETERS TO BE DOCUMENTED IN PATIENT'S FILE AFTER RUSSIAN CURRENT THERAPY

- *Stimulator type:* portable or cabinet
- *Current waveform type:* sinusoidal, square, or rectangular
- *Burst duration:* ms
- *Interburst duration:* ms
- *Burst frequency:* bups
- *Training contraction level:* % of MVC
- *Ramp-up time:* ms
- *Ramp-down time:* ms
- *ON time; OFF time:* ON:OFF time ratio
- *Duty cycle:* %
- *Electrode placement:* monopolar, bipolar, quadripolar, or multipolar
- *Stimulation mode when 2 channels used:* synchronous, reciprocal, or overlapping
- *Number of bouts of contractions per training session*
- *Number of training sessions per day*

Case Study 17-1 Quadriceps Weakness after ACL Reconstruction

A 26-year-old man is referred by his treating orthopedic surgeon for lasting problems related to decreased quadriceps muscle strength and function following right anterior cruciate ligament (ACL) knee reconstruction, done 12 weeks ago, following a ski accident. At discharge from hospital, the patient was given a full home quadriceps muscle strengthening program. Questioned about his compliance with the program over the past 8 weeks, the patient readily admits very poor compliance thinking that doing his regular daily activities will be enough to regain full knee extension strength. The patient's chief complaints are right quadriceps muscle weakness and atrophy, combined with difficulty squatting, climbing stairs, and running. He is also frustrated with not being able to ski. Physical examination of the injured knee shows no sign of inflammation, and complete range of motion. Measurements reveal a quadriceps force deficit of 40% and a thigh girth deficit of 1.5 cm on the affected side. The patient's goal is to rebuild the bulk and strength in his right quadriceps so he can ski safely and effectively once again. He is now well motivated, realizing that just doing his daily activities will not restore full knee strength and function. You propose Russian current therapy using the electrical stimulation plus volition, or superimposed method of strength training.

Evidence-Based Steps Toward the Resolution of This Case

1. List medical diagnosis.

Complete right-ACL rupture

2. List key impairment(s).

■ Quadriceps muscle weakness
■ Thigh muscle atrophy

3. List key functional limitation(s).

■ Difficulty squatting
■ Difficulty climbing stairs
■ Difficulty running

4. List key disability/disabilities.

■ Unable to ski

5. Justification for Russian current therapy.

Is there justification to use Russian current therapy in this case? This chapter has established that there is *moderate-to-strong* strength of evidence and *good* justification for the use of Russian therapy for enhancing muscle strength (see Section VI,). This textbook recommends the use of this EPA for the following reasons. First, there is strong evidence (Eriksson et al., 1979; Delitto et al., 1986a,b; Wigerstad-Lossing et al., 1988; Anderson et al., 1989; Draper et al., 1991; Snyder-Mackler et al., 1991, 1994, 1995; Lieber et al., 1996; Delitto et al., 1988a,b; Fitzgerald et al., 2003) to suggest that Russian current therapy can strengthen human quadriceps muscle following surgical ACL reconstruction by enhancing MU action and promoting muscle hypertrophy. Second, there is evidence to suggest that superimposing Russian current stimulation on top of volitional quadriceps will help to accomplish full voluntary MU recruitment, which will induce the desired muscle hypertrophy, which will in turn translate into increased muscle strength. Because EPAs should not be used in isolation or as a sole intervention, Russian current therapy is used here concomitantly with a home regimen of functional training involving squatting exercises, climbing stairs, and running on the treadmill.

6. Search for contraindications.

None is found.

7. Search for dangers and precautions.

None is found.

8. List the therapeutic goal(s) you and your patient wish to achieve.

■ Increase quadriceps muscle force
■ Decrease muscle atrophy
■ Increase ability to squat, climb, and run
■ Accelerate return to skiing

9. List outcome measurement(s) used to assess treatment effectiveness.

■ Muscle force: dynamometry
■ Thigh atrophy: measuring tape
■ Knee function: Patient-Specific Functional Scale (PSFS)

10. Instruct patient about what he/she should experience, do, and not do during the treatment session.

■ Feel sensation of strong muscle contraction
■ Do maximum voluntary muscle contraction during electrically evoked contraction (electrical stimulation plus volition stimulating method)
■ Do not resist knee extension during electrical stimulation

11. Outline your therapeutic prescription based on the best sources of evidence available.

The prescription suggested below is based on the following publications: Eriksson et al., 1979; Wigerstad-Lossing et al., 1988; Delitto et al., 1986a,b; Anderson et al., 1989; Draper et al., 1991; Snyder-Mackler et al., 1991, 1994, 1995; Lieber et al., 1996; Delitto, Rose et al., 1988a,b; Fitzgerald et al., 2003.

■ *Russian stimulator type:* cabinet
■ *Waveform type:* 2500 Hz carrier balanced sinusoidal
■ *Number of stimulating channel:* 2
■ *Burst duration:* 10 ms
■ *Burst interval:* 10 ms
■ *Burst frequency:* 50 bups
■ *Ramp-up time:* 1 s
■ *Ramp-down time:* 2 s
■ *Training level:* set at 70% of MVC torque measured on healthy knee, by adjusting the current amplitude
■ *Stimulating method:* electrical stimulation with voluntary motion (superimposed)
■ *Electrode placement:* quadripolar
■ *Electrode type, shape, and size:* carbon rubber; square; 4×4 cm (2×2 in)
■ *Electrode coupling:* electroconductive gel
■ *Stimulation mode:* synchronous
■ *Treatment protocol:* 10c/50s/10s, meaning a bout of consecutive 10 evoked tetanic contractions, each lasting 10 s and separated by a 50-s rest period. This is equivalent to an ON:OFF time ratio of 10s:50s which corresponds to a duty cycle of 16.6%
■ *Number of evoked exercise bouts per training session:* 4 bouts, each separated by a 5-min rest period
■ *Number of treatment sessions per week:* 3
■ *Total treatment duration:* 3 weeks

(Continued)

Case Study 17-1   Continued

12. Collect outcome measurements.

Pre- and posttreatment comparison:

- Quadriceps force: 30% gain (from 40 to 10% deficit)
- Thigh atrophy: gain of 1.0 cm (from 1.5 to 0.5 deficit)
- Knee function: improved PSFS score (from 6 to 9)

13. Assess therapeutic effectiveness based on outcome measures.

The results show that Russian current therapy, delivered concomitantly with voluntary muscle contraction (superimposed method) and combined with a home functional training program, conducted over a 9-week period, led to a significant gain of force and hypertrophy in the right quadriceps in addition to significantly improving knee function. Electrically evoked muscle contraction in addition to voluntary contraction helped the patient to achieve better MU activation and,

consequently, greater muscle force. Moreover, the use of this EPA helped the patient to resume his recreational skiing activity now that his right knee is strong enough to sustain the demand put on it during this activity. Overall, this treatment approach was beneficial in acting on the patient's disablement status created by the pathology, as illustrated in the **figure below**.

14. State the prognosis.

The prognosis is excellent if this young active man performs his home quadriceps muscle-strengthening program until he can achieve full right quadriceps force (force level equivalent to the contralateral healthy side). To minimize the risk of reinjuring his right knee, the patient is strongly advised to resume his home quadriceps-strengthening program before and during his skiing season.

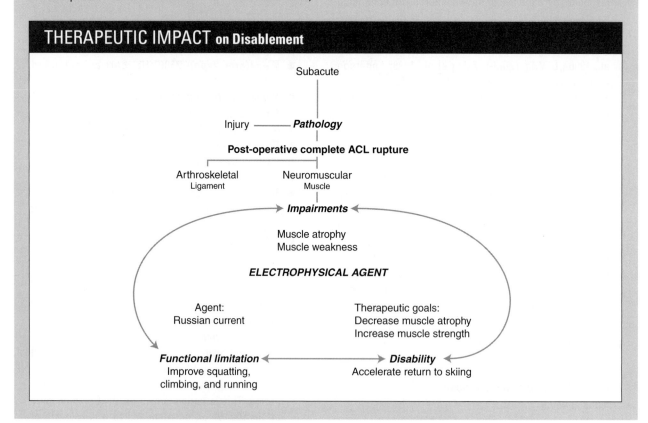

THERAPEUTIC IMPACT on Disablement

CRITICAL THINKING QUESTIONS

Clarification: What is meant by Russian current therapy?

Assumptions: Many of your colleagues assume that the use of Russian current stimulation causes less discomfort

and generates greater tetanic force than other non-burst-modulated stimulating currents. How would you verify or disprove this assumption?

Reasons and evidence: What led you to believe that motor unit recruitment during electrical stimulation is synchronous and occurs in a reverse-size order?

Viewpoints or perspectives: How would you respond to a colleague who says that Russian current therapy is as effective as any voluntary muscle exercise program for enhancing muscle strength?

Implications and consequences: What are the potential implications and consequences of the following parameter settings: (1) increasing the ON time while keeping the OFF time the same during the course of the training program; (2) using 30 bups as opposed to 50 bups; (3) setting no ramp-up and ramp-down time?

About the question: Why is it that the use of Russian current therapy for muscle strengthening is perceived, by both patients and healthy subjects, to be as painful as the application of other stimulating currents used to deliver NMES? Why do you think I ask this question?

References

Articles

Anderson AF, Lipscomb AB (1989) Analysis of rehabilitation technique after anterior cruciate reconstruction. Am J Sports Med, 17: 154–160

Balogun JA (1986) Pain complaint and muscle soreness associated with high-voltage electrical stimulation: Effect of ramp time. Percept Mot Skills, 62: 799–804

Behm DG, St-Pierre DM, Perez D (1996) Muscle inactivation: Assessment of interpolated twitch technique. J Appl Physiol, 81: 2267–2273

Belanger AY, Allen ME, Chapman AE (1992) Cutaneous versus muscular perception of electrically evoked tetanic pain. J Orthop Sports Phys Ther, 16: 162–168

Belanger AY, McComas AJ (1981) Extent of motor unit activation during effort. J Appl Physiol Respir Environ Exerc, 51: 1131–1135

Boutelle D, Smith B, Malone T (1985) A strength study utilizing the Electro-Stim 180. J Orthop Sports Phys Ther, 7: 50–53

Brooks ME, Smith EM, Currier DP (1990) Effect of longitudinal versus transverse electrode placement on torque production by the quadriceps femoris muscle during neuromuscular electrical stimulation. J Orthop Sports Phys Ther, 11: 530–534

Caggiano E, Emrey T, Shirley S (1994) Effects of electrical stimulation or voluntary contraction for strengthening the quadriceps femoris muscles in an aged male population. J Orthop Sports Phys Ther, 20: 22–28

Callaghan MJ, Oldham JA, Winstanley J (2001) A comparison of two types of electrical stimulation of the quadriceps in the treatment of patellofemoral pain syndrome. A pilot study. Clin Rehabil, 15: 637–646

Crevenna R, Wolzt M, Fialka-Moser V, Keilani M, Nurh M, Paternostro-Sluga T, Pacher R, Mayr W, Quittan M (2004) Long-term transcutaneous neuromuscular electrical stimulation in patients with bipolar sensing implantable cadioverter defibrillators: A pilot safety study. Artif Organs, 28: 99–102

Crevenna R, Mayr W, Keilani M, Pleiner J, Nurh M, Quittan M, Pacher R, Pialka-Moser V, Wolzt M (2003) Safety of a combined strength and endurance training using neuromuscular electrical stimulation of thigh muscles in patients with heart failure and bipolar sensing cardiac pacemakers. Wien Klin Wochenschr, 115: 710–714

Currier DP, Mann R (1983) Muscle strength development by electrical stimulation in healthy individuals. Phys Ther, 63: 915–921

Currier DP, Mann R (1984) Pain complaint: Comparison of isometric stimulation with conventional isometric exercise. J Orthop Sports Phys Ther, 5: 318–323

Curwin S, Stanish WD, Valinat G (1980) Clinical applications and biochemical effects of high frequency electrical stimulation. Can Athl Assoc J, 7: 15–16

Daichman J, Johnston TE, Evans K, Tecklin JS (2003) The effects of a neuromuscular electrical stimulation home program on impairments and functional skills of a child with spastic diplegic cerebral palsy: A case report. Pediatr Phys Ther, 15: 153–158

Delitto A (2002) Russian electrical stimulation: Putting this perspective into perspective. Phys Ther, 82: 1017–1018

Delitto A, McKowen JM, McCarthy JA, Shively RA, Rose SJ (1988a) Electrically elicited co-contraction of a thigh muscular after anterior cruciate ligament surgery. A description and single-case experiment. Phys Ther, 68: 45–50

Delitto A, Rose SJ (1986a) Comparative comfort of three waveforms used in electrically eliciting quadriceps femoris muscle contractions. Phys Ther, 66: 1704–1707

Delitto A, Rose SJ (1986b) Electrically eliciting quadriceps femoris muscle contractions. Phys Ther, 66: 1704–1707

Delitto A, Rose SJ, McKowen JM, Lehman RC, Thomas JA, Shively RA (1988b) Electrical stimulation versus voluntary exercise in strengthening thigh musculature after anterior cruciate ligament surgery. Phys Ther, 68: 663–666

Delitto A, Snyder-Mackler L (1990) Two theories of muscle strength augmentation using percutaneous electrical stimulation. Phys Ther, 70: 158–164

Delitto A, Strube MJ, Shulman AD, Minor SD (1992) A study of discomfort with electrical stimulation. Phys Ther, 72: 410–421

Dobsak P, Novakova M, Fiser B, Siegelova J, Balcarkova P, Spinarova L, Vitovec J, Minami N, Nagasaka M, Kohzuki M, Yambe T, Imachi K, Nitta S, Eicher JC, Wolf JE (2006) Electrical stimulation of skeletal muscles. An alternative to aerobic exercise training in patients with chronic heart failure? Int Heart J, 47: 441–453

Dowling JJ, Konert E, Ljucovic P, Andrews DM (1994) Are humans able to voluntary elicit maximum force? Neurosci Lett, 179: 25–28

Draper V, Ballard L (1991) Electrical stimulation versus electromyographic biofeedback in the recovery of quadriceps femoris muscle function following anterior cruciate ligament surgery. Phys Ther, 71: 455–461

Eriksson E, Haggmark T (1979) Comparison of isometric muscle training and electrical stimulation supplementing isometric muscle training in the recovery after major knee ligament surgery. Am J Sports Med, 17: 169–171

Fahey TD, Harvey M, Schroeder RV (1985) Influence of sex differences and knee joint position on electrical stimulated strength increases. Med Sci Sports Exerc, 17: 144–177

Farragher D, Kidd GL, Tallis R (1987) Eutrophic electrical stimulation for Bell's palsy. Clin Rehabil, 1: 265–271

Ferguson JP, Blackley MW, Knight RD, Sutlive TG, Underwood FB, Greathouse DG (1989) Effects of varying electrode site placements on the torque output of an electrically stimulated involuntary quadriceps femoris muscle contraction. J Orthop Sports Phys Ther, 11: 24–29

Fitzgerald GK, Piva SR, Irrgang JJ (2003) A modified neuromuscular electrical stimulation protocol for quadriceps strength training following anterior cruciate ligament reconstruction. J Orthop Sports Phys Ther, 492–501

Franklin ME, Currier DP, Smith ST, Mitts K, Werrell LM, Chenier TC (1991) Effect of varying the ratio of electrically induced muscle contraction time to rest time on serum creatine kinase and perceived soreness. J Orthop Sports Phys Ther, 13: 310–315

Gaines JM, Metter EJ, Talbot LA (2004) The effect of neuromuscular electrical stimulation on arthritis knee pain in older adults with osteoarthritis of the knee. Appl Nurs Res, 17: 201–206

Grimby G, Wigerstad-Lossing I (1989) Comparison of high- and low-frequency muscle stimulators. Arch Phys Med Rehab, 70: 835–838

Harris S, LeMaitre JP, Mackenzie G, Fox KA, Denvir MA (2003) A randomized study of home-based electrical stimulation of the legs and conventional bicycle exercise training for patients with chronic heart failure. Eur Heart J, 24: 871–878

Hartsell HD, Kramer JK (1992) A comparison of the effects of electrode placement, muscle tension, and isometric torque of the knee extensors. J Orthop Sports Phys Ther, 15: 168–174

Henneman E, Somjen G, Carpenter DG (1965) Functional significance of cell size spinal motoneurons. J Neurophysiol, 28: 560–580

Hortobagyi T, Lambert NJ, Tracy C (1992) Voluntary and electromyostimulation forces in trained and untrained men. Med Sci Sports Exerc, 24: 702–707

Kerr C, McDowell B, Cosgrove A, Walsh D, Bradbury I, McDonough S (2006) Electrical stimulation in cerebral palsy: A randomized controlled trial. Dev Med Child Neurol, 48: 870–876

Kubiak RJ, Whitman KM, Jonhson RM (1987) Changes in quadriceps femoris muscle strength using isometric exercise versus electrical stimulation. J Orthop Sports Phys Ther, 8: 537–541

Laufer Y, Ries JD, Leininger PM, Alon G (2001) Quadriceps femoris muscle torques and fatigue generated by neuromuscular electrical stimulation with three different waveforms. Phys Ther, 81: 1307–1316

Laughman RK, Youdas JW, Garrett TR, Chao EY (1983) Strength changes in the normal quadriceps femoris muscle as a result of electrical stimulation. Phys Ther, 63: 494–499

Lewek M, Stevens J, Snyder-Mackler L (2001) The use of electrical stimulation to increase quadriceps femoris muscle force in an elderly patient following a total knee arthroplasty. Phys Ther, 81: 1565–1571

Lieber RL, Silva PD, Daniel DM (1996) Equal effectiveness of electrical and volitional strength training for quadriceps femoris muscles after anterior cruciate ligament surgery. J Orthop Res, 14: 131–138

Lyons CL, Robb JB, Irrgang JJ, Fitzgerald GK (2005) Differences in quadriceps femoris torque when using a clinical electrical stimulator versus a portable electrical stimulator. Phys Ther, 85: 44–51

Man IO, Morrissey MC, Cywinski JK (2007) Effect of neuromuscular electrical stimulation on ankle swelling in the early period after ankle sprain. Phys Ther, 87: 53–65

McMiken DF, Todd-Smith M, Thompson C (1983) Strengthening of human quadriceps muscles by cutaneous electrical stimulation. Scand J Rehabil Med, 15: 25–28

Mintken PE, Carpenter KJ, Eckhoff D, Kohrt WM, Stevens JE (2007) Early neuromuscular electrical stimulation to optimize quadriceps muscle function following total knee arthroplasty: A case report. J Orthop Sports Phys Ther, 37: 364–371

Nitz AJ, Dobner JJ (1987) High-intensity electrical stimulation effect on thigh musculature during immobilization for knee sprain. A case report. Phys Ther, 67: 219–222

Noel G, Belanger AY (1987) Relation entre la force maximale volontaire, force tetanique et douleur lors de l'electrostimulation du quadriceps femoris. Physiother Can, 39: 377–383

Nuhr MJ, Pette D, Berger R, Quittan M, Crevenna R, Huelsman M, Wiesinger GF, Moser P, Fialka-Moser V, Pacher R (2004) Beneficial effects of chronic low-frequency stimulation of thigh muscles in patients with advanced chronic heart failure. Eur Heart J, 25: 136–143

Owens J, Malone T (1983) Treatment parameters of high frequency electrical stimulation as established on the Electro-Stim 180. J Orthop Sports Phys Ther, 4: 162–168

Paniora L (1994) The treatment of Bell's palsy using the Respond unit—A case study. Aus J Physiother, 40:30–32

Parker MG, Bennett MJ, Hieb MA, Hollar AC, Roe AA (2003) Strength response in human femoris muscle during 2 neuromuscular electrical stimulation programs. J Orthop Sports Phys Ther, 33: 719–726

Parker MG, Keller L, Evenson J (2005) Torque responses in human quadriceps to burst-modulated alternating current at 3 carrier frequencies. J Orthop Sports Phys Ther, 35: 239–245

Paternostro-Sluga T, Fialka C, Alacamiiogliu Y, Saradeth T, Fialka-Moser V (1999) Neuromuscular electrical stimulation after anterior cruciate ligament surgery. Clin Orthop Relat Res, 368: 166–175

Petterson S, Snyder-Mackler L (2006) The use of neuromuscular electrical stimulation to improve activation deficits in a patient with chronic quadriceps strength impairments following total knee arthroplasty. J Orthop Sports Phys Ther, 36: 678–685

Pfeifer AM, Cranfield T, Wagner S, Craik RL (1997) Muscle strength: A comparison of electrical stimulation and volitional isometric contractions in adults over 65 years. Physiother Can, 49: 32–39

Quittan M, Wiesinger GF, Sturm B, Puig S, Mayr W, Sochor A, Paternostro T, Resch KL, Pacher R, Fialka-Moser V (2001) Improvement of thigh muscles by neuromuscular electrical stimulation in patients with refractory heart failure. Am J Phys Med Rehabil, 80: 206–214

Romero JA, Sanford TL, Schroeder RV (1982) The effects of electrical stimulation on normal quadriceps on strength and girth. Med Sci Sports Exerc, 14: 194–197

Rooney JG, Currier DP, Nitz AJ (1992) Effect of variation in the burst and carrier frequency modes of neuromuscular electrical stimulation on pain perception of healthy subjects. Phys Ther, 72: 800–806

Rutherford O, Jones DA, Newham DJ (1986) Clinical and experimental application of the percutaneous twitch superimposition technique for the study of human muscle activation. J Neurol Neurosurg Psych, 49: 1288–1291

Selkowitz DM (1985) Improvement in isometric strength of the quadriceps femoris muscle after training with electrical stimulation. Phys Ther, 65: 186–196

Sinacore DR, Delitto A, King DS, Rose SJ (1990) Type II fiber activation with electrical stimulation: A preliminary report. Phys Ther, 70: 416–422

Sisk TD, Stralka SW, Deering MB, Griffin JW (1987) Effect of electrical stimulation on quadriceps strength after reconstructive surgery of the anterior cruciate ligament. Am J Sports Med, 15: 215–220

Snyder-Mackler L, Delitto A, Baily SL, Stralka SW (1995) Strength of the quadriceps femoris muscle and functional recovery after reconstruction of the anterior cruciate ligament. A prospective, randomized clinical trial of electrical stimulation. J Bone Joint Surg (A), 77: 1166–1173

Snyder-Mackler L, Delitto A, Stralka SW, Bailey SL (1994) Use of electrical stimulation to enhance recovery of quadriceps femoris muscle production in patients following anterior cruciate ligament reconstruction. Phy Ther, 74: 901–907

Snyder-Mackler L, Garrett M, Roberts M (1989) A comparison of torque generating capabilities of three different electrical stimulating currents. J Orthop Sports Phys Ther, 10: 297–301

Snyder-Mackler L, Ladin Z, Schepsis AA, Young JC (1991) Electrical stimulation of the thigh muscles after reconstruction of the anterior cruciate ligament. Effects of electrically elicited contraction of the quadriceps femoris and hamstring muscles on gait and on strength of the thigh muscles. J Bone Joint Surg (A), 73: 49–54

Soo CL, Currier DP, Threlkeld AJ (1988) Augmenting voluntary torque of healthy muscle by optimization of electrical stimulation. Phys Ther, 68: 333–337

Stevens JE, Mizner RL, Snyder-Mackler L (2004) Neuromuscular electrical stimulation for quadriceps muscle strengthening after bilateral total knee arthroplasty: A case series. J Orthop Sports Phys Ther, 34: 21–29

St-Pierre D, Taylor AW, Lavoie M, Sellers W, Kots YM (1986) Effects of 2500 Hz sinusoidal current on fiber area and strength of the quadriceps femoris. J Sports Med Phys Fitness, 26: 60–66

Targan RS, Alon G, Kay SL (2000) Effect of long-term electrical stimulation on motor recovery and improvement of clinical residuals in patients with unresolved facial nerve palsy. Otolaryngol Head Neck Surg, 122: 246–252

Trimble MH, Enoka RM (1991) Mechanisms underlying the training effects associated with neuromuscular electrical stimulation. Phys Ther, 71: 273–280

Underwood FB, Kremser GL, Finstuen K, Greathouse DG (1990) Increasing involuntary torque production by using TENS. J Orthop Sports Phys Ther, 12: 101–104

Weiss MH (1976) Case report: Successful treatment of Bell's palsy. Dent Surg, 22: 32–33

Wigerstad-Lossing I, Grimby G, Jonsson T, Morelli B, Peterson L, Renstrom P (1988) Effects of electrical muscle stimulation combined with voluntary contraction after knee ligament surgery. Med Sci Sports Exerc, 20: 93–98

Williams RA, Morrissey MC, Brewster CE (1986) The effect of electrical stimulation on quadriceps strength and thigh circumference in meniscectomy patients. J Orthop Sports Phys Ther, 8: 143–146

Review Articles

Bax L, Staes F, Verhagen A (2005) Does neuromuscular electrical stimulation strengthen the quadriceps femoris? A systematic review of randomized controlled trials. Sports Med, 35: 191–212

Belanger AY (1991) Neuromuscular electrostimulation in physiotherapy: A critical appraisal of controversial issues. Physiother Theory Pract, 7: 83–89

Glinsky J, Harvey L, van Es P (2007) Efficacy of electrical stimulation to increase muscle strength in people with neurological conditions: A systematic review. Phys Res Int, 12: 175–194

Kramer JF (1989) Muscle strengthening via electrical stimulation. Crit Rev Phys Med Rehab, 1: 97–133

Kramer JF, Mendryk SW (1982) Electrical stimulation as a strength improvement technique: A review. J Orthop Sports Phys Ther, 4: 91–98

Lake DA (1992) Neuromuscular electrical stimulation. Sports Med, 13: 320–336

Paillard T, Noe F, Passelergue P, Dupui P (2005) Electrical stimulation superimposed onto voluntary muscular contraction. Sports Med, 35: 951–966

Peckham PH, Knutson JS (2005) Functional electrical stimulation for neuromuscular applications. Annu Rev Biomed Eng, 7: 327–360

Quinn R, Cramp F (2003) The efficacy of electrotherapy for Bell's palsy: A systematic review. Phys Ther Rev, 8: 151–164

Selkowitz DM (1989) High frequency electrical stimulation in muscle strengthening: A review and discussion. Am J Sports Med, 17: 103–111

Ward AR, Shkuratova N (2002) Russian electrical stimulation: The early experiments. Phys Ther, 82: 1019–1030

Chapters of Textbooks

Alon G (1999) Principles of electrical stimulation. In: Clinical Electrotherapy, 3rd ed. Nelson RM, Hayes KW, Currier DR (Eds). Appleton & Lange, Stamford, pp 85–87

Baker LL (1999) Electrical stimulation to increase functional activity. In: Clinical Electrotherapy, 3rd ed. Nelson RM, Hayes KW, Currier DR (Eds). Appleton & Lange, Stamford, pp 355–410

Cohn JC, Mullin C (2006) Neuromuscular electrical stimulation. In: Physical Agents: Theory and Practice, 2nd ed. Behrens BJ, Michlovitz SL (Eds), FA Davis Co, Philadelphia, pp 175–189

Farquhar SJ, Snyder-Mackler L (2008) Electrical stimulation of muscle: Techniques and applications. In: Clinical Electrophysiology: Electrotherapy and Electrophysiological Testing, 3rd ed. Robinson AJ, Snyder-Mackler L (Eds). Lippincott Wiliams & Wilkins, Baltimore, MD, pp 197–237

Gerleman DG, Barr JO (1999) Instrumentation and product safety. In: Clinical Electrotherapy, 3rd ed. Nelson RM, Hayes KW, Currier DR (Eds). Appleton & Lange, Stamford, pp 15–53

Greathouse DG, Matulionis DH (1992) Effects of neuromuscular electrical stimulation on skeletal muscle ultrastructure. In: Dynamics of Human Biologic Tissues. Currier DP, Nelson RM (Eds). FA Davis Co., Philadelphia, pp 114–133

Hayes KW (2000) Electrical stimulation. In: Manual for Physical Agents, 5th ed. Prentice Hall Health, Upper Saddle River, pp 103–119

Hooker DN (2002) Electrical stimulation currents. In: Therapeutic Modalities for Physical Therapists, 2nd ed. Prentice WE (Ed). McGraw-Hill, New-York, pp 72–132

Johnson TE (2005) Muscle weakness and loss of motor performance. In: Modalities for Therapeutic Intervention, 4th ed. Michlovitz SL, Nolan TP (Eds). FA Davis Co, Philadelphia, pp 247–270

McDonough S, Kitchen S (2002) Neuromuscular and muscular electrical stimulation. In: Electrotherapy: Evidenced-Based Practice, 11th ed. Kitchen S (Ed), Churchill Livingstone, London, pp 241–257

Prentice WE (1998) Location of the motor points. In: Therapeutic Modalities for Allied Health Professionals. Prentice WE (Ed). McGraw-Hill, St. Louis, pp 506–508

Selkowitz DM (1999) Electrical currents. In: Physical Agents in Rehabilitation: From Research to Practice. Cameron MH (Ed). WB Saunders Co., Philadelphia, pp 345–427

Shapiro S (2003) Electrical currents. In: Physical Agents in Rehabilitation: From Research to Practice, 2nd ed. Cameron MH (Ed). Saunders, Philadelphia, pp 219–259

Speilholz NI (1999) Electrical stimulation of denervated muscle. In: Clinical Electrotherapy, 3rd ed. Nelson RM, Hayes KW, Currier DR (Eds). Appleton & Lange, Stamford, pp 411–446

Stackhouse S (2008) Electrical stimulation of muscle for control of movement and posture. In: Clinical Electrophysiology: Electrotherapy and Electrophysiological Testing, 3rd ed. Robinson AJ, Snyder-Mackler L (Eds). Lippincott Wiliams & Wilkins, Baltimore, MD pp 239–274

Starkey C (2004) Electrical stimulation techniques. In: Therapeutic Modalities, 3rd ed. FA Davis Co, Philadelphia, pp 200–239

Van Swearingen J (1999) Electrical stimulation for improving muscle performance. In: Clinical Electrotherapy, 3rd ed. Nelson RM, Hayes KW, Currier DR (Eds). Appleton & Lange, Stamford, pp 143–182

Special Reports

Kots YM (1971) Training with the method of electric tetanic stimulation of muscle by orthogonal impulses. Theory Pract Phys Cult, 4: 66–72 (Translated from Russian and French)

Kots YM (1977) Electrostimulation. Babkin I, Timentsko N (Translators). Paper presented at the Symposium on Electrostimulation of Skeletal Muscles. Canadian–Soviet Exchange Symposium, Concordia University, December 6–10

Interferential Current Therapy

Learning Objectives

Knowledge: List and describe each of the four methods to deliver interferential current (IFC) therapy.
Comprehension: Compare each method of IFC delivery.
Application: Show how the application of one method of delivery over another can enlarge the area of stimulation.

Analysis: Explain the interference principle.
Synthesis: Describe the rationale behind the claim that IFC decreases soft-tissue impedance.
Evaluation: Discuss the role of IFC therapy in the field of neuromuscular electrical stimulation.

I. RATIONALE FOR USE

A. DEFINITION AND DESCRIPTION

Interferential current, designated under the acronym IFC, is defined and described as a low-frequency, amplitude-modulated electrical current that results from the *interference* (hence the word *interferential*) caused by crossing two or more medium-frequency alternating sine-wave currents with different carrier frequencies (De Domenico, 1981, 1987; Savage, 1984; Nikolova, 1987; Alon, 1999). The carrier frequency of these medium alternating sine-wave currents ranges between 3000 and 5000 cycles per second (cps).

B. INTERFERENTIAL STIMULATORS

Figure 18-1 shows typical portable- **(A)** and cabinet-type **(B)** interferential current stimulators. Portable-type stimulators are powered by batteries, offer two stimulation channels, and usually come in a plastic carrying case containing lead wires, reusable plate electrodes, and electroconductive gel. Cabinet-type stimulators may come with more than two stimulation channels. IFC delivery to the tissues using such cabinet-type devices is usually done using regular *plate* electrodes, as shown in **Figure 18-1B** and, occasionally, using *suction-type* electrodes. In the latter case, the interferential stimulator is linked to or mounted with a vacuum device.

C. VACUUM UNIT

IFC devices may be used in combination with vacuum devices, mounted with pairs of *suction* electrodes. The vacuum pump produces the suction force necessary to keep the IFC stimulating suction electrodes in place. In other words, IFC is delivered via the suction electrodes, which are kept in place by the suction force generated by the vacuum device.

D. RATIONALE FOR USE

Interferential current was discovered in Austria in the 1950s. At that time practitioners were circumscribed in their choice of electrical currents to treat soft-tissue pathologies because their patients felt that all the available currents (e.g., traditional pulsed rectangular, square, and sinusoidal currents) were painful. The rationale behind the development and application of IFC was to provide practitioners with yet another type of electrical current that could penetrate deeper into the layers of soft tissue with minimum discomfort or pain for the patients.

II. HISTORICAL PERSPECTIVE

A. DISCOVERY

The discovery of IFC is attributed to an Austrian inventor named Hans Nemec, who in the 1950s patented a concept that led to the creation of the first IFC therapy device (Nemec, 1959; Kloth, 1991; Hooke, 1998). IFC therapy was first introduced in Europe during the 1960s, and then in Australia, Canada, and the United States in the 1980s.

B. INFLUENTIAL TEXTS

The introduction of this new electrophysical agent (EPA) in North America coincided with the publication of four influential texts on IFC therapy, two by Canadian Giovanni De Domenico (1981, 1987) and the other two by Margaret Savage (1984) from Great Britain and Lilyana Nikolova (1987) from Bulgaria. A recent critical appraisal reviewed the uses and beliefs associated with IFC therapy and attests to the importance that most practitioners have attributed to the several unsubstantiated theoretical concepts and empirical protocols of treatment found in the above texts (Johnson, 1999).

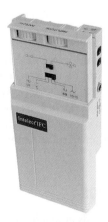

A

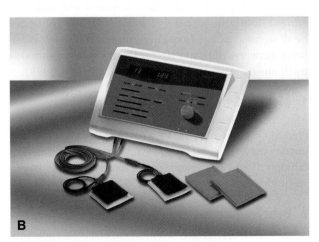

B

FIGURE 18-1 Typical portable **(A)** and cabinet-type **(B)** IFC stimulators (A: Courtesy of Chattanooga Group; B: Courtesy of Metron Medical.)

C. WIDESPREAD USE

Several studies have attested to the fact that IFC therapy is widely and frequently used by physical therapists in England and Ireland (Mantle et al., 1991; Pope et al., 1995; Foster et al., 1999), Australia (Lindsay et al., 1990; Robertson et al., 1998), and in Canada (Lindsay et al., 1995; Nussbaum et al., 2007). No study could be found on the use of this EPA in the United States.

D. BODY OF LITERATURE

IFC therapy has been the topic of a few *review articles* (De Domenico, 1982; Goats, 1990; Gerleman et al., 1999; Noble et al., 2000) and *chapters of textbooks* (Wadsworth et al., 1988; Kloth, 1991; Martin, 1996; Hooke, 1998; Starkey, 1999; Hayes, 2000; Palmer et al., 2002; Stephenson et al., 2008). Brief *coverage* of IFC is also offered in more recent textbooks (Knight et al., 2008; Robinson, 2008).

III. BIOPHYSICAL CHARACTERISTICS

A. INTERFERENCE PRINCIPLE

The biophysical principle underlying the creation of an IFC is the *interference* caused by superimposing two (and sometimes three; see below) medium-frequency sinusoidal currents generated by independent oscillatory circuits incorporated into the interferential devices (De Domenico, 1981, 1987; Goats, 1990; Kloth, 1991; Lambert et al., 1993; Martin, 1996; Hooke, 1998; Alon, 1999; Starkey, 1999). Before considering the following paragraphs, readers are *urged to review* Chapter 5, which presents an illustrated glossary of electrophysical terminology pertinent to the use of IFC.

B. LOW VERSUS MEDIUM FREQUENCY

The terms low frequency and medium frequency refer to a traditional and arbitrary classification stipulating that current output frequencies of less than 1000 Hz or cps be designated as low-frequency currents and those oscillating between 1001 and 10,000 Hz or cps be classified as medium-frequency currents (Kloth, 1991; Alon, 1999).

1. Medium Carrier Frequency

Medium-frequency sinusoidal currents used today to generate IFC, as illustrated in **Figure 18-2**, have a carrier frequency range of 3000–5000 cycles per second (cps). For example, the first (C1) and second (C2) circuit may have a carrier frequency of 3000 and 3050 cps, respectively.

2. Beat Frequency

The carrier frequencies of one or both circuits are programmable so as to deliver low, amplitude-modulated frequency (AMF), or *beat* frequency, IFC in the range of

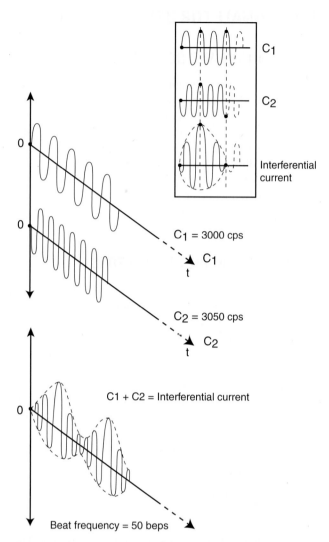

FIGURE 18-2 The bipolar, or premodulated, method results from the interference within the device circuitry of two medium-frequency sinusoidal currents with different frequencies. Illustrated here is the interference of a 3000 cps current with a 3050 cps current, leading to the characteristic oval-shaped field of IFC with a beat frequency of 50 beps. The inset shows the characteristic rhythmic rise and fall in the current amplitude (or amplitude modulation) resulting from mixing together the two medium-frequency currents.

1–200 beats per second (beps). The term *beat* is borrowed from the acoustic literature to designate the characteristic "beat of sound" that can be heard when two acoustic waves of different frequencies interfere with each other (Hooke, 1998). For example, the beat frequency, as shown in **Figure 18-2**, resulting from the interference of two circuits, one set at 3000 cps and the other at 3050 cps, is 50 beps.

C. DELIVERY METHODS

There are four basic methods available to practitioners for delivery of IFC to soft tissues: premodulated or bipolar, quadripolar or true interferential, quadripolar with automatic vector scan, and stereodynamic methods. Each method has its unique biophysical characteristics.

1. Premodulated or Bipolar Method

This first method is illustrated in **Figure 18-2**. The term *bipolar* means that this method is delivered using two (bi) electrodes applied over the target tissue. The term *premodulated* means that the electronic interference between the two medium-frequency sine-wave currents occurs at the level of the electronic circuitry within the device, not at the soft tissue level, as is the case with the other methods (see below). Therefore, the resulting IFC is modulated before (thus the word premodulated) being delivered to the electrodes.

a. Premodulated Current Interference

Figure 18-2 shows the electronic interference caused by superimposing, within the device's circuitry, one medium-frequency sinusoidal current set at 3000 cps (circuit 1; C1) on another medium-frequency sinusoidal current set at 3050 cps (circuit 2; C2). The constructive and destructive interferences occurring between these two medium-frequency sine-wave currents lead to the formation of a low-frequency amplitude-modulated IFC (Kloth, 1991; Alon, 1999). The beat frequency associated with IFC is defined as the net difference between the carrier frequencies of each of these two medium-frequency sinusoidal currents (C2 − C1; 3050 cps − 3000 cps = 50 beps).

b. Oval-Shaped Field

Each beat of IFC is composed of polyphasic sinusoidal pulses of varying amplitudes. The theoretical current field associated with each premodulated beat is pictured to have an *oval shape* (**Fig 18-2**).

2. Quadripolar or True Interferential Method

This second method, illustrated in **Figure 18-3**, refers to the use of four (quadri-) electrodes, each pair of electrodes connected to its respective circuit or channel of stimulation. The quadripolar method is commonly known as the *true method* to deliver IFC therapy because current interference occurs within the targeted soft tissues as opposed to the level of the electronic circuitry within the device console, as was the case with the premodulated method described.

a. True Current Interference

As with the premodulated method, two unmodulated medium-frequency sinusoidal currents are generated through the first (C1) and second (C2) circuits of the IFC stimulator, as shown in **Figure 18-3**. Contrary to the premodulated method, current interference occurs *externally* to the device, at the level of the treated area. Current interference at the tissue level is said to be *true* interference. The resulting beat frequency is also 50 beps because the net difference between the two medium frequencies is 50 cps.

b. Four Leaf Clover–Shaped Field

When the two medium-frequency sine-wave currents intersect at 90° to each other, the maximum resultant amplitude of the IFC field is halfway between these two lines of current (in this case, at 45° from each circuit). The theoretical current field associated with this configuration is pictured having a *four leaf clover shape* (**Fig 18-3**).

3. Quadripolar With Automatic Vector Scan Method

As with the quadripolar method, this third method is also generated using two unmodulated medium-frequency sine-wave currents delivered using four (quadri-) electrodes. This method differs from the basic quadripolar method, as illustrated in **Figure 18-4**, by allowing the current amplitude in one circuit to slowly vary between 50% and 100% of the maximum set value, with the current amplitude of the second circuit set automatically at a fixed value (e.g., 75% of its maximum amplitude).

a. Vector Current Scan

This automatic and periodic current amplitude variation in one circuit relative to the other creates an electronic phenomenon described as *vector scan*. With this method, the vector or field pattern (fourleaf clover shape) observed using the quadripolar method automatically rotates back and forth between the two lines of current, as illustrated in **Figure 18-4**, thus scanning the treatment surface within this area.

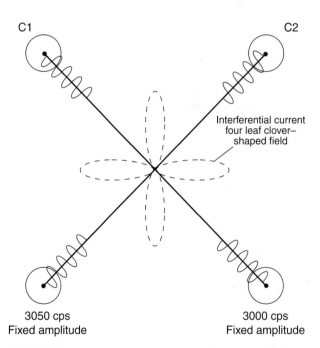

C1   C2

Interferential current four leaf clover–shaped field

3050 cps
Fixed amplitude   3000 cps
Fixed amplitude

FIGURE 18-3 The quadripolar, or true, method results from the interference, at the level of the targeted tissue, of two medium-frequency sinusoidal currents with different frequencies. Illustrated here is the interference of a 3000 cps current with a 3050 cps current, leading to the characteristic four leaf clover–shaped field of IFC.

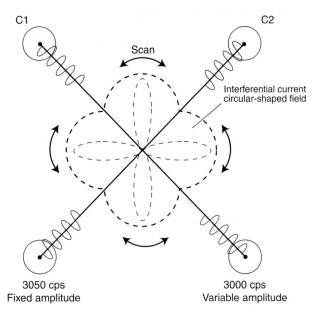

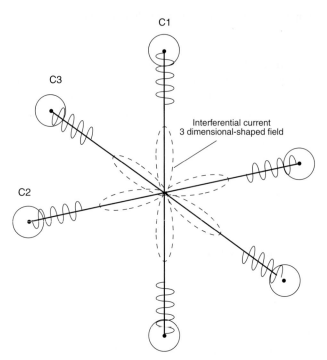

FIGURE 18-4 The quadripolar with automatic vector scan method is identical to the quadripolar method described in the legend of Figure 18-3, except that the four leaf clover–shaped field is now automatically rotating or scanning back and forth. This vector scanning leads to the enlarged field of IFC with the characteristic circular shape.

FIGURE 18-5 The stereodynamic method refers to the interference, at the level of the targeted tissue, of three medium-frequency sinusoidal currents, leading to the characteristic 3-D, six-petal flower–shaped field of IFC. This method requires the use of six electrodes, which are presented as a pair of star- or Y-shaped electrodes. Each star or Y electrode has three poles or three electrodes, and each pair is connected to their respective channels.

b. Enlarged Stimulated Area

This scanning action results in an enlarged treatment area due to the enlarged field of IFC, as shown in **Figure 18-4**. The purpose of using this method over the quadripolar method is, therefore, to *enlarge* the stimulating treatment area. Because the carrier frequency of each circuit remains the same as with the two previous methods (3000 and 3050 cps), the beat frequency remains the same at 50 beps.

c. Circular-Shaped Field

The characteristic four leaf clover–shaped field seen in the quadripolar method is replaced, in the quadripolar with automatic vector scan method, by a larger, more *circular-shaped field* (**Fig 18-4**).

4. Stereodynamic Method

This fourth and last delivery method is much less common than the three already described and requires the use of a special type interferential current stimulator. The stereodynamic method, as shown in **Figure 18-5**, is created by adding a third circuit (C3), or a third medium-frequency sinusoidal current, to the device output generator. It is called stereodynamic because of the *three-dimensional (3-D)* effect achieved within the targeted tissues as these three sinusoidal currents interfere with each other within the tissue.

a. Electrodes

Because this method requires simultaneous use of three medium-frequency sinusoidal circuits, six electrodes

(or three pairs) are required for application. Two pairs of Y-shaped electrodes, each made of three poles, are commonly used to apply this delivery method.

b. Enlarged 3-D Stimulated Area

The stereodynamic method allows the effective IFC field, or stimulated area, to be *enlarged three-dimensionally*, contrary to the quadripolar method with automatic vector scan, which allows enlargement of the treatment field only two-dimensionally.

c. Six-Petal Flower–Shaped Field

The theoretical interference field pattern caused by mixing three medium-frequency circuits is pictured to have a *six-petal flower* shape (**Fig 18-5**).

5. Key Characteristics

The four IFC delivery methods, with their respective numbers of output circuits and electrode requirements, are represented in **Figure 18-6**. This figure reveals the following key characteristics: (1) only the quadripolar with vector scan method offers a dynamic (i.e., rotating or scanning) interferential field; the other three methods offer a static field only; (2) the stereodynamic method is the only method that offers a 3-D interferential field; (3) the premodulated, quadripolar, quadripolar with vector scan, and stereodynamic methods require two, four, four, and six electrodes, respectively.

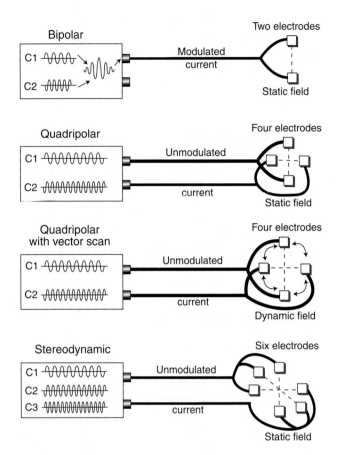

FIGURE 18-6 Summary of delivery methods for interferential current therapy.

D. POSSIBLE CONFUSION

Readers should not confuse the terms bipolar and quadripolar delivery methods of IFC with the terms bipolar and quadripolar electrode placement techniques, commonly used for neuromuscular electrical stimulation (see Chapter 17).

IV. PHYSIOLOGICAL AND THERAPEUTIC EFFECTS

A. NEMEC'S CLAIMS

Before addressing the proposed physiological and therapeutic effects associated with IFC therapy, it is crucial to consider Nemec's claims related to his newly discovered current (Nemec, 1959).

1. Interference and Beating Effect

Nemec's first claim was that crossing and superimposing two medium-frequency alternating sine-wave currents of different frequencies will cause the two currents to interfere with each other, producing a low-frequency, amplitude-modulated, beating effect on soft tissues.

2. Decreased Skin Impedance

Nemec's second claim was that using sine-wave currents with medium carrier frequencies (i.e., between 3000 and 5000 cps) will decrease skin impedance, leading to deeper tissue stimulation with less current amplitude.

a. Skin Impedance

Denoted by the symbol Z, skin impedance is measured in ohms and refers to three sources of resistance to alternating current flow offered by the outer layer (stratum corneum) of the skin. Because the skin, biophysically speaking, is composed of different electrical elements, such as resistors, inductors, and capacitors, these sources of resistance are labeled as follows: resistance (R), capacitive reactance (X_C), and inductive reactance (X_L). For more details on the concept of skin impedance, readers can consult Gerleman et al. (1999) and Alon (1999), as well as Chapter 5, Section E, Impedance.

i. Reactance. This term refers to the resistance offered by the skin's inductive (X_L) and capacitive (X_C) elements to the passage of an alternating current.

ii. Resistance. The term refers to the resistance offered by the skin's resistive (R) element to the passage of continuous and alternating current.

b. Basis for Claims

Nemec's claim that his IFC decreases skin impedance is based on the capacitive reactance (X_C) component of skin being inversely related to alternating current carrier frequency (f), as represented by the formula $X_C = 1/f$. This formula dictates that the higher the alternating current carrier frequency, the lower the skin X_C, and thus the greater the current capacity to penetrate deeper into the tissues (Alon, 1999).

B. NEMEC'S CLAIMS TESTED

Presented here is the body of evidence available that either supports or refutes Nemec's claims.

1. Interference and Beating Effect: Supported

There is clear biophysical evidence to support (see **Fig 18-2**) the claim that superimposing two medium-frequency alternating sine-wave currents, each with different frequencies, will cause output interference, resulting in a newly formed IFC, with a beating sound (Alon, 1999; Palmer et al., 2002).

2. Decrease in Skin Impedance: Supported

There is also clear biophysical evidence, based on the formula $X_C = 1/f$, to support the claim that the higher the alternating sine-wave carrier frequency, the lower the skin's capacitive reactance (X_C) to the passage of such an alternating current.

C. CORPORATE CLAIMS

As part of a global marketing strategy of IFC therapy, several manufacturers claimed that interferential stimulators were *unique* in offering less skin impedance to current flow, meaning that only IFC-type stimulators could penetrate deeper into soft tissues when compared with other types of nerve-depolarizing electrical stimulators on the market.

1. Misleading and Inaccurate Claim

To claim that only an IFC can lower the skin's capacitive reactance is *inaccurate and misleading*. The higher the alternating current frequency (f), the shorter the period (P), as expressed in the formula f = 1/P. For example, if the carrier frequency is 4000 cps, the resulting period duration will be 250 μs. In this example, the period duration is equal to the cycle or pulse duration because the sine-wave current is continuously delivered. It follows that any alternating current, or pulsed biphasic current, with pulse durations in the range of 250 μs, is theoretically capable of decreasing skin impedance. Biophysics teaches us that any medium-frequency alternating or biphasic current, whether resulting from interference or not, will have a short period and consequently a short pulse duration. To sum up, all such current stimulators, not only IFC stimulators, have the capacity to decrease skin impedance by decreasing its capacitive reactance, regardless of interference.

D. PROPOSED EFFECTS

Shown in **Figure 18-7** are the proposed physiological and therapeutic effects associated with IFC therapy. This EPA is used primarily in the management of urinary incontinence (pelvic floor muscle weakness), muscle weakness affecting other skeletal muscles, and pain. The effect of this EPA on pain is presumed to be modulated by the spinal gate and descending endogenous opiate system (see Chapter 14).

1. Nerve Depolarization

The practice of IFC therapy falls within the field of transcutaneous nerve electrical stimulation, as is the case with other EPAs such as TENS (Chapter 14), HVPC (Chapter 16), Russian current (Chapter 17), and diadynamic current (Chapter 19) therapies. It follows that electrically evoked nerve depolarization is the key physiological effect behind the use of IFC therapy. Readers are *urged to review* Chapter 14 for details related to the process of *electrically, evoked nerve depolarization.*

2. Increased Blood Circulation

It has been theorized that the therapeutic effects of IFC therapy may also be attributed to increased blood circulation in the affected and treated area (De Domenico, 1982, 1987; Savage, 1984; Nikolova, 1987). The present body of evidence, based on experiments conducted on humans, *fails* to support such a proposal (Bersglien et al., 1988; Nussbaum et al., 1990; Indergand et al., 1995; Olson et al., 1999). Noble et al. (2000) used suction electrodes on healthy subjects and showed a significant increase in blood flow in the stimulated quadriceps muscle. This finding raises the question regarding the specific effect that a particular electrode type (i.e., pad vs. suction electrodes) may have on blood circulation after IFC therapy.

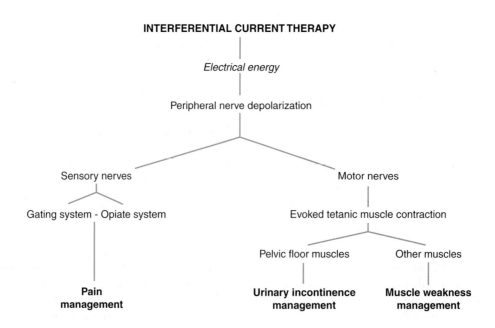

FIGURE 18-7 Proposed physiological and therapeutic effects of interferential current therapy.

3. Low-Frequency-Dependant Effect

IFC is characterized by delivering beats of current at low frequency (1–200 beps) based on the interference between medium-frequency alternating currents. Delivery of such low frequencies, which mimics the traditional low-frequency stimulation achieved with other low-frequency electrical stimulators, was originally claimed by many authors and manufacturers to be the stimulating parameter responsible for the physiological and therapeutic effects (De Domenico, 1981, 1987; Savage, 1984; Nikolova, 1987).

E. PREMODULATED VERSUS TRUE IFC

There has been an ongoing debate in the literature about whether the premodulated (or bipolar) or the true (quadripolar) method of delivery is best in terms of depth efficiency, muscle torque production, and patient comfort during stimulation. The present claim is that true IFC *may be superior* because the current interference takes place within the targeted tissues.

1. Claim Tested

The recent study by Ozcan et al. (2004) on 12 healthy human subjects provides the first element of evidence related to this important question. The authors compared two fundamental differences between true and premodulated IFCs: (1) the current type applied to the electrodes (constant versus modulated amplitude) and (2) the current path within the tissue (crossed versus parallel).

2. Premodulated Delivery May Be Better

Results reported by Ozcan et al. (2004) showed that (1) crossed currents did not have greater depth efficiency than parallel currents and that (2) premodulated applied currents produced higher muscle torque values with less discomfort than true or constant-amplitude currents. These findings suggest that premodulated IFC, delivered via two large electrodes, may be more clinically effective in terms of depth efficiency, muscle torque production, and patient's comfort than true IFC delivered using four smaller electrodes.

V. DOSIMETRY

A. PARAMETERS

The dosimetry associated with IFC therapy requires setting specific parameters to achieve the desired level of evoked sensory and motor stimulation to achieve its two main therapeutic effects: pain modulation and muscle strengthening (see **Fig 18-7**).

B. FOR PAIN MODULATION

Key parameters are current amplitude, beat frequency, method of delivery, and electrode placement.

1. Current Amplitude

Setting the current amplitude will determine the desired level of sensory or motor nerve stimulation required for pain management. This is done by adjusting the stimulator's current amplitude, calibrated as peak (A_{pk}, for square or rectangular waveform) or as root-mean-square (A_{rms}, for sinusoidal waveform) amperage. A_{rms} is equivalent to 70.7% of the peak value (Gerleman et al., 1999). For example, setting the current amplitude at 80 A_{pk} is equivalent to setting it at 56 A_{rms}.

2. Beat Frequency

The body of literature on TENS therapy (Chapter 14) has shown that pain modulation can be achieved using low (1–10) as well as high (greater than 80) beat frequencies. Practitioners may select within a range of 1–200 beps.

3. Delivery Method

Selecting one delivery method over another is an arbitrary decision since no method has been found to be better than the others. The most common methods used are the premodulated and quadripolar methods.

4. Electrode Placement

Based on the body of literature on TENS (Chapter 14), the electrodes should be positioned in one of the following arrangements: over the painful area, along the dermatome(s) within the painful area, or over acupuncture points.

C. FOR MUSCLE STRENGTHENING

Key parameters for NMES using IFC are current amplitude, beat frequency, method of delivery, ON and OFF times and duty cycle, and ramp-up and ramp-down times. Note that *recent* IFC stimulators, such as the one shown in **Figure 18-1B**, incorporate ON and OFF time, as well as ramp-up and ramp-down time controls, making them more suitable than earlier models for NMES applications.

1. Current Amplitude

Based on the evidence on Russian current therapy (Chapter 17), which is used primarily for muscle strengthening, this parameter is set such as to obtain electrically evoked muscle force training levels between 40% and 70% of maximal voluntary contraction (MVC).

2. Beat Frequency

In keeping with the application of Russian current (Chapter 17), this parameter is set between 40 and 60 beps so as to evoke a fused tetanic muscle contraction.

3. Delivery Method

Selecting one method over another is a matter of preference. Practitioners should keep in mind, however, the results of Ozcan et al. (2004), which suggest that premodulated IFC, delivered via two large electrodes, may be more clinically effective for muscle strengthening purpose than true IFC delivered using four smaller electrodes.

4. ON:OFF Time Ratio and Duty Cycle

In keeping with the application of Russian current therapy (Chapter 17), ON and OFF times such as 10 second ON and 50 seconds OFF may be used (10s:50s ratio), which is equivalent to a duty cycle of 16.7%. This ratio may be adjusted during the course of therapy.

5. Ramp-Up and Ramp-Down Times

Again in keeping with Russian current therapy, the ramp-up and ramp-down times may be set between 1 and 2 seconds, so as to mimic the physiological time course of a voluntary muscle contraction.

6. Electrode Placement

Practitioners may select between the monopolar, bipolar, quadripolar, and multipolar electrode placement techniques (see Chapter 17). Recall that to obtain an electrically evoked muscle contraction with the minimum current amplitude, the stimulating electrodes should be placed preferably over the muscle's motor point(s).

VI. EVIDENCE FOR INDICATIONS

A. GUIDED BY EVIDENCE

Dictionaries generally define *evidence* as anything that establishes a fact or gives reason to believe something. The aim of this textbook is to present scientific evidence on therapeutic EPAs. To be guided by evidence is the process of integrating the evidence from research, however imperfect or scarce this evidence may be, with clinical experience and patients' preferences. In other words, the *evidence-based practice* of EPA requires that practitioners consider the evidence from research, in addition to their own clinical experience and patient's own preference and beliefs about a given EPA, when the time comes to justify, prescribe, and apply the therapeutic agent. To be guided by evidence is a process, not a search for the absolute truth. Finally, a lack of evidence from research in support of any given EPA does not mean that this EPA should never be used. What it means is that no statement can be made about its therapeutic effectiveness and that until more evidence from research is presented, its routine use cannot be recommended.

B. EVIDENCE FROM HUMAN RESEARCH

Box 18-1 provides evidence for IFC therapy based on an exhaustive search of published English-language, peer-reviewed studies on humans. The term *indication* is used in reference to a list of pathologies for which IFC therapy is employed. Ratings of therapeutic benefit (Yes or No) and grading of strength of scientific evidence (I, II, or III),

including the reference, are included for each pathological condition. The stronger the evidence for a given pathology, the better the justification for using that agent.

1. Rating Therapeutic Benefit

The rating, expressed as Yes or No, is based on the overall conclusion(s) reached on the issue of therapeutic effectiveness by the author(s) who conducted the peer-reviewed study.

2. Grading Strength of Evidence

The grading, numerically classified as I, II, and III, is based on the type of research methodology or experimental design used by the author(s). All those listed are studies on humans published in English-language, peer-reviewed journals. It follows that the evidence in studies graded I is stronger than in those graded II, and the evidence in studies graded II is stronger than in those graded III.

a. Grade I

Evidence based on *controlled* studies on humans, regardless of their level of randomization and blindness.

b. Grade II

Evidence based on *non-controlled* studies on humans, regardless of their level of randomization and blindness.

c. Grade III

Evidence based on *case* studies on humans, regardless of their level of randomization and blindness.

3. Strength of Evidence Behind the Agent

The strength of evidence in support of the agent, as presented in the research-based indication box, is arbitrarily assessed in this textbook as *weak*, *moderate*, or *strong*. For example, the larger the number of studies graded I, regardless of therapeutic benefit, the stronger the scientific evidence in support the agent.

4. Evidence Justifying Usage of Agent

The strength of evidence justifying the usage of an agent for an individual pathology or groups of pathologies, as listed in the research-based indication box, is arbitrarily assessed in this textbook as *poor*, *fair*, *good*, or *conflicting*. For example, where the number of grade I studies showing therapeutic benefit (Yes), for any given pathology, is larger than that of similar studies showing no benefit, the justification for usage of this agent for that pathology is assessed as *good*. A *conflicting* usage is reported when about an equal number of studies with similar grades show therapeutic benefit (Yes) and no benefit (No).

C. STRENGTH OF EVIDENCE AND JUSTIFICATION FOR USAGE

The results presented in **Box 18-1** show *moderate* strength of evidence for the use of IFC therapy for the management of urinary incontinence (pelvic muscle weakness), and for

Box 18-1   Research-Based Indications for the Use of Interferential Current Therapy

PATHOLOGY	BENEFIT	GRADE	REFERENCE
Pelvic muscle weakness—urinary incontinence	Yes	I	Laycock et al., 1993
	Yes	I	Vahtera et al., 1997
	Yes	II	Dougall, 1985
	Yes	II	McQuire, 1975
	Yes	II	Laycock et al., 1988
	Yes	II	Dumoulin et al., 1995a
	Yes	II	Dumoulin et al., 1995b
	Yes	II	Olah et al., 1990
	Yes	II	Wilson et al., 1987
	Yes	II	Turkan et al., 2005
	Yes	III	Henella et al., 1987
	No	III	Sylvester et al., 1987
Osteoarthritis pain	Yes	I	Adedoyin et al., 2002
	Yes	I	Hurley et al., 2001
	Yes	II	Shafshak et al., 1991
	Yes	II	Ni Chiosig et al., 1994
	No	II	Quirk et al., 1985
Bone-fracture healing	Yes	II	Ganne, 1988
	Yes	II	Ganne et al., 1979
	No	I	Fourie et al., 1997
	No	I	Christie et al., 1990
Low-back pain	Yes	I	Zambito et al., 2007
	Yes	I	Zambito et al., 2006
	Yes	II	Hurley et al., 2001
	No	II	Werners et al., 1999
Palmar psoriasis	Yes	II	Philipp et al., 2000
Psoriasic arthritis	Yes	III	Walker et al., 2006
Jaw pain	No	I	Taylor et al., 1987
Shoulder pain	No	I	Van der Heijden et al., 1999
Peripheral vascular disease	Yes	III	Belcher, 1974
Migraine	Yes	III	Truscott, 1984
Detrusor muscle hyperreflexia	Yes	II	Van Poppel et al., 1985
Postsurgical knee pain	Yes	I	Jarit et al., 2003
Quadriceps femoris weakness	Yes	I	Bircan et al., 2002
Dysmenorrheal pain	Yes	II	Tugay et al., 2007

osteoarthritis pain and low-back pain, with a large majority of studies graded II showing benefit. These results also show that the *justification for usage* of IFC therapy is *good* for urinary incontinence and *fair* for osteoarthritis and low-back pain. Until more evidence from research is provided with regard to the remaining pathologies listed, or any other pathology, the *routine use* of IFC therapy for such pathologies *cannot be recommended*.

D. EXPERIMENTAL PAIN ON HEALTHY SUBJECTS

The evidence as to the effectiveness of IFC for the management of experimentally induced pain in healthy subjects is *conflicting*. Beneficial results have been reported by some authors (Stephenson et al., 1995; Johnson et al., 1997, 2003b; Cheing et al., 2003; McManus et al., 2006; Shanahan et al., 2006), while others have reported no benefit (Johnson et al., 1999; Minder et al., 2002; Stephenson et al., 2003; Johnson et al., 2003a,c).

VII. CONTRAINDICATIONS

Table 18-1 describes the contraindications associated with the practice of IFC therapy. These contraindications are similar to those listed for TENS (Chapter 14) and Russian current (Chapter 17) therapy.

VIII. RISKS, PRECAUTIONS, AND RECOMMENDATIONS

The practice of IFC therapy is not without risk for the patient. The major risks associated with this EPA, as well as some precautions and recommendations designed to improve safety and effectiveness, are listed in **Table 18-2**. These are identical to those listed for TENS (Chapter 14) and Russian current (Chapter 17) therapy.

IX. CONSIDERATIONS FOR APPLICATION AND DOCUMENTATION

A. CONSIDERATIONS AND PROCEDURES

Safe, effective, and optimal application of IFC requires that clinicians run through a systematic set of considerations and procedures for every single application. The following is a list of such considerations and procedures.

TABLE 18-1	CONTRAINDICATIONS TO INTERFERENTIAL CURRENT THERAPY
CONTRAINDICATIONS	**RATIONALE**
Over the anterior cervical area	Risk of stimulating key organs, such as the vagus nerve, phrenic nerve, and carotid sinuses, resulting in adverse effects such as hypotensive reaction and laryngeal spasm.
Over the thoracic region	Risk of affecting normal heart function. Stimulation over intercostal muscles led to a respiratory failure in one cardiac patient.
Over the cranial area	Risk of affecting normal brain function.
With patients wearing rate-responsive pacemakers or implanted cardioverter defibrillators (ICDs)	Risk of electronic interference with units (for more details see Chapters 14 and 17). *Important note*: NMES may be use with these patients *only* if the ICU unit is *turned off* during therapy.
Over the abdominal, pelvic, or lumbar areas of pregnant women in their first trimester	Risk of inducing labor.
Over metal implants	Risk of causing unnecessary pain due to electrical current-induced overheating of implants.
With epileptic patients	Risk of causing an epileptic episode.
Over hemorrhagic area	Risk of enhanced bleeding due to increased blood flow in the treated area.
Over malignant area	Risk of increasing and spreading the tumor due to increased blood flow in the treated area.
Over damaged skin	Risk of causing unnecessary and severe pain.

TABLE 18-2	RISKS, PRECAUTIONS, AND RECOMMENDATIONS FOR INTERFERENTIAL CURRENT THERAPY

RISKS	RATIONALE
Prolonged use of electrode, electroconductive gel, and adhesive tape over the same skin areas	Risk of causing contact dermatitis related to the materials that the electrode, gel, or adhesive tape are made of (see Chapter 14).
Usage near functioning shortwave diathermy (SWD) device	Risk of causing electronic interference. A patient reporting a sudden and variable surge of current output when an SWD unit is functioning in the neighborhood may be indicative of such electronic interference.
Use of vacuum electrode over fragile skin	Risk of causing temporary hematoma, or ecchymosis, due to the suction force (negative pressure) exerted on fragile skin (Kloth, 1991).
Variety of unexpected adverse effects, such as fainting, nausea, skin rashes, increased swelling, and pain	Risk of inducing such adverse effects found to be greater with IFC than with other common electrophysical agents, such as TENS and ultrasound (Partridge et al., 1999; Kitchen, 2000). Stimulation of the autonomic system may account for some of these adverse effects.

PRECAUTIONS	RATIONALE
With confused and unreliable patients	May result in unreliable information, which may have a negative impact on treatment effectiveness.
Home IFC therapy	Instruct patients to keep the portable IFC unit out of the reach of children at all times.

RECOMMENDATIONS	RATIONALE
Clean and dry exposed skin surface areas before each treatment	Wiping the skin surface with alcohol will reduce its impedance significantly, in addition to removing impurities, thus allowing an optimal electrical coupling at the skin–electrode interface.
Clip hair over exposed skin areas	To ensure optimal electrode–skin coupling (Kloth, 1991).
Wash and dry reusable electrodes after each treatment	To ensure optimal performance; follow the manufacturers' instructions.
Check cables and electrodes regularly for visible wear and tear	To ensure optimal efficacy. Prevent macroshock if line-powered stimulators are used.
Check electrode impedance monthly	To ensure appropriate electrode impedance for optimal conduction, because electrodes will deteriorate with use and time. Use an ohmmeter to check impedance.
Keep all IFC units at least 3 m (10 ft) away from any functioning SWD device	Minimize the risk of electronic interference.
Discard all electrodes after 6 months of usage	Material deterioration will increase electrode impedance, thus reducing efficacy.
Disinfect suction electrodes and sponges	Because transmission of microorganisms is likely if suction electrodes and sponges are used, these should be disinfected with 70% isopropyl alcohol after treatment of each patient to avoid cross-infection from one patient to another (Lambert et al., 2000).
Monitor patients for adverse effects during therapy	Prevent the occurrence of major adverse effects.
Plug line-powered stimulater into GFCI receptacle	Prevent the risk of electrocution (see Chapter 27 for details).
Conduct regular maintenance and calibration	To ensure optimal treatment efficacy. Follow the manufacturer's recommendations and schedule.

1. Checklists

Before proceeding with treatment, always go through the list of contraindications (**Table 18-1**) and the list of risks, precautions, and recommendations (**Table 18-2**).

2. Skin Preparation

Before each application, cleanse the skin on the stimulation area with rubbing alcohol to remove impurities and reduce skin impedance.

3. Electrode Type

Clinicians can choose from *plate-type* (i.e., carbon-silicone, mesh) and *suction-type* electrodes. To use suction electrodes, IFC devices must be used concomitantly with a vacuum device. Suction electrodes are indicated over anatomical areas where plate electrode placement is difficult or impossible, such as in the pelvic area.

4. Electrode Preparation

For plate electrodes, make sure that a thin and evenly distributed coating of electroconductive gel is applied to each electrode to optimize conduction at the electrode–skin interface. For suction electrodes, adjust the vacuum pressure level to ensure adequate fixation on the body.

5. Electrode Spacing and Penetration Depth

The distance between a pair of electrodes influences current dispersion within the tissues, which in turn affects the current's penetration depth. The wider the interelectrode distance is, the deeper the current penetration into the tissue. In contrast, the closer the two electrodes, the more superficial the stimulating effect.

6. Set Dosimetry

IFC therapy is used for muscle strengthening and pain. Select the appropriate dosimetric parameters according to the therapeutic goal (see Section V, Dosimetry).

7. Electrode Orientation

Electrode orientation, whether it is parallel, crossed, or mixed, depends on the delivery method used.

a. Parallel

With the premodulated method, the lines of current run parallel between the two electrodes.

b. Crossed

With quadripolar and quadripolar plus vector scan methods, each pair of electrodes is positioned so that the current lines of the first circuit cross those of the second circuit, allowing for interference to occur at the tissue level.

c. Mixed

With the stereodynamic method, which requires six electrodes, the electrode orientation is said to be mixed, as some electrodes run parallel and other electrodes cross each other.

8. Electrode Attachment

Plate electrodes are mechanically attached to the skin with hypoallergic tape or self-adhesive patches. Suction electrodes are kept in place by the vacuum pressure exerted by the vacuum pump. Because suction electrodes are kept in place without using tapes or straps, they are the preferred choice for stimulation in specific body areas such as the pelvic area (i.e., pelvic muscle weakness in urinary incontinence).

9. End of Treatment

Inspect the skin under each plate or suction electrode. Document any unusual sensation the patient felt during treatment in the patient's file.

B. DOCUMENTATION

Table 18-3 shows the key parameters to be documented in the patient's file with regard to the application of IFC therapy.

TABLE 18-3	**KEY TREATMENT PARAMETERS TO BE DOCUMENTED IN PATIENT'S FILE AFTER INTERFERENTIAL CURRENT THERAPY**

- *IFC stimulator type:* portable or cabinet; with or without vacuum unit
- *Carrier frequency for each circuit:* cps
- *Beat frequency:* beps
- *Current amplitude:* mA or A_{RMS}
- *Delivery method:* premodulated; quadripolar, quadripolar with vector scan; stereodynamic
- *Electrode type:* plate; suction
- *Electrode size:* description
- *Electrode orientation:* parallel or crossed
- *ON: OFF time ratio and duty cycle:* time in seconds; duty cycle in %
- *Ramp-up and ramp-down times:* seconds
- *Treatment duration:* minutes

Case Study 18-1   Genuine Stress Incontinence

A 42-year-old healthy female, the mother of three young children, is referred by her gynecologist for the management of her genuine stress incontinence problem. This condition began 2 years ago after the birth of her third child. Her main complaint, over the past 6 months, is frequent urine loss, particularly with sneezing, coughing, or laughing and also during more strenuous physical home and recreational activities. Physical examination reveals severe pelvic floor muscle (PFM) weakness (grade force of 1/5 on palpation), leading to incomplete urethral closure. The recruitment is slow and the ability to hold is poor. The patient's goal is to regain control of her micturition without the use of medication and intravaginal cone or electrode.

Evidence-Based Steps Toward the Resolution of This Case

1. **List medical diagnosis.**

    Genuine stress incontinence

2. **List key impairment(s).**

    ■ Urethral sphincter weakness
    ■ Pelvic floor muscle weakness

3. **List key functional limitation(s).**

    ■ Urine loss while performing activities of daily living.

4. **List key disability/disabilities**

    ■ Difficulty performing recreational activities without urine loss.

5. **Justification for IFC therapy.**

    Is there justification to use IFC current therapy in this case? This chapter has established that there is *moderate-to-strong* strength of evidence and *good* justification for the use of this EPA for enhancing PFM strength in cases of urinary incontinence (see Section VI). This textbook recommends the use of this EPA for the following reasons. First, there is moderate-to-strong evidence (Dougall, 1985; Laycock et al., 1988; Olah et al., 1990; Laycock et al., 1993; Dumoulin et al., 1995a,b; Turkan et al., 2005; Stephenson et al., 2008) to suggest that IFC current therapy can strengthen human pelvic floor muscle by enhancing motor unit action. Second, there is evidence that electrically evoked PFM contraction, using suction electrodes, is possible if one uses an IFC stimulator mounted with a vacuum unit. Third, the patient's preference is to avoid using intravaginal electrode for muscle stimulation. Because EPAs should not be used in isolation as a sole intervention, IFC therapy is used here *concomitantly* with a regimen of home pelvic floor muscle (PFM) strengthening exercises.

6. **Search for contraindications.**

    None is found.

7. **Search for risks and precautions.**

    None is found.

8. **Outline the therapeutic goal(s) you and your patient wish to achieve.**

    ■ Increase PFM strength
    ■ Increase sphincter strength and control, enhance urethral closure
    ■ Decrease episodes and severity of incontinence
    ■ Accelerate return to normal home, work, and recreational activities

9. **List outcome measurement(s) used to assess treatment effectiveness.**

    ■ Pelvic floor muscle/sphincter strength: Palpation (force grading /5)
    ■ Urinary incontinence: Continence chart (daily voiding diary)

10. **Instruct patient about what he/she should experience, do, and not do during the treatment session.**

    ■ Sensation of moderate-to-strong sensation of muscle contraction in the pelvic area

11. **Outline your therapeutic prescription based on the best sources of evidence available.**

    The IFC prescription suggested below is based on the following publications: Dougall, 1985; Laycock et al., 1988; Olah et al., 1990; Laycock et al., 1993; Dumoulin et al., 1995a,b; Turkan et al., 2005; and Stephenson et al., 2008.

    ■ *IFC device:* cabinet type mounted with a vacuum unit
    ■ *Stimulation method:* quadripolar
    ■ *Beat frequency:* 50 beps; carrier frequency of 4000–4050 cps
    ■ *Current amplitude:* maximum level tolerated (mA)
    ■ *ON:OFF ratio and duty cycle:* 10 s:40 s; duty cycle 20%
    ■ *Ramp up and down time:* up—1 s; down—1 s
    ■ *Patient position:* semi-supine, with the hips and knee flexed
    ■ *Electrode type and size:* 4 circular vacuum electrodes; 4 cm (2 in) diameter
    ■ *Electrode placement:* 2 placed on the abdomen, 2 placed on the inside of the thighs; crisscross arrangement

(Continued)

Case Study 18-1   Continued

- **Electrode cover:** enclosed in sterile cellulose sponge pads soaked in warm tap water
- **Vacuum electrode suction force:** high enough to secure the electrodes
- **Treatment session duration:** 30 min
- **Treatment frequency:** 5 consecutive days over a 2-week period
- **Total number of treatments:** 10

12. Collect outcome measurements.

Pre- and posttreatment comparison:

- PMF strength: from 1/5 to 4/5 (palpation grading)
- Continence chart: improved by 90%

13. Assess therapeutic effectiveness based on outcome measures.

The results show that 10 applications of IFC therapy, delivered daily for 5 days over a 2-week period, in combination with a home PMF exercise program, led to a significant increase of PMF strength and to a significant decrease in the number of episodes of urine loss per day. The electrically evoked muscle contraction has made the patient again aware of her pelvic floor muscle. She can now feel and command at will the contraction of these muscles. This patient can now sneeze, cough, and laugh at will, as well as perform her normal home, work, and recreational activities, with minimal urine loss. Overall, IFC therapy had a beneficial impact on the patient's disablement status created by this condition, as illustrated in the **figure below**.

14. State the prognosis.

The prognosis is excellent if the patient continues her daily home PFM strengthening program. Her condition should still improve over the next weeks until full recovery occurs.

THERAPEUTIC IMPACT on Disablement

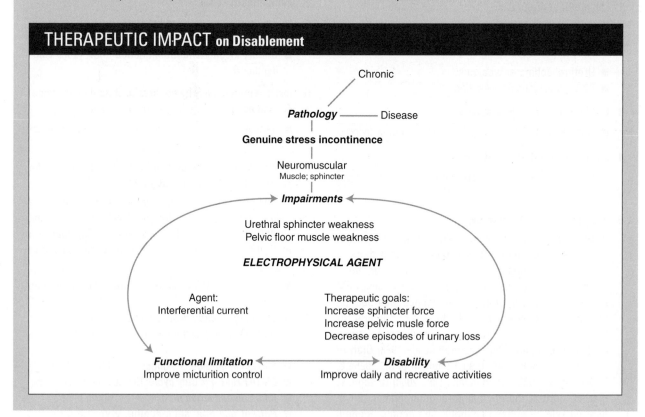

CRITICAL THINKING QUESTIONS

Clarification: What is meant by interferential current (IFC) therapy?

Assumptions: You have assumed that the physiological and therapeutic effects of IFC are similar to those of Russian current therapy (see Chapter 17). How do you justify making that assumption?

Reasons and evidence: What led you to believe that the application of IFC reduces skin impedance?

Viewpoints or perspectives: How would you respond to a colleague who says that the quadripolar method (true

IFC) is better than the premodulated method for muscle strengthening?

Implications and consequences: What are the implications and consequences of applying IFC therapy over a metallic implant and operating such a device in close proximity to a functioning shortwave diathermy unit?

About the question: Is it true that IFC is the only current type capable of deep penetration within soft tissues? Why do you think I ask this question?

References

Articles

Adedoyin RA, Olaogun MO, Fagbeja OO (2002) Effects of interferential current stimulation in management of osteoarthritic knee pain. Physiotherapy, 88: 493–499

Belcher J (1974) Interferential therapy. N Z J Physiother, 6: 29–34

Bergslien O, Thoresen M, Odemark H (1988) The effects of three electrotherapeutic methods on blood velocities in human peripheral arteries. Scand J Rehab Med, 20: 29–33

Bircan S, Senocak O, Kaya PO, Tamci SA, Gulbahar A, Akalin E (2002) Efficacy of two forms of electrical stimulation in increasing quadriceps strength: A randomized controlled trial. Clin Rehabil, 16: 194–199

Cheing GL, Hui-Chan CW (2003) Analgesic effects of transcutaneous electrical nerve stimulation and interferential currents on heat pain in healthy subjects. J Rehabil Med, 35: 15–19

Christie AD, Willoughby GL (1990) The effect of interferential therapy on swelling following open reduction and internal fixation of ankle fractures. Physiother Theory Pract, 6: 3–7

Dougall D (1985) The effects of interferential therapy in incontinence and frequency of micturition. Physiotherapy, 71: 135–136

Dumoulin C, Seabore DE, Quirion-de-Girardi C, Sullivan SJ (1995a) Pelvic-floor rehabilitation. Part 1: Comparison of two surface electrode placements during stimulation of the pelvic-floor musculature in women who are continent using bipolar interferential currents. Phys Ther, 75: 1067–1074

Dumoulin C, Seabore DE, Quirion-de-Girardi C, Sullivan SJ (1995b) Pelvic-floor rehabilitation. Part 2: Pelvic-floor reeducation with interferential currents and exercise in the treatment of genuine stress incontinence in postpartum women—A cohort study. Phys Ther, 75: 1075–1081

Foster NE, Thompson KA, Baxter GD, Allen JM (1999) Management of nonspecific low back pain by physiotherapists in Britain and Ireland. A descriptive questionnaire of current clinical practice. Spine, 24: 1332–1342

Fourie JA, Bowerbank P (1997) Stimulation of bone healing in new fractures of tibial shaft using interferential currents. Physiother Res Int, 2: 255–268

Ganne JM (1988) Stimulation of bone healing with interferential therapy. Aust J Physiother, 34: 9–20

Ganne JM, Speculand B, Mayne LH, Goss AN (1979) Interferential therapy to promote union of mandibular fractures. Aust N Z J Surg, 49: 81–83

Henella SM, Hutchins CJ, Castleden CM (1987) Conservative management of urethral sphincter incompetence. Neurourol Urodyn, 6: 191–192

Hurley DA, Minder PH, McDonough SM, Walsh DM, Moore AP, Baxter DG (2001) Interferential therapy electrode placement technique in acute low back pain: A preliminary investigation. Arch Phys Med Rehabil, 82:485–493

Indergand NJ, Morgan BJ (1995) Effect of interference current on forearm vascular resistance in asymptomatic humans. Phys Ther, 75: 306–312

Jarit GK, Mohr KJ, Waller R, Glousman RE (2003) The effects of home interferential therapy on postoperative pain, edema, and range of motion of the knee. Clin J Sports Med, 13: 16–20

Johnson MI (1999) The mystique of interferential currents when used to manage pain. Physiotherapy, 85: 294–296

Johnson MI, Tabasam G (1999) A double blind placebo-controlled investigation into the analgesic effects of interferential effects (IFC) and transcutaneous electrical nerve stimulation (TENS) on cold-induced pain in healthy subjects. Physioth Theor Pract, 15: 217–233

Johnson MI, Tabasam G (2003a) A single blind investigation into the hypoanalgesic effects of different swing patterns of interferential currents on cold-induced pain in healthy subjects. Arch Phys Med Rehabil, 84: 350–357

Johnson MI, Tabasam G (2003b) An investigation into the analgesic effects of interferential currents and transcutaneous electrical nerve stimulation on experimentally induced ischemic pain in otherwise pain-free volunteers. Phys Ther, 83: 208–223

Jonhson MI, Tabasan G (2003c) An investigation into the analgesic effects of different frequencies of the amplitude-modulated wave of interferential current therapy on cold-induced pain in normal subjects. Arch Phys Med Rehabil, 84: 1387–1394

Johnson MI, Wilson H (1997) The analgesic effects of different swing patterns of interferential currents on cold-induced pain. Physiotherapy, 83: 461–467

Kitchen S (2000) Audit of the unexpected effects of electrophysical agents. Physiotherapy, 86: 152–155

Lambert I, Tebbs SE, Hill D, Moss HA, Davies AJ, Elliott TS (2000) Interferential therapy machines as possible vehicles for cross-infection. J Hosp Infect, 44: 59–64

Lambert JL, Vanderstreaten GG, De Cuyper HJ (1993) Electric current distribution during interferential therapy, Eur J Phys Med Rehab 3: 6–10

Laycock J, Green RJ (1988) Interferential therapy in the treatment of incontinence. Physiotherapy, 74: 161–164

Laycock J, Jerwood D (1993) Does premodulated interferential therapy cure genuine stress incontinence? Physiotherapy, 79: 553–560

Lindsay D, Dearness J, Richardson C, Chapman A, Cuskelly G (1990) A survey of electromodality usage in private physiotherapy practices. Aust J Physiother, 36: 249–256

Lindsay DM, Dearness J, McGinley CC (1995) Electrotherapy usage trends in private physiotherapy practice in Alberta. Physiother Can, 47: 30–34

Mantle J, Versi E (1991) Physiotherapy for stress incontinence: A national survey. Br Med J, 302: 753–755

McManus FJ, Ward AR, Robertson VJ (2006) The analgesic effects of interferential therapy on two experimental pain models: Cold and mechanically induced pain. Physiotherapy, 92: 95–102

McQuire WA (1975) Electrotherapy and exercises for stress incontinence and urinary frequency. Physiotherapy, 61: 305–307

Minder PM, Noble JG, Alves-Guerreiro J, Hill ID, Lowe AS, Walsh DM, Baxter GD (2002) Interferential therapy: Lack of effect upon experimentally induced delayed onset muscle soreness. Clin Physiol Funct Imaging, 22: 339–347

Nemec H (1959) Interferential therapy: A new approach in physical medicine. Br J Physiother, 12: 9–12

Ni Chiosig F, Hendricks O, Malone J (1994) A pilot study of the therapeutic effects of bipolar and quadripolar interferential therapy, using bipolar osteoarthritis as a model. Physiotherapy Ireland, 15: 3–7

Noble JG, Henderson G, Cramp AF, Walsh DM, Lowe AS (2000) The effect of interferential therapy upon cutaneous blood flow in humans. Clin Physiol, 20: 2–7

Nussbaum EL, Burke S, Johnstome L, Lahiffe G, Robitaille E, Yoshida K (2007) Use of electrophysical agents: Findings and implications of a survey of practice in Metro Toronto. Physioth Can, 59: 118–131

Nussbaum E, Rush P, Disenhaus L (1990) The effects of interferential therapy on peripheral blood flow. Physiotherapy, 76: 803–807

Olah KS, Bridges N, Denning J, Farrar DJ (1990) The conservative management of patients with symptoms of stress incontinence: A randomized, prospective study comparing weighted vaginal cones and interferential therapy. Am J Obstet Gynecol, 162: 87–92

Olson SL, Perez JV, Stacks LN, Walsh MH (1999) The effects of TENS and interferential current on cutaneous blood flow in healthy subjects. Physiother Can, 51: 27–31

Ozcan J, Ward AR, Robertson VJ (2004) A comparison of true and premodulated interferential currents. Arch Phys Med Rehabil, 85: 409–415

Partridge CJ, Kitchen SS (1999) Adverse effects of electrotherapy used by physiotherapists. Physiotherapy, 85: 298–303

Philipp A, Wolf GK, Rzany B, Dertinger H, Jung EG (2000) Interferential current is effective in palmar psoriasis: An open prospective trial. Eur J Dermatol, 10: 195–198

Pope GD, Mockett SP, Wright JP (1995) A survey of electrotherapeutic modalities ownership and use in the NHS in England. Physiotherapy, 82: 82–91

Quirk A, Newham RJ, Newham KJ (1985) An evaluation of interferential therapy, shortwave diathermy and exercise in the treatment of osteoarthrosis of the knee. Physiotherapy, 71: 55–57

Robertson VJ, Spurritt D (1998) Electrophysical agents: implications of their availability and use in undergraduate clinical placements. Physiotherapy, 84: 335–334

Shafshak TS, El-Sheshai AM, Soltan, HE (1991) Personality traits in the mechanisms of interferential therapy for osteoarthritic knee pain. Arch Phys Med Rehab, 72: 579–581

Shanahan C, Ward AR, Robertson VJ (2006) Comparison of the analgesic efficacy of interferential therapy and transcutaneous electric nerve stimulation. Physiotherapy, 92: 247–253

Stephenson R, Johnson M (1995) The analgesic effects of interferential therapy on cold-induced pain in healthy subjects: A preliminary report. Physiother Theory Pract, 11: 89–95

Stephenson R, Walker EM (2003) The analgesic effects of interferential (IF) current on cold-pressor pain in healthy subjects: A single blind trial of three IF currents against sham IF and control. Physiother Theory Pract, 19: 99–107

Sylvester KL, Keilty SEJ (1987) A pilot study to investigate the use of interferential in the treatment of anorectal incontinence. Physiotherapy, 73: 207–208

Taylor K, Newton R, Personius W, Bush F (1987) Effect of interferential current stimulation for treatment of subjects with recurrent jaw pain. Phys Ther, 67: 346–350

Truscott B (1984) Interferential therapy as a treatment for classical migraine: Case reports. Aust J Physiother, 30: 33–35

Tugay N, Akbayrak T, Demirturk F, Karakaya IC, Kocaacar O, Tugay U, Karakaya MG, Demirturk F (2007) Effectiveness of transcutaneous electrical nerve stimulation and interferential current in primary dysmenorrhea. Pain Med, 8: 295–300

Turkan A, Inci Y, Fazli D (2005) The short-term effects of physical therapy in different intensities of urodynamic stress incontinence. Gynecol Obstet Invest, 59: 43–48

Vahtera T, Haaranen M, Viramo-Koskela AL, Ruutiainen J (1997) Pelvic floor rehabilitation is effective in patients with multiple sclerosis. Clin Rehab, 11: 211–219

Van der Heijden G, Leffers P, Wolters P, Verheijden J, van Mameren H, Houben JP, Bouter LM, Knipschild PG (1999) No effect of bipolar interferential electrotherapy and pulsed ultrasound for soft tissue shoulder disorders: A randomized controlled trial. Ann Rheum Dis, 58: 530–540

Van Poppel H, Ketelaer P, Van-Deweerd A (1985) Interferential therapy for detrusor hyperreflexia in multiple sclerosis. Urology, 25: 607–612

Walker UA, Uhl M, Weiner SM, Warnatz K, Lange-Nolde A, Dertinger H, Peter HH, Jurenz SA (2006) Analgesic and disease modifying effects of interferential current in psoriatic arthritis. Rheumatol Int, 26: 904–907

Werners R, Pynsent PB, Bulstrode CJ (1999) Randomized trial comparing interferential therapy with motorized lumbar traction and massage in the management of low back pain in a primary care settings. Spine, 24: 1579–1584

Wilson PD, Al-Samarrai T, Deakin M, Kolbe E, Brown AD (1987) An objective assessment of physiotherapy for female genuine stress incontinence. Br J Obstet Gynaecol, 94: 575–582

Zambito A, Bianchini D, Gatti D, Rossini M, Adami S, Viapiana O (2007) Interference and horizontal therapies in chronic low back pain due to multiple vertebral fractures: A randomized, double blind, clinical study. Osteoporos Int, 18: 1541–1545

Zambito A, Bianchini D, Gatti D, Viapiana O, Rossini M, Adami S (2006) Interferential and horizontal therapies in chronic low back pain: a randomized, double blind, clinical study. Clin Exp Rheumatol, 24: 534–539

Review Articles

De Domenico G (1982) Pain relief with interferential therapy. Aust J Physiother, 28: 14–18

Goats GC (1990) Interferential current therapy. Br J Sports Med, 24: 187–192

Noble JG, Lowe AS, Walsh DM (2000) Interferential therapy review: 1. Mechanism of analgesics action and clinical usage. Phys Ther Rev, 5: 239–245

Chapters of Textbooks

Alon G (1999) Principles of electrical stimulation. In: Clinical Electrotherapy, 3rd ed. Nelson RM, Hayes, KW, Currier DP (Eds). Appleton & Lange, Stamford, pp 82–85, 108–109

Gerleman DG, Barr JO (1999) Instrumentation and product safety. In: Clinical Electrotherapy, 3rd ed. Nelson RM, Hayes, KW, Currier DP (Eds). Appleton & Lange, Stamford, pp 15–53

Hayes KW (2000) Interferential stimulation. In: Manual for Physical Agents, 5th ed. Appleton & Lange, Norwalk, pp 149–155

Hooke DN (1998) Electrical estimulating currents. In: Therapeutic Modalities for Allied Health Professionals. Prentice WE (Ed). McGraw Hill Corp, New York, pp 114–117

Kloth LC (1991) Interference current. In: Clinical Electrotherapy, 2nd ed. Nelson RM, Currier DP (Eds). Appleton and Lange, Norwalk, pp 221–260

Knight KL, Draper DO (2008) Application Procedures: Electrotherapy. In: Therapeutic Modalities. The Art and Science. Lippincott Williams & Wilkins, Philadelphia, pp 158–165

Martin D (1996) Interferential therapy. In: Clayton's Electrotherapy, 10th ed. Kitchen S, Bazin S (Eds). WB Saunders Co., London, pp 306–315

Palmer S, Martin D (2002) Interferential current for pain control. In: Electrotherapy Evidence-Based Practice, 11th ed. Kitchen S (Ed). Churchill Livingstone, London, pp 2287–2300

Robinson AJ (2008) Instrumentation in electrotherapy. In: Clinical Electrophysiology. Electrotherapy and Electrophysiological Testing, 3rd ed. Robinson AJ, Snyder-Mackler L (Eds). Lippincott Williams & Wilkins, Philadelphia. pp 57–58

Starkey C (1999) Electrical agents. In: Therapeutic Modalities, 2nd ed. FA Davis Co., Philadelphia, pp 236–244

Stephenson RG, Shelly ER (2008) Electric stimulation and biofeedback for genitourinary dysfunction. In: Clinical Electrophysiology. Electrotherapy and Electrophysiological Testing, 3rd ed. Robinson AJ, Snyder-Mackler L (Eds). Lippincott Williams & Wilkins, Philadelphia. pp 301–349

Wadsworth H, Chanmugam APP (1988) Interferential currents. In: Electrophysical Agents in Physiotherapy: Therapeutic and Diagnostic Use, 2nd ed. Science Press, Marrickville, pp 274–289

Textbooks

De Domenico G (1981) Basic Guidelines for Interferential Therapy. Theramed Boors, Sydney

De Domenico G (1987) New Dimensions in Interferential Therapy. A Theoretical and Clinical Guide. Reid Medical Books, Lindfield

Nikolova L (1987) Treatment with Interferential Currents. Churchill Livingstone, Edinburgh

Savage B (1984) Interferential Therapy. Faber & Faber, London

Diadynamic Current Therapy

Learning Objectives

Knowledge: List and describe the five (DF, MF, CP, LP, and RS) diadynamic current waveforms.

Comprehension: Compare the proposed physiological effect of DC application with those associated with the five diadynamic current waveforms.

Application: Illustrate the five diadynamic current waveforms.

Analysis: Explain how the use of diadynamic current may lead to pain modulation.

Synthesis: Formulate the distinctions, based on electric parameters such as waveform and pulse duration, between the diadynamic current waveforms and those generated by modern TENS devices used to modulate pain.

Evaluation: Discuss the body and strength of the English-language, scientific evidence behind the use of diadynamic current therapy and decide if this EPA is presently justified for the treatment of soft-tissue pathology.

I. RATIONALE FOR USE

A. DEFINITION AND DESCRIPTION

The term *diadynamic current* was first proposed, in the early 1950s, by its inventor, a French dentist named Pierre Bernard. The exact meaning of the word *diadynamic* remains obscure. According to Bernard (1950), his empirically discovered current is presumed to have an *analgesic effect* on a wide variety of soft-tissue and systemic disorders. This current is defined as a pulsed rectified alternating sinusoidal current. It is described as a monophasic current made of half-sine waveforms. Like many other types of therapeutic electrical currents considered in this textbook—TENS, HVPC current, Russian current, and interferential current—diadynamic current also falls into the broad category of transcutaneous electrical nerve stimulation.

B. DIADYNAMIC STIMULATOR

Modern cabinet-type therapeutic electrical stimulators, commonly named combo stimulators, are manufactured so as to be able to generate multi-currents and multi-current waveforms. **Figure 19-1** shows a typical cabinet line-powered electrical stimulator, mounted on a movable cart, capable of generating a diadynamic current.

C. ELECTRODES AND COUPLING GEL

The delivery of diadynamic current to soft tissues, as was the case with other nerve depolarizing currents covered in this textbook (see Chapters 14, 16, 17, and 18), is usually done using reusable surface electrodes covered with electroconductive gel and made of various materials and sizes. Examples of such electrodes, with coupling gel, are presented in Chapter 17.

D. RATIONALE FOR USE

Most pathologies resulting from injuries and diseases cause pain. The rationale behind the development of this diadynamic current was to provide practitioners with an alternative therapy to medication and thermal agents for the management of pain. In retrospect, diadynamic current, first used in the 1950s, may be considered as the ancestor of TENS therapy, first used in the 1970s, for the management of pain. As shown in this textbook, diadynamic current therapy is one of several EPAs practitioners can use today for the management of pain resulting from soft-tissue pathology.

II. HISTORICAL PERSPECTIVE

A. DISCOVERY

The discovery of diadynamic current is credited to Pierre Bernard, a French dentist. In his textbook, Bernard (1950) details the technical nature of his newly discovered

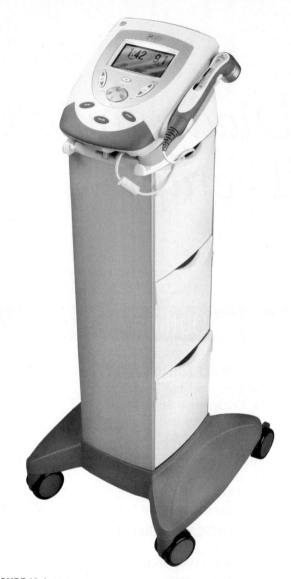

FIGURE 19-1 Multi-current electrical stimulator system, mounted on a therapy system cart, capable of generating a diadynamic current. (Courtesy of Chattanooga Group.)

current and describes its therapeutic effects based on his own clinical observations.

B. WORLD PRACTICE

The practice of diadynamic current therapy, pioneered during the 1940s by Bernard himself in France, later spread to Russia, Germany, Finland, and Poland during the 1960s and eventually reached Canada and Australia during the late 1960s and early 1970s. This current, although available in most U.S.-made combo-type stimulators, still remains unknown to most American practitioners working with EPAs, as would appear from the contents of recently published EPA textbooks.

C. BODY OF LITERATURE

Diadynamic current therapy, unlike all other EPAs covered in this textbook, has been the object of a *very limited* number of English-language publications. An exhaustive search of the scientific literature identified only a handful of human research–oriented, English-language *articles* (Theron et al., 1983; Hamalainen et al., 1990; Can et al., 2003), *chapters of textbooks* (Rennie, 1988; Wadsworth et al., 1988), and *paragraphs* written by American (Robinson et al., 2008) and British authors (Low et al., 1990), in addition to Bernard's own *textbook* (Bernard, 1950).

III. BIOPHYSICAL CHARACTERISTICS

A. PRINCIPLE

The biophysical principle underlying the production of diadynamic current is the *electronic modulation* of a symmetrical biphasic sinusoidal current, the carrier frequency of which is derived from the stimulator's own main-line power supply of either 50 (most European countries) or 60 (North America) cycles per second (cps). Before considering the following paragraphs, readers are *urged to review* Chapter 5, which presents an illustrated glossary of terms related to electricity.

B. CURRENT WAVEFORMS

Illustrated in **Figure 19-2** are the five diadynamic current waveforms originally described by Bernard (1950) and generated by present-day therapeutic electrical stimulators. These diadynamic current waveforms are all monophasic sinusoidal currents bearing their original French names: *diphasé fixe* (DF), *monophasé fixe* (MF), *courtes périodes* (CP), *longues périodes* (LP), and *rythme syncopé* (RS). The equivalent English translations are *fixed diphase* (DF), *fixed monophase* (MF), *short periods* (CP), *long periods* (LP), and *syncopal rhythm* (RC), respectively.

1. DF and MF

Both DF and MF current waveforms are obtained through the full-wave (DF) and half-wave (MF) rectification of the original symmetrical biphasic sinusoidal current.

2. CP, LP, and RS Waveforms

The CP, LP, and RS current waveforms are obtained from different combinations of DF and MF current waveforms.

a. CP

Alternate delivery of DF and MF currents leads to production of the CP current waveform.

b. LP

Alternate delivery of DF, the current amplitude of which is ramped up and down over time, plus MF, leads to creation of the LP current waveform.

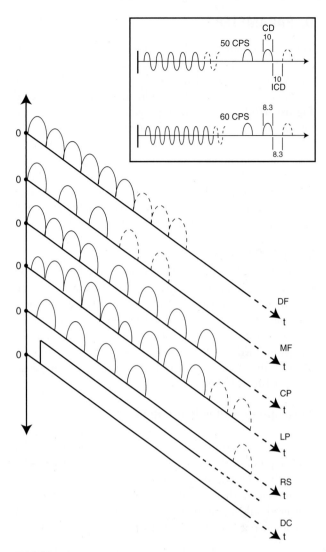

FIGURE 19-2 The five original diadynamic current waveforms (DF, MF, CP, LP, and RS) and associated continuous DC current waveform. Shown in the upper right is the basic symmetrical biphasic sine-wave current, from which all diadynamic current waveforms are extracted, as well as the cycle duration (CD) and intercycle duration (ICD) related to the stimulator's own carrier frequency.

c. RS

Delivery of MF for a fixed duration, followed by an equal duration of rest, leads to creation of the RS current waveform.

C. DIRECT CURRENT

The practice of diadynamic current therapy requires the use of a direct current (DC) in addition to the basic diadynamic waveforms (**Fig 19-2**). According to Bernard (1950), DC must always be applied *before* any of the listed diadynamic currents (see Section V, Dosimetry). Bernard (1950) hypothesized that flowing a low-amplitude DC before delivering diadynamic currents will decrease the transmembrane nerve potential, thus minimizing the current amplitude levels associated with the subsequent delivery of either DF, MF, CP, LP, or RS necessary for sensory and motor nerve depolarization. No experimental scientific evidence, however, was provided by Bernard to support his hypothesis.

D. PARAMETERS

The cycle duration (CD) and intercycle duration (ICD) associated with all diadynamic waveforms are fixed, and their values are determined by the main-line power frequency of the stimulator. Illustrated in the inset of **Figure 19-2** is the carrier frequency of a symmetrical biphasic sine wave, from which all diadynamic currents are derived, with the corresponding CD and ICD. If the sine-wave carrier frequency powering the stimulator is 50 cps, then both CD and ICD will be 10 msec (50 cps = 1000 / [10 + 10]). If the carrier frequency powering the device is 60 cps, as is the case in North America, then both CD and ICD will be 8.3 msec (60 cps = 1000 / [8.3 + 8.3]).

1. Cycle Duration

The term cycle duration (CD) is synonymous here with the term phase duration, because the current waveforms are all monophasic in nature. Diadynamic CDs are extremely long, ranging from 8.3 to 10 msec, depending on the carrier or line-powered frequency of the stimulator (see above), compared with cycle or pulse durations generated by modern therapeutic electrical stimulators, which range from 0.01 to 1.0 msec.

2. Longer Pulse/Cycle Duration

There is a consensus in the literature that the longer the pulse or cycle duration for a fixed current waveform and amplitude, the more painful the electrical stimulation. This observation may explain why Bernard (1950) recommended that each diadynamic current waveform be delivered only for short periods of time (often <120 sec) and at current amplitudes comfortable for the patient.

E. MODERN DIADYNAMIC STIMULATORS

Newer electrical stimulators, such as the one illustrated in **Figure 19-1**, are generating diadynamic current waveforms that are slightly different from the original current waveforms described by Bernard (1950). For example, the LP mode described in the device illustrated in **Figure 19-1** results from the rhythmical fluctuation between two MF waveforms; this mode significantly differs from the original LP made of the alternative delivery of DF plus MF. Clinicians are invited to check the technical sheet of modern electrical stimulators to determine whether the diadynamic current generated is original (i.e., as described by Bernard) or not.

IV. PHYSIOLOGICAL AND THERAPEUTIC EFFECTS

A. PAUCITY OF RESEARCH

Although diadynamic current stimulation has been practiced for more than 60 years in many countries around the

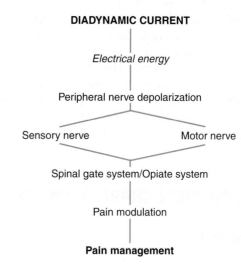

FIGURE 19-3 Proposed physiological and therapeutic effects of diadynamic current therapy.

world, the proposed physiological and therapeutic effects reported here and originally postulated by Bernard (1950) remain highly hypothetical and poorly understood due to the *paucity* of basic and clinical research found in the English-language, scientific literature (see References).

B. PROPOSED EFFECTS

Illustrated in **Figure 19-3** are the physiological and therapeutic effects of diadynamic current therapy, as proposed by Bernard (1950).

1. Physiological Effect

Delivery of the five diadynamic waveforms over the skin surface leads to depolarization of sensory and/or motor nerve fibers, depending on the current amplitude used (i.e., sensory versus motor threshold). The process of electrically evoked nerve depolarization is described in Chapter 14.

2. Therapeutic Effect

Bernard (1950) theorized that this nerve depolarization induces a pain-modulating or analgesic effect. This form of pain modulation, at the threshold for sensory and motor nerve fiber depolarization, resembles that achieved by the use of TENS therapy (Chapter 14). An important difference, however, is that TENS therapy is delivered using short (microsecond range) biphasic balanced pulses as opposed to the characteristically long (millisecond range) monophasic and obviously unbalanced diadynamic pulses.

3. Effect of DC Current

The delivery of DC *before* any of the five diadynamic currents, as well as during the entire treatment session, has no added therapeutic effect according to Bernard (1950). Its sole purpose, as hypothesized by Bernard, is physiological—that is, to *reduce the resting nerve membrane*, thus facilitating depolarization by requiring smaller diadynamic current amplitudes. No evidence can be found in the English-language literature to support this hypothesis.

V. DOSIMETRY

A. BERNARD'S APPROACH

There is no scientific evidence on which to base the dosimetry associated with diadynamic current therapy. The only dosimetric approach known, which is empirically based, is that of Bernard (1950). The steps underlying this dosimetric approach are as follows. Each application usually last a few seconds to a maximum of 3 minutes.

1. Dosimetric Steps

Always begin therapy with a DC application. Immediately follow this DC application with a DF application. Follow the previous DC and DF applications with a combination of MF, CP, LP, or RS. Deliver MF, CP, LP, or RS for periods ranging from 2 to 5 minutes. Set all diadynamic current amplitudes between the threshold of perception and the threshold of pain. Reverse current polarity regularly during treatment to avoid any polar or electrolytic effects on the skin under the electrodes.

2. Dosage Example

A given dose may be made of one application of DC lasting 3 minutes followed by one application of DF (2 minutes), one of MF (3 minutes), and one of CP (3 minutes), in that order.

B. EMPIRICAL DOSIMETRY

The selection of one diadynamic current over the other for any given pathological condition is totally arbitrary because it stems from Bernard's own clinical empirical observations and suggestions reported in his textbook (1950).

VI. EVIDENCE FOR INDICATIONS

A. GUIDED BY EVIDENCE

Dictionaries generally define *evidence* as anything that establishes a fact or gives reason to believe something. The aim of this textbook is to present scientific evidence

behind therapeutic EPAs. To be guided by the evidence is the process of integrating the evidence from research, however imperfect or scarce this evidence may be, with clinical experience and patient's preferences. In other words, the *evidence-based practice* of EPA requires that practitioners consider the evidence from research, in addition to their own clinical experience and the patient's own preference and beliefs about a given EPA, when the time comes to justify, prescribe, and apply the therapeutic agent. To be guided by the evidence is a process, not a search for the absolute truth. Finally, a lack of evidence from research in support of any given EPA does not mean that this EPA should never be used. What it means is that no statement can be made about its therapeutic effectiveness and that until more evidence from research is presented, its routine use cannot be recommended.

B. EVIDENCE FROM HUMAN RESEARCH

Box 19-1 provides evidence for diadynamic therapy based on an exhaustive search of published English-language, peer-reviewed studies on humans. The term *indication* is used with regard to a list of pathologies for which cryotherapy is employed. Ratings of therapeutic benefit (Yes or No) and grading of strength of scientific evidence (I, II, or III), including the reference, are included for each pathological condition.

1. Rating Therapeutic Benefit

The rating, expressed as Yes or No, is based on the overall conclusion(s) reached on the issue of therapeutic effectiveness by the author(s) who conducted the peer-reviewed study.

2. Grading Strength of Evidence

The grading, numerically classified as I, II, and III, is based on the type of research methodology, or research design, used by the author(s). All those listed are studies on humans published in English-language peer-reviewed journals. It follows that the evidence in studies graded I is stronger than in those of graded II, and evidence in studies graded II is stronger than in those graded III.

a. Grade I

Evidence based on *controlled* studies on humans, regardless of their level of randomization and blindness.

Box 19-1	Research-Based Indications for the Use of Diadynamic Current Therapy		
PATHOLOGY	**BENEFIT**	**GRADE**	**REFERENCE**
Postoperative ileus (intestinal mobility)	Yes	II	Theron et al., 1983
Patellofemoral pain	Yes	II	Can et al., 2003

b. Grade II

Evidence based on *noncontrolled* studies on humans, regardless of their level of randomization and blindness.

c. Grade III

Evidence based on *case* studies on humans, regardless of their level of randomization and blindness.

3. Strength of Evidence Behind the Agent

The evidence behind the agent, as presented in the research-based indication box, is arbitrarily assessed in this textbook as *weak, moderate,* or *strong.* For example, the larger the number of studies graded I, regardless of therapeutic benefit, the stronger the scientific evidence behind the agent.

4. Evidence to Justify Usage of Agent

The evidence to justify the use of the agent for an individual pathology or groups of pathologies, as listed in the research-based indication box, is arbitrarily assessed in this textbook as *poor, fair, good,* or *conflicting.* For example, where a larger number of grade I studies show therapeutic benefit (Yes) than no benefit, for any given pathology, the justification for usage of the agent for that pathology is assessed as *good. Conflicting* usage is reported when about an equal number of studies with similar grades show therapeutic benefit (Yes) and no benefit (No).

C. STRENGTH OF EVIDENCE AND JUSTIFICATION FOR USAGE

The results presented in **Box 19-1** show *weak* evidence for the use of diadynamic current therapy with only two clinical studies (Theron et al., 1983; Can et al., 2003) and one study on experimental pain in healthy subjects (Hamalainen et al., 1990). These results suggest that the *justification for usage* of diadynamic current therapy is *poor.* Until more evidence from research is provided with regard to therapeutic effectiveness of this EPA, its use *cannot be recommended.*

D. CAUSE FOR SERIOUS CONCERN

The fact that only a handful of clinical studies on the therapeutic effect of diadynamic current can be found in published English-language, peer-reviewed studies on humans is of particular concern, in view of the fact that this EPA has been used in many English-speaking countries over the past six decades. This strongly suggests that the practice of diadynamic current therapy has been based, in these English-speaking countries, solely on the original observations and dictum of Bernard (1950), and that of corporate literature, rather than on evidence provided by scientific literature. This textbook reemphasizes the opinion that until more evidence from research on humans is provided with regard to therapeutic effectiveness of this EPA, its use *cannot be recommended.*

VII. CONTRAINDICATIONS

Table 19-1 describes the contraindications associated with diadynamic current therapy. Because this current falls into the category of transcutaneous nerve electrical stimulation, the contraindications are *similar* to those listed for TENS (Chapter 14), HVPC (Chapter 16), Russian current (Chapter 17), and interferential current (Chapter 18).

TABLE 19-1	CONTRAINDICATIONS TO DIADYNAMIC CURRENT THERAPY
CONTRAINDICATIONS	**RATIONALE**
Over the anterior cervical area	Risk of stimulating key organs, such as the vagus nerve, phrenic nerve, and carotid sinuses, resulting in adverse effects such as hypotensive reaction and laryngeal spasm.
Over the thoracic region	Risk of affecting normal heart function. Stimulation over intercostal muscles led to respiratory failure in one cardiac patient.
Over the cranial area	Risk of affecting normal brain function.
With patients wearing rate-responsive pacemakers or implanted cardioverter defibrillators (ICDs)	Risk of electronic interference with units (for more details see Chapter 14). *Important note*: Stimulators may be used with these patients *only* if the ICU unit is turned off during therapy.
Over the abdominal, pelvic, or lumbar areas of pregnant women in their first trimester	Risk of inducing labor.
Over superficial metal implants	Risk of causing unnecessary pain due to electrical current-induced overheating of implants.

(Continued)

TABLE 19-1	CONTINUED
CONTRAINDICATIONS	**RATIONALE**
With epileptic patients	Risk of causing an epileptic episode.
Over hemorrhagic areas	Risk of enhanced bleeding due to increased blood flow in the treated area.
Over malignant areas	Risk of increasing and spreading the tumor due to increased blood flow in the treated area.
Over damaged skin	Risk of causing unnecessary and severe pain.

VIII. RISKS, PRECAUTIONS, AND RECOMMENDATIONS

Table 19-2 is presented with the purpose of increasing the safety and effectiveness of diadynamic current therapy. Special attention should be given to skin inspection after therapy considering the monophasic nature of this current, which may dispose the skin to irritation and possible burn.

IX. CONSIDERATIONS FOR APPLICATION AND DOCUMENTATION

A. PROCEDURES

Safe, effective, and optimal application of diadynamic current therapy requires that clinicians go through a systematic set of procedures for each and every application. The following is a list of such procedures, beginning with checklists and ending with the documentation of key treatment parameters.

1. Checklists
Before proceeding with treatment, *always* go through the list of contraindications (**Table 19-1**) and the list of risks, precautions, and recommendations (**Table 19-2**).

2. Skin Preparation
Clean the skin area under the electrode with rubbing alcohol. If necessary, cut or trim excess hair. These skin areas should be free of open wounds.

3. Electrode Selection, Preparation, and Fixation
Select the electrode type and size, coupling medium, and fixation that best match the treatment area.

TABLE 19-2	RISKS, PRECAUTIONS, AND RECOMMENDATIONS FOR DIADYNAMIC CURRENT THERAPY
RISK	**RATIONALE**
Usage near functioning shortwave diathermy (SWD) device	Risk of causing electronic interference. A patient reporting a sudden and variable surge of current output when an SWD unit is functioning in the neighborhood may be indicative of such electronic interference.
PRECAUTIONS	**RATIONALE**
With confused and unreliable patients	May result in unreliable information, which may have a negative impact on treatment effectiveness.
Home therapy	Instruct patients to keep the portable stimulator out of the reach of children at all times.

(Continued)

TABLE 19-2	CONTINUED
RECOMMENDATIONS	**RATIONALE**
Clean and dry exposed skin surface areas before each treatment	Wiping the skin surface with alcohol will reduce its impedance significantly in addition to removing impurities, thus allowing an optimal electrical coupling at the skin–electrode interface.
Clip hair over exposed skin areas	To ensure optimal electrode–skin coupling.
Wash and dry reusable electrodes after each treatment	To ensure optimal performance; follow the manufacturer's instructions.
Check cables and electrodes regularly for visible wear and tear	To ensure optimal efficacy.
Check electrode impedance monthly	To ensure appropriate electrode impedance for optimal conduction because electrodes will deteriorate with use and time. Use an ohmmeter to check impedance.
Keep the stimulator at least 3 m (10 feet) away from any functioning SWD device.	To minimize the risk of electronic interference.
Plug line-powered stimulators into GFCI receptacles	Prevent the risks of electrocution (see Chapter 27 for details).
Conduct regular maintenance and calibration	To ensure optimal treatment efficacy. Follow the manufacturer's recommendations and schedule.
Discard all electrodes after 6 months of usage.	Material deterioration will increase electrode impedance thus reducing efficacy.

4. Electrode Placement

The main proposed therapeutic effect of diadynamic current is to modulate pain. Consequently, the electrode placement is same as in TENS therapy (Chapter 15). Electrode may be placed over the painful area, along the dermatomes(s) covered by the painful area, or over specific acupuncture points.

5. During Treatment

Inform the patient that he or she will experience some tingling and light muscle contraction during therapy, as well as a light sensation of heat under the electrodes.

6. Dosimetry

Apply DC current before diadynamic current. From the five diadynamic current waveforms, select the most

appropriate combination of waveforms for the pathological condition under treatment (see Section V, Dosimetry, for details).

7. End of Treatment

Carefully remove the electrodes and immediately inspect the skin under the electrodes for any lesion. If present, inform the patient and document these in the patient's file. Clean reusable electrode surfaces with warm water and let dry over a towel on a flat surface.

B. DOCUMENTATION

Table 19-3 shows the key treatment parameters to be documented in the patient's file.

TABLE 19-3	KEY TREATMENT PARAMETERS TO BE DOCUMENTED IN PATIENT'S FILE AFTER DIADYNAMIC CURRENT THERAPY

- Diadynamic stimulator: model
- DC application: current amplitude, mA; duration of application, sec
- Diadynamic waveform application: for each waveform used (DF, MF, CP, LP, RS) current amplitude, mA; application duration, sec
- Sequence of DC and diadynamic current waveforms applications during treatment: description
- Electrode type and size: description and measurement
- Electrode placement: description

Case Study 19-1   Cervicalgia

Note: This chapter reveals that the evidence behind the practice of diadynamic current therapy, based on English-language, peer-reviewed scientific studies on humans, is weak and that, consequently, the justification for its use is poor. One is thus forced to conclude that the clinical usage of this EPA has not been driven by scientific evidence. The following case study and its resolution, therefore, are not based on evidence. The resolution of the following case is based on clinical experience and recommendations drawn from Bernard's book and corporate literature.

A 52-year-old male taxi driver, with no history of neck pain, consults for treatment. He reports first experiencing neck pain after having played in a friendly bowling tournament a week ago. His main complaint is neck pain associated with, and a lack of, head rotation movement, bilaterally. Physical examination reveals a moderate muscle spasm affecting the right and left upper trapezius muscle as well as the lack of a 20-degree range of motion during left and right head rotation. The patient reports a tingling and burning sensation in the neck area. He is worried about his being able to drive safely and effectively for long periods of time because, as a taxi driver, he is at the wheel 12 hours a day. He mentions a chronic heart condition for which he receives regular medical treatment. He also mentions suffering from chronic gastric irritation, forcing him to seek a conservative treatment first, before considering drug treatment (analgesics, anti-inflammatory agents, and muscle relaxers) offered by his physician. The patient's goals are to return to his taxi driver job full-time in addition to resuming bowling.

Arbitrary Steps Toward the Resolution of This Case

1. **Establish medical diagnosis.**
   Cervicalgia of mechanical origin

2. **List key impairment(s).**
   - Cervical pain
   - Cervical muscle spasm
   - Lack of 20-degree left and right ROM—head rotation

3. **List key functional limitation(s).**
   - Limited bilateral head rotation

4. **List key disability.**
   - Difficulty driving a car
   - Difficulty bowling

5. **Justification of selected EPA and other therapeutics.**
   Is there justification to use diadynamic therapy in this case? As previously mentioned, the use of diadynamic current therapy is poorly justified based on the available body of scientific evidence. Selecting diadynamic current therapy for this patient is, therefore, justified strictly on the basis of clinical experience and because of the patient's desire to try a conservative treatment first. Considering the evidence, TENS therapy (Chapter 14) should have been the first EPA to be selected for this case. Diadynamic current therapy is selected here because it is hypothesized that it may modulate pain. It is also selected because its application, in the context of a case study, needs to be described. This EPA is used concomitantly with a home therapeutic exercise program.

6. **Search for contraindications.**
   None is found. Recall that the application is over the posterior cervical area, not over the anterior cervical area, where it is contraindicated.

7. **Search for risks and precautions.**
   None is found. Because this patient is diagnosed with a heart condition, the clinician should take the necessary time to explain the use of electrical current as a treatment, and thus decrease the level of anxiety the patient may have, considering that electricity will pass through the back of his neck.

8. **Outline the therapeutic goal(s) you and your patient wish to achieve.**
   - Decrease neck pain
   - Improve head rotation

9. **List outcome measurement(s) used to assess treatment effectiveness.**
   - Pain: Short-Form McGill Pain Questionnaire (SF-MPQ)
   - Head ROM: goniometry (CROM—cervical range of motion)
   - Ability to bowl/drive: Patient-Specific Functional Scale (PSF)

10. **Advise patient about what he/she should experience, do, and not do during the treatment session.**
    - Mild sensation of heat under the electrodes
    - Weak-to-moderate neck muscle contraction

11. **Outline your therapeutic prescription based on the best sources of evidence available**
    Considering the serious lack of scientific evidence behind this EPA (**Box 19-1**), the following prescription is empirically based on and is in keeping with Bernard's (1950) empirical dosimetric approach.
    - ***Diadynamic stimulator type:*** cabinet
    - ***Electrode type and size:*** carbon rubber—2.5 × 2.5 cm (1 × 1 in)
    - ***Total number of electrodes used:*** 4 (2 pairs)
    - ***Coupling medium:*** electroconductive gel

(Continued)

Case Study 19-1   Continued

- **Electrode fixation:** precut tape patches
- **Electrode arrangements:**
  - **First pair:** over left and right upper cervical muscle
  - **Second pair:** over left and right upper trapezius muscle
- **DC current:** 2 mA for a period of 400 sec
- **Diadynamic waveforms applied consecutively after DC application:**
  - DF: 30 mA for 100 sec
  - CP: 25 mA for 90 sec
  - RS: 40 mA for 120 sec
- **Total number of treatments:** 10 treatments, delivered over two periods of 5 days, each separated by a weekend.

12. Collect outcome measurements.

Pre- and posttreatment comparison:

- Pain:
  - Sensory score decreased by 50%
  - Affective score decreased by 45%
  - Intensity score decreased by 60%
- Head rotation: gain of 15 degrees on both sides— 5 degrees bilateral deficit
- Ability to drive: increased PSFS score by 65%

13. Assess therapeutic effectiveness based on outcome measures.

The results show that 10 consecutive treatments of diadynamic current therapy over a 2-week period, combined with a home-based active neck exercise program, led to an increase in head rotation and a decrease of neck pain. The patient now feels more confident driving his car as reflected in the PSFS score. He is much less worried about his work. He is happy that his condition improved without having to take the drug treatment proposed by his physician. Overall, this treatment had a beneficial impact on the *patient's disablement status* created by the pathology, as illustrated in the **figure below.**

14. State the prognosis.

The pain-spasm cycle observed in this patient should gradually disappear over the next few days if the patient continues his home exercise program. Meanwhile, he is advised to move his head, within the limit of pain, daily. He is also advised to gradually increase the amount of time he spends driving, and to gradually return to bowling.

THERAPEUTIC IMPACT on Disablement

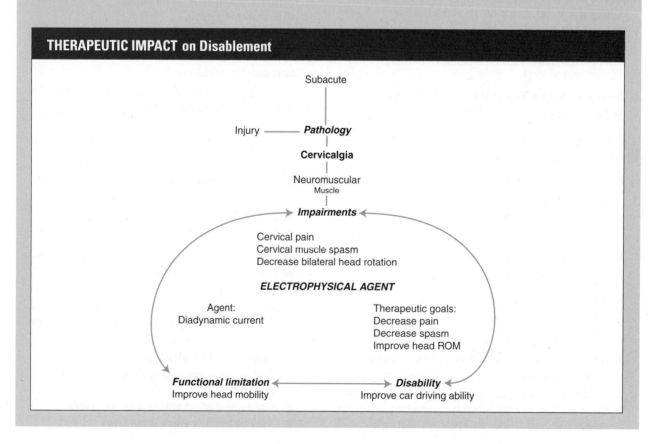

CRITICAL THINKING QUESTIONS

Clarification: What is meant by diadynamic current therapy?

Assumptions: You have assumed that the application of diadynamic current waveforms is effective in modulating pain. How do you justify making that assumption?

Reasons and evidence: What led you to believe that diadynamic current is capable of depolarizing sensory and motor nerve fibers?

Viewpoints or perspectives: How would you respond to a colleague who says that the use of diadynamic current is still justified today for the treatment of soft-tissue pathologies?

Implications and consequences: What are the implications of an electrophysical agent, such as diadynamic current therapy, presenting an extreme lack of scientific evidence in the practice of health care today?

About the question: How much scientific evidence is needed before a therapeutic treatment or agent is justifiable in the actual context of health-care delivery? Why do you think I ask this question?

References

Articles

Can F, Tandoan R, Yilman I, Dolunay E, Erden Z (2003) Rehabilitation of patellofemoral pain syndrome: TENS versus diadynamic current therapy for pain relief. The Pain Clinic, 15: 61–68

Hamalainen O, Kemppainen P (1990) Experimentally induced ischemic pain and so-called diaphase fix current. Scand J Rehab Med, 22: 25–27

Theron EJ, Vermeulen AM (1983) The utilization of transcutaneous nerve stimulation in postoperative ileus. S Afr Med J, 63: 971–972

Chapters of Textbooks

Rennie S (1988) Diadynamic current therapy. In: Current Physical Therapy. Peat M (Ed). BC Decker, Philadelphia, pp 207–211

Wadsworth H, Chanmugan APP (1988) Diadynamic currents. In: Electrophysical Agents in Physiotherapy, 2nd ed. Science Press, Marrickville, pp 268–270

Sections in Textbook Chapters

Low J, Reed A (1990) Nerve and muscle stimulation. In: Electrotherapy Explained: Principles and Practice. Butterworth Heinemann, London, pp 82–84

Robinson AJ (2008) Instrumentation for Electrotherapy. In: Clinical Electrophysiology: Electrotherapy and Electrophysiologic Testing, 3rd ed. Robinson AJ, Snyder-Mackler L (Eds). Lippincott Williams & Wilkins, Philadelphia, pp 58–59

Textbook

Bernard PA (1950) La Therapie Diadynamique. Les Editions Naim, Paris

Ultrasound Therapy

Chapter Outline

Learning Objectives

Knowledge: Define and describe ultrasound (US) and its conventional, LIPUS, and MIST types of therapy.

Comprehension: Compare the biophysical parameters associated with the delivery of conventional versus LIPUS therapy.

Application: Explain dosimetric calculations, delivery modes, and application techniques for both conventional and LIPUS therapy.

Analysis: Explain the thermal and mechanical effects associated with US therapy.

Synthesis: Explain the difference between conventional and LIPUS therapy.

Evaluation: Discuss the body of English-language, scientific evidence supporting the use of conventional, LIPUS, and MIST therapy.

I. RATIONALE FOR USE

A. DEFINITION AND DESCRIPTION

The term *ultrasound*, designated by the acronym US, is broadly defined as acoustic or mechanical energy travelling through a medium at frequencies above the limit of human hearing. *Ultrasound* is described as ultrasonic pressure or mechanical or acoustic waves at frequencies beyond the upper limit of human audibility, which is measured to be approximately 20,000 Hz (Leighton, 2007; O'Brien, 2007; ter Harr, 2007).

B. THERAPEUTIC ULTRASOUND

The field of US therapy refers to the use of mechanical energy delivered for the purpose of treating a variety of soft-tissue pathologies, including bone fractures and wounds. More specifically, US therapy used today in the field of physical medicine and rehabilitation may be classified,

as shown in **Table 20-1**, into three *types*: Conventional, low-intensity pulsed US (LIPUS), and MIST therapy.

C. CONVENTIONAL THERAPY

Introduced in the early 1950s, this first type, labeled as *conventional* in this chapter because it is the oldest and most traditional therapeutic type used in the world today, is characterized by ultrasonic energy delivered at high frequency (1–3 MHz) and intensity (0.1–3 W/cm²). Acoustic energy is delivered to soft tissues with a movable (dynamic) applicator, which makes contact with the skin on the area being treated, through a coupling medium—ultrasonic gel. In the noncontact method tap water is used as the coupling medium. The proposed physiological and therapeutic effects of this type of US therapy are mechanical and thermal in nature. Conventional US therapy is used for the treatment of a wide variety of soft-tissue pathologies, with the exception of bone fractures (**Table 20-1**).

TABLE 20-1	SPECTRUM OF THERAPEUTIC ULTRASOUND		
CHARACTERISTIC		**TYPE**	
	CONVENTIONAL	**LIPUS**	**MIST**
Frequency	1–3 MHz	1–1.5 MHz	40 KHz
Intensity	0.1–3 W/cm²	0.03 mW/cm²	0.1–0.8 W/cm²
Application method	Contact/noncontact	Contact/noncontact	Noncontact
Application technique	Dynamic	Stationary	Dynamic
Coupling agent	Gel/tap water	Gel	Saline water
Effect	Mechanical/thermal	Mechanical	Mechanical
Usage	Soft-tissue pathology	Bone fracture	Open wound

D. LIPUS THERAPY

Introduced in the 1980s, the second type, labeled as *low-intensity pulsed US*, or LIPUS, is characterized by ultrasonic energy delivered at a lower frequency (1–1.5 MHz) and at much lower intensity (0.03 mW/cm^2), producing only mechanical effect. The therapy is provided using a stationary applicator, which makes contact with the skin surface overlying the bone fracture site. Ultrasonic gel is required as the coupling medium. When used in in-cast or over-cast applications, the noncontact method is employed. LIPUS therapy is used for the treatment of fresh and slow-to-heal bone fractures (**Table 20-1**)

E. MIST THERAPY

First introduced in the early 2000s, this third and most recent type of US therapy, commercialized under the brand name *MIST therapy system*®, is characterized by ultrasonic energy delivered at a much lower frequency (40 KHz) than for the previous two types, with an intensity in the middle range. This system uses sterile saline water contained in a bottle as the coupling medium. It is applied in a dynamic fashion (with treatment head movements over the wound) and by the noncontact mode. In other words, this system creates US waves that produce and propel a gentle mist of sterile saline water to the wound bed. This mist facilitates the transfer of ultrasonic energy to the wound bed without direct contact. MIST therapy is used to promote wound healing through wound cleansing, debridement, and antibacterial effect. More precisely, MIST therapy is indicated for wound cleaning, and debridement of wounds containing yellow slough, fibrin, tissue exudates, or bacteria, the removal of which is important for the healing process (**Table 20-1**).

F. ULTRASOUND DEVICES

Presented in **Figure 20-1** are typical therapeutic US devices used worldwide to deliver US therapy. Shown in

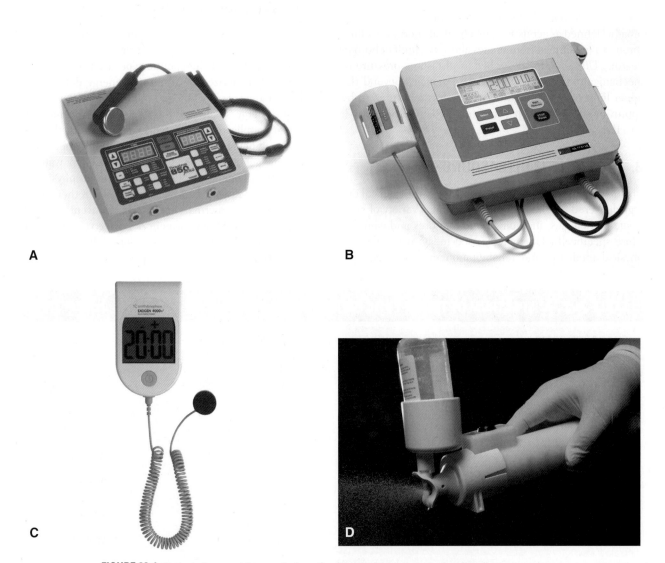

A

B

C

D

FIGURE 20-1 Typical ultrasound therapy devices. Conventional devices and related applicators (**A**, **B**); low-intensity pulsed ultrasound (LIPUS) device (**C**), and MIST therapy system (**D**). (A: Courtesy of Dynatronics; B: Courtesy of Rich-Mar; C: Courtesy of Smith & Nephew Inc.; D: Courtesy of Celleration.)

A and **B** are line-powered conventional devices made of an electrical generator to which is attached a manually operated (**A**) or automated, hands-free (**B**) applicator. The piezoelectric transducer is housed in the applicator. Shown in **C** is a typical battery-powered portable LIPUS device with its applicator, which may be applied in-cast, on-cast, or directly on the skin overlying the bone fracture site using a specially designed assembly system. Illustrated in **D** is a MIST therapy system, which consists of an electrical generator (not shown) and its applicator or treatment head. The handheld treatment head houses the piezoelectric transducer and is made of an applicator assembly holding a sterile saline water bottle. Finger pressure on the US control button of the treatment head releases an ultrasonic flow of mist water over the wound.

G. ACCESSORIES

Different accessories are needed to deliver these types of US therapy. Shown in **Figure 20-2** are common accessories used for the delivery of conventional US therapy.

1. Conventional

This type of therapy requires an ultrasonic coupling gel (**A**) between the applicator and the skin overlying the treatment area. This gel may be spread directly on the skin by squeezing it from a plastic bottle (**A**, **right**). A larger flexible gel container (**A**, **left**) is used to refill the bottle when empty. The ultrasonic gel may also be kept in a sealed pad (**B**) that is positioned between the applicator and the skin overlying the treatment area. When there

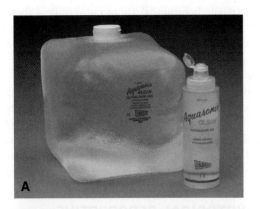
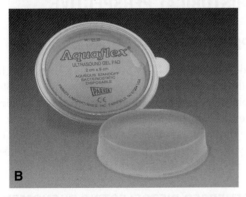
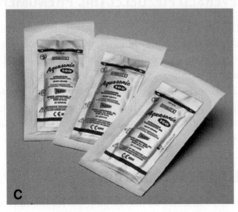
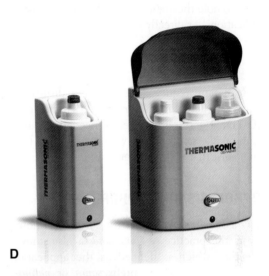
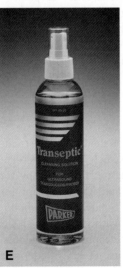

FIGURE 20-2 Typical accessories used with conventional devices: (**A**) ultrasonic gel bottles and dispensers; (**B**) disposable gel pad; (**C**) disposable gel sterile pouches; (**D**) gel bottle warmer; (**E**) soundhead cleansing solution. (Courtesy of Parker Laboratories Inc.)

is risk of infection, sterile ultrasonic gel may be used (**C**). The gel temperature may be kept constant using a bottle warmer (**D**). To minimize the risk of cross-infection from using the same applicator for several patients (conventional and LIPUS therapy), applicators must be cleansed with an antimicrobial solution (**E**) after each application. A common commercial plastic water bath is also needed if the water immersion technique of application is used.

2. LIPUS

This type of therapy also requires ultrasonic gel between the applicator and the skin overlying the fracture site, in addition to a retaining and alignment fixture/snap-on cap/strap assembly system (see manufacturer's Web site for details—for example, www.celleration.com). Such a system is needed to hold the applicator in place for in-cast or on-cast applications, or directly over the skin area overlying the bone fracture site.

3. MIST

This type of therapy requires the use of a disposable applicator and sterile saline water bottle, as shown in **Figure 20-1D**. No ultrasonic gel is needed because the applicator makes no contact with the wound bed; it is the water mist that makes direct contact with it.

H. SONOPHORESIS/PHONOPHORESIS

Traditionally associated with the use of conventional US therapy is the practice of *sonophoresis*, also known as *phonophoresis*, which is defined as the application of acoustic energy (hence the prefix *sono-* or *phono-*) for the transfer (*phoresis*) of drug ions through the skin for therapeutic purposes. In other words, sonophoresis (phonophoresis) is a form of drug iontophoresis (Chapter 13), where acoustic energy is substituted for electrical energy.

I. SCOPE OF CHAPTER

This chapter covers conventional US therapy for the treatment of pathologies in soft tissues such as tendons, ligaments, joint capsules, and muscles; LIPUS therapy for the treatment of bone fractures; and MIST therapy for the treatment of open wounds. Sonophoresis (phonophoresis), traditionally associated with conventional US therapy, is *beyond the scope* of this chapter. The evidence today points to the fact that the use of US frequencies much lower than (less than 100 KHz) and well above (up to 16 MHz) frequencies used in conventional US therapy (i.e., 1 and 3 MHz) may be more effective in enhancing drug uptake (see **Table 20-1**). To learn more about sonophoresis/phonophoresis, readers are requested to refer to the following articles: Mitragori et al., 2004; Vranic, 2004; Lavon et al., 2004; Mitragori, 2005, ter Haar, 2007; and Saliba et al., 2007.

J. CLINICAL USAGE

Surveys on the use of therapeutic electrophysical agents (EPAs) in physical medicine and rehabilitation, conducted in several countries (United States, Canada, England, Australia, and the Netherlands), have all concluded that conventional US therapy is by far the most widely used EPA (ter Harr et al., 1988; Robinson et al., 1988; Lindsay et al., 1990, Lindsay et al., 1995; Robertson et al., 1998; Roebroeck et al., 1998; Nussbaum et al., 2007; Wong et al., 2007). LIPUS and MIST therapy are, however, used more frequently today (see References) as there is an expanding body of evidence showing therapeutic benefits for the management of bone fractures and wounds with these therapies.

K. RATIONALE FOR USE

The rationale behind the use of conventional therapeutic US is to induce thermal and mechanical effects in pathological soft tissues, particularly in tissues rich in proteins, such as tendons, ligaments, joint capsules, and muscles, while inducing minimal effect on the overlying skin and subcutaneous tissues. The rationale for LIPUS therapy, on the other hand, is to promote and accelerate bone growth, through its mechanical effects, in cases of fresh and slow-to-heal bone fractures. Finally, the rationale for MIST therapy is to facilitate wound debridement through its mechanical effect, and thus promote wound healing.

II. HISTORICAL PERSPECTIVE

A. PIEZOELECTRIC PHENOMENON

The development of US waves as a means to treat human disorders dates back to the discovery, in the 1880s, of the piezoelectric phenomenon by two French scientists, Pierre and Paul-Jacques Curie. This phenomenon refers to the development of electrical energy on certain natural and synthetic crystals by applying mechanical pressure on them (O'Brien, 2007).

B. REVERSED PIEZOELECTRIC PHENOMENON

In 1910, another French scientist, Paul Langevin, discovered the reverse piezoelectric phenomenon. This phenomenon refers to the development of mechanical energy on these crystals by applying electrical energy across them (O'Brien, 2007). This discovery is the fundamental biophysical principle behind the manufacture of modern therapeutic and industrial US devices (see Section III, Biophysical Characteristics).

C. CLINICAL FOUNDATION

The basic foundation of therapeutic US for humans was laid down in the early 1950s at the first symposium on Ultrasound in Biology and Medicine (O'Brien, 2007). This period coincides with the first use of conventional US therapy.

1. First Application of Conventional Therapy

The work of Justus Lehmann and colleagues, in the early 1960s, led to the use of conventional US, through its heating and mechanical effects, for the treatment of soft tissues, such as tendons, ligament, joint capsules, and muscles (Lehmann et al., 1990).

2. First Application of LIPUS Therapy

The use of LIPUS for treating bone fractures originated in the early 1980s from the pioneering work of Duarte on animals (Duarte, 1983). Xavier and Duarte (1983) are recognized as the authors of the first study dealing with the application of LIPUS to human bone fractures. Other applications of LIPUS for the treatment of fresh and difficult-to-heal fractures in humans followed in the 1990s (Warden, 2003; Claes et al., 2007).

3. First Application of MIST Therapy

The use of MIST for treating open wounds originated in the early 2000s from the studies of Ennis et al. on humans (2005, 2006).

D. BODY OF LITERATURE

Over the past two decades, US therapy has been the topic of numerous *articles* (see References), *review articles* (Dyson, 1987; Falconer et al., 1990; Kitchen et al., 1990a,b; Gam, 1991; Holmes et al., 1991; Hayes, 1992; Maxwell, 1992; Cole et al., 1994; Gam et al., 1995; Nussbaum, 1997, 1998; Hadjiargyrou et al., 1998; van der Windt et al., 1999; Baker et al., 2001; Robertson et al., 2001; Rubin et al., 2001; Busse et al., 2002; Robertson, 2002; Warden, 2003; Babba-Akbari et al., 2006; Kimmel, 2006; Malizos et al., 2006; Claes et al., 2007; Leighton, 2007; O'Brien, 2007; ter Harr, 2007; Walker et al., 2007), and *chapters in textbooks* (Dunn et al., 1990; Frizzell et al., 1990; Lehmann et al., 1990; Low et al., 1990, 1994; Dyson, 1995; McDiarmid et al., 1996; ter Haar, 1996; Hayes, 2000; Khan, 2000; Draper et al., 2002; Young, 2002; Cameron, 2003; Starkey, 2004a,b; Sparrow, 2005; Nussbaum et al., 2006; Sweitzer, 2006; Knight et al., 2008).

III. BIOPHYSICAL CHARACTERISTICS

A. ACOUSTIC WAVE FORMATION

Figure 20-3 illustrates the formation of an ultrasonic beam of energy, characterized by mechanical waves, based on the reverse piezoelectric phenomenon.

1. Reverse Piezoelectric Phenomenon

This phenomenon states that when a high-frequency, alternating electrical current (AC) is applied to the surface of a piezoelectric material or crystal, called a *transducer*, mechanical deformations of this transducer follow in the

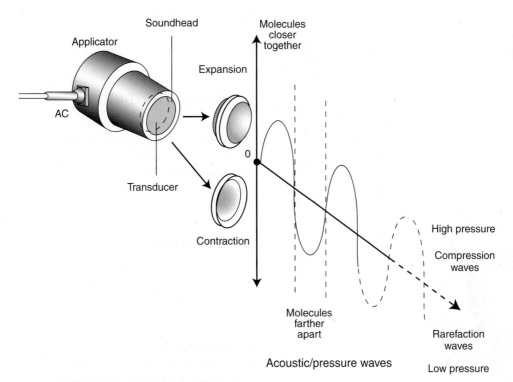

FIGURE 20-3 Production of an ultrasonic beam. Applying a high-frequency alternating current (AC) to the piezoelectric transducer, housed in the applicator and bound to the soundhead faceplate, causes it to expand and contract, thus creating cycles of compression waves (during expansion) and rarefaction waves (during contraction) directed at the tissues. Compression waves are high-pressure waves that push molecules closer together, whereas rarefaction waves are low-pressure waves that allow molecules to move farther apart.

form of oscillations, or cycles of expansion and contraction, of this material.

2. Acoustic/Mechanical/Pressure Waves

These repeated cycles of micro-expansion and micro-contraction of the transducer create the ultrasonic beam of energy seen as acoustic, mechanical, or pressure waves with a sinusoidal shape, traveling in time in a medium (**Fig 20-3**).

3. Compression/Rarefaction

During the expansion phase of the transducer, high pressure develops in the soft tissues, bringing molecules closer together. During the contraction phase, however, low pressure develops, which sends molecules farther apart (**Fig 20-3**).

B. ULTRASONIC BEAM

The schematic in **Figure 20-4** is an upper and lateral view of an ultrasonic beam emitted from a typical therapeutic applicator. The *applicator* is made of two parts: *transducer* and *soundhead*. The *transducer* is a natural or synthetic piezoelectric crystal embedded into the applicator. The transducer converts electrical energy applied

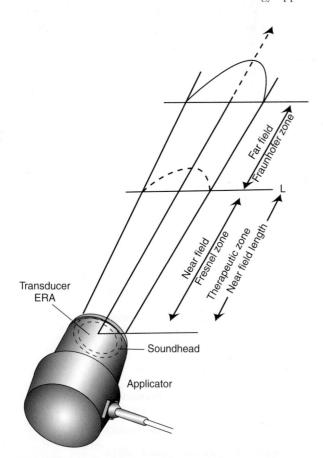

FIGURE 20-4 An ultrasonic beam emitted from the soundhead. Shown are the near field (Fresnel zone) and the far field (Fraunhofer zone). Note that the intensity of the ultrasonic beam is much more focused in the near field than in the far field.

against the crystal into mechanical or acoustic energy. The *soundhead*, on the other hand, is the metal plate, or faceplate, attached to the transducer; it is often called the applicator's faceplate. The soundhead's role is to transfer the acoustic energy from the transducer to soft tissues.

1. Near Field Versus Far Field

The ultrasonic beam region closest to the transducer faceplate is termed the *near field* or *Fresnel zone*. The region that immediately follows is termed the *far field* or *Fraunhofer zone* (Frizzell et al., 1990). Biophysics has shown that the near field corresponds to the less divergent, or more focused, region of the beam emitted from the soundhead or faceplate. The far field, in contrast, corresponds to the more divergent, or less focused, region of the beam (**Fig 20-4**).

2. Near-Field Length

The length (L) of the near field, relative to the soundhead faceplate, corresponds to the boundary line separating these two fields or zones (**Fig 20-4**). This length (L) is directly related to the squared radius (r^2) of the transducer's effective radiating area (ERA) and is inversely related to the ultrasonic beam's wavelength ($L = r^2/wavelength$; ter Haar, 1996). Acoustic waves travel in aqueous media (e.g., gel, water, human tissues) at a speed (C) of approximately 1500 m/s. For example, the near-field length (L) of an ultrasonic beam emitted at 1 MHz from a transducer ERA of 10 cm^2 is 21.1 cm. This value is calculated as follows: First, wavelength (0.15 cm) = C (1500 m/s) ÷ frequency (1,000,000). Second, the radius of a 10 cm^2 circular transducer is 1.78 cm. Third, $L = (1.78^2/0.15) = 21.1$ cm.

C. THERAPEUTIC ZONE

The near field or Fresnel zone is recognized as the region of the ultrasonic beam where the therapeutic effects occur in the tissues, because the distances separating the piezoelectric transducer from the targeted tissues, in most applications, are well within the length (L) of the near field (Lowe et al., 1990; ter Haar, 1996).

D. DELIVERY MODE

Practitioners may select, for conventional therapy, from two delivery modes: *continuous* or *pulsed*. LIPUS devices offer only the pulsed mode, while MIST devices offer only the continuous mode.

1. Continuous Mode

This mode refers to the continuous, or uninterrupted, flow of acoustic energy during the whole treatment duration.

2. Pulsed Mode

This mode refers to the periodic interruption, or rhythmic flow, of acoustic energy. US energy is delivered for a given duration (ON time), followed by a period of no delivery (OFF time).

a. Pulse Frequency

The pulse frequency is the frequency with which ultrasonic pulses are delivered and is calculated as follows: f = 1/ON time + OFF time. For example, a pulsation frequency of 1000 Hz will result from the combination of an ON time of 0.2 ms and an OFF time of 0.8 ms (1000 Hz = 1000/0.2 + 0.8). This mode is further characterized by the expression and calculation of a parameter called the duty cycle.

b. Duty Cycle

The duty cycle is the period of time, measured in percentage, during which the acoustic energy is delivered. Duty cycle is calculated using the following formula: Duty cycle (%) = (ON time / ON time + OFF time) $\times$ 100.

c. Preset Duty Cycle

Most conventional US devices are equipped with a range of preset duty cycles ranging between 10% and 50%. Where a duty cycle of 20%, for example, is selected, it means that ultrasonic acoustic energy is being delivered for a period equivalent to 20% of the total treatment duration. In other words, if the total treatment duration is 6 minutes, acoustic energy is being delivered for a total of 1.2 minutes only (1.2 min = 6 min $\times$ 20%), which is equivalent to 1/5, or 20%, of the total application duration.

E. TRANSDUCER ERA

A US applicator is made of two parts: transducer (piezoelectric crystal) and soundhead (steel plate attached to the transducer faceplate). The term effective radiating area (ERA) refers to the surface or area, measured in square centimeters, of the transducer faceplate over which the ultrasonic beam is generated. This surface area is always smaller than the faceplate area and varies in size.

F. INTENSITY

Intensity is the amount of acoustic power, measured in watts (W), delivered through the transducer ERA, measured in square centimeters, used to deliver this energy to the tissues. Intensity (I) is thus measured in watts per square centimeter (W/cm^2). Because US energy can be delivered using transducers with different ERAs (space), in both continuous and pulsed modes (time), the concept of intensity must be clarified further in relation to these two elements. The terms *spatial* and *temporal* are thus used to describe US intensity in terms of space and time, respectively.

1. Spatial

The term *spatial* describes acoustic intensity in relation to space, that is, in relation to the transducer ERA. Biophysics has shown that the beam of intensity delivered at the transducer faceplate is irregular or nonuniform, meaning that the intensity is greater in the center than at the edges of the transducer, as illustrated in **Figure 20-5** (Dunn et al., 1990; Frizzell et al., 1990; Lehmann et al., 1990). This implies that both spatial average intensity (I_{SA}) and spatial peak intensity (I_{SP}) should be defined and taken into consideration to determine the ultrasonic beam nonuniformity ratio, or BNR (see Section III G).

a. Spatial Peak Intensity (I_{SP})

This measurement represents the maximum intensity output, as illustrated in **Figure 20-5**, delivered over the transducer faceplate ERA.

b. Spatial Average Intensity (I_{SA})

This measurement represents the average intensity output delivered over the transducer ERA. For example, a power output of 8 W delivered through a transducer with an ERA of 5 cm^2 will give an I_{SA} of 1.6 W/cm^2 (1.6 W/cm^2 = 8 W/5 cm^2).

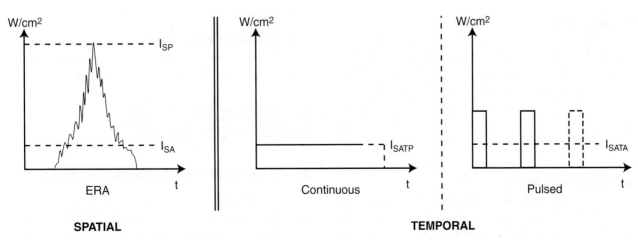

FIGURE 20-5 Spatial and temporal concept of ultrasound intensity.

2. Temporal

The term, *temporal,* describes acoustic intensity in relation to time, that is, in relation to the modes of delivery used (continuous vs. pulse mode), as illustrated in **Figure 20-5**.

a. Spatial Average Temporal Peak Intensity (I_{SATP})

This term refers to the peak intensity output, expressed in W/cm^2, delivered during the ON time of the pulse, and is restricted to the continuous mode. Because the ON time is maximal when using this delivery mode (there is no OFF time), I_{SATP} corresponds to the peak intensity output delivered by the device during the entire treatment duration. In other words, I_{SATP} corresponds to I_{SP}.

b. Spatial Average Temporal Average Intensity (I_{SATA})

This term is used to express the average intensity output delivered when the pulsed mode is used. Because there is an OFF time in between the ON time of each pulse, the intensity output is averaged out over time. I_{SATA} is calculated by taking the I_{SATP} times the duty cycle, expressed in percentage. For example, the spatial average temporal average intensity output (I_{SATA}) delivered using an I_{SATP} of 1.5 W/cm^2, combined with a duty cycle of 30%, equals 0.45 W/cm^2.

c. Two Meanings for "Peak"

Readers may easily be confused by the term *peak,* as it is used in two ways. The first relates to the concept of space (surface area); the second relates to the concept of time (continuous or pulsed mode). In other words, the initial use of peak is synonymous with the maximum crest intensity, whereas the second is to differentiate between peak (continuous) and average (pulsed) intensity.

G. BEAM NONUNIFORMITY RATIO

The nonuniformity of the ultrasonic beam intensity is measured as the beam nonuniformity ratio, or BNR. **Figure 20-6** shows this nonuniformity of acoustic intensity within the near field.

1. Calculation

The BNR is calculated as the ratio of the spatial peak intensity (I_{SP}), which corresponds to the highest peak intensity, to the spatial average intensity (I_{SA}) of all peaks, which is normalized to unity, or 1 as shown in **Figure 20-6** . For example, a BNR value of 5, also expressed as 5:1, means that the spatial peak intensity generated by the device is 5 times larger than the spatial average intensity (5 = 5 W/cm² / 1 W/cm²).

2. Transducer's Quality

The BNR is determined by the intrinsic biophysical properties of the piezoelectric transducer. The higher the piezoelectric quality of the transducer, the more uniform the beam intensity across its ERA, and the lower its BNR

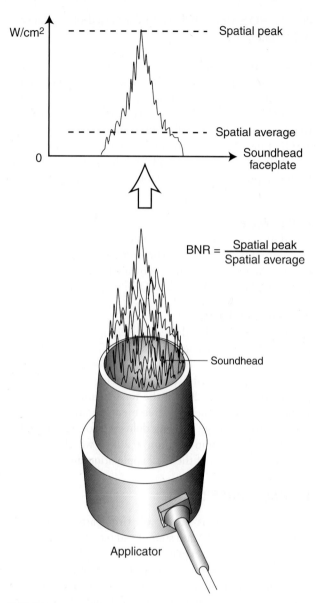

FIGURE 20-6 Ultrasonic beam nonuniformity ratio.

value. This means that the quality of an US device depends, above all, on the biophysical quality of its piezoelectric transducer.

3. BNR Recommended Values

There is a consensus that the BNR values found on therapeutic US devices should range between 2 and 8.

IV. PHYSIOLOGICAL AND THERAPEUTIC EFFECTS

A. THERMAL VERSUS MECHANICAL EFFECTS

Shown in **Figure 20–7** are the proposed physiological and therapeutic effects of conventional, LIPUS, and MIST therapeutic US. Biophysics has shown that acoustic energy can be induced in human soft tissues, including bones,

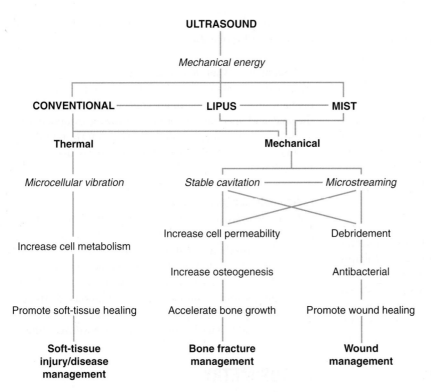

FIGURE 20-7 Proposed physiological and therapeutic effects of ultrasound therapy.

triggering thermal as well as mechanical (or nonthermal), physiological, and therapeutic effects (see Baker et al., 2001; Robertson et al., 2001; Robertson, 2002; Warden, 2003; Cleas et al., 2007). Research has shown that the physiological and therapeutic effects behind conventional US may be both thermal and mechanical in nature, while those attributed to LIPUS and MIST are only mechanical in nature.

B. THERMAL EFFECT

When acoustic energy is absorbed as it penetrates soft tissues, molecules are caused to vibrate under repeated cycles of compression waves (i.e., molecules moving closer together) and rarefaction waves (i.e., molecules moving farther apart). The higher the intensity of the ultrasonic beam and the more continuous the emission of acoustic waves are, the more vigorous the molecular vibration or kinetic energy. The more intense the molecular vibration is, the more vigorous the resulting microfriction between those millions of irradiated molecules. The more vigorous the microfriction is, the more frictional heat generated in the tissue (Dyson, 1987, 1995). Tissue heating is presumed to enhance tissue cell metabolism, which in turn is believed to promote soft-tissue healing.

1. Heating Depth

Research has shown that the application of conventional US energy, especially at 1 MHz, and using the continuous mode, can produce thermal effect to a depth of approximately 5 cm (2.5 in) in soft tissues (see Gallo et al., 2004; Morrisette et al., 2004).

2. Lumbar Area

A study by Morrissette et al. (2004) on healthy adult subjects has shown that a continuous 1-MHz US application over the lumbar zygapophyseal joints lead to a joint temperature elevation of approximately 3°C.

C. MECHANICAL EFFECTS

The mechanical, or nonthermal, effects induced in soft tissues by US therapy are attributed, as shown in **Figure 20-7**, to two interrelated biophysical phenomena: stable cavitation and microstreaming (Kimmel, 2006; O'Brien, 2007).

1. Cavitation

The word *cavitation* is derived from the Latin word *cavus*, meaning hollow, and refers to the formation, in fluids or solids, of empty spaces or cavities resulting from the formation of microbubbles.

2. Acoustic Cavitation

This phenomenon, triggered by the absorption of acoustic energy, begins when minute gas pockets that infiltrate most biological fluids, termed nuclei, develop into microscopic bubbles, thus causing cavities in these fluids and the surrounding soft tissues. Under the sustained influence of acoustic radiation, these microscopic bubbles expand and contract (pulsate or oscillate) at the same carrier frequency at which the acoustic waves are produced.

3. Acoustic Cavitation Type

Depending on the frequency and intensity level of these acoustic waves, two types of cavitation can occur in soft tissues: *stable* or *unstable cavitation.*

a. Stable Cavitation

This phenomenon occurs when the bubbles begin to pulsate, that is, compress during the high-pressure waves and expand during the low-pressure waves. Stable cavitation triggers molecular motion, and the molecules move closer together during the compression phase and farther apart during the rarefaction phase of the acoustic waves.

b. Unstable Cavitation

This phenomenon occurs when the bubbles, subjected to strong cycles of compression and expansion, collapse or implode, releasing very high temperature and pressure changes in their vicinity, in the fluid. Biophysics has shown that therapeutic US devices do not have the energy output, or carrier frequency, necessary to produce unstable cavitation; therefore this response should pose no therapeutic concern.

c. Microstreaming

This phenomenon, characterized by a minute flow of fluid in the vicinity of the pulsating bubbles, is triggered by stable cavitation, as shown in **Figure 20-7.**

d. Therapeutic Effects

Together, stable cavitation and microstreaming are presumed to cause mechanical, or nonthermal, therapeutic effects within soft tissues, promoting wound healing and accelerating bone growth through increased osteogenesis as shown in **Figure 20-7.**

e. Concomitant Therapeutic Effects

Although the physiological and therapeutic effects of conventional US treatment are traditionally separated into thermal and mechanical effects, growing evidence suggests that both effects occur concomitantly, one dominating the other, depending on the dosimetry used (Baker et al., 2001).

f. Acoustic Energy Absorption

For physiological and therapeutic effects to occur, a percentage of the acoustic energy emitted at the applicator–skin interface must be absorbed by the targeted tissues. Biophysics has established that acoustic energy is better absorbed by tissues with high density, such as bone, and high protein content, such as tendons, cartilage, ligaments, and joint capsules (e.g., Draper et al., 2002; Cameron, 2003; Nussbaum et al., 2006; Sweitzer, 2006).

V. DOSIMETRY

A. PARAMETERS

Shown in **Table 20-2** are key biophysical parameters related to the dosimetry of conventional, LIPUS, and MIST therapy. These parameters are *frequency, delivery mode, transducer's ERA, intensity, application duration,* and *treatment frequency.*

TABLE 20-2	DOSIMETRIC PARAMETERS FOR ULTRASOUND THERAPY		
PARAMETERS	**CONVENTIONAL**	**LIPUS**	**MIST**
Frequency	1 MHz or 3 MHz	1.0–1.5 MHz	40 KHz
Delivery mode	Continuous or pulsed	Pulsed	Continuous
If pulse mode			
Frequency	Variable	100–1000 Hz	NA
ON time	Variable	Fixed: 0.2; 2 ms	NA
OFF time	Variable	Fixed: 0.8; 8 ms	NA
Duty cycle	Variable	Fixed: 20%	NA
Transducer ERA	1–5–10 cm^2	3–5 cm^2	1–2 cm^2
I_{SATP}	Variable: Up to 3 W/cm^2	NA	0.1–0.8 W/cm^2
I_{SATA}	Variable	0.03 mW/cm^2	NA
Application duration	5–10 min	15–20 min	5–10 min
Treatment frequency	Every second day	Daily	Daily

1. Frequency

Practitioners may select, for conventional therapy, from two frequency settings: *1 MHz* or *3 MHz*. The body of literature reviewed in this chapter suggests that ultrasonic energy emitted at 1 MHz penetrates soft tissues *deeper* than that emitted at 3 MHz. LIPUS devices may be set at 1 MHz or 1.5 MHz, while MIST devices usually emit at a preset frequency of 40 KHz.

2. Delivery Mode

For conventional therapy, practitioners may select from two delivery modes: *continuous* or *pulsed*. The continuous mode, for a given intensity, is preferred over the pulsed mode when thermal effect is needed. If the pulsed mode is selected, practitioners may select variable frequencies and ON and OFF times that will yield variable duty cycle values. For LIPUS therapy, only the pulsed mode is available. For each of the two frequencies available (100 or 1000 Hz), the ON and OFF times are preset, giving a fixed and preset duty of 20%. For MIST therapy, only the continuous mode is available.

3. Transducer ERA

It is important to differentiate between the transducer faceplate ERA and the soundhead faceplate area (**Figs 20-3** and **20-4**). Technically speaking, the transducer ERA of conventional US devices may be 10% to 20% smaller than the soundhead area. Unfortunately, not all manufacturers report both surface areas, which creates confusion in clinical practice because several practitioners are led to believe that the transducer ERA is the same as the soundhead faceplate area. Conventional US therapy is commonly delivered using one of three transducer ERAs, that is, 1, 5, or 10 cm^2 in size. Transducer ERA selection for LIPUS therapy may range between 3 and 5 cm^2. The transducer ERA of MIST device is fixed and may range between 1 and 2 cm^2. The selection of one transducer ERA rather than the other, for the application of conventional and LIPUS therapy, depends on the surface area (S) under treatment. The larger the treatment surface area is, the larger the transducer ERA.

4. Intensity

The ultrasonic beam intensity used to deliver conventional therapy is greater than the one used for MIST therapy, with LIPUS therapy delivered using the lowest intensity

5. Application Duration

The application duration per session, as listed in **Table 20-2**, is similar for conventional and MIST therapy (approximately 5–10 min) and about twice as long for LIPUS therapy (approximately 20 min).

6. Treatment Frequency

Unlike conventional therapy, which is commonly delivered every second day, both LIPUS and MIST therapy are applied on a daily basis (**Table 20-2**).

B. DOSIMETRIC CALCULATIONS EXAMPLES

Presented in **Table 20-3** are key parameters on which the dosimetry for US therapy is based. Also presented are

TABLE 20-3	EXAMPLES OF DOSIMETRIC CALCULATIONS FOR ULTRASOUND THERAPY			
PARAMETERS	**CONVENTIONAL**		**LIPUS**	**MIST**
	CONTINUOUS	**PULSED**	**PULSED**	**CONTINUOUS**
Power (P)	10 W	10 W	0.6 W	1 W
Transducer ERA	5 cm^2	5 cm^2	4 cm^2	2 cm^2
Treatment surface area (S)	10 cm^2	10 cm^2	1.5 cm^2	25 cm^2
Duty cycle	100%	20%	20%	NA
I_{SATP}	2 W/cm^2	NA	NA	0.5 W/cm^2
I_{SATA}	NA	0.4 W/cm^2	0.03 W/cm^2	NA
Application duration (T)	480 s	480 s	1200 s	360 s
Total energy (E_t)	4800 J	960 J	144 J	360 J
Therapeutic dose (D)	480 J/cm^2	96 J/cm^2	96 J/cm^2	14.4 J/cm^2

examples of calculation that distinguish between each of them. From the intensity (i.e., I_{SATP} or I_{SATA}) and the application duration (T), two other important parameters can be calculated: the total energy delivered by the device (E_t) and the actual therapeutic dose (D) or total energy delivered per square centimeter of tissue.

1. I_{SATP}

Spatial average temporal peak intensity is calculated by dividing power (P), measured in watts (W), by the transducer faceplate effective area (ERA), measured in cm^2.

2. I_{SATA}

Spatial average temporal average intensity is calculated by multiplying the spatial average temporal peak intensity (I_{SATP} or P/ERA) by the duty cycle, which is determined by the ON and OFF times, and is calculated as follows: duty cycle (%) = ON time / (ON time + OFF time) × 100.

3. Simplification

The terms I_{SATP} and I_{SATA} correspond to spatial peak and spatial average intensity, respectively. For the sake of simplifying the terminology, these two terms may be abbreviated as I_{SP} and I_{SA}, respectively.

4. Application Duration

This parameter corresponds to the absolute amount of time (T), measured in seconds, during which the treatment is delivered.

5. Total Energy (E_t)

This parameter or measurement refers to the total amount of acoustic energy, expressed in Joules (J), delivered under the transducer ERA during the application duration (T). It is calculated as follows: $\mathbf{E_t = I \times ERA \times S}$, where $J/cm^2 = (W/cm^2 \times cm^2) \times s$; J = W.s. For example, an E_t of 4800 J is calculated for conventional US therapy delivered using the continuous mode (480 J = 2 W/cm^2 × 5 cm^2 × 480 s).

6. Therapeutic Dose (D)

This parameter refers to the amount of acoustic energy delivered at the applicator–skin interface *per square centimeter of tissue*, and is thus measured in J/cm^2. The dose (D) takes into account the relationship between the total acoustic energy delivered at the transducer ERA, that is, E_t, and the treated surface area (S). It is calculated as follows: $\mathbf{D = E_t/S}$, where $J/cm^2 = J/cm^2$. In keeping with the above example, a D value of 480 J/cm^2 is calculated for the continuous mode.

C. CONCEPT OF DOSE

The concept of dose is, unfortunately, confusing to many clinicians and authors of textbooks on EPAs. Theoretically speaking, the therapeutic ultrasonic dose used to manage a given soft-tissue pathology refers to the amount of acoustic energy delivered, expressed in *Joules per square centimeter of tissue* (J/cm^2), at the transducer–skin interface. This dose, as shown in **Table 20-3**, depends on four parameters: intensity, application duration, transducer ERA, and the treatment surface area.

1. Confusion

According to current practice the concept of dose is often limited to only two parameters: intensity and application duration. If only these two parameters—for example, *2 W/cm² SATP for 8 minutes*—are considered, it simply means that a total of 980 J/cm^2 of acoustic energy is delivered per transducer square centimeter (2 W/cm^2 × 480 s) during treatment. It does not inform clinicians about the therapeutic dose delivered to the *tissues*, that is, the total amount of energy per square centimeter of tissue which corresponds to 480 J/cm^2. Failure to account for the treatment surface area (S) in determining therapeutic dose is *misleading*.

2. Recommendation

Biophysics has established that the physiological and therapeutic effects of US treatment applied on soft tissues are caused by the amount of acoustic energy absorbed by the tissues. Consequently, it is *strongly recommended* that the therapeutic US dose, for both conventional and LIPUS therapy, be expressed in *units of energy per square centimeter of tissue* (J/cm^2), as illustrated in **Table 20-3**, and not in terms of the intensity (W/cm^2) delivered per square centimeter of soundhead ERA for the duration of the application.

VI. EVIDENCE FOR INDICATIONS

A. GUIDED BY EVIDENCE

Dictionaries generally define *evidence* as anything that establishes a fact or gives reason to believe something. The aim of this textbook is to present scientific evidence behind therapeutic EPAs. To be guided by evidence is the process of integrating the evidence from research, however imperfect or scarce it may be, with clinical experience and the patient's wishes. In other words, the *evidence-based practice* of EPA requires that practitioners consider the evidence from research, in addition to their own clinical experience and the patient's own preference and beliefs about a given EPA, when the time comes to justify, prescribe, and apply the therapeutic agent. To be guided by evidence is a process, not a search for the ultimate truth. Finally, a lack of evidence from research in support of any given EPA does not mean that this EPA should never be used. What it means is that no statement can be made about its therapeutic effectiveness and that until more evidence from research is presented, its routine use cannot be recommended.

B. EVIDENCE FROM HUMAN RESEARCH

Box 20-1 provides evidence for conventional, LIPUS, and MIST US therapy based on an exhaustive search of published English-language, peer-reviewed studies on humans. The term *indication* is used in reference to a list of pathologies for which US therapy is employed. Ratings of therapeutic benefit (Yes or No) and the grading of scientific evidence (I, II, or III), including the reference, are included for each pathological condition.

1. Rating Therapeutic Benefit

The rating, expressed as Yes or No, is based on the overall conclusion(s) reached on the issue of therapeutic

effectiveness by the author(s) who conducted the peer-reviewed study.

2. Grading Strength of Evidence

The grading, numerically classified as I, II, and III, is based on the type of research methodology, or experimental design, used by the author(s). All those listed are studies on humans, published in English-language, peer-reviewed journals. It follows that the evidence in studies graded I is stronger than in those graded II, and the evidence in studies graded II is stronger than in those graded III.

a. Grade I

Evidence based on *controlled* studies on humans, regardless of their level of randomization and blindness.

Box 20-1	Research-Based Indications For the Use of Ultrasound Therapy		
PATHOLOGY	**BENEFIT**	**GRADE**	**REFERENCE**
CONVENTIONAL			
Shoulder disorders	Yes	I	Ebenbichler et al., 1999
	Yes	I	Munting, 1978
	Yes	II	Ebenbichler et al., 1997
	Yes	II	Aldes et al., 1954a
	Yes	II	Aldes et al., 1954b
	Yes	II	Cline, 1963
	Yes	II	Roden, 1952
	Yes	II	Grynbaum, 1954
	Yes	II	Flax, 1964
	Yes	II	Herrera-Lasso et al., 1993
	Yes	II	Shehab et al., 2000
	Yes	III	Bundt, 1958
	Yes	III	Bearzy, 1953
	Yes	III	Gorkiewicz, 1984
	No	I	Downing et al., 1986
	No	I	Ainsworth et al., 2007
	No	I	Perron et al., 1997
	No	I	Inaba et al., 1972
	No	II	Nykänen, 1995
	No	II	Hamer et al., 1976
Dermal ulcers	Yes	I	McDiarmid et al, 1985
	Yes	I	Callam et al., 1987
	Yes	I	Dyson et al., 1976
	Yes	I	Roche et al., 1984
	Yes	II	Nussbaum et al., 1994
	Yes	II	Paul et al., 1960
	No	I	Ericksson et al., 1991
	No	I	ter Riet et al., 1996
	No	II	Lundeberg et al., 1990

(Continued)

Box 20-1   **Continued**

PATHOLOGY	BENEFIT	GRADE	REFERENCE
Arthritic disorders	Yes	I	Huang et al., 2005
	Yes	II	Kazanoglu et al., 2003
	Yes	II	De Preux, 1952
	Yes	II	Svarcova et al., 1988
	Yes	II	Swartz, 1953
	Yes	II	Lehmann et al., 1954
	No	I	Falconer et al., 1992
	No	I	Mueller et al., 1954
	No	II	Aldes et al., 1952
Mix of soft-tissue disorders	Yes	II	Patrick, 1978
	Yes	II	Middlemast et al., 1978
	Yes	II	Soren, 1965
	Yes	II	Klaiman et al., 1998
	No	I	Roman, 1960
	No	I	Van der Heijden et al., 1999
Epicondylitis	Yes	I	Binder et al., 1985
	Yes	II	Aldes, 1956
	Yes	II	Davidson et al., 2001
	No	I	Haker et al., 1991
	No	II	Lundeberg et al., 1988
Perineal lesions	Yes	I	McLaren, 1984
	Yes	III	Fieldhouse, 1979
	No	I	Everett et al., 1992
	No	I	Creates, 1987
	No	I	Grant et al., 1989
Postexercise muscle soreness	No	I	Hasson et al., 1990
	No	I	Craig et al., 1999
	No	I	Stay et al., 1998
	No	I	Plaskett et al., 1999
	No	I	Brock Symons et al., 2004
Ankle sprain	Yes	II	Makuloluwe et al., 1977
	No	I	Williamson et al., 1986
	No	I	Nyanzi et al., 1999
	No	I	Zammit et al., 2005
Plantar warts	Yes	I	Cherup et al., 1963
	Yes	II	Vaughn, 1973
	Yes	II	Kent, 1959
Carpal tunnel syndrome	Yes	I	Ebenbichler et al., 1998
	Yes	II	Bakhtiary et al., 2004
	No	I	Ortas et al., 1998
Post-extraction dental pain	No	I	Hashish et al., 1986
	No	I	Hashish et al., 1988
Prolapsed intervertebral disc	Yes	I	Nwuga, 1983
	Yes	II	Aldes et al., 1958

(Continued)

Box 20-1 Continued

PATHOLOGY	BENEFIT	GRADE	REFERENCE
Herpes zoster	Yes	II	Garret et al., 1982
	Yes	II	Jones, 1984
Breast engorgement	No	I	McLachlan et al., 1991
Postherpetic neuralgia	Yes	II	Payne, 1984
Plantar fasciitis	Yes	II	Clarke et al., 1976
Tibial periostitis	Yes	II	Smith et al., 1986
Myofascial pain	Yes	II	Talaat et al. 1995
Tenosynovitis	Yes	II	Lanfear et al., 1972
Bicipital tendinitis	Yes	II	Echternach, 1965
Trigger points	No	I	Gam et al., 1998
Myofascial pain	Yes	II	Esenyel et al., 2000
Scar tissue	Yes	II	Bierman, 1954
Fibrotic muscles	No	I	Klemp et al., 1982
Dupuytren's contracture	Yes	III	Markham et al., 1980
Hip contracture	Yes	II	Lehmann et al., 1961
Phantom pain	Yes	II	Tepperberg et al., 1953
Reflex sympathetic dystrophy	Yes	III	Portwood et al., 1987
Surgical wounds	Yes	II	Ferguson, 1981
Neuroma and neurofibroma	Yes	II	Uygur et al., 1995
Post-hemiplegia spasticity	No	III	Ansari et al., 2006a
Low-back pain	Yes	I	Ansari et al., 2006b
Meniscus tear	Yes	III	Muche, 2003
Patellar tendinopathy	No	II	Stasinopoulos et al., 2004
Chronic maxillary and frontal sinusitis	Yes	II	Ansari et al., 2007

LIPUS

PATHOLOGY	BENEFIT	GRADE	REFERENCE
Bone fracture—fresh and delayed union cases	Yes	I	Heckman et al., 1994
	Yes	I	Kristiansen et al., 1997
	Yes	I	Leung et al., 2004

(Continued)

Box 20-1   Continued

PATHOLOGY	BENEFIT	GRADE	REFERENCE
	Yes	II	Xavier et al., 1983
	Yes	II	Mayr et al., 2000
	Yes	II	Cook et al., 1997
	Yes	II	Gebauer et al., 2005a
	Yes	II	Jingushi et al., 2007
	Yes	II	Gebauer et al., 2005b
	Yes	II	Nolte et al., 2001
	Yes	II	Lerner et al., 2004
	Yes	II	Handolin et al., 2005
	Yes	III	Stein et al., 2005
	Yes	III	Gold et al., 2005
	No	I	Emani et al., 1999
Calcaneal osteoporosis	No	II	Warden et al., 2001
Chronic epicondylitis	No	I	D'Vaz et al., 2006
Congenital pseudoarthrosis	Yes	III	Okada et al., 2003
MIST			
Open wounds	Yes	I	Ennis et al., 2005
	Yes	II	Kavros et al., 2007a
	Yes	II	Kavros et al., 2007b
	Yes	II	Ennis et al., 2006
	Yes	III	Gehling et al., 2007

b. Grade II
Evidence based on *non-controlled* studies on humans, regardless of their level of randomization and blindness.

c. Grade III
Evidence based on *case* studies on humans, regardless of their level of randomization and blindness.

3. Strength of Evidence Behind the Agent
The evidence behind an agent, as presented in the research-based indication box, is arbitrarily assessed in this textbook as *weak, moderate,* or *strong.* For example, the larger the number of studies graded I, regardless of therapeutic benefit, the stronger the scientific evidence behind the agent.

4. Evidence to Justify Usage of Agent
The evidence to justify the usage of an agent for an individual pathology or groups of pathologies, as listed in the research-based indication box, is arbitrarily assessed in this textbook as *poor, fair, good,* or *conflicting.* For example, where the number of grade I studies showing therapeutic benefit (Yes), for any given pathology, is larger than that of similar studies showing no benefit, the evidence

that justifies the usage of the agent for that pathology is assessed as *good. Conflicting* evidence is reported when about an equal numbers of studies, with similar grades, show therapeutic benefit (Yes) and no benefit (No).

C. STRENGTH OF EVIDENCE AND JUSTIFICATION FOR USAGE
The body of research on humans, as presented in **Box 20-1**, shows major differences, as far as the strength of evidence and the justification of usage are concerned, between conventional, LIPUS, and MIST therapy.

1. Conventional Therapy
Results presented in **Box 20-1** show *moderate* strength of evidence behind the use of this therapy, with the majority of studies graded as II. The evidence to justify its usage for shoulder disorders, dermal ulcers, arthritic disorders, and for various soft tissue disorders is *fair-to-good.* Evidence for both epicondylitis and perineal lesions is *conflicting.* There is *no* evidence to support use of conventional US for postexercise muscle soreness. Finally, the evidence for justification of this type of US therapy is *poor* for all the other pathological conditions listed.

2. LIPUS Therapy

The results show *strong* evidence and *good* justification for the usage of LIPUS therapy for the management of fresh and delayed-union bone fractures, with the exception of spinal and skull fractures (**Box 20-1**).

3. MIST Therapy

Results presented in **Box 20-1** show that the strength of evidence for MIST therapy is *moderate* and the justifica-

tion for its use is *good* for the management (cleansing and debridement) of open wounds.

VII. CONTRAINDICATIONS

A. CONTEXT

Table 20-4 lists the contraindications associated with the practice of conventional, LIPUS, and MIST US therapy.

TABLE 20-4	CONTRAINDICATIONS TO ULTRASOUND THERAPY
CONTRAINDICATIONS	**RATIONALE**
CONVENTIONAL	
Over malignant areas	Risk of promoting tumor growth (Sicard-Rosenbaum et al., 1995).
Over hemorrhagic areas	Risk of enhancing the hemorrhagic response.
Over ischemic areas	Risk of enhancing ischemia because of the vascular system's inability to meet the increased metabolic demand induced by the induced-heat response.
Over thrombosis areas	Risk of thrombus detachment, leading to embolism.
Over infected lesions	Risk of enhancing and spreading the infection to surrounding regions because of increased blood circulation.
Over gonads	Risk of infertility.
Over the eye	Risk of inducing cavitation into the humors of the eye and destroying the retina.
Over the pelvic abdominal and lumbar area of a pregnant woman	Risk of inducing cavitation into the amniotic fluid and disrupting fetal development.
Over the pelvic and lumbar area of a menstruating woman	Risk of increasing menstrual flow.
Over the spinal cord after laminectomy	Increased risk of cavitation within the cerebrospinal fluid.
Over plastic implants	Risk of damaging the implant because most plastic materials have high coefficients of ultrasound absorption. Risk of cement overheating leading to soft-tissue damage (Draper et al., 2002).
Over all electronic implants	Risk of electronic malfunction and possible death (Medtronic of Canada, Ltd., 2001).
LIPUS	**RATIONALE**
No contraindication	NA
MIST	
Near or over electronic implants	Risk of electronic malfunction of implants.
Over lower back and abdomen during pregnancy	Risk of complications during pregnancy.
Over malignant areas	Risk of growing and spreading the tumor.

Note that there is no contraindication for LIPUS therapy according to the clinical literature cited in this chapter and manufacturers' brochures consulted (see, www. exogen.com).

B. ELECTRONIC IMPLANTS

Acoustic energy transfer to an implanted system can cause heating at the stimulation electrode–tissue interface, which under certain circumstances can result in permanent tissue or nerve damage that could lead to severe injury or death. The exact nature of potential tissue damage depends on the location of the implanted stimulation electrodes and the extent of exposure to US treatment (Medtronic of Canada, Ltd., 2001).

1. Medtronic Neurostimulation System

This contraindication applies regardless of where the US treatment is targeted, on the patient's body, in relation to the implanted stimulation system, whether it is used in continuous or pulsed mode, and whether the Medtronic system is turned on or off. It also applies if any individual component of the neurostimulation system remains implanted in the body (Medtronic of Canada, Ltd, 2001).

2. Severe Damages

The manufacturer has received two case reports of patients implanted with deep brain stimulation systems who received diathermy therapy (US, SWD, and MWD). In both cases, severe and permanent brain damage occurred; both patients remain comatose since receiving diathermy treatment (Medtronic of Canada, Ltd, 2001). It is unclear to the author whether these unfortunate events resulted from the application of conventional US therapy programmed to induce thermal effects.

VIII. RISKS, PRECAUTIONS, AND RECOMMENDATIONS

The practice of US therapy is not without risks for the patient. The main risks associated with this EPA, as well as some precautions and recommendations designed to improve safety and effectiveness, are listed in **Table 20-5**.

IX. CONSIDERATIONS FOR APPLICATION AND DOCUMENTATION

A. CONSIDERATIONS AND PROCEDURES

The safe, effective, and optimal application of therapeutic US therapy requires that practitioners go through a systematic set of considerations and procedures for each and every application. These considerations and procedures are discussed in this section.

B. CONVENTIONAL APPLICATION

The application of this type of US therapy is complex when compared to the other two types of US therapy.

1. Checklists

Before going ahead with treatment, always go through the list of contraindications (**Table 20-4**) and list of risks, precautions, and recommendations (**Table 20-5**).

2. Skin Heat Discrimination Testing

If thermal effect is needed, conduct test as described in Chapter 25, and record result.

3. Skin Preparation

Cleanse the skin overlying the targeted area with rubbing alcohol. Clip or shave excessive hair if required.

4. Tissue Lesion Location, Depth, and Surface Area

Locate the pathological soft tissue lesion (e.g., a tendon or ligament) and estimate its depth (in centimeters) from the skin surface as well its surface area (in square centimeters). Information about tissue depth will guide the selection of frequency. Likewise, if the practitioner knows the lesion surface area, it will help him or her select the right applicator size.

5. Therapeutic Effects Desired

Determine whether more thermal than mechanical effects (or vice versa) are required, on the basis of the acuity of the pathology and your therapeutic goals. The more acute the lesion, the lesser the thermal effect should be.

6. Delivery Mode

Select either the continuous or pulsed mode. Theoretically, the continuous mode will always deliver more acoustic energy to the tissues, and consequently more thermal effects, because its duty cycle corresponds to 100%. Pulse mode implies the selection of a duty cycle; modern devices offer a choice of 50%, 20%, and 10%. The lower the duty cycle, the lesser the thermal effect, because a significant portion of heat will dissipate in between pulses.

7. Therapeutic Dose

Determine the dose (J/cm^2), at the applicator–skin interface, that you want to deliver to the tissues. Determining this therapeutic dose remains arbitrary because, to date, there is no known dose–response relationship (Robertson, 2002). Recall that the dose (D) is derived by specifying the quantities of four parameters: intensity, application duration, transducer ERA, and treatment surface area. Recall that expressing dosage in terms of only intensity and application duration, such as *1.5 W/cm² for 5 minutes,* is *misleading* and no longer acceptable in the context of evidence-based practice of EPAs, because it provides no

TABLE 20-5	RISKS, PRECAUTIONS, AND RECOMMENDATIONS FOR ULTRASOUND THERAPY

RISKS	RATIONALE
Unsupervised use (home self-treatment) and abusive use (great number of treatments)—conventional therapy	Risk of severe pain and bleeding in the treated region (Levenson et al., 1983).
Spreading of infection—conventional therapy	Risk of nocosomial infection from the soundhead faceplate. This risk can be eliminated by cleaning the faceplate with 70% alcohol between patients (Schabrun et al., 2006).

PRECAUTIONS	RATIONALE
Impaired ability to discriminate skin sensory heat—conventional therapy	Risk of cutaneous burn and inadequate dosimetry if thermal heat ultrasound is used.
Over epiphyseal plates in children—conventional therapy	Risk of altering normal bone growth; use low dose (De Forrest et al., 1953; Vaughen et al., 1959; Nussbaum et al., 2006).
Over back area in cases of radicular pain—conventional therapy	Risk of increased pain (Gnatz, 1989).
Blisters—conventional therapy	Risk of blisters during treatment; emphasize the need for regular device calibration (Frye et al., 2007).

RECOMMENDATIONS	RATIONALE
Wait at least 6 months after the last radiotherapy treatment (when applicable) before initiating ultrasound therapy—conventional therapy	Minimize risk of triggering new cancerous response in the previous cancerous target tissue.
Conduct skin sensory thermal discrimination testing—conventional therapy	Prevent skin irritation or burn.
With obese patients—conventional therapy	Expect comparable increases in muscle temperature using ultrasound on patients with varying thicknesses of adipose tissue, because fat is not a barrier to ultrasound (Draper et al., 1993a).
Keep **all** ultrasound devices at least 5 meters (15 feet) away from functioning shortwave diathermy	Prevent electromagnetic interference.
Wipe off air bubble formation over the soundhead during treatment—conventional therapy	Ensure maximum absorption of acoustic energy.
Use plastic tubs for water immersion technique—conventional therapy.	Plastic tubs are highly recommended. Stainless steel tubs should not be used because of their high capacity to reflect acoustic waves over other body areas
No hot pack therapy before ultrasound therapy—conventional therapy	Hot pack and ultrasound have an additive effect on intramuscular temperature; so caution is advised (Draper et al., 1998). Preheating the treated surface with a hot pack does not affect the deep-heating capacity of ultrasound (Lehmann et al., 1978).
Keep the treated surface area less than 3 times the transducer ERA—conventional therapy	The treated surface area should be no more than 3 times the transducer ERA for optimal results (McDiarmid et al., 1996; Chan et al., 1998).

(Continued)

TABLE 20-5	CONTINUED

RECOMMENDATIONS	RATIONALE
Keep the applicator close to the treated surface area—conventional therapy with water immersion technique	The farther away the soundhead faceplate from the treated skin surface, the less the temperature elevation in the tissues (Robertson et al., 1996). To compensate for thermal energy loss to water, increase dosage with distance (Draper et al., 1993b; Robertson et al., 1996).
Keep ultrasonic coupling media at room temperature—conventional therapy	Room-temperature coupling medium is more efficient than cooled or heated gel in achieving maximal thermal effects at a 5-cm depth intra-muscularly (Oshikoya et al., 2000). There is no apparent additive benefit when using a cooled or heated gel during standard ultrasound treatment (Oshikoya et al., 2000).
Use ultrasound devices with low BNR ratios (1:2 to 1:8)	Minimize the presence of hot spots during therapy.
Use over metallic implants—conventional therapy	Ultrasound can be safely used over or around metallic implants (Gersten, 1958; Lehmann et al., 1958, 1959, 1961; Skoubo-Kristensen et al., 1982).
No cryotherapy before ultrasound therapy—conventional therapy	Skin cooling prior to ultrasound leads to significantly less heating of deeper tissues (Draper et al., 1995b).
Always use commercial ultrasonic coupling media	Many noncommercial media may significantly diminish therapeutic efficacy due to poor acoustic energy transmission (Klucinec et al., 2000). Avoid gel and degassed water in latex gloves or condoms (Klucinec, 1997).
Shave or clip excess hair over treatment area	Air bubbles tend to cling to them, thus reducing ultrasound transmission.
Keep applicator displacement speed between 2 and 7 cm/s—conventional therapy	Similar thermal effects were observed using applicator speed ranging from 2 to 7 cm/s when the treatment area was twice the size of the transducer ERA (Weaver et al., 2006).
Plug line-powered ultrasound devices into ground fault circuit interrupter (GFCI) receptacles	Eliminate the risk of electrical macroshock (see Chapter 27 for details).
Perform regular maintenance of calibration	Ensure devices' optimal performance. Because US devices used to deliver conventional therapy are particularly susceptible to rapid de-calibration, more frequent maintenance and calibration schedules are recommended (Artho et al., 2002; Daniel et al., 2003; Johns et al., 2007; Straub et al., 2008). LIPUS and MIST therapy devices also need regular maintenance and calibration. Follow manufacturers' recommendations.

information about the therapeutic dose delivered to the tissues (see Section V, Dosimetry).

8. Frequency

Select the higher frequency (3 MHz) if the lesion is su-perficial and the lower frequency (1 MHz) if the lesion is located deeper within the tissues (Draper et al., 1995a). However, there is some evidence to suggest that delivery at 3 MHz may extend heat deeper into soft tissues than originally theorized (Hayes et al., 2004).

9. Delivery Mode

Select the continuous mode when optimal thermal effects are required. To optimize mechanical effects, use the pulsed mode with a duty cycle as low as possible.

10. Transducer ERA Versus Treatment Surface Area

Transducer ERA is directly related to the treatment surface area (S) under consideration, which in turn is re-lated to the size or surface area of the lesion. The bigger the lesion, the larger the treatment surface area (S) and transducer ERA should be. Transducers with different ERAs are available for purchase. The recommendation is to maintain a ratio of less than 3 between these two surface areas, such that the treated surface area (S) is no more than 3 times greater than the transducer ERA. For example, the maximum surface area that can be treated with a transducer of 5-cm^2 ERA is 15 cm^2.

11. Delivery Method

Three methods are used to deliver conventional US therapy: *direct contact*, *cushion*, and *water immersion*. The optimal selection, as discussed below, is based on the geometry and tenderness of the treated surface area.

a. Direct Contact

In this method, the applicator's soundhead faceplate is applied directly to the skin surface, separated from it by only a thin gel coupling layer (see below). It is the most convenient and efficient method, provided that the treated surface is relatively flat and not sensitive to pressure exerted by the soundhead faceplate during treatment.

b. Cushion Contact

This method consists of cushioning the contact between the soundhead faceplate and the skin surface overlying the treatment area with a soft, ultrasonic gel-filled pad (see **Fig 20-2B**). A thin layer of ultrasonic gel is required at both the soundhead faceplate–pad interface and the pad–skin interface. This method is used when the treated surface area is irregular and sensitive to pressure.

c. Water Immersion

In this noncontact method, both the treated surface area and the applicator are immersed in a plastic bath filled with tap water, which is used as the coupling agent. The soundhead faceplate is positioned over and close to the skin overlying the treatment area. Stainless-steel baths or tubs should be *avoided* because of their high capacity to reflect ultrasonic waves back to the operator's immersed hand during therapy, thus exposing it to an unwanted overdose of ultrasonic radiation over repeated applications. This method is less convenient and less effective than the two previous methods; it is used when the other two methods cannot be used. If tap water is used, air bubbles will accumulate on the soundhead faceplate and on the irradiated skin surface during treatment. These bubbles should be wiped off periodically, using a stick or with a brush of one's finger, to ensure maximum transmission at all times during the application.

d. Coupling Media

Biophysics has established that acoustic energy does not travel well in air, so a coupling medium is required to facilitate transmission of the acoustic energy between the soundhead faceplate and the treated soft tissue. There is a substantial body of literature on the topic of ultrasonic

coupling media (Reid et al., 1973, 1977; Warren et al., 1976; Griffin, 1980; Docker et al., 1982; Balmaseda et al., 1986; Brueton et al., 1987; Forrest et al., 1989, 1992; Draper et al., 1993b; Klucinec, 1997; Klucinec et al., 2000; Oshikoya et al., 2000; Myrer et al., 2001; Merrick et al., 2002; Casarotto et al., 2004; Gulick et al., 2005). The evidence from these sources indicates that clinicians *should use commercially certified acoustic coupling agents*, such as sonic gel and gel pads, rather than any other generic gels, lotions, or creams.

12. Application Techniques

The techniques for delivering US therapy to soft tissues are either *stationary* or *dynamic*. In the stationary technique, the applicator is kept immobile, or at the same place, during the whole treatment session. In the dynamic technique, the applicator is constantly moved, either manually or automatically (hands-free), at a certain speed and with a certain pressure, over the treatment area, throughout treatment.

a. Dynamic Technique

Select the dynamic technique. There is a consensus that the stationary technique should *be avoided* because it tends to create unwanted and often painful hot spots under the soundhead, especially if the piezoelectric transducer has a relatively high beam nonuniformity ration, or BNR (Draper et al., 2002).

i. Manual displacement. Practitioners can manually displace the applicator (**Fig 20-1A**) over the surface area under treatment in a series of relatively slow up-and-down, side-to-side, and overlapping circular movements, while attempting to (1) cover the whole treated surface area evenly, (2) maintain a light pressure on the skin surface, and (3) keep the soundhead faceplate perpendicular to the treated surface to minimize reflection.

ii. Automated displacement. Applicators are available that allow completely automated manipulation of the soundhead faceplate (**Fig 20-1B**) over the surface area being treated. This hands-free approach has important advantages over traditional manual manipulation. For example, the movement of the transducer faceplate, buried in the ultrasonic applicator, is done at the recommended speed (4 cm/s or 1.75 in/s), evenly, over the whole treated surface area, while a constant contact force (450 g or 1 pound) is maintained between the transducer and the skin overlying the treatment area. Another advantage is that the soundhead faceplate is always kept perpendicular to the treatment area, thus minimizing acoustic beam reflection (Klucinec et al., 1997). A disadvantage of this automated application is that its use is limited to relatively flat and normal (not pathologic) skin surfaces.

iii. Speed and force of application. The movement of these applicators should not be too fast, because the faster the movements, the less the absorption of ultrasonic energy into the soft tissues per unit of time (Draper et al., 2002).

13. Posttreatment Skin Inspection

Inspect the patient's exposed skin areas after every treatment, and record any unusual reaction.

14. End of Treatment Session

After using direct contact, wipe off excess ultrasonic gel and clean the soundhead faceplate to ensure optimal hygiene and prevent cross-contamination between patients.

15. Maintenance and Calibration

There is strong evidence to support the view that conventional US devices are highly susceptible to *decalibration* after use (Stewart et al., 1974; Allen et al., 1978; Stewart et al., 1980; Snow, 1982; Hekkenberg et al., 1986; Rivest et al., 1987; Chartered Society of Physiotherapy, 1990; Pye et al., 1994; Pye, 1996; Kimura et al., 1998; Artho et al., 2002; Johns et al., 2007). This situation may explain why different clinical outcomes are observed in human controls treated with seemingly identical devices and similar dosimetry (Holcomb et al., 2003; Merrick et al., 2003). On the basis of his extended survey of US device performance, Pye (1996) strongly recommends that all devices be inspected and calibrated several times a year, and weekly if used frequently. This author further recommends that all new US devices be tested before their first use to verify that the biophysical parameters (e.g., BNR, ERA, carrier frequency, power, and intensity) outlined in the manufacturer's technical brochure are properly set and calibrated. Finally, Artho et al. (2002) stress that further improvements in the accuracy of US devices is desperately needed.

C. LIPUS APPLICATION

Compared to the application of conventional therapy, the application of LIPUS therapy is much simpler.

1. Checklists

There is no contraindication to LIPUS therapy (**Table 20-4**). Before going ahead with treatment, always go through the list of risks, precautions, and recommendations (**Table 20-5**).

2. Skin Preparation

Cleanse the skin overlying the targeted fracture site area with rubbing alcohol. Clip or shave excessive hair if required.

3. Applicator Placement

The applicator may be placed in-cast, or over-cast, using a specially designed fixation system, or directly (noncast) over the skin area overlying the fracture site as marked by the orthopedic surgeon, using a permanent dermatological pen. The application is by contact method, and the application technique is stationary. For technical details on in-cast and on-cast applications, which are done by orthopedic surgeons during casting procedures, readers are advised to consult manufacturers' Web sites (see www.exogen.com).

4. Dosimetry

Set the frequency (1–1.5 MHz), pulsed frequency (100; 1000 Hz), intensity, application duration, and treatment frequency needed.

5. End of Treatment

Remove the transducer from the fixation assembly system. Remove the gel from the treated site and clean the transducer.

D. MIST APPLICATION

Unlike in the other two types of therapy, ultrasonic energy is used to produce and propel a gentle *mist* of sterile saline to the wound bed. This water *mist* improves the transfer of acoustic energy from the device to the wound bed without contact or pain to the patient.

1. Checklists

Before going ahead with the treatment, always go through the list of contraindications (**Table 20-4**) and list of risks, precautions, and recommendations (**Table 20-5**).

2. Wound Preparation

Undress and irrigate the wound bed with saline.

3. Distance Between Applicator Leading Edge and Wound Bed

Keep the applicator's leading edge at a distance of 0.5–1.5 cm from the wound. Audible and visual bubbling denotes optimal distance from the wound.

4. Applicator Displacement

Move the applicator in slow, even strokes, vertically, then horizontally, across the wound, with multiple passes.

5. Application Duration

Select a time span for the device console. Treatment duration is automatically or manually calculated on the basis of the wound bed size. For example, if the wound bed is less than 15 cm^2, it may be treated for 4 minutes (Ennis et al., 2005). Larger wound beds will require longer treatment durations.

6. Treatment Frequency

Fix a schedule, between daily to 3 times a week.

7. End of Treatment

Discard the plastic applicator and saline bottle. Wipe transducer faceplate and generator with antimicrobial wipes. Dress the wound.

E. DOCUMENTATION

Table 20-6 shows the key parameters that should be documented in the patient's file for conventional, LIPUS, and MIST therapy.

TABLE 20-6	KEY TREATMENT PARAMETERS TO BE DOCUMENTED IN PATIENT'S FILE AFTER ULTRASOUND THERAPY

CONVENTIONAL	LIPUS	MIST
■ *Frequency:* 1 MHz; 3 MHz ■ *BNR:* from 2 to 8 ■ *Delivery mode:* continuous; pulsed ■ *If pulsed mode used:* ON time and OFF time, and duty cycle (%) ■ *Transducer faceplate (ERA):* cm^2 ■ *Treatment surface area (s):* cm^2 ■ *Intensity:* I$_{SATP}$ for continuous mode or I$_{SATA}$ for pulsed mode—W/cm^2 ■ *Application duration:* min ■ *Application method:* direct contact; cushion contact; water immersion ■ *Application technique:* dynamic (speed cm/s)—manual or automated ■ *Coupling medium:* gel; gel pad; tap water ■ *Therapeutic dose (D):* J/cm^2	■ *Frequency:* 1–1.5 MHz ■ *BNR:* from 2 to 8 ■ *Delivery mode:* pulsed—ON time and OFF time, plus duty cycle ■ *Transducer faceplate (ERA):* cm^2 ■ *Treatment surface area(s):* cm^2 ■ *Intensity:* I$_{SATA}$—W/cm^2 ■ *Application duration:* min ■ *Application method:* contact ■ *Application technique:* static ■ *Coupling medium:* gel ■ *Therapeutic dose (D):* J/cm^2	■ *Frequency:* 40 KHz ■ *BNR:* from 2 to 8 ■ *Delivery mode:* continuous ■ *Intensity:* I$_{SATA}$—W/cm^2 ■ *Wound size:* cm^2 ■ *Application duration:* min ■ *Therapeutic dose (D):* J/cm^2

Case Study 20-1   Conventional US Therapy for Shoulder Tendinosis

A 44-year-old right-handed commercial painter, diagnosed with a rotator cuff tendonitis to his right shoulder four months ago, is referred by his orthopaedic surgeon for conservative treatment before considering surgery. The shoulder condition has evolved, over this four-month period, from a state of tendinitis to tendinosis. Radiological imaging reveals no calcification. This patient has a surgical history related to this right shoulder; there is metallic implant associated with a past injury to his acromioclavicular joint. Past treatments include oral and injected analgesic and anti-inflammatory drugs; this therapeutic approach gave less-than-satisfactory results. The patient continues taking analgesic drugs to control his chronic shoulder pain. His main complaint is pain during movement and at palpation, and restricted right shoulder function. Goniometric evaluation reveals deficits in range of motion (ROM) of 20 degrees in abduction and 30 degrees in elevation. He is currently working 3 days a week, and with his right arm, doing only those painting tasks that are below shoulder height. His goal is to resume full work with no functional limitation as soon as possible and without having to undergo surgical treatment. You propose the use of conventional US therapy.

Evidence-Based Steps Toward the Resolution of This Case

1. **List medical diagnosis.**

   Right shoulder tendinosis

2. **List key impairment(s).**

   ■ Pain
   ■ Decreased shoulder abduction and elevation range of motion

3. **List key functional limitation(s).**

   ■ Difficulty with shoulder mobility

4. **List key disability.**

   ■ Inability to resume full-time work

5. **Justification for conventional ultrasound therapy.**

   Is there justifiction for the use of conventional US therapy in this case? This chapter has established that there is *moderate* strength in the evidence and *fair* justification for the use of conventional US for shoulder disorders (see Section VI). The selection of conventional therapy is based primar-

(Continued)

Case Study 20-1   Continued

ily on the body of evidence found in the following publications: Ebenbichler et al., 1997, 1999; Herrara-Lasso et al., 1993; Munting, 1978; Robertson et al., 2001; Aldes et al., 1954a, b; Flax, 1964; Cline, 1963. The use of this agent through its thermomechanical effects is expected to enhance the proliferative and maturation phase of tendon healing, thus facilitating normal function. Because EPAs should not be used in isolation or as a sole intervention, conventional US therapy is used here *concomitantly* with a home-based program focused on maintaining shoulder movements.

6. **Search for contraindications.**

   None is found, although metallic implants are present in the right shoulder area. Recall that plastic implants, **not** metallic implants, present a contraindication to conventional US therapy.

7. **Search for risks and precautions.**

   None is found.

8. **Outline the therapeutic goal(s) you and your patient wish to achieve.**

   - Decrease pain
   - Increase shoulder range of motion
   - Facilitate full return to work

9. **List the outcome measurement(s) used to assess treatment effectiveness.**

   - Pain: Visual Analog Scale (VAS)
   - Shoulder ROM: goniometry

10. **Instruct the patient about what he/she should experience, do, and not do during US treatment.**

    - Light pressure caused by the contact of the applicator against the skin.

11. **Outline the prescription of conventional US based on the evidence available.**

    This prescription is based on the following articles: Ebenbichler et al., 1997, 1999, and Robertson et al., 2001.

    - *Ultrasound device:* cabinet-type conventional
    - *Frequency:* 1 MHz
    - *BNR:* 4
    - *Delivery mode:* pulsed
    - *ON:OFF time:* 1 s : 4 s
    - *Duty cycle:* 20%
    - *Applicator type:* handheld
    - *Treatment surface area (S):* 15 cm^2
    - *Transducer ERA:* 5 cm^2

- *Application method:* contact
- *Coupling agent:* ultrasonic pad (pressure tenderness over treated surface area)
- I_{SATA}: 0.5 W/cm^2
- *Application duration:* 600 s (10 min)
- *Therapeutic dose:* 100 J/cm^2, calculated as follows:
  - $D = E_t / S$
  - $E_t = I_{SATA} \times ERA \times T = 0.5$ W/cm^2 $\times 5$ cm^2 $\times 600$ s $= 1500$ J
  - $D = E_t / S = 1500$ J / 15 cm^2 $= 100$ J/cm^2
- *Total number of treatments:* 12
- *Treatment schedule:* 3 per week for 3 consecutive weeks

12. **Analyze outcome measurements.**

    Pre- and posttreatment comparison:

    - Pain: decreased VAS score, from 6 to 2
    - Shoulder ROM: full range achieved
    - Work: resumed full-time work

13. **Assess therapeutic effectiveness based on outcome measures.**

    The results show that 12 conventional US treatments, each lasting 10 minutes, delivered over 4 consecutive weeks, decreased the patient's pain level, while improving his shoulder function, allowing him to resume full abduction and elevation with a tolerable level of pain at work. The patient is satisfied with the results. He is now working full time, without functional limitations. Overall, this regimen of conventional US therapy had a beneficial effect on the patient's disablement status created by the pathology, as illustrated in the **figure shown** on the next page.

14. **State the prognosis.**

    The short- and medium-term prognosis is good, considering that this treatment allowed him to resume full-time work, keeping in mind the *instruction to minimize the use of his right upper limb* for painting tasks above shoulder height. The long-term prognosis, however, is not so good if one considers the high risk of aggravation of his shoulder condition because of the nature of his employment (repeated use of his right upper limb for painting commercial buildings). This patient will need to strengthen his right shoulder and make a judicious use (using the left upper limb more often) of his right shoulder at work. Otherwise, the need for additional conventional US treatments is very likely over the months or years to come. Surgery as a last resort cannot be ruled out if further conservative treatments fail, and if the patient is then willing to accept it.

THERAPEUTIC IMPACT on Disablement

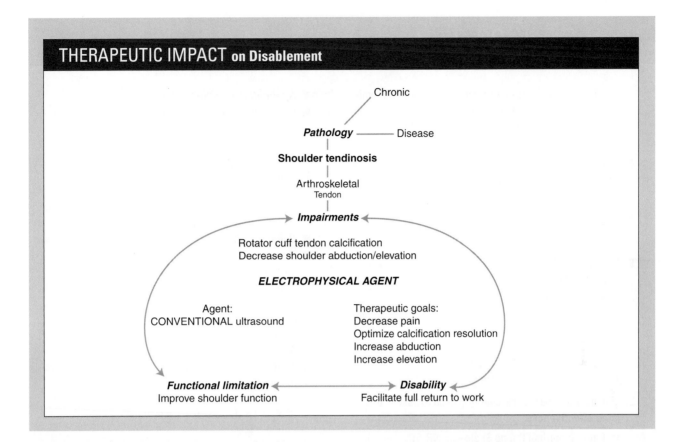

Chronic

Pathology ——— Disease

Shoulder tendinosis

Arthroskeletal
Tendon

Impairments

Rotator cuff tendon calcification
Decrease shoulder abduction/elevation

ELECTROPHYSICAL AGENT

Agent:
CONVENTIONAL ultrasound

Therapeutic goals:
Decrease pain
Optimize calcification resolution
Increase abduction
Increase elevation

Functional limitation
Improve shoulder function

Disability
Facilitate full return to work

Case Study 20-2   LIPUS Therapy for Nonunion Humerus Fracture

An active 57-year-old woman broke her left humerus about 11 months ago in a bad fall while skiing. Despite traditional orthopaedic management and regular follow-up of her condition (surgery involving metallic rod, plates, and screws, followed by cast immobilization), she is diagnosed today with nonunion of her fracture. Her main complaint is residual pain, combined with the limited use of her upper right arm in the course of her daily activities. She is eager to resume her daily activities, including skiing. Her goal is to achieve complete union or resolution of her fracture without further surgery. To accelerate bone healing and the complete resolution of this fracture, the orthopaedic surgeon refers this patient for LIPUS therapy. The purpose is to initiate treatment at the hospital and then to instruct and train her for home therapy for the remaining weeks of treatment. The patient is asked to come to the hospital for periodic radiographs to monitor the resolution of her bone fracture.

Evidence-Based Steps Toward the Resolution of This Case

1. List medical diagnosis.

Nonunion humeral fracture

2. List key impairment(s).

- Pain
- Bone nonunion at site of fracture

3. List key functional limitation(s).

- Limited use of upper right arm
- Limited ability to do activities of daily living

4. List key disabilities.

- Inability to resume skiing

5. Justification for LIPUS therapy.

Is there justification for the use of LIPUS therapy in this case? This chapter has established that there is *strong* evidence and *good* justification for the use of LIPUS therapy for nonunion bone fractures (see Section IV,). The selection of this agent is based on the body of evidence found in the following studies: Xavier et al., 1983; Heckman et al., 1994; Cook et al., 1997; Kristiansen et al., 1997; Mayr et al., 2000; Leung et al., 2004; Gebauer et al., 2005a,b: Jingushi et al., 2007. The use of LIPUS is expected to promote osteogenesis, thus building the necessary callus for complete union of the bones. Because EPAs should not be used in isolation or as a

(Continued)

Case Study 20-2   Continued

sole intervention, LIPUS therapy is used here concomitantly with a home-based program focusing on maintaining upper limb function through activities of daily living.

6. **Search for contraindications.**

   None is found. Recall that there is no known contraindication to the use of LIPUS therapy.

7. **Search for risks and precautions.**

   None is found.

8. **Outline the therapeutic goal(s) you and your patient wish to achieve.**

   - Reduce pain
   - Achieve complete bone calcification and complete union of bones
   - Resume full use of upper right arm
   - Resume full activities of daily living
   - Resume full skiing activities

9. **List the outcome measurement(s) used to assess treatment effectiveness.**

   - Pain: Numerical Rating Scale—5 (NR-5)
   - Bone calcification and fracture resolution: serial radiography
   - Upper arm function: Patient-Specific Functional Scale (PSFS)

10. **Instruct the patient about what he/she should experience, do, and not do during the LIPUS treatment.**

    - No sensation is felt

11. **Outline the prescription of LIPUS based on the evidence available.**

    This prescription is based on the following articles: Xavier et al., 1983; Heckman et al., 1994; Kristiansen et al., 1997; Cook et al., 1997; Mayr et al., 2000; Leung et al., 2004; Sakurakichi et al., 2004; Gebauer et al., 2005a,b; Jingushi et al., 2007. Contrary to conventional US therapy, where several prescriptions can be used, LIPUS therapy requires a single standardized prescription, described below.

    - *Ultrasound device:* portable LIPUS device
    - *Frequency:* 1.5 MHz
    - *BNR:* 4
    - *Delivery mode:* pulsed
      - Fixed pulse rate: 1000 Hz
      - Fixed ON time: 0.2 ms; OFF time: 0.8 ms
      - Fixed duty cycle: 20%
    - *Application method:* contact—directly on the skin, over the surgeon's skin marking

    - *Application technique:* stationary
    - *Fracture site surface area (S):* 3 cm^2; site marked on the skin by the orthopaedic surgeon, using a dermatological pen
    - *Transducer ERA:* 5 cm^2
    - *Transducer fixation:* The transducer is kept in place with a plastic retaining and alignment fixture strapped in position over the marking on the skin that identifies the nonunion fracture site.
    - *Coupling agent:* ultrasonic gel
    - *Device alert signals:* Audible signals alert the patient if the device is not operating properly. The device monitors the treatment time and automatically turns off the treatment session after 20 minutes.
    - I_{SATA}: 0.03 mW/cm^2
    - *Application duration:* 1200 s (20 min)
    - *Therapeutic dose (D):* 48 J/cm^2, calculated as follows:
      - $D = E_t / S$
      - $E_t = I \times ERA \times T = 0.03$ W/cm$^2 \times 4$ cm$^2 \times 1200$ s $= 144$ J
      - $D = E_t / S = 144$ J/3cm$^2 = 48$ J/cm^2
    - *Total number of treatments:* 90
    - *Treatment schedule:* daily, for 90 consecutive days

12. **Analyze outcome measurements.**

    Pre- and posttreatment comparison:

    - Pain: decreased NRS-5 score, from 2 to 0
    - Bone fracture resolution: complete, based on radiographs
    - Upper arm use at home: full usage
    - Recreational activity: full skiing activity

13. **Assess therapeutic effectiveness based on outcome measures.**

    The results show that 90 applications of LIPUS therapy on the skin overlying the nonunion fracture site, delivered daily for a period of 20 minutes, led to complete resolution of this fracture. This EPA also allowed the patient full use of her upper right arm, without pain, at home and while skiing. The patient is overwhelmed with the result. Overall, this regimen of LIPUS therapy had a beneficial impact on the patient's disablement status created by the pathology, as illustrated in the **figure shown** on the next page.

14. **Outline your prognosis.**

    The prognosis is excellent because complete bone fracture resolution was achieved.

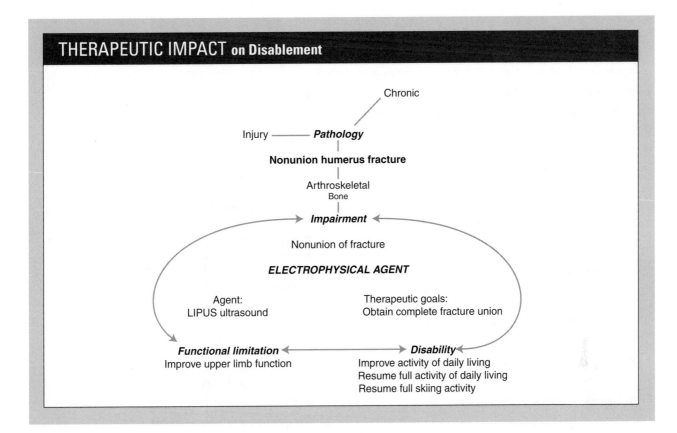

THERAPEUTIC IMPACT on Disablement

Chronic

Injury ——— *Pathology*

Nonunion humerus fracture

Arthroskeletal
Bone

Impairment

Nonunion of fracture

ELECTROPHYSICAL AGENT

Agent:
LIPUS ultrasound

Therapeutic goals:
Obtain complete fracture union

Functional limitation
Improve upper limb function

Disability
Improve activity of daily living
Resume full activity of daily living
Resume full skiing activity

Case Study 20-3   MIST US Therapy for Recalcitrant Diabetic Ankle Ulcer

A 54-year-old diabetic man, diagnosed 5 months ago with a right ankle ischemic ulcer, is referred by his dermatologist for treatment. Physical examination reveals the presence of yellow slough, fibrin, tissue exudates, and bacteria in the wound bed. The wound has been recalcitrant to standard care (manual debridement and dressing), which has delayed healing. The therapeutic goal is for wound cleansing and debridement so as to promote healing. The ulcer is located below the medial malleola. The wound size is irregular, with a surface area corresponding to 15 cm^2. The patient has difficulty wearing shoes and walking, both of which have a negative impact on his activities of daily living and work (no car; must use public transportation to commute to work). Pain is always present and is aggravated by ankle joint movement. The patient is anxious. He desperately wants to keep his ability to walk such as to keep his ability to commute to work.

Evidence-Based Steps Toward the Resolution of This Case

1. **List medical diagnosis.**

   Diabetic right ischemic ankle ulcer

2. **List key impairment(s).**

   ■ Pain
   ■ Open infected wound
   ■ Bacterial infection

3. **List key functional limitation(s).**

   ■ Difficulty walking

4. **List key disabilities.**

   ■ Difficulty commuting (walking) to work

(Continued)

Case Study 20-3 Continued

5. Justification for MIST therapy.

Is there justification for the use of MIST US therapy in this case? This chapter has established that there is *moderate* strength in the evidence and *fair-to-good* justification for the use of MIST therapy for cutaneous wounds (see Section IV). The selection of this agent is based on the body of evidence found in the following clinical studies: Ennis et al., 2005, 2006; Kavros et al., 2007a,b; Gehling et al., 2007. MIST therapy is expected to cleanse and disinfect the wound through effective debridement, and thus facilitate and accelerate wound healing. Because EPAs should not be used in isolation or as a sole therapeutic intervention, a standard home wound care (dressing) is used, in addition to a slight shoe modification to prevent unwanted pressure on the wound.

6. Search for contraindications.

None is found.

7. Search for risks and precautions.

None is found.

8. Outline the therapeutic goal(s) you and your patient wish to achieve.

- Decrease pain
- Eliminate wound infection
- Close the wound
- Resume full activities of daily living
- Resume full work and commuting activities

9. List the outcome measurement(s) used to assess treatment effectiveness.

- Pain: Visual Analog Scale (VAS)
- Wound infection: serial bacterial cultures
- Wound healing: serial digital photographs
- Walking performance (home and commuting to work): Patient-Specific Functional Scale (PSFS)

10. Instruct the patient about what he/she should experience, do, and not do during the LIPUS treatment.

- Light water mist over wound

11. Outline the prescription of MIST based on the evidence available.

This prescription is based on the following articles: Ennis et al., 2005, 2006; Kavros et al., 2007a,b; and Gehling et al., 2007.

- **Ultrasound device:** MIST therapy system
- **Frequency:** 40 KHz

- **BNR:** 4
- **Delivery mode:** continuous
- **Application method:** noncontact—water mist
- **Application technique:** dynamic (vertical and horizontal passes)
- **Wound size:** 15 cm^2
- **Transducer ERA:** 2 cm^2
- **Coupling agent:** sterile water contained in a bottle
- **I_{SATP}:** 0.8 W/cm^2
- **Application duration:** 420 s (7 min)
- **Therapeutic dose (D):** 44.8 J/cm^2, calculated as follows:
  - $D = E_t/S$
  - $E_t = I_{SATP} \times ERA \times T = 0.8$ W/cm$^2 \times 2$ cm$^2 \times 420$ s $= 672$ J
  - $D = E_t/S = 672$ J/15 cm$^2 = 44.8$ J/cm^2
- **Total number of treatments:** 15
- **Treatment schedule:** 3 per week over 5 consecutive weeks

12. Analyze outcome measurements.

Pre- and posttreatment comparison:

- Pain: decreased VAS score, from 6 to 2
- Infection: bacterial count of 0—bacterial infection eliminated
- Wound healing: complete, based on serial digital radiographs
- Walking performance at home and to work: complete, based on PSFS score.

13. Assess therapeutic effectiveness based on outcome measures.

The results show that 15 applications of MIST therapy over the infected wound bed, delivered 3 times a week for a period of 7 minutes over 5 consecutive weeks combined with nursing care and a slight shoe modification led to complete healing. This EPA also allowed the patient to resume full walking activities at home and for commuting to work. Overall, this regimen of MIST therapy had a beneficial impact on the patient's disablement status created by the pathology, as illustrated in the **figure** shown next page.

14. Outline your prognosis.

The prognosis is excellent because complete wound closure was achieved. To prevent reoccurrence, the patient needs to control his diabetic condition and wear adequate shoes.

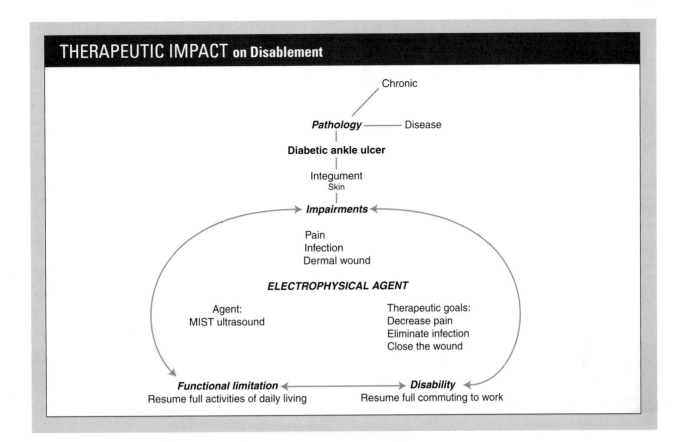

THERAPEUTIC IMPACT on Disablement

Chronic

Pathology ———— Disease

Diabetic ankle ulcer

Integument
Skin

Impairments

Pain
Infection
Dermal wound

ELECTROPHYSICAL AGENT

Agent:
MIST ultrasound

Therapeutic goals:
Decrease pain
Eliminate infection
Close the wound

Functional limitation
Resume full activities of daily living

Disability
Resume full commuting to work

CRITICAL THINKING QUESTIONS

Clarification: What is meant by conventional, LIPUS, and MIST ultrasound (US) therapy?

Assumptions: You have assumed that LIPUS therapy is more effective than conventional therapy for managing soft tissue pathologies. How do you justify making that assumption?

Reasons and evidence: What led you to believe that the reverse piezoelectric phenomenon is responsible for the production of acoustic waves?

Viewpoints or perspectives: How would you respond to a colleague who says that the use of LIPUS therapy is similar to using conventional US therapy in its pulse mode and at low intensity?

Implications and consequences: What are the implications and consequences of using conventional US for its thermal effect on a patient wearing an implanted Medtronic neurostimulation system?

About the question: What is the difference between intensity and therapeutic dose? Why do you think I ask this question?

References

Articles

Ainsworth R, Dziedzic K, Hiller L, Daniels J, Bruton A, Broadfield J (2007) A prospective double blind placebo-controlled randomized trial of US in the physiotherapy treatment of shoulder pain. Rheumatology, 48: 815–820

Aldes JH (1956) Ultrasonic radiation in the treatment of epicondylitis. Gen Pract, 13: 89–96

Aldes JH, Grabin S (1958) Ultrasound in the treatment of intervertebral disc syndrome. Am J Phys Med, 37: 199–202

Aldes JH, Jadeson WJ (1952) Ultrasonic therapy in the treatment of hypertrophic arthritis in elderly patients. Ann West Med Surg, 6: 545–550

Aldes JH, Jadeson WJ, Grabinsky S (1954a) A new approach to the treatment of subdeltoid bursitis. Am J Phys Med, 33: 79–88

Aldes JH, Klaras T (1954b) Use of ultrasonic radiation in the treatment of subdeltoid bursitis with and without calcareous deposits. West J Surg Obstet Gynecol, 62: 369–376

Allen KG, Battye CK (1978) Performance of ultrasonic therapy instruments. Physiotherapy, 64: 174–179

Ansari NN, Adelmanesh F, Nafhdi S, Tabtabaei A (2006a) The effect of physiotherapeutic ultrasound on muscle spasticity in patients with hemiplegia: A pilot study. Electromyogr Clin Neurophysiol, 46: 247–252

Ansari NN, Ebadi S, Talebian S, Naghdi S, Mazaheri H, Olyaei G, Jalaie S (2006b) A randomized single blind placebo controlled clinical trial on the effect of continuous ultrasound on low back pain. Electromyogr Clin Neurophysiol, 46: 329–336

Ansari NN, Haghdi S, Farhadi M, Jalaie S (2007) A preliminary study into the effect of low-intensity pulsed ultrasound on chronic maxillary and frontal sinusitis. Physioth Theory Pract, 23: 211–218

Artho PA, Thyme JG, Warring BP, Willis CD, Brismee JM, Latman NS (2002) A calibration study of therapeutic ultrasound units. Phys Ther, 82: 257–263

Bakhtiary AH, Rashid-Pour A (2004) Ultrasound and laser therapy in the treatment of carpal tunnel syndrome. Aust J Physiother, 50: 147–151

Balmaseda MT, Fatehi MT, Koozekanani SH (1986) Ultrasound therapy: A comparative study of different coupling media. Arch Phys Med Rehab, 67: 147–150

Bearzy HJ (1953) Clinical applications of ultrasonic energy in treatment of acute and chronic subacromial bursitis. Arch Phys Med Rehab, 34: 228–231

Bierman W (1954) Ultrasound in the treatment of scars. Arch Phys Med Rehabil, 35: 209–214

Binder A, Hodge G, Greenwood AM, Hazelman BL, Page TD (1985) Is therapeutic ultrasound effective in treating soft tissue lesions? Br Med J, 290: 512–514

Brock Symons T, Clasey JL, Gater DR, Yates JW (2004) Effects of deep heat as a preventive mechanism on delayed onset muscle soreness. J Strength Cond Res, 18: 155–161

Brueton RN, Campbell B (1987) The use of geliperm as a sterile coupling agent for therapeutic ultrasound. Physiotherapy, 73: 653–654

Bundt FB (1958) Ultrasound therapy in supraspinatus bursitis. Phys Ther Rev, 38: 826–827

Callam MJ, Harper DR, Dale JJ, Ruckley CV, Prescott RJ (1987) A controlled trial of weekly ultrasound therapy in chronic leg ulceration. Lancet, ii (8552): 204–206

Casarotto RA, Adamowski JC, Fallopa F, Bacanelli F (2004) Coupling agents in therapeutic ultrasound: Acoustic and thermal behavior. Arch Phys Med Rehabil, 85: 162–165

Chan AK, Myer JW, Measom GJ, Draper DO (1998) Temperature changes in human patellar tendon in response to therapeutic ultrasound. J Athl Train, 33: 130–135

Chartered Society of Physiotherapy (1990) Guide lines for the safe use of ultrasound physiotherapy equipment. Physiotherapy, 76: 683–684

Cherup N, Urben J, Bender LF (1963) Treatment of plantar warts with ultrasound. Arch Phys Med Rehabil, 44: 602–604

Clarke GR, Stenner L (1976) Use of therapeutic ultrasound. Physiotherapy, 62: 185–190

Cline PD (1963) Radiographic follow-up of ultrasound therapy in calcific bursitis. Phys Ther, 43: 16–18

Cook SD, Ryaby JP, McCabe J, Frey JJ, Heckman JD, Kristiansen TK (1997) Acceleration of tibial and distal radius fracture healing in patients who smoke. Clin Orthop, 337: 198–207

Craig JA, Bradley J, Walsh DM, Baxter GD, Allen JM (1999) Delayed onset muscle soreness: Lack of effect of therapeutic ultrasound. Arch Phys Med Rehabil, 80: 318–323

Creates V (1987) Study of ultrasound treatment to the painful perineum after childbirth. Physiotherapy, 73: 162–165

Davidson JH, Vandervoort A, Lessard L, Miller L (2001) The effect of acupuncture versus ultrasound on pain level, grip strength and disability in individuals with lateral epicondylitis: A pilot study. Physiother Can, 53: 195–202

De Forrest RE, Herrick JF, Janes JM, Krusen FH (1953) Effects of ultrasound on growing bone. Arch Phys Med Rehab, 34: 21–31 (animal study)

De Preux T (1952) Ultrasonic wave therapy in osteoarthritis of the hip joint. Br J Phys Med, 15: 14–19

Docker MF, Foulkes DJ, Patrick MK (1982) Ultrasound couplants for physiotherapy. Physiotherapy, 68. 124–125

Downing DS, Weinstein A (1986) Ultrasound therapy of subacromial bursitis: A double blind trial. Phys Ther, 66: 194–199

Draper DO, Castel JC, Castel D (1995a) Rate of temperature increase in human muscle during 1 MHz and 3 MHz continuous ultrasound. J Orthop Sports Phys Ther, 22: 142–150

Draper DO, Harris ST, Schulthies S, Durrant E, Knight KL, Ricard M (1998) Hot-pack and 1 MHz ultrasound treatments have an additive effect on muscle temperature increase. J Athl Train, 33: 21–24

Draper DO, Shulthies S, Sorvisto, P, Hautala AM (1995b) Temperature changes in deep muscles of humans during ice and ultrasound therapies: An in-vivo study. J Orthop Sports Phys Ther, 21: 153–157

Draper DO, Sunderland (1993a) Examination of the law of Grotthus-Draper: Does ultrasound penetrate subcutaneous fat in humans? J Athl Train, 28: 246–250

Draper DO, Sunderland S, Kirkendall DT, Ricard MD (1993b) A comparison of temperature rise in human calf muscles following applications of underwater and topical gel ultrasound. J Orthop Sports Phys Ther, 17: 247–251

Duarte LR (1983) The stimulation of bone growth by ultrasound. Orthop Trauma Surg, 101: 153–159

D'Vaz AP, Ostor AJ, Speed CA, Jenner JR, Bradley M, Prevost AT, Hazleman BL (2006) Pulsed low-intensity ultrasound therapy for chronic lateral epicondylitis: A randomized controlled trial. Rheumatol, 45: 566–570

Dyson M, Franks C, Suckling J (1976) Stimulation of healing of varicose ulcers by ultrasound. Ultrasonics, 14: 232–236

Ebenbichler GR, Erdogmus CB, Resh KL, Funovics MA, Kainberger F, Barisani G, Aringer M, Nicolakis P, Wiesinger GF, Baghestanian M, Preisinger E, Fialka-Moser V (1999) Ultrasound therapy for calcific tendonitis of the shoulder. N Engl J Med, 340: 1533–1538

Ebenbichler GR, Resch, KL, Graninger WB (1997) Resolution of calcium deposits after ultrasound of the shoulder. J Rheumatol, 24: 235–236

Ebenbichler GR, Resch, KL, Nicolakis P, Wiesinger GF, Uhl F, Ghanem AH, Filaka, V (1998) Ultrasound treatment for treating the carpal tunnel syndrome: Randomized sham controlled trial. Br Med J, 316: 731–735

Echternach JL (1965) Ultrasound: An adjunct treatment for shoulder disabilities. Phys Ther, 45: 865–869

Emani A, Petren-Mallmin M, Larsson S (1999) No effect of low-intensity ultrasound on healing time of intramedullary fixed tibial fractures. J Orthop Trauma, 13: 252–257

Ennis WJ, Foremann P, Mozen N, Massey J, Conner-Kerr T, Meneses P (2005) Ultrasound therapy for recalcitrant diabetic foot ulcers: Results of a randomized, double-blind, controlled, multicenter study. Ostomy Wound Manage, 51; 24–59

Ennis WJ, Valdes W, Gainer M, Meneses P (2006) Evaluation of clinical effectiveness of MIST ultrasound therapy for the healing of chronic wounds. Adv Skin Wound Care, 19: 437–446

Esenyel M, Caglar N, Aldemir T (2000) Treatment of myofascial pain. Am J Phys Med Rehabil, 79: 48–52

Ericksson SV, Lundeberg T, Malm M (1991) A placebo-controlled trial of ultrasound therapy in chronic leg ulceration. Scand J Rehab Med, 23: 211–213

Everett T, McIntosh J, Grant A (1992) Ultrasound therapy for persistent post-natal perineal pain and dyspareunia: a randomized placebo-controlled trial. Physiotherapy, 78: 263–267

Falconer J, Hayes KW, Chang RW (1992) Effect of ultrasound on mobility in osteoarthritis of the knee. A randomized clinical trial. Arthritis Care Res, 5: 29–35

Ferguson HN (1981) Ultrasound in the treatment of surgical wounds. Physiotherapy, 67: 43

Fieldhouse C (1979) Ultrasound for relief of painful episiotomy scars. Physiotherapy, 65: 217

Flax HJ (1964) Ultrasound treatment of peritendonitis calcerea of the shoulder. Am J Phys Med, 43: 117–124

Forrest G, Rosen K (1989) Ultrasound: Effectiveness of treatment given under water. Arch Phys Med Rehabil, 70: 28–29

Forrest G, Rosen K (1992) Ultrasound treatment in degassed water. J Sports Rehab, 1: 284–289

Frye JL, Johns LD, Tom JA, Ingersoll CD (2007) Blisters on the anterior shin of 3 research subjects after 1-MHz, 1.5-W/cm^2, continuous ultrasound treatment: A case series. J Athl Train, 42: 425–430

Gallo JA, Draper DO, Brody LT, Fellingham GW (2004) A comparison of human muscle temperature increases during 3-MHz continuous and pulsed ultrasound with equivalent temporal average intensities. J Orthop Sports Phys Ther, 34: 395–401

Gam AM, Warming S, Larsen LH, Jensen B, Hoydolsmo O, Alloni, Anderson B, Gotzchen E, Petersen M, Mathiesen B (1998) Treatment of myofascial trigger-points with ultrasound combined with massage and exercise: A randomized controlled trial. Pain, 77: 73–79

Garrett AS, Garrett M (1982) Ultrasound therapy for herpes zoster pain. J R Coll Gen Pract, 32: 709–711

Gebauer D, Correl J (2005a) Pulsed low-intensity ultrasound: A new salvage procedure for delayed unions and nonunions after leg lengthening in children. J Pediatr Orthop, 25: 750–754

Gebauer D, Mayr E, Orthner E, Ryaby JP (2005b) Low-intensity pulsed ultrasound: Effects on nonunions. Ultrasound Med Biol, 31: 1391–1402

Gehling ML, Samies JH (2007) The effect of noncontact, low-intensity, low frequency therapeutic ultrasound on lower-extremity chronic wound pain: a retrospective chart review. Ostomy Wound Manage, 53: 44–50

Gersten JW (1958) Effects of metallic objects on temperature rises produced in tissue by ultrasound. Am J Phys Med, 37: 75–82 (animal study)

Gnatz SM (1989) Increased radicular pain due to therapeutic ultrasound applied to the back. Arch Phys Med Rehabil, 70: 493–494

Gold SM, Wasserman R (2005) Preliminary results of tibial bone transports with pulsed low intensity ultrasound (Exogen). J Orthop Traum, 19: 10–16

Gorkiewicz R (1984) Ultrasound for subacromial bursitis. Phys Ther, 64: 46–47

Grant A, Sleep J, McIntosh J, Ashurst H (1989) Ultrasound and pulsed electromagnetic energy treatment for perineal trauma: A randomized placebo-controlled trial. Br J Obstet Gynaecol, 96: 434–439

Griffin JE (1980) Transmissiveness of ultrasound through tap water, glycerin and mineral oil. Phys Ther, 60: 1010–1016

Grynbaum BB (1954) An evaluation of the clinical use of ultrasonics. Am J Phys Med, 33: 75–78

Gulick DT, Ingram N, Krammes T, Wilds C (2005) Comparison of tissue heating using 3 MHz ultrasound with T-Prep versus Aquasonic gel. Phys Ther Sports, 6: 131–136

Haker E, Lundeberg T (1991) Pulsed ultrasound treatment in lateral epicondylalgia. Scand J Rehab Med, 23: 115–118

Hamer J, Kirk JA (1976) Physiotherapy of the frozen shoulder: A comparative trial of ice and ultrasonic therapy. N Z Med J, 83: 191–192

Handolin L, Kiljunen V, Arnala I, Kiuru MJ, Pajarinen J, Pertio EK, Rokkanen P (2005) Effect of ultrasound therapy on bone healing of lateral malleolar fractures of the ankle joint fixed with bioarsorbable screws. J Orthop Sci, 10: 391–395

Hashish I, Hai H, Harvey W (1988) Reproduction of postoperative pain and swelling by ultrasound treatment: A placebo effect. Pain, 33: 303–311

Hashish I, Harvey W, Harris M (1986) Anti-inflammatory effects of ultrasound therapy: Evidence for a major placebo effect. Br J Rheumatol, 25: 77–81

Hasson S, Mundorf R, Barnes W, Williams J, Fijii M (1990) Effect of pulsed ultrasound versus placebo on muscle soreness perception and muscular performance. Scand J Rehab Med, 22: 199–205

Hayes BT, Merrick MA, Sandrey MA, Cordova ML (2004) Three-MHz ultrasound heats deeper into tissues than originally theorized. J Athl Train, 39: 230–234

Hekkenberg RT, Oosterbaan WA, van Beckum WT (1986) Evaluation of ultrasound therapy devices. Physiotherapy, 72: 390–395

Heckman JD, Ryabi JP, Mccabe J, Frey JJ, Kilcoyne RF (1994) Acceleration of tibial fracture-healing by noninvasive, low-intensity pulsed ultrasound. J Bone Joint Surg (Am), 76: 26–34

Herrera-Lasso I, Mobarak L, Fernandez-Dominguez L, Cardiel MH, Alargon-Segovia D (1993) Comparative effectiveness of pack-

ages of treatment including ultrasound or transcutaneous electrical nerve stimulation in painful shoulder syndrome. Physiotherapy, 79: 251–253

Holcomb WR, Joyce CJ (2003) A comparison of temperature increases produced by 2 commonly used ultrasound units. J Athl Train, 38: 24–27

Huang MH, Lin YS, Lee CL, Yang RC (2005) Use of ultrasound to increase effectiveness of isokinetic exercise for knee osteoarthritis. Arch Phys Med Rehabil, 86; 1545–1551

Inaba MK, Piorkowski M (1972) Ultrasound in treatment of painful shoulders in patients with hemiplegia. Phys Ther, 52: 737–741

Johns LD, Straub SJ, Howard SM (2007) Analysis of effective radiation area, power, intensity, and field characteristics of ultrasound transducers. Arch Phys Med Rehabil, 88: 124–129

Jones RJ (1984) Ultrasonic therapy: Report on a series of twelve patients. Physiotherapy, 70: 94–96

Jingushi S, Mizuno K, Matsushita T, Itoman M (2007) Low-intensity pulsed ultrasound treatment for postoperative delayed union or nonunion of long bone fracture. J Orthop Sci, 12: 35–41

Kavros CJ, Miller JL, Hanna SW (2007a) Treatment of ischemic wound with noncontact, low-frequency ultrasound: The Mayo Clinic experience, 2004–2006. Adv Skin Wound Care, 20: 221–226

Kavros SJ, Schenck EC (2007b) Use of noncontact low-frequency ultrasound in the treatment of chronic foot and leg ulcerations: A 51-patient analysis. J Am Podiatr Med Assoc, 97: 95–101

Kazanoglu E, Basaran S, Guzel R, Guler-Uysal F (2003) Short term efficacy of ibuprofen phonophoresis versus continuous ultrasound therapy in knee osteoarthritis. Swiss Med Wkly, 133: 333–338

Kent H (1959) Plantar wart treatment with ultrasound. Arch Phys Med Rehab, 40: 15–18

Kimura IF, Gulick DT, Shelly J, Ziskin MC (1998) Effects of two ultrasound devices and angles of application on the temperature of tissue phantom. J Orthop Sports Phys Ther, 27: 27–31

Klaiman MD, Shrader JA, Danoff JV, Hicks JE, Pesce WJ, Ferland J (1998) Phonophoresis vers ultrasound in the treatment of common musculoskeletal conditions. Med Sci Sports Exerc, 30: 1349–1355

Klemp P, Staberg B, Korsgård J, Nielsen HV, Crone P (1982) Reduced blood flow in fibromyotic muscles during ultrasound therapy. Scand J Rehab Med, 15: 21–23

Klucinec B (1997) The effectiveness of the aquaflex gel pad in the transmission of acoustic energy. J Athl Train, 31: 313–317

Klucinec B, Denegar C, Mahmood R (1997) The transducer pressure variable: Its influence on acoustic energy transmission. J Sports Rehab, 6: 47–53

Klucinec B, Scheidler M, Denegar C, Dohmholdt E, Burgess S (2000) Transmissivity of coupling agents used to deliver ultrasound through indirect methods. J Orthop Sports Phys Ther, 30: 263–269

Kristiansen TK, Ryaby JP, McCabe J, Frey JJ, Roe LR (1997) Accelerated healing of distal radial fractures with the use of specific, low-intensity ultrasound. J Bone Joint Surg (Am), 79: 961–973

Lanfear RT, Clarke WB (1972) The treatment of tenosynovitis in industry. Physiotherapy, 58: 128–129

Lehmann JF, Brunner GD, Martinis AJ, McMillan JA (1959) Ultrasonic effects as demonstrated in live pigs with surgical metallic implants. Arch Phys Med Rehabil, 40: 483–488 (animal study)

Lehmann JF, Brunner GD, McMillan JA (1958) Influence of surgical metal implants on temperature distribution in thigh specimen exposed to ultrasound. Arch Phys Med Rehab, 39: 692–695 (animal study)

Lehmann JF, Erickson DJ, Martin GM, Krusen FH (1954) Comparison of ultrasonic and microwave diathermy in the physical treatment of periarthritis of the shoulder. Arch Phys Med Rehabil, 35: 627–634

Lehmann JF, Fordyce WE, Rathbun LA, Larson, RE, Wood DH (1961) Clinical evaluation of a new approach in the treatment of contracture associated with hip fracture after internal fixation. Arch Phys Med Rehabil, 42: 95–100

Lehmann JF, Stonebridge JB, de Lateur B, Warren CG, Halar E (1978) Temperature of human thighs after hot pack treatment followed by ultrasound. Arch Phys Med Rehabil, 59: 472–475

Leung KS, Lee WS, Tsui HF, Liu PP, Cheung WH (2004) Complex tibial fracture outcome following treatment with low-intensity pulsed ultrasound. Ultrasound Med Biol, 30: 389–395

Lerner A, Stein H, Soudry M (2004) Compound high-energy limb fractures with delayed union: Our experience with adjuvant ultrasound stimulation (Exogen). Ultrasonics, 42: 915–917

Levenson JL, Weissberg MP (1983) Ultrasound abuse: Case report. Arch Phys Med Rehabil, 64: 90–91

Lindsay D, Dearnes J, Richardson C, Chapman A, Cuskelly G (1990) A survey of electromodality usage in private physiotherapy practices. Aust J Physiother, 36: 348–356

Lindsay DM, Dearnes J, McGinley CC (1995) Electrotherapy usage trends in private physiotherapy practice in Alberta. Physiother Can, 47: 30–34

Lundeberg T, Abrahamsson P, Haker E (1988) A comparative study of continuous ultrasound, placebo ultrasound and rest in epicondylalgia. Scand J Rehab Med, 20: 99–101

Lundeberg T, Nordström F, Brodda-Jensen G, Ericksson SV, Kjartansson J, Samuelson VE (1990) Pulsed ultrasound does not improve healing of venous ulcers. Scand J Rehab Med, 22: 195–197

Makuloluwe RTB, Mouzas GL (1977) Ultrasound in the treatment of sprained ankles. Practitioner, 218: 586–588

Markham DE, Wood MR (1980) Ultrasound for Dupuytren's contracture. Physiotherapy, 66: 55–58

Mayr E, Frankel V, Ruter A (2000) Ultrasound—an alternative healing method for nonunions? Arch Orthop Trauma Surg, 120: 1–8

McDiarmid T, Burns PN, Lewith GT, Machin D (1985) Ultrasound and the treatment of pressure sores. Physiotherapy, 71: 66–70

McLachlan Z, Milne EJ, Lumley J, Walker BL (1991) Ultrasound treatment for breast engorgement: A randomized double blind trial. Aust J Physiother, 37: 23–28

McLaren J (1984) Randomized controlled trial of ultrasound therapy for the damaged perineum. Clin Phys Physiol Meas, 5: 40–46

Merrick MA, Bernard KD, Devor ST, Williams JM (2003) Identical 3-MHz ultrasound treatments with different devices produce different intramuscular temperatures. J Orthop Sports Phys Ther, 33: 379–385

Merrick MA, Mihalyov MR, Roethemeier JL, Cordova ML, Ingesoll CD (2002) A comparison of intramuscular temperatures during ultrasound treatments with coupling gel or gel pads. J Orthop Sports Phys Ther, 32: 216–220

Middlemast S, Chatterjee DS (1978) Comparison of ultrasound and thermography for soft-tissue injuries. Physiotherapy, 64: 331–332

Morrissette DA, Brown D, Saladin ME (2004) Temperature change in lumbar periarticular tissues with continuous ultrasound. J Orthop Sports Phys Ther, 34: 754–760

Mueller EE, Mead S, Schulz BF, Vaden MR (1954) A placebo-controlled study of ultrasound treatment for periarthritis. Am J Phys Med, 33: 31–35

Muche JA (2003) Efficacy of therapeutic ultrasound treatment of a meniscus tear in a severely disabled patient: A case report. Arch Phys Med Rehabil, 84: 1558–1559

Munting E (1978) Ultrasonic therapy for painful shoulders. Physiotherapy, 64: 180–181

Myrer JW, Measom GJ, Fellingham GW (2001) Intramuscular temperature rises with topical analgesics used as coupling agents during therapeutic ultrasound. J Athl Train 36: 20–26

Nolte PA, Van der Krans A, Patka P, Janssen IM, Ryaby JP, Albers GH (2001) Low-intensity pulsed ultrasound in the treatment of nonunions. J Trauma, 51: 693–702

Nussbaum EL, Blemann I, Mustard B (1994) Comparison of ultrasound/ultraviolet-C and laser treatment of pressure ulcers in patient with spinal cord injury. Phys Ther, 74: 812–823

Nussbaum EL, Burke S, Johnstone L, Lahiffe G, Robitaille E, Yoshida K (2007) Use of electrophysical agents: Findings and implications of survey of practice in Metro Toronto. Physioth Can, 59: 118–131

Nwuga VC (1983) Ultrasound in treatment of back pain resulting from prolapsed intervertebral disc. Arch Phys Med Rehabil, 64: 88–89

Nyanzy CS, Landgride J, Heyworth JR, Mani R (1999) Randomized controlled study of ultrasound therapy in the management of acute lateral ligament sprains of the ankle joint. Clin Rehab, 13: 16–22

Nykänen M (1995) Pulsed ultrasound treatment of the painful shoulder: A randomized, double-blind, placebo-controlled study. Scand J Rehab Med, 27: 105–108

Okada K, Miyakoshi N, yalahashi S, Ishigaki S, Nishida J, Itoi E (2003) Congenital pseudoarthrosis of the tibia treated with low-intensity pulsed ultrasound stimulation (LIPUS). Ultrasound Med Biol, 29: 1061–1064

Ortas O, Turan B, Bora I, Karakaya MK (1998) Ultrasound therapy effect in carpal tunnel syndrome. Arch Phys Med Rehabil, 79: 1540–1544

Oshikoya CA, Shultz SJ, Mistry D, Perrin DH, Arnold BL, Gansneder BM (2000) Effect of coupling medium temperature on the rate of intramuscular temperature rise using continuous ultrasound. J Athl Train, 35: 417–421

Patrick MK (1978) Applications of therapeutic pulsed ultrasound. Physiotherapy, 64: 103–104

Paul BJ, Lafratta CW, Dawson AR, Baab E, Bullock F (1960) Use of ultrasound in the treatment of pressure sores in patients with spinal cord injury. Arch Phys Med Rehab, 41: 438–440

Payne C (1984) Ultrasound for post-herpetic neuralgia: A study to investigate the results of treatment. Physiotherapy, 70: 96–97

Perron M, Malouin F (1997) Acetic acid iontophoresis and ultrasound for the treatment of calcifying tendinitis of the shoulder: A randomized control trial. Arch Phys Med Rehabil, 78: 379–384

Plaskett C, Tiidus P, Livingston L (1999) Ultrasound treatment does not affect postexercise muscle strength recovery or soreness. J Sport Rehabil, 8: 1–9

Portwood MM, Lieberman JS, Taylor RG (1987) Ultrasound treatment of reflex sympathetic dystrophy. Arch Phys Med Rehab, 68: 116–118

Pye S (1996) Ultrasound therapy equipment—Does it perform? Physiotherapy, 82: 39–44

Pye SD, Milford C (1994) The performance of ultrasound therapy machines in Lothian region. 1992. Ultrasound Med Biol, 20: 347–359

Reid DC, Cummings GE (1973) Factors in selecting the dosage of ultrasound: With particular reference to the use of various coupling agents. Physiother Can, 25: 5–9

Reid DC, Cummings GE (1977) Efficiency of ultrasound coupling agents. Physiotherapy, 63: 255–257

Reobroeck ME, Dekker J, Oostendorp RAB (1998) The use of therapeutic ultrasound by physical therapists in Dutch primary health care. Phys Ther, 78: 470–478

Rivest M, Quirion-DeGirardi C, Seaborne D, Lambert J (1987) Evaluation of therapeutic ultrasound devices: Performance stability over 44 weeks of clinical use. Physiother Can, 39: 77–86

Robertson VJ, Spurritt D (1998) Electrophysical agents: Implications of EPA availability and use in private practices. Physiotherapy, 84: 335–344

Robertson VJ, Ward AR (1996) Limites interchangeability of methods of applying 1 MHz ultrasound. Arch Phys Med Rehabil, 77: 379–383

Robinson AJ, Snyder-Mackler L (1988) Clinical application of electrotherapeutic modalities. Phys Ther, 68: 1235–1238

Roche C, West J (1984) A controlled trial investigating the effect of ultrasound on venous ulcers referred from general practitioners. Physiotherapy, 70: 475–477

Roden D (1952) Ultrasonic waves in the treatment of chronic adhesive subacromial bursitis. J Irish Med Assoc, 30: 85–88

Roman MP (1960) A clinical evaluation of ultrasound by use of a placebo technique. Phys Ther Rev, 40: 649–652

Sakurakichi K, Tsuchiya H, Uehara K, Yamashiro T, Tomita K, Azuma Y (2004) Effects of timing of low-intensity pulsed ultrasound on distraction osteogenesis. J Orthop Res, 22: 395–403

Saliba S, Mistry DJ, Perrin DH, Gieck J, Weltman A (2007) Phonophoresis and the absorption of dexamethasone in the presence of an occlusive dressing. J Athl Train, 42: 349–354

Schabrun S, Chipchase L, Rikard H (2006) Are therapeutic ultrasound units a potential vector for nocosomial infection? Physiother Res Int, 11: 61–71

Shehab D, Adham N (2000) Comparative effectiveness of ultrasound and transcutaneous electrical stimulation in treatment of periarticular shoulder pain. Physiother Can, 52: 208–210

Sicard-Rosenbaum, Lord D, Danoff JV, Thom AK, Eckhaus MA (1995) Effects of continuous therapeutic ultrasound on growth and metastasis of subcutaneous murine tumors. Phys Ther, 75: 3–11 (animal study)

Skoubo-Kristensen E, Sommer J (1982) Ultrasound influence on external fixation with a rigid plate in dogs. Arch Phys Med Rehabil, 63: 371–373 (animal study)

Smith W, Winn F, Parette R (1986) Comparative study versus four modalities in shinsplint treatments. J Orthop Sports Phys Ther, 8: 77–82

Snow CJ (1982) Ultrasound therapy units in Manitoba and Northwestern Ontario: Performance evaluation. Physiother Can, 34: 185–189

Soren A (1965) Evaluation of ultrasound treatment in musculoskeletal disorders. Physiotherapy, 51: 214–217

Stasinopoulos D, Stasinopoulos I (2004) Comparison of effects of exercise programme, pulsed ultrasound and transverse friction in the treatment of chronic patellar tendinopathy. Clin Rehabil, 18: 347–352

Staub SJ, Johns LD, Howard SM (2008) Variability in effective radiating area at 1 MHz affects ultrasound treatment intensity. Phys Ther, 88: 5057

Stay JC, Ricard MD, Draper DO, Schulties SS, Durrant E (1998) Pulsed ultrasound fails to diminish delayed-onset muscle soreness symptoms. J Athl Train, 33: 341–346

Stein H, Lerner A (2005) How does pulsed low-intensity ultrasound enhance fracture healing? Orthopedics, 28: 1161–1163

Stewart HF, Abzug JL, Harris GR (1980) Considerations in ultrasound therapy and equipment performance. Phys Ther, 60: 424–428

Stewart HF, Harris GR, Herman BA, et al. (1974) Survey of use and performance of ultrasonic therapy equipment in Pinellas County, Florida. Phys Ther, 54: 707–714

Svarcova J, Trnavsky K, Zvarova J (1988) The influence of ultrasound, galvanic currents and shortwave diathermy on pain intensity with osteoarthritis. Scand J Rheumatol (Suppl), 67: 83–85

Swartz FZ (1953) Ultrasonics in osteoarthritis. J Med Assoc Al, 22: 182–185

Talaat AM, El-Dibany MM, El-Garf A (1995) Physical therapy in the management of myofascial pain dysfunction syndrome. Ann Otol Rhinol Laryngol, 95: 225–228

Tepperberg I, Marjey E (1953) Ultrasound therapy of painful postoperative neurofibromas. Am J Phys Med, 32: 27–30

Ter Harr G, Dyson M, Oakley EM (1988) Ultrasound in physiotherapy in the United Kingdom: Results of a questionnaire. Physiother Theory Pract, 4: 69–72

Ter Riet G, Kessels AG, Knipschild P (1996) A randomized clinical trial of ultrasound in the treatment of pressure ulcers. Phys Ther, 76: 1301–1312

Uygur F, Sener G (1995) Application of ultrasound in neuromas: Experience with seven below-knee strumps. Physiotherapy, 81: 758–762

Van der Heijden GJMC, Leffers P, Wolters PH, Verheijden JJ, van Mameren H, Hoiber JP, Bouter LM, Knipscheild, PG (1999) No effect of bipolar interferential electrotherapy and pulsed ultrasound for soft tissue shoulder disorders: A randomized controlled trial. Ann Rheum Dis, 58: 530–540

Vaughen JL, Bender LF (1959) Effects of ultrasound on growing bone. Arch Phys Med Rehabil, 34: 158–160 (animal study)

Vaughn DT (1973) Direct method versus underwater method in the treatment of plantar warts with ultrasound. Phys Ther, 53: 396–397

Warden SJ, Bennel KL, Matthews DJ, Brouwn DJ, McMeeken JM, Wark JD (2001) Efficacy of low-intensity pulsed ultrasound in the prevention of osteoporosis following spinal cord injury. Bone, 29: 431–436

Warren GC, Koblanski JN, Sigelmann RA (1976) Ultrasound coupling media: Their relative transmissivity. Arch Phys Med Rehabil, 57: 218–222

Weaver SL, Demchak TJ, Stone MB, Brucker JB, Burr PO (2006) Effect of transducer velocity on intramuscular temperature during a 1-MHz ultrasound treatment. J Orthop Sports Phys Ther, 36: 320–325

Williamson JB, George TK, Simpson DC, Hannah B, Bardbury E (1986) Ultrasound in the treatment of ankle sprains. Injury, 17: 176–178

Wong RA, Schumann B, Twonsend R, Phelps CA (2007) A survey of therapeutic ultrasound by physical therapists who are orthopaedic certified specialists. Phy Ther, 87: 986–994

Xavier CA, Duarte LR (1983) Ultrasonic stimulation on bone callus: Clinical application. Rev Brazil Orthop, 18: 73–80

Zammit E, Herrington L (2005) Ultrasound therapy in the management of acute lateral ligament sprains of the ankle joint. Phys Ther Sports, 6; 116–121

Review Articles

Babba-Akbari SA, Flemming K, Cullum NA, Wollina U (2006) Therapeutic ultrasound for pressure ulcers. Cochrane Database Syst Rev: 3: CD001275

Baker KG, Robertson VJ, Duck FA (2001) A review of therapeutic ultrasound: Biophysical effects. Phys Ther, 81: 1351–1358

Busse JW, Bhandari M, Kulkarni AV, Tunks E (2002) The effects of low-intensity pulsed ultrasound therapy on time to fracture healing: A meta-analysis. CMAJ, 166: 437–341

Claes L, Willie B (2007) The enhancement of bone regeneration by ultrasound Prog Biophys Mol Biol, 93: 384–398

Cole AJ, Eagleston RA (1994) The benefit of deep therapy. Phys Sportmed, 22: 77–86

Dyson M (1987) Mechanisms involved in the therapeutic ultrasound. Physiotherapy, 73: 116–120

Falconer J, Hayes KW, Chang RW (1990) Therapeutic ultrasound in the treatment of musculoskeletal conditions. Arthritis Care Res, 3: 85–91

Gam AN, Johannsen F (1995) Ultrasound therapy in musculoskeletal disorders: A meta-analysis. Pain, 63: 85–91

Gann N (1991) Ultrasound: Current concepts. Clin Manage, 11: 64–69

Hadjiargyrou M, McLeod K, Ryaby JP, Rubin C (1998) Enhancement of fracture healing by low intensity ultrasound. Clin Orthop Relat Res, 355: S216–229

Hayes KW (1992) The use of ultrasound therapy to decrease pain and improved mobility. Crit Rev Phys Med Rehabil, 3: 271–287

Holmes MA, Rudland JR (1991) Clinical trials of ultrasound treatment in soft tissue injury: A review and critique. Physiother Theory Pract, 7: 163–175

Kimmel E (2006) Cavitation bioeffects. Crit Rev Biomed Eng, 34: 105–161

Kitchen SS, Partridge CJ (1990a) A review of therapeutic ultrasound. Part 1: Background and physiological effects. Physiotherapy, 76: 593–595

Kitchen SS, Partridge CJ (1990b) A review of therapeutic ultrasound. Part 2: The efficacy of ultrasound. Physiotherapy, 76: 595–599

Lavon I, Kost J (2004) Ultrasound and transdermal drug delivery. Drug Discov Today, 9: 670–676

Leighton TG (2007) What is ultrasound? Prog Biophys Mol Biol, 93: 1–83

Malizos KN, Hantes ME, Protopappas V, Papachristos A (2006) Low-intensity pulsed ultrasound for bone healing: An overview. Injury, 37: S56–62

Maxwell L (1992) Therapeutic ultrasound. Physiotherapy, 78: 421–426

Mitragotri S, Kost J (2004) Low-frequency sonophoresis: A review. Adv Drug Deliv Rev, 27: 589–601

Mitragotri S (2005) Healing sound: The use of ultrasound in drug delivery and other therapeutic applications. Nat Rev Drug Discov, 4: 255–260

Nussbaum EL (1998) The influence of ultrasound on healing tissues. J Hand Ther, 11: 140–147

Nussbaum EL (1997) Ultrasound: To heat or not to heat—That is the question. Phys Ther Rev, 2: 59–72

O'Brien WD (2007) Ultrasound-biophysics mechanisms. Prog Biophys Mol Biol, 93: 212–255

Robertson VJ (2002) Dosage and treatment response in randomized clinical trials of therapeutic ultrasound. Phys Ther Sports, 3: 124–133

Robertson VJ, Baker KG (2001) A review of therapeutic ultrasound: Effective studies. Phys Ther, 81: 1339–1350

Rubin C, Bolander M, Ryaby JP (2001) The use of low-intensity pulsed ultrasound to accelerate the healing of fractures. J Bone Joint Surg (Am), 83: 170– 259

Ter Haar G (2007) Therapeutic applications of ultrasound. Prog Biophys Mol Biol, 93: 111–129

Van der Windt D, van der Heijden G, van den Berg S, ter Riet G, de Winter A, Bouter LM (1999) Ultrasound therapy for musculoskeletal disorders: A systematic review. Pain, 81: 257–271

Vranic E (2004) Sonophoresis-mechanisms and application. Bosn J Basic Med Sci, 4: 25–32

Walker NA, Denegar CR, Preische J (2007) Low-intensity pulsed ultrasound and pulsed electromagnetic field in the treatment of tibial fractures. A systematic review. J Athl Train, 42: 530–535

Warden SJ (2003) A new direction for ultrasound therapy in sports medicine. Sports Med, 33: 95–107

Chapters of Textbooks

Cameron MH (2003) Ultrasound. In: Physical Agents in Rehabilitation: From Research to Practice, 2nd ed. pp 185–217

Draper DO, Prentice WE (2002) Therapeutic ultrasound. In: Therapeutic Modalities for Physical Therapists. Prentice WE (Ed). McGraw-Hill, St. Louis, pp 270–316

Dunn F, Frizzell LA (1990) Bioeffects of ultrasound. In: Therapeutic Heat and Cold, 4th ed. Lehmann JF (Ed). Williams & Wilkins, Baltimore, pp 398–416

Dyson M (1995) Role of ultrasound in wound healing. In: Wound Healing: Alternatives in Managements, 2nd ed. McCulloch JM, Kloth LC, Feedar JA (Eds). FA Davis Co., Philadelphia, pp 318–345

Frizzell LA, Dunn F (1990) Biophysics of ultrasound. In: Therapeutic Heat and Cold, 4th ed. Lehmann JF (Ed). Williams & Wilkins, Baltimore, pp 362–397

Hayes KW (2000) Ultrasound. In: Manual for Physical Agents, 5th ed. Prentice-Hall Health, Upper Saddle River, pp 43–56

Kahn J (2000) Ultrasound. In: Principles and Practice of Electrotherapy, 4th ed. Churchill Livingstone, New York, pp 49–68

Knight KL, Draper DO (2008) Therapeutic ultrasound. In: Therapeutic Modalities. The Art and Science. Lippincott Williams & Wilkins, Philadelphia, pp 254–283

Lehmann JF, De Lateur BJ (1990) Therapeutic heat. In: Therapeutic Heat and Cold, 4th ed. Lehmann JF (Ed). Williams & Wilkins, Baltimore, pp 504–581

Low J, Reed A (1990) Therapeutic ultrasound. In: Electrotherapy Explained. Butterworth-Heineman, London, pp 133–162

Low J, Reed A (1994) Sonic energy, sound and ultrasound. In: Physical Principles Explained. Butterworth-Heinemann, London, pp 132–147

McDiarmid T, Ziskin MC, Michlovitz SL (1996) Therapeutic ultrasound. In: Thermal Agents in Rehabilitation 3rd ed. Michlovitz SL (Ed). FA Davis Co., Philadelphia, pp 168–212

Nussbaum EL, Berhens BJ (2006) Therapeutic ultrasound. In: Physical Agents: Theory and Practice, 2nd ed. In: Behrens BJ, Michlovitz SL (Eds). FA Davis Co., Philadelphia, pp 56–79

Sparrow KJ (2005) Therapeutic ultrasound. In: Modalities for Therapeutic Interventions, 4th ed. Michlovitz SL, Nolan PN (Eds). FA Davis Co., Philadelphia, pp 79–96

Starkey C (2004a) Therapeutic ultrasound. In: Therapeutic Modalities, 3rd ed. FA Davis Co, Philadelphia, pp 156–173

Starkey C (2004b) Clinical application of therapeutic ultrasound. In: Therapeutic Modalities, 3rd ed. FA Davis Co, Philadelphia, pp 174–183

Sweitzer RW (2006) Ultrasound. In:Integrating Physical Agents in Rehabilitation, 2nd ed. Hecox B, Mehreteab TA, Weisberg J, Sanko J (Eds). Pearson Prentica-Hall, Upper Saddle River, pp 179–214

Ter Harr G (1996) Electrophysical principles. In: Clayton's Electrotherapy, 10th ed. Kitchen S, Bazin S (Eds). WB Saunders Co., London, pp 3–30

Young S (2002) Ultrasound therapy. In: Electrotherapy—Evidence-Based Practice, 11th ed. Kitchen S (Ed). Churchill Livingstone, London, pp 211–230

Corporate Report

Medtronic of Canada, Ltd. (2001) Medtronic Safety Reminder. Contraindication to diathermy for patients implanted with any type of Medtronic neurostimulation system. May 2001.

Spinal Traction Therapy

Learning Objectives

Knowledge: List and describe the various methods of spinal traction practitioners can use to deliver spinal traction therapy.

Comprehension: Compare the static and intermittent traction modes.

Application: Illustrate the applications of cervical and lumbar traction.

Analysis: Explain the proposed physiological and therapeutic effects associated with spinal traction therapy.

Synthesis: Distinguish between various methods of spinal traction.

Evaluation: Discuss the body and strength of the English-language-based scientific evidence supporting the use of spinal traction therapy to manage cervical and lumbar pathologies.

I. RATIONALE FOR USE

A. DEFINITION AND DESCRIPTION

The term *spinal traction* is defined as the use of static and intermittent traction forces applied to the cervical and lumbar spine via various mechanical systems. *Spinal traction therapy* refers to any method of elongating the spine for the purpose of increasing intervertebral spaces in cases of cervical and low back pain disorders.

B. SPINAL TRACTION METHODS

Spinal traction therapy is delivered today, as described in **Box 21-1**, using nine methods of traction: *weighted, motorized, pneumatic, manual, auto-tractive, positional, gravitational, self-tractive,* and *inverted*. In these methods, the traction force is exerted by dead weight (*weighted*), electric motor (*motorized*), air pump (*pneumatic*), practitioner's own manual force (*manual*), or by the patients themselves, using the strength of their upper limbs or the weight of their body segments (*auto-tractive, positional, gravitational, self-tractive,* and *inverted*).

1. Most Commonly Used Methods

The body of literature on spinal traction therapy presented in this chapter indicates that *weighted, motorized, pneumatic,* and *manual* are the most common traction methods used today by clinicians.

2. Less Commonly Used Methods

The *auto-tractive, positional, gravitational,* and *self-traction* methods of spinal traction are less commonly used. When used, these traction methods are usually applied in the context of a home therapy program.

3. Not Recommended

The *inverted* method, which implies suspending the patient by the ankles or thighs in the *head-down* position, is not recommend because of its major side effects, including increased blood pressure (Haskvitz et al., 1986) and ocular problems (Zito, 1988). Moreover, this traction

Box 21-1	Spinal Traction Methods

METHODS	TRACTION FORCE AND USAGE
Weighted	Traction force is applied by hanging dead weights. Requires a cable, pulleys, and either a halter (for cervical spine) or harnesses (for lumbar spine). Use in static mode. Use for cervical spine or lumbar spine.
Motorized	Traction force is applied by an electric traction generator. Requires a commercial split table mounted with an electric traction generator and related cable, halter, and harnesses. Use in static or intermittent mode. Use for cervical spine or lumbar spine.
Pneumatic	Traction force is applied with a manual inflatable air pump. Requires a specialized cervical and lumbar pneumatic traction device. Use in static or intermittent mode. Use for cervical spine or lumbar spine.
Manual	Traction force is applied by the clinician manually. Requires the use of a regular or commercially designed table. Requires that the treating clinician be present during the entire treatment session. Use in intermittent mode. Use for cervical spine.
Auto-tractive	Traction force is applied by the patient via a pulling or pushing action. Requires a commercially designed table with sections that move apart during treatment. Use in intermittent mode. Use for lumbar spine.

(Continued)

Box 21-1	Continued

METHODS	TRACTION FORCE AND USAGE
Positional	Traction force is applied by the patient's own body segment weights. Requires a regular table and a circular pillow. The patient adopts a body position with the pillow placed to cause a positional traction that stretches or distracts the spinal area under treatment. The patient keeps this position for a prolonged period of time. Use in static mode. Use for cervical spine or lumbar spine.
Gravitational	Traction force is applied by the weight of the patient's suspended body segment. Requires a tilting table and a thoracic harness. The chest harness secures the patient as the treatment table is tilted to a vertical position. The suspended lower-body segment provides the traction force. Use in static mode. Use for lumbar spine.
Self-tractive	Traction force is applied by the suspended patient's segment weight The patient uses his or her upper arms to suspend his or her lower body segment. This type of traction is gravitational, so that the suspended lower-body segment provides the traction force. The patient can use the armrest of a chair, an overhead bar, or parallel bars to create this traction. Use in intermittent mode. Use for lumbar spine.
Inverted	Traction force is applied by the suspended patient's segment weight The patient is suspended by the ankles or thighs, in a head-down position. This type of traction is gravitational; so the suspended upper-body segment provides the traction force. Use in static mode. Use for lumbar spine.

method is the most uncomfortable, with the head down, especially if the position is maintained for any substantial amount of time.

C. SCOPE OF CHAPTER

This chapter focuses on the use of the most commonly used methods, that is, weighted, motorized, and pneumatic. The manual traction method is *beyond* the scope of this chapter because it falls within the broad field of *manual therapy* about which several textbooks have been written. The remaining five traction methods are also beyond the scope of this chapter because they are less commonly used or are not recommended.

D. SPINAL TRACTION DEVICES

Some common weighted (**A**) and motorized (**B**) spinal traction devices are shown in **Figure 21-1**.

1. Weighted Device
Figure 21-1A shows the classic over-the-door weighted cervical system. This system is composed of a portable mechanical pulley system mounted on a door. A rope is attached at one end to a cervical harness or halter and at the other end to a plastic bag filled with water, which serves as a dead weight.

2. Motorized Device
Figure 21-1B shows an electric motorized traction device, which can be used for both the lumbar and the cervical spine. The figure shows a setup for lumbar traction, with the lumbar harness attached to the traction cable and the thoracic harness holding the thoracic segment of the spine in place during traction. In this system, an electric motor pulls the traction cable, which is embedded in a programmable console, all of which are mounted on a specially designed (split) table.

3. Pneumatic Device
This device consists of an air cushion positioned between the occipital and the upper trapezius area that can be inflated using a manual rubber bulb and deflated using an air release valve. Contrary to the classic gravitational over-the-door system (**Fig 21-1A**), the pneumatic cervical system generates no pressure on the temporomandibular

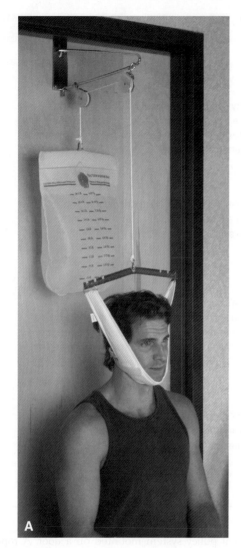

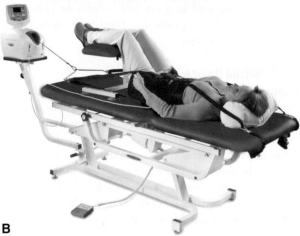

FIGURE 21-1 Common spinal traction devices. (**A**) weighted; (**B**) motorized. (Courtesy of Chattanooga Group.)

joint and hence no jaw pain and interference with the patient's normal jaw function during therapy.

E. RATIONALE FOR USE

Neck and back disorders are common, disabling to various degrees, and costly to treat. A wide variety of therapeutic interventions are used today to treat these disorders, often resulting from disc herniation, degenerative disc diseases, and nerve root compression (Philadelphia Panel, 2001a,b). Among the conservative treatments available, mechanical spinal traction plays an important role by providing either static or intermittent passive spinal elongation, the key purpose of which is to increase intervertebral spaces. Vertebral distraction, or decompression, is thought to increase the foraminal area, which in turn would decrease the peripheral nerve and nucleus pulposus pressure, thus reducing pain and disability.

II. HISTORICAL PERSPECTIVE

A. EARLY PROMOTION

The driving force behind the use of spinal traction therapy for spinal disorders began with James Cyriax in the 1950s. Cyriax later wrote two textbooks on the diagnosis and treatment of soft tissues, promoting traction as one of many therapeutic interventions (Cyriax, 1982, 1984).

B. FIRST HUMAN STUDIES

Mechanical traction therapy gained further support in the 1950s and 1960s based on the first studies on humans, conducted by Judovich and colleagues (1954, 1955, 1957) and Colachis and Strohm (1965a,b, 1966, 1969). These studies showed that human vertebral separation can be achieved by exerting a traction force on the vertebral column.

C. CLINICAL SURVEYS

Recent studies indicate that physical therapists use spinal traction to manage cervical and lumbar disorders at the following rates: 41% in the United Kingdom (Harte et al., 2005), 30% in Canada (Li et al., 2001), 21% in the United States (Jette et al., 1997), 14% in Northern Ireland (Gracey, 2002), and 7% in the England, Southern Ireland (Foster et al., 1999), and the Netherlands (van der Heijden et al., 1995). Cheatle et al. (1991), who surveyed 534 orthopedic surgeons and physiatrists to evaluate their decision-making process in considering the use of lumbar traction, reported that 28% responded that they would prescribe traction for radicular low-back pain.

D. BODY OF LITERATURE

Spinal traction therapy has been the subject of several *articles* (see Reference), *review articles* (Pellecchia, 1994; van der Heijden et al., 1995; Aker et al., 1996; Shterenshis, 1997; Saunders, 1998; Kjellman et al., 1999; Krause et al., 2000; Hoving et al., 2001; Philadelphia Panel, 2001a,b; Harte et al., 2003; Clarke et al., 2006; Graham et al., 2006; Macario et al., 2006; Gay et al., 2008), *chapters of textbooks* (Hooker, 2002; Cameron, 2003; Starkey, 2004; Lowe et al., 2005; Weisberg et al., 2006; Knight et al., 2008), including one *textbook* (Saunders et al., 2003).

III. BIOPHYSICAL CHARACTERISTICS

A. MECHANICAL PRINCIPLE

The principle behind spinal traction, regardless of the methods and modes used to deliver it (see below), lies in the application of a *mechanical force*, the aim of which is to exert a traction effect on the vertebral column that will result in the separation of cervical, or lumbar, vertebrae.

B. EFFECTIVE TRACTION FORCE

To be therapeutically effective, this traction force must be sufficient to overcome the sum of the resistive forces offered by the body segment under therapy (i.e., head/neck and lumbar segments).

1. Cervical Resistive Force

During cervical traction, these resistive forces may correspond to either the weight of the head (vertical gravitational system) or to the friction force resulting from the head being in contact with the traction table (horizontal motorized table or pneumatic system), plus the tensile force exerted by soft tissues surrounding the neck region, such as ligaments, muscles, and tendons.

2. Lumbar Resistive Force

During lumbar traction, which is practically always delivered in the horizontal position using a motorized table, the resistive force corresponds to the friction force exerted between the hip/lower limb segment and the surface of the traction table, plus the tensile force exerted by soft tissues surrounding the lumbar region.

3. Nonfrictional Rolling Lumbar Section

The frictional force observed during lumbar traction is significantly decreased, but not eliminated, when the traction table is split, that is, when it is mounted with a nonfrictional rolling lumbar section. The weight of the lower lumbar/hip segment rests on this rolling or sliding section of the table during traction. The weight of the lower limbs, however, still rests on the non-rolling distal section of the table, creating residual frictional force during traction.

C. TRACTION FORCE UNITS

Traction force is expressed in units of kilogram (kg) or pound (lb). It is also expressed in units of percentage body weight (% BW). For example, using a lumbar traction force of 40 kg (88 lbs) on an 80-kg (176 lbs) patient is equivalent to using a 50% BW traction force. Conversely, using a 30% BW traction force on the same patient is equivalent to a traction force of 24 kg (53 lbs).

D. TRACTION MODES

Spinal traction using the weighted, motorized, and pneumatic methods can be delivered using two traction modes known as static and intermittent.

1. Static Mode

Static mode denotes the steady or continuous application of a fixed traction force for the entire treatment session duration. This mode corresponds, for example, to the application of a traction force of 30 kg (66 lbs) for a period of 20 minutes.

2. Intermittent Mode

Intermittent mode refers to the alternating application of a *fixed* or *fluctuating* [ranging between preset maximum (MAX) and minimum (MIN) levels] traction force applied through a preset cycle of application (ON time) and rest period (OFF time), which is repeated for the entire treatment session duration.

a. Example of Fixed Traction Force

The application of a traction force of 20 kg (44 lb) for 20 seconds followed by a rest period of 10 seconds (ON: OFF time = 20s:10s), for a total treatment duration of 20 minutes. In this case, 2 cycles of traction per minute (i.e., 30s × 2) are delivered, for a total of 40 cycles of traction during the entire treatment session duration.

b. Example of Fluctuating Traction Force

The application of a traction force fluctuating between a maximum (MAX) of 15 kg (33 lb) and a minimum (MIN) of 10 kg (22 lb) for 60 seconds followed by a rest period of 30 seconds (ON:OFF time = 60s:30s), for a total treatment duration of 30 minutes. In this case, 1 cycle of traction is delivered every 90 seconds, for a total of 20 traction cycles during the entire treatment session duration.

IV. PHYSIOLOGICAL AND THERAPEUTIC EFFECTS

A. GENERAL EFFECTS

Figure 21-2 summarizes the proposed physiological and therapeutic effects of spinal traction therapy.

1. Spinal Elongation

The main physiological effect of exerting a tractive force on the vertebral column is to elongate the spine to increase the spacing between the vertebrae.

2. Related Effects

This spine elongation effect then triggers two related effects: it widens the intervertebral foramen and tenses or stretches several perivertebral anatomical structures (e.g., ligaments, muscles, and facet joints).

B. THERAPEUTIC EFFECTS

Together, these physiological effects are presumed to decrease pain and enhance spinal mobility through various anatomo-physiological responses such as reduced nerve root compression, released subluxated facet joints,

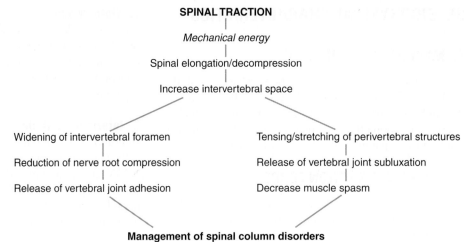

FIGURE 21-2 Proposed physiological and therapeutic effects of spinal traction therapy.

released adhesions around vertebral joints and discs, and decreased muscle spasm.

V. DOSIMETRY

A. PARAMETERS

The dosimetry associated with spinal traction consists of setting the following parameters, which will vary depending on whether the application is for the cervical spine or for the lumbar spine: *traction method, patient position, traction mode, traction force, application duration,* and *treatment frequency.*

1. Traction Methods

Practitioners may choose between nine traction methods (**Box 21-1**). The most common methods are the weighted, motorized, and pneumatic methods. Selecting one method over the other may be dictated by the availability of equipment of the patient's preference. There is no evidence to show that one method is more effective than any other for managing cervical and lumbar disorders.

a. Cervical Traction Harnesses

Cervical traction is applied using either the traditional mandibular-occipital harness or the newly developed occipital harness. The latter harness (or halter) has the advantage of placing the traction force on the skull's occipital bone rather than on the temporomandibular joint, thus greatly improving comfort during therapy.

b. Lumbar Traction Harnesses

Lumbar traction is applied using two types of harness: *pelvic* and *thoracic.* Traction is applied to the lower movable body segment (i.e., pelvis and lower limbs) using a pelvic harness, while the upper nonmoveable segment (i.e., trunk, upper limb, and head) is stabilized using a thoracic harness. These harnesses are adjustable to accommodate various body sizes and shapes.

2. Patient's Position

Spinal traction using the weighted, motorized, or pneumatic method is delivered in the *seated* or *supine position.* Cervical traction may be delivered in the seated or supine position, whereas lumbar traction is delivered only in the supine position because relaxation of the big trunk and back muscle is optimized in this position. Cervical traction with the patient in the supine position has the advantage of reducing the resistive force offered because it reduces the gravitational force acting on the head while promoting muscle relaxation. This position, in contrast to the seated position, implies that a lower, more comfortable, traction force can be used for treatment.

3. Traction Mode

Practitioners may select between the *static* or *intermittent* mode. Note that the weighted method can only be done in the static mode (see Section IIID). There is no evidence to show that one mode is more effective than the other for managing cervical and lumbar disorders.

4. Traction Force

Selecting the most appropriate traction force, measured in units of kilogram (kg) or pound (lb), or in percentage of body weight (% BW), is directly related to the magnitude of the resistive forces exerted by the body segment against the traction table (i.e., friction force) and that exerted by the body's soft tissues during traction. Anthropometric research has shown that the human head accounts for approximately 8.3% of the total BW, meaning that the head of a 90-kg (198 lb) man weighs approximately 7.5 kg (16.5 lb). Anthropometric research also indicates that the human pelvis/lower limbs segment accounts for approximately 30% of the total BW, meaning a weight of approximately 27 kg (60 lb) for a man weighing 90 kg (198 lb).

a. Optimal Selection

The traction force used for treatment *should be based on the patient's weight.* There is a *consensus* in the literature (see References) that, to be effective in elongating the *cervical spine* in the supine position, the traction force used in treatment should be in the range of *20–30% BW*. There is also consensus in the literature that this traction force should be in the range of *30–60% BW* to be effective in elongating the *lumbar spine* in the supine position. Force adjustment will be guided by the patient's response during treatment and by the evolution of the spinal disorder.

b. Static Versus Intermittent Application

The applied traction force may be static (i.e., it is kept constant for the entire treatment session duration) or intermittent, allowing the traction force to fluctuate in magnitude between minimum (MIN) and maximum (MAX) values throughout the entire application duration.

c. Traction Force Angle of Pull

The traction force angle of pull is the angle with which the traction is applied. An angle of pull of 0 degree means that the traction force pulls the cervical or lumbar segment *in line* with the vertebral column; a 0 angle of pull is referred to as the neutral position. An angle of pull greater than 0 degree means that the cervical or lumbar segment is pulled offline—with a certain degree of flexion or lateral flexion. There is evidence to show that when using motorized traction for the cervical spine in a supine position in healthy people, the neutral position (0 degree) yields greater percentages of posterior intervertebral separation and facet joint separation when compared with an angle of pull of 30 degrees of flexion (Wong et al., 1992). Spinal traction therapy is usually delivered with the cervical and lumbar segment in the neutral position.

5. Application Duration

The duration can range between 10 and 30 minutes depending of the patient's condition, traction method, and mode used.

6. Treatment Frequency

Treatment frequency can range between daily to every other day.

B. DOSAGE

The magnitude of traction force exerted on the spine depends of two key factors. The *patient's weight* is the first factor; traction force needs to be large enough to overcome the friction or gravity. The second factor is the patient's tolerance to traction; for this therapy to be effective, the traction force should always be larger than the friction or gravity force acting on the spinal segments.

VI. EVIDENCE FOR INDICATIONS

A. GUIDED BY EVIDENCE

Dictionaries generally define *evidence* as anything that establishes a fact or gives reason to believe something.

The aim of this textbook is to present scientific evidence behind therapeutic EPAs. To be guided by evidence is the process of integrating the evidence from research, however imperfect or scarce this evidence may be, with clinical experience and patients' preferences. In other words, the *evidence-based practice* of EPA requires that practitioners consider the evidence from research, in addition to their own clinical experience and the patient's own preference and beliefs about a given EPA, when the time comes to justify, prescribe, and apply the therapeutic agent. To be guided by evidence is a process, not a search for the absolute truth. Finally, lack of evidence from research in support of any given EPA does not mean that this EPA should never be used. What it means is that no statement can be made about its therapeutic effectiveness and that until more evidence from research is presented, its routine use cannot be recommended.

B. EVIDENCE FROM HUMAN RESEARCH

Box 21-2 provides evidence for spinal traction therapy based on an exhaustive search of published English-language, peer-reviewed studies on humans. The term *indication* is used in reference to a list of pathologies for which spinal traction therapy is employed. Ratings of clinical benefit (Yes or No) and grading of strength of scientific evidence (I, II, or III), including the reference, are included for each pathological condition.

1. Rating Therapeutic Benefit

The rating, expressed as Yes or No, is based on the overall conclusion(s) reached on the issue of therapeutic effectiveness by the author(s) who conducted the peer-reviewed study.

2. Grading Strength of Evidence

The grading, numerically classified as I, II, and III, is based on the type of research methodology, or experimental design, used by the author(s). All those listed are studies on humans published in English-language, peer-reviewed journals. It follows that the evidence in studies graded I is stronger than in those graded II and the evidence in studies graded II is stronger than in those graded III.

a. Grade I

Evidence based on *controlled* studies on humans, regardless of their level of randomization and blindness.

b. Grade II

Evidence based on *non-controlled* studies on humans, regardless of their level of randomization and blindness.

c. Grade III

Evidence based on *case* studies on humans, regardless of their level of randomization and blindness.

Box 21-2   **Research-Based Indications for the Use of Spinal Traction Therapy**

PATHOLOGY	BENEFIT	GRADE	REFERENCE
Low-back pain	Yes	II	Larsson et al., 1980
	Yes	II	Beattie et al., 2008
	Yes	II	Macario et al., 2008
	Yes	II	Lidstrom et al., 1970
	Yes	II	Sherry et al., 2001
	Yes	II	Tesio et al., 1993
	Yes	II	Letchuman et al., 1993
	Yes	II	Oudenhoven, 1978
	Yes	II	Harrison et al., 2002a
	Yes	II	Gionis et al., 2003
	Yes	II	Gose et al., 1998
	Yes	II	Naguszewski et al., 2001
	Yes	II	Onel et al., 1989
	Yes	II	Tesio et al., 1989
	Yes	II	Guevenol et al., 2000
	Yes	II	Ljunggren et al., 1984
	Yes	II	Moret et al., 1998
	Yes	III	Meszaros et al., 2000
	Yes	III	Corkery, 2001
	Yes	III	Gupta et al., 1978
	Yes	III	Hood et al., 1968
	No	I	Mathews et al., 1975
	No	II	Mathews et al., 1987
	No	II	Coxhead et al., 1981
	No	II	Borman et al., 2003
	No	II	Beurskens et al., 1995
	No	II	Beurskens et al., 1997
	No	II	Pal et al., 1986
	No	II	Werners et al., 1999
	No	II	Sweetman et al., 1993
	No	II	van der Heijden et al., 1995
	No	II	Weber, 1973
	No	II	Weber et al., 1984
	No	II	Ljunggren et al., 1992
Cervical pain	Yes	I	Harrison et al., 2002b
	Yes	II	Lee et al., 1996
	Yes	II	Swezey et al., 1999
	Yes	II	Valtonen et al., 1970
	Yes	II	Hattori et al., 2002
	Yes	II	Zylbergold et al., 1985
	Yes	III	Walker, 1986
	Yes	III	Chung et al., 2002
	Yes	III	Constantoyannis et al., 2002
	Yes	III	Browder et al., 2004
	Yes	III	Olson, 1997
	Yes	II	Moeti et al., 2001
	No	II	Goldie et al., 1970
	No	II	Klaber-Moffett et al., 1990
	No	II	Wong et al., 1997
	No	II	Pennie et al., 1990
	No	III	Jette et al., 1985
Cervical spondylosis	Yes	II	Shakoor et al., 2002
	No	II	Loy, 1983
Scoliosis	Yes	III	Hales et al., 2002

3. Strength of Evidence Behind the Agent

The evidence behind the agent, as presented in the research-based indication box, is arbitrarily assessed in this textbook as *weak*, *moderate*, or *strong*. For example, the larger the number of studies graded I, regardless of therapeutic benefit, the stronger the scientific evidence in support of the agent.

4. Evidence Justifying Usage of Agent

The evidence justifying the usage of the agent for an individual pathology or groups of pathologies, listed in the research-based indication box, is arbitrarily assessed in this textbook as *poor*, *fair*, *good*, or *conflicting*. For example, where the number of grade I studies showing therapeutic benefit (Yes), for any given pathology, is larger than that of similar studies showing no benefit, the justification for the usage of this agent for that pathology is assessed as good. A *conflicting* justification is reported when about an equal number of studies with similar grades show therapeutic benefit (Yes) and no benefit (No).

C. STRENGTH OF EVIDENCE AND JUSTIFICATION FOR USAGE

The results presented in **Box 21-2** show moderate strength of evidence behind spinal traction therapy, with the majority of studies graded II. These results also show *conflicting* justification for usage of this EPA for cervical and lumbar pain, with almost equal number of clinical studies demonstrating benefit (Yes) and no (No) benefit. They also show *poor* justification of usage for all the remaining pathologies listed. Until more evidence is provided, the *routine* use of spinal traction for all of the other pathologies listed *cannot be recommended*.

VII. CONTRAINDICATIONS

Table 21-1 describes the contraindications associated with therapeutic spinal traction. Thorough physical and radiological examinations of the cervical or lumbar spine are *mandatory* before this therapeutic agent can be used.

VIII. RISKS, PRECAUTIONS, AND RECOMMENDATIONS

The practice of spinal traction therapy is not without risks for the patient. The main risks associated with this EPA, as well as some precautions and recommendations designed to improve safety and effectiveness, are listed in **Table 21-2**.

TABLE 21-1	CONTRAINDICATIONS TO SPINAL TRACTION THERAPY
CONTRAINDICATIONS	**RATIONALE**
Vertebral fracture or dislocation	Risk of damaging the spinal cord due to increased joint mobility.
Osteoporosis	Risk of vertebral fracture.
Diseases, infections, or tumors affecting the integrity of the vertebral column	Risk of further enhancing the gravity of these conditions.
Severe disc herniation including displaced disc fragment	Risk of further disrupting the damaged tissues (Starkey, 2004).
Rheumatoid arthritis and osteoarthritis	Risk of enhancing the vertebral inflammatory process.
When traction increases pain	Risk of worsening the condition.
Vertebral artery dysfunction (cervical traction only)	Risk of vascular damage.
Aortic aneurysm	Risk of hemorrhaging.
Spinal instability or hypermobility	Risk of damaging the spinal cord due to increased joint mobility.
Spinal cord compression	Risk of further compressing the spinal cord.
Pregnancy (lumbar traction only)	Risk of complications.
Temporomandibular dysfunction (cervical traction only)	Risk of aggravating the condition if a halter is used.
Hernia—hiatal and abdominal	Risk of aggravating the condition.

TABLE 21-2	RISKS, PRECAUTIONS, AND RECOMMENDATIONS FOR SPINAL TRACTION THERAPY

RISKS	RATIONALE
Hypertension (inverse traction only)	Risk of aggravating the condition.
Internal jugular vein thrombosis	Risk using the weight and pulley system (Simmers et al., 1997).
Acute spinal condition	Risk of aggravating the condition.

PRECAUTIONS	RATIONALE
Patients with history of spinal surgery	May lead to complications.
Patients with respiratory and hypertensive disorders	May enhance the conditions; these patients should be observed for signs of distress during initial application (Quain et al., 1985; Balogun et al., 1990; Podein et al., 1998).
Patients with dentures	May cause undue pressure on the dentures if a mandibular halter is used. Use only an occipital halter.
Patients with temporomandibular dysfunction	May aggravate the condition if a mandibular halter is used. Use only an occipital halter.
Plug line-powered device into GFCI receptacle	Prevent the occurance of macroshock (see Chapter 28 for details)
Patients with history of breathing problems (lumbar traction only)	May cause breathing discomfort during treatment.

RECOMMENDATIONS	RATIONALE
Use spinal traction therapy only after thorough physical and radiological examinations—**mandatory**	Because sensitive spinal cord tissues may be exposed to significant traction force, spinal traction therapy should be considered only after the patient's condition has been thoroughly examined.
Ask patients to empty their bladder before treatment	Traction force exerted by pelvic belts may trigger urgency for micturition on a relatively full bladder.
Position the patient in a the most comfortable position (supine or seated)	Allows maximum body relaxation thus allowing maximum elongation and vertebral separation.
Position patient's hips at 90° flexion (lumbar traction only)	Maximum posterior vertebral interspace achieved (Reilly et al., 1979).
Plug line-powered device into GFCI receptacle	Prevent the occurance of macroshocks (see Chapter 27 for details)
Conduct regular maintenance and calibration schedule	Ensures optimal efficiency. Follow the manufacturers' recommendations.

IX. CONSIDERATIONS FOR APPLICATION AND DOCUMENTATION

A. PROCEDURES

The safe, effective, and optimal application of this therapeutic agent requires that clinicians go through a systematic set of considerations and procedures for each and every application. The following is a list of these considerations and procedures.

1. Checklists

Before proceeding with treatment, always go through the list of contraindications (**Table 21-1**) and the list of risks, precautions, and recommendations (**Table 21-2**).

2. Traction Method

Select the weighted, motorized, or pneumatic method. Other methods (**Box 21-1**), although less frequent, can also be used.

3. Body Positioning

Select the seated or supine position. Ensure that the patient adopt the most comfortable position, so as to ensure maximal body relaxation during therapy.

4. Traction Mode

Choose between the static or intermittent mode. If intermittent, select ON:OFF time ratio and MAX:MIN force ratio.

5. Traction Force

For cervical spine therapy, select a traction force ranging between 20% and 30% BW. For lumbar traction therapy, select a traction force ranging between 30% and 60% BW.

6. Traction Force Angle of Pull

The neutral (0°) angle is recommended. An angle of pull may be used for cervical therapy, which may range between 1° and 30°.

7. Application Duration

Durations may range between 5 and 30 minutes.

8. Treatment Frequency

Treatment frequency may be daily to every second day.

9. End of Treatment

Inspect the skin where the harnesses were positioned and question the patient on the level of spinal elongation he or she has perceived during treatment. Document any unusual sensation the patient felt during treatment in the patient's file.

B. DOCUMENTATION

Table 21-3 shows the key parameters that should be documented in the patient's file during spinal traction therapy.

TABLE 21-3	KEY TREATMENT PARAMETERS TO BE DOCUMENTED IN PATIENT'S FILE AFTER SPINAL TRACTION THERAPY

- *Traction method:* description
- *Traction mode:*
  - Static
  - Intermittent: ON: OFF time: fixed or fluctuating force (MAX: MIN)
- *Body position:* seated; supine
- *Traction force:* kg, lb, or, % BW
- *When applicable, traction force angle of pull:* degrees
- *Application duration:* minutes

Case Study 21-1 Cervical Radiculopathy

A 36-year-old woman, who fell on ice 4 weeks ago while ice skating, is referred for treatment by her physician. Magnetic resonance imaging, taken 2 weeks ago, indicates the presence of a C5–C6 paracentral herniated disc, with mild neural foraminal narrowing. Medical examination revealed that this patient is suffering from a moderate case of cervical radiculopathy caused by this C5–C6 herniated disc. The medical file reveals no history or presence of atherosclerotic obstruction of the carotid and vertebral arteries. The patient is complaining, today, of pain radiating to the upper extremities that is provoked or exacerbated by cervical active range of motion (ROM). She also complains of limited ROM in her neck, and occasional headaches. Physical examination now reveals the presence of a paracervical spasm. There is also myotomal muscle weakness and paresthesia related to the C5–C6 spinal level. This woman has a history of temporomandibular dysfunction, which is currently under control following therapy. Her body weight is 50 kg (110 lb). This patient is limited in her activities of daily living and is presently able to work only part-time. Her past 4-week drug treatment, which consisted of analgesic, anti-inflammatory, and antispasmodic drugs, provided some pain relief. She definitively wants to be treated conservatively before considering surgery as the ultimate therapeutic option. Her goal is to be able to resume her normal daily activities and return to full-time work.

Evidence-Based Steps Toward the Resolution of This Case

1. **List medical diagnosis.**
   Cervical C5–C6 radiculopathy.

2. **List key impairment(s).**
   - Bilateral upper limb radicular pain
   - Paracervical muscle spasm
   - Myotomal weakness
   - Dermatomal paresthesia

(Continued)

Case Study 21-1 Continued

3. **List key functional limitation(s).**
   - Difficulty with head movements

4. **List key disability/disabilities.**
   - Inability to work full time

5. **Justification for spinal traction therapy.**

   Is there justification to use spinal traction therapy in this case? This chapter has established that there is moderate strength but *conflicting* justification for the use of spinal traction for cervical pathologies (see Section VI). The selection of spinal traction therapy is based on the body of evidence found in the following studies on human subjects: Browder et al., 2004; Chung et al., 2002; Hattori et al., 2002; and Moeti et al., 2001. The use of spinal traction is expected to decrease the narrowing of, or increase, the intervertebral space at the C5–C6 level to reduce the nerve root compression that is causing the radicular pain and spasm. Because EPAs should not be used in isolation or as a sole intervention, spinal traction therapy is *used here concomitantly* with a home-based program focusing on maintaining proper neck and head posture.

6. **Search for contraindications.**

   None is found.

7. **Search for risks and precautions.**

   The fact that this patient has a medical history of temporomandibular dysfunction emphasizes the need to use the occipital halter as opposed to the traditional temporomandibular type to deliver the cervical traction.

8. **Outline the therapeutic goal(s) you and your patient wish to achieve.**
   - Decrease radicular pain
   - Decrease paracervical muscle spasm
   - Increase cervical ROM
   - Accelerate return to full-time work

9. **List the outcome measurement(s) used to assess treatment effectiveness.**
   - Pain: Visual Analog Scale (VAS)
   - Neck range of motion: Cervical range of motion goniometry (CROM)
   - Neck function: Neck Disability Index (NDI)

10. **Instruct the patient about what he/she should experience, do, and not do during the SWD treatment.**
    - Sensation of intermittent neck traction.
    - Symptoms may disappear during the traction phase and reappear during the resting phase of treatment.

    - If symptoms increase **significantly** during treatment, **stop** the traction immediately by pushing the **stop** button in your hand and call for immediate help.

11. **Outline the prescription of SWD based on the evidence available.**

    This prescription is based on the following sources of evidence: Browder et al., 2004; Chung et al., 2002; Hattori et al., 2002; and Moeti et al., 2001.

    - *Traction method:* motorized
    - *Patient's position:* supine because relaxation of paracervical muscle is optimized
    - *Cervical halter type:* occipital because of history of temporomandibular dysfunction
    - *Traction force angle of pull:* neutral (0 degree)
    - *Traction force:* 20% BW (this patient weighs 50 kg [110 lb], thus 10 kg [22 lb]
    - *Traction mode:* intermittent with fixed force
    - *Traction ON:OFF cycle:* 2:1 (ON: 20 s, OFF: 10 s)
    - *Traction force:* 10 kg (22 lbs)
    - *Application duration:* 30 minutes
    - *Frequency of treatments per week:* 3 treatments per week
    - *Total treatment period:* 4 weeks

12. **Analyze outcome measurements.**
    - Pre- and posttreatment comparison:
    - Pain: VAS score reduced from 6 to 1
    - Cervical ROM: Complete range of motion achieved
    - Neck function: NDI score improved by 75%
    - Work status: Resumed full-time work.

13. **Assess therapeutic effectiveness based on outcome measures.**

    The results show that the delivery of 12 cervical spinal traction treatments, spread over a 4-week period, combined with a home-based head postural program, led to a significant improvement of radicular pain, to the recovery of full cervical ROM, to a 75% increase in neck ROM, and to a return to work, full time. The patient is very pleased with the results of this conservative approach. Overall, the spinal traction treatment had a beneficial impact on the patient's disablement status created by the pathology, as illustrated in the **figure shown** on the next page.

14. **State the prognosis.**

    The prognosis is excellent because a post-therapeutic follow-up magnetic resonance image revealed complete regression of the herniated intervertebral disc. The patient is instructed to fully mobilize her neck at home and, if possible, engage in a cervical muscle-strengthening program under the supervision of a health care practitioner until normal muscle strength is achieved.

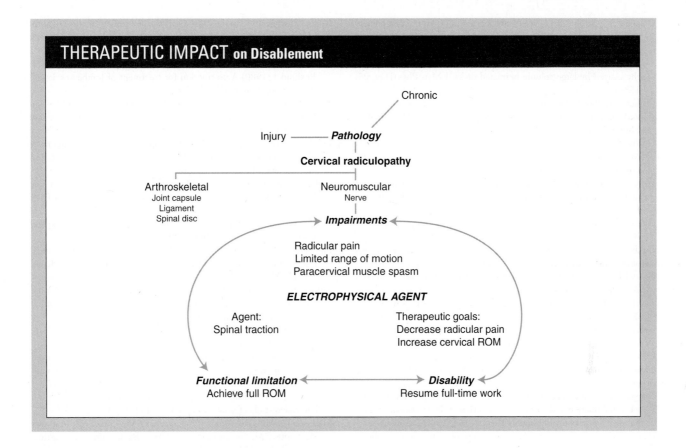

THERAPEUTIC IMPACT on Disablement

Chronic

Injury ——— *Pathology*

Cervical radiculopathy

Arthroskeletal
Joint capsule
Ligament
Spinal disc

Neuromuscular
Nerve

→ *Impairments* ←

Radicular pain
Limited range of motion
Paracervical muscle spasm

ELECTROPHYSICAL AGENT

Agent:
Spinal traction

Therapeutic goals:
Decrease radicular pain
Increase cervical ROM

Functional limitation ←——→ *Disability* ←
Achieve full ROM   Resume full-time work

CRITICAL THINKING QUESTIONS

Clarification: What is meant by spinal traction therapy?

Assumptions: You have assumed that spinal traction therapy is more effective for managing cervical disorders than lumbar disorders. How do you justify making that assumption?

Reasons and evidence: What led you to believe that spinal traction force can elongate the vertebral column?

Viewpoints or perspectives: How would you respond to a colleague who says that spinal traction therapy is contraindicated in cases of disc herniation?

Implications and consequences: What are the implications of using spinal traction therapy without initially carrying out thorough physical and radiologic examinations?

About the question: What is the rationale for choosing the occipital versus the temporomandibular halter to deliver cervical traction? Why do you think I ask this question?

References

Articles

Balogun JA, Abereoje OK, Olaogun MO, Obajuluwa VA, Okonofua FE (1990) Cardiovascular responses of healthy subjects during cervical traction. Physioth Can, 42: 16–22

Beattie PF, Nelson RM, Michener LA, Cammarata J, Donley J (2008) Outcomes after a prone lumbar traction protocol for patients with activity-limiting low back pain: A prospective case series studies. Arch Phys Med Rehabil, 89: 269–274

Beurskens AJ, de Vet HC, Koke AJ, Lindeman E, Regtop W, van der Heijden GJ, Knipschield PG (1995) Efficacy of traction for non specific low back pain: A randomized clinical trial. Lancet, 346: 1596–1600

Beurskens AJ, de Vet HC, Koke AJ, Regtop W, van der Heijden GJ, Lindeman E, Knipschield PG (1997) Efficacy of traction for nonspecific low back pain: 12-week and 6-month results of a randomized clinical trial. Spine, 22: 2756–2762

Borman P, Kerskin D, Bodur H (2003) The efficacy of lumbar traction in the management of patients with low back pain. Rheumatol Int, 23: 82–86

Browder DA, Erhard RE, Piva SR (2004) Intermittent cervical traction and thoracic manipulation for management of mild cervical compressive myelopathy attributed to cervical herniated disc: A case series. J Orthop Sports Phy Ther, 34: 701–712

Cheatle MD, Esterhai JL (1991) Pelvic traction as treatment for acute back pain. Efficacious, benign, or deleterious? Spine, 16: 1379–1381

Chung TS, Lee YJ, Kang SW, Park CJ, Kang WS, Shim YM (2002) Reducibility of cervical disk herniation: Evaluation at MR imaging during cervical traction with a nonmagnetic traction device. Radiology, 225: 895–900

Colachis SC, Strohm BR (1965a) Cervical traction relationship of time to varied tractive force with constant angle of pull. Arch Phys Med Rehab, 46: 815–819

Colachis SC, Strohm BR (1965b) A study of tractive forces and angle of pull on vertebral interspaces in the cervical spine. Arch Phys Med Rehab, 46: 820–830

Colachis SC, Strohm BR (1966) Effect of duration of intermittent cervical traction on vertebral separation. Arch Phys Med Rehab, 47: 353–359

Colachis SC, Strohm BR (1969) Effects of intermittent traction on separation of lumbar vertebrae. Arch Phys Med Rehab, 50: 251–258

Constantoyannis C, Konstantinou D, Kourtopoulos H, Papadakis N (2002) Intermittent cervical traction for cervical radiculopathy caused by large-volume herniated disks. J Man Phys Ther, 25: 188–192

Corkery M (2001) The use of lumbar harness traction to treat a patient with lumbar radicular pain: A case report. J Manual Manipulative Ther, 9: 191–197

Coxhead CE, Inskip H, Meade TW, North WR, Troup JD (1981) Multicentre trial of physiotherapy in the management of sciatic symptoms. Lancet, 1: 1065–1068

Foster NE, Thompson KA, Baxter GD, Allen JM (1999) Management of non-specific low back pain by physiotherapists in Britain and Ireland. Spine, 24: 1332–1342

Gionis TA, Groteke E (2003) Spinal decompression. Orthopedic Technol Rev, 5: 36–39

Goldie I, Landquist A (1970) Evaluation of the effect of different forms of physiotherapy in cervical pain. Scand J Rehab Med, 2: 117–121

Gose EE, Naguzewski WK, Naguzewski RK (1998) Vertebral axis decompression therapy for pain associated with herniated or degenerated discs or facet syndrome: An outcome study. Neurol Res, 20: 186–190

Gracey JH, McDonough SM, Baxter GD (2002) Physiotherapy management of low back pain: A survey of current practice in Northern Ireland. Spine, 27: 406–411

Gupta R, Ramarao S (1978) Epidurography in reduction of lumbar disc prolapsed by traction. Arch Phys Med Rehab, 59: 322–327

Guevenol K, Tuzun C, Peker O, Goktay Y (2000) A comparison of inverted spinal traction and conventional traction in the treatment of lumbar disc herniations. Physiother Theory Pract, 16: 151–160

Hales J, Larson P, Iaizzo PA (2002) Treatment of adult lumbar scoliosis with axial spinal unloading using the LTX3000 Lumbar Rehabilitation System. Spine, 27: E71–E79

Harrison DE, Caillet R, Harrison DD, Janik TJ, Holland B (2002a) Changes in sagittal lumbar configuration with a new method of extension traction: Nonrandomized clinical controlled trial. Arch Phys Med Rehab, 83: 1585–1591

Harrison DE, Caillet R, Harrison DD, Janik TJ, Holland B (2002b) A new 3-point bending traction method of restoring cervical lordosis and cervical manipulation: A nonrandomized clinical controlled trial. Arch Phys Med Rehab, 83: 447–453

Harte AA, Gracey JH, Baxter GD (2005) Current use of lumbar traction in the management of low back pain: Results of a survey of physiotherapists in the United Kingdom. Arch Phys Med Rehabil, 86: 1164–1169

Haskvitz EM, Hanten WP (1986) Blood pressure response to inversion traction. Phys Ther, 66: 1361–1364

Hattori M, Shirai Y, Aoki T (2002) Research on the effectiveness of intermittent cervical traction therapy, using short-latency somatosensory evoked potentials. J Orthop Sci, 7: 208–216

Hood LB, Chrisman D (1968) Intermittent pelvic traction in the treatment of the ruptured intervertebral disc. Phys Ther, 48: 21–30

Hood CJ, Hart DL, Smith HG, Davis H (1981) Comparison of electromyographic activity in normal lumbar sacrospinalis musculature during continuous and intermittent pelvic traction. J Orthop Sports Phys Ther, 2: 137–141

Jette AM, Delitto A (1997) Physical Therapy treatment choice for musculoskeletal impairments. Phys Ther, 77: 145–154

Jette DU, Flakel JE, Trombly C (1985) Effect of intermittent, supine cervical traction on the myoelectric activity of the upper trapezius muscle in subjects with neck pain. Phys Ther, 65: 1173–1176

Judovich BD (1954) Lumbar traction therapy and dissipated force factors. Lancet, 74: 411–414

Judovich BD (1955) Lumbar traction therapy. Elimination of physical factors that prevent lumbar stretch. JAMA, 159: 549–550

Judovich BD, Nobel GR (1957) Traction therapy: A study of resistance forces. Preliminary report on a new method of lumbar traction. Am J Surg, 93: 108–114

Klaber-Moffett JA, Hughes GI, Griffiths P (1990) An investigation of the effects of cervical traction. Part 2: The effects on the neck musculature. Clin Rehab, 4: 287–290

Larsson U, Choler U, Lindstrom A, Lind G, Nachemson A, Nilsson B, Roslund J (1980) Auto-traction for treatment of lumbago-sciatica. Acta Orthop Scand, 51: 791–798

Lee MY, Wong MK, Tang FT, Chang WH, Chiou WK (1996) Design and assessment of an adaptive intermittent cervical traction modality with EMG biofeedback. J Biomech Eng, 118: 597–600

Letchuman R, Deusinger R (1993) Comparison of sacrospinalis myoelectric activity and pain levels in patients undergoing static and intermittent lumbar traction. Spine, 18: 1361–1365

Li LC, Bombardier C (2001) Physical therapy management of low back pain: An exploratory survey of therapist approaches. Phys Ther, 81: 1018–1028

Lidstrom A, Zachrisson M (1970) Physical therapy on low back pain and sciatica. Scand J Rehab Med, 2: 37–42

Ljunggren AE, Weber H, Larssen S (1984) Autotraction versus manual traction in patients with prolapsed lumbar intervertebral discs. Scand J Rehab Med, 16: 117

Ljunggren AE, Walker L, Weber H, Amundsen T (1992) Manual traction versus isometric exercises in patients with herniated lumbar discs. Physioth Theory Pract, 8: 207–213

Loy T (1983) Treatment of cervical spondylosis: Electroacupuncture versus physiotherapy. Med J Aust, 2: 32–34

Macario A, Richmond C, Auster M, Pergolizzi JV (2008) Treatment of 94 outpatients with chronic discogenic low back pain with the DRX9000: A retroscpetive chart review. Pain Pract, 8: 11–17

Mathews JA, Hickling J (1975) Lumbar traction: A double blind controlled study of sciatica. Rheumatol Rehab, 14: 222–225

Mathews JA, Mills SB, Jenkins VM, Grimes SM, Morkel MJ, Mathews W, Scott CM, Sittampalam Y (1987) Back pain and sciatica: Controlled trial of manipulation, traction, sclerosant and epidural injections. Br J Rheumatol, 26: 416–423

Meszaros TF, Olson R, Kulig K, Creighton D, Czarnecki E (2000) Effect of 10%, 30%, and 60% body weight traction on the straight leg raise test of symptomatic patients with low back pain. J Orthop Sports Phys Ther, 30: 595–601

Moeti P, Marchetti G (2001) Clinical outcome from mechanical intermittent cervical traction for the treatment of cervical radiculopathy: A case series. J Orthop Sports Phys Ther, 31: 207–213

Moret MC, van der Stap M, Hagmeijer R, Molenaar A, Koes BW (1998) Design and feasibility of a randomized clinical trial to evaluate the effect of vertical traction in patients with a lumbar radicular syndrome. Man Ther, 3: 203–211

Naguszewski WK, Naguszewski RK, Gose EE (2001) Dermatomal somatosensory evoked potential demonstration of nerve root decompression after VAX-D therapy. Neurol Res, 23: 706–714

Olson VL (1997) Whiplash-associated chronic headache treated with home cervical traction. Phys Ther, 77: 417–424

Onel D, Tuzlaci M, Sari H, Demir K (1989) Computed tomographic investigation of the effect of traction on lumbar disc herniations. Spine, 14: 82–90

Oudenhoven RC (1978) Gravitational lumbar traction. Arch Phys Med Rehab, 59: 510–512

Pal B, Mangion P, Hossain MA, Diffey BL (1986) A controlled trial of continuous lumbar traction in the treatment of back pain and sciatica. Br J Rheumatol, 25: 181–183

Pennie B, Agambar L (1990) Wiplash injuries: A trial of early management. J Bone Joint Surg (B), 72: 277–279

Podein RJ, Iaizzo PA (1998) Applied forces and associated physiological responses induced by axial spinal unloading with the LTX 3000 lumbar rehabilitation system. Arch Phys Med Rehabil, 79: 505–513

Quain MC, Tecklin JS (1985) Lumbar traction: Its effect on respiration. Phys Ther, 65: 1343–1346

Reilly JP, Gersten JW, Clinkingbeard JR (1979) Effect of pelvic-femoral position on vertebral separation produced by lumbar traction. Phys Ther, 59: 282–286

Shakoor MA, Ahmed MS, Kibria G, Khan AA, Mian MA, Hasan SA, Nahar S, Hossain MA (2002) Effect of cervical traction and exercises therapy in cervical spondylosis. Bengladesh Med Res Counc Bull, 28: 61–69

Sherry E, Kitchener P, Smart R (2001) A prospective randomized controlled study of VAX-D and TENS for the treatment of chronic low back pain. Neurol Res, 23: 780–784

Simmers TA, Bekkenk MW, Vidakovic-Vukic M (1997) Internal jugular vein thrombosis after cervical traction. J Int Med Res, 241: 333–335

Sweetman BJ, Heinrich I, Anderson JA (1993) A randomized controlled trial of exercises, short wave diathermy, and traction for low back pain, with evidence of diagnosis-related response to treatment. J Orthop Rheumatol, 6: 159–166

Swezey RL, Swezey AM, Warner K (1999) Efficacy of home cervical traction therapy. Am J Phys Med Rehabil, 78: 30–32

Tesio L, Luccarelli G, Fornari M (1989) Natchev's auto-traction for lumbago-sciatica: Effectiveness in lumbar disc herniation. Arch Phys Med Rehabil, 70: 831–834

Tesio L, Merlo A (1993) Autrotraction versus passive traction: An open controlled study in lumbar disc herniation. Arch Phys Med Rehabil, 74: 871–876

Valtonen EJ, Kiuru E (1970) Cervical traction as a therapeutic tool. A clinical analysis based on 212 patients. Scand J Rehabil Med, 2: 29–36

Van der Heijden GJ, Beurskens AJ, Dirx MJ, Bouter LM, Lindeman E (1995) Efficacy of lumbar traction: A randomized clinical trial. Physiotherapy, 81: 29–35

Walker GL (1986) Gooldley polyaxial cervical traction: A new approach to a traditional treatment Phys Ther, 66: 1255–1259

Weber H (1973) Traction therapy in sciatica due to disc prolapse. J Oslo City Hosp, 23: 167–176

Weber H, Ljunggren E, Walker L (1984) Traction therapy in patients with herniated lumbar intervertebral discs. J Oslo City Hosp, 34: 61–70

Werners R, Pynsent PB, Bulstrode CJ (1999) Randomized trial comparing interferential therapy with motorized lumbar traction and massage in the management of low back pain in a primary care setting. Spine, 24: 1579–1584

Wong AM, Leong C, Chen C (1992) The traction angle and cervical intervertebral separation. Spine, 17: 136–138

Wong AM, Lee M, Chang W, Tang F (1997) Clinical trial of a cervical traction modality with electromyographic biofeedback. Am J Phys Med Rehabil, 76: 19–25

Zito M (1988) Effect of two gravity inversion methods on heart rate, systolic brachial pressure, and ophthalmic artery pressure. Phys Ther, 68: 20–25

Zylbergold RS, Piper MC (1985) Cervical spine disorders: A comparison of three types of traction Spine, 10: 867–871

Review Articles

Aker PD, Gross AR, Goldsmith PP, Peloso P (1996) Conservative management of mechanical neck pain: Systematic overview and meta-analysis. BMJ, 313: 1291–1296

Clarke JA, van Tulder MW, Blomberg SE, de Vet HC, van der Heijden GJ, Bronfort G (2006) Traction for low-back pain with or without sciatica. Cochrane Library, Issue 3: 1–55

Gay RE, Brault JS (2008) Evidenced-informed management of chronic low back pain with traction therapy. Spine Journal, 8: 234–242

Graham N, Gross AR, Goldsmith C (2006) Mechanical traction for mechanical neck disorders: A systematic review. J Rehab Med, 38: 145–152

Harte AA, Baxter GD, Gracery JH (2003) The efficacy of traction for back pain: A systematic review of randomized controlled trials. Arch Phys Med Rehab, 84: 1542–1553

Hoving JL, Gross AR, Gasner D, Kay T, Kennedy C, Hondras MA, Haines T, Bouter LM (2001) A critical appraisal of review articles on the effectiveness of conservative treatment for neck pain. Spine, 26: 196–205

Kjellman GV, Skargren EI, Oberg BE (1999) A critical analysis of randomized clinical trials on neck pain and treatment efficacy, A review of the literature. Scand J Rehabil Med, 31: 139–152

Krause M, Refshauge KM, Dessen M, Boland R (2000) Lumbar spine traction: Evaluation of effects and recommended application for treatment. Man Ther, 5: 72–81

Macario A, Pergolizzi JV (2006) Systematic literature review of spinal decompression via motorized traction for chronic discogenic low back pain. Pain Pract, 6: 171–178

Pellecchia GL (1994) Lumbar traction: A review of the literature. J Orthop Sports Phys Ther, 20: 262–267

Philadelphia Panel (2001a) Evidence-based clinical practice guidelines on selected rehabilitation interventions for low back pain. Phys Ther, 81: 1641–1674

Philadelphia Panel (2001b) Evidence-based clinical practice guidelines on selected rehabilitation interventions for neck pain. Phys Ther, 81: 1701–1717

Saunders HD (1998) The controversy over traction for neck and low-back pain. Physiotherapy, 84: 285–288

Shterenshis MV (1997) The history of modern spinal traction with particular reference to neural disorders. Spinal Cord, 35: 139–146

van der Heijden GJ, Beurskens AJ, Koes BW, Assendelft WJ, de Vet HC, Bouter LM (1995) The efficacy of traction for back and neck pain: A systematic, blinded review of randomized clinical trial methods. Phys Ther, 75: 93–104

Chapters of Textbooks

Cameron MH (2003) Traction. In: Physical Agents in Rehabilitation: From Research to Practice, 2nd ed. Saunders, Philadelphia, pp 307–340

Hooker DN (2002) Spinal traction. In: Therapeutic Modalities for Physical Therapists, 2nd ed. Prentice WE (Ed). McGraw-Hill, New York, pp 363–393

Knight KL, Draper DO (2008) Spinal traction. In: Therapeutic Modalities: The Art and Science. Lippincott Williams & Wilkins, Philadelphia, pp 319–333

Lowe E, Smith W, Nolan TP (2005) Mechanical modalities. Traction and intermittent pneumatic compression. In: Modalities for Therapeutic Intervention, 4th ed. Michlovitz SL, Nolan TP (Eds). FA Davis Co, Philadelphia, pp 165–181

Starkey C (2004) Cervical and lumbar traction. In: Therapeutic Modalities, 3rd ed. FA Davis Co, Philadelphia, pp 308–325

Weisberg J, Schmidt TA (2006) Spinal traction. In: Integrated Physical Agents in Rehabilitation, 2nd ed. Hecox B, Mehreteab TA, Weisberg J, Sanko J (Eds). Pearson Prentice Hall, Upper Saddle River, pp 363–385

Textbooks

Cyriax J (1982) Textbook of Orthopedic Medicine. Vol I: Diagnosis of Soft Tissue Lesions. Bailliere Tindall, London

Cyriax J (1984) Textbook of Orthopedic Medicine. Vol II: Treatment by Manipulation, Massage and Injection. Bailliere Tindall, London

Saunders HD, Saunders R (2003) Spinal Traction. Evaluation, Treatment and Prevention of Musculoskeletal Disorders. The Saunders Group, Chaska

Intermittent Pneumatic Compression Therapy

Learning Objectives

Knowledge: List the key parameters related to the dosimetry of intermittent pneumatic compression (IPC) therapy.

Comprehension: Compare the uniform and sequential methods of compression.

Application: Illustrate the mechanical principle behind IPC therapy.

Analysis: Explain the mechanical and biochemical effects attributed to IPC therapy.

Synthesis: Explain the rationale for using IPC therapy, as opposed to a traditional drug therapy regimen, for the prevention of or prophylaxis against deep vein thrombosis (DVT).

Evaluation: Discuss the contraindications, risks, and precautions associated with the use of IPC therapy.

I. RATIONALE FOR USE

A. DEFINITION AND DESCRIPTION

Intermittent pneumatic compression, known by the acronym IPC, is defined as the application of intermittent external compressive forces, generated by air or pneumatic compressor units, which pump air into custom-made inflatable garments for the purpose of compressing veins and arteries in the upper and lower limbs. IPC devices can be described as mechanical forces that intermittently pump body fluids (blood and lymph) from the peripheral to the central circulation. IPC therapy is the use of compressive force to simulate the muscle pump mechanism, thus encouraging blood flow.

B. IPC DEVICES AND ACCESSORIES

Shown in **Figure 22-1** are typical IPC devices and accessories available on the market today for treating *upper* and *lower* extremities. IPC devices consist essentially of an inflatable garment and a programmable pneumatic pump that fills the garment with compressed air. The garment is intermittently inflated and deflated, with cycle times and pressures that vary between devices. The garment may have a single chamber (**A**), which is inflated to a single pressure, or multiple chambers (**B**), which are individually inflated in sequential order. IPC devices are designated, in the scientific and corporate literature, on the basis of number of chambers within the garment and on the basis of the name of the compressed body segment. For the lower extremities we have a one-chambered foot device (IPC_{foot}) and a two-chambered calf-and-foot device ($IPC_{calf-foot}$), as well as a three-chambered device for the thigh, calf, and foot ($IPC_{thigh-calf-foot}$). Shown in **Figure 22-1-C** is a typical IPC_{foot} device. For the upper extremities we have a two-chambered device for the forearm and hand ($IPC_{forearm-hand}$) as well as a three-chambered device for the arm, forearm, and hand ($IPC_{arm-forearm-hand}$).

C. SCOPE OF CHAPTER

This chapter focuses solely on IPC therapy. Other therapeutic interventions designed to exert compressive forces on the extremities, such as compressive stockings, taping, or massage, are beyond the scope of this chapter.

D. RATIONALE FOR USE

The rationale behind the development and clinical application of IPC therapy was to provide practitioners with a therapeutic means, other than voluntary muscle contraction, elastic compression (stocking and band), and massage, to enhance peripheral blood and lymphatic circulation after injuries and surgery, as well as in the presence of diseases. For example, IPC may be used to reduce

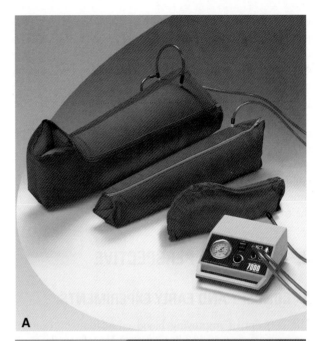

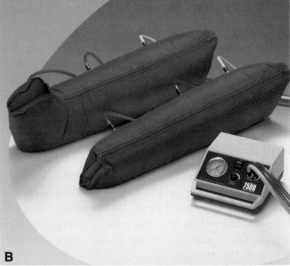

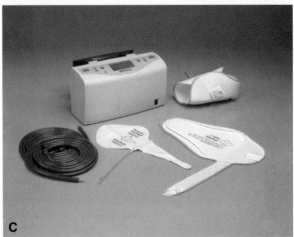

FIGURE 22-1 Typical intermittent pneumatic compression devices and garments. **A**: (left to right) single-chambered $IPC_{thigh-calf-foot}$, $IPC_{arm-forearm-hand}$, and IPC_{foot} devices. **B**: left to right), three-chambered $IPC_{thigh-calf-foot}$, and $IPC_{arm-forearm-hand}$ devices. **C**: Single-chambered IPC_{foot} device. (A,B: Courtesy of KCI Licensing, Inc., 2008; C: Courtesy of Covidien.)

venous stasis by exerting a pumping effect on a patient's impaired venous circulation in order to prevent deep venous thrombosis (DVT) after lower extremity orthopedic surgical procedures, and thus minimize the risk of pulmonary embolus. Likewise, it may be used to enhance blood flow into the lower extremities and thus promote the development of collateral circulation, leading to improved oxygenation, in patients suffering from vascular intermittent claudication. In contrast to the therapies mentioned above, IPC devices can be programmed to deliver a desired compressive force on the limbs for extended periods of time, without requiring physical effort by the patient or the treating clinician.

II. HISTORICAL PERSPECTIVE

A. CONCEPT AND EARLY EXPERIMENTS

The concept of improving blood circulation by exerting external pressure on the extremities dates from the early 1800s (Chen et al., 2001). In the early 1930s, a group of investigators noted that cycles of positive and negative pressures applied to the lower limbs of patients suffering from various peripheral vascular diseases such as Raynaud's disease, vascular claudication, and foot ulcers had a beneficial therapeutic effect, by improving arterial circulation (Landis et al., 1933; Reid et al., 1934; Landis, 1935).

B. RENEWED INTEREST

According to Delis et al. (2005), clinical interest in IPC therapy remained dormant for approximately four decades until a study by Gaskell et al. (1978), which showed a significant improvement in the walking ability of patients with vascular stable intermittent claudication, after treatment with IPC therapy.

C. IPC USE TODAY

According to the body of scientific literature available, IPC devices are clinically used today primarily to *prevent* DVT in patients undergoing lower limb surgery and for the management of vascular intermittent claudication, venous ulcers, lymphedema and posttraumatic lower limb edema.

D. BODY OF LITERATURE

A substantial body of evidence has been accumulated from studies on healthy subjects and patients to support the claim that most IPC devices on the market today enhance arterial and venous blood flow in the upper and lower extremities (Eze et al., 1996; Flam et al., 1996; Westrich et al., 1998; Malone et al., 1999; Westrich et al., 2000; Delis, et al., 2000a; Delis, et al., 2000; Whitelaw et al., 2001; Masri et al., 2004; Iwama et al., 2004). IPC

therapy has been the subject, over the past two decades, of several *articles* (see Reference), *review articles* (Alguire et al., 1997; O'Neil, 1997; Brennan et al., 1998; Choucair et al., 1998; Imperiale, et al. 1994; Meegens et al., 1998; Vanek, 1998; Freedman et al., 2000; Westrich et al., 2000; Chen et al., 2001; Kunimoto et al., 2001; Vowden, 2001; Hopkins, 2002; Kumar et al., 2002; Berliner et al., 2003; Morris et al., 2004; Boudouroglou et al., 2004; Ramzi et al., 2004; Delis, 2005; Roderick et al., 2005; Urbankova et al., 2005; Illingworth et al., 2007; MacLellan et al., 2007), and a few *chapters in textbooks* (Cameron, 2003; Starkey, 2004; Lowe et al., 2005; Hecox et al., 2006).

III. BIOPHYSICAL CHARACTERISTICS

A. ARTIFICIAL VASCULAR PUMP

The important physiological role played by the lower limbs' natural muscle pumps to enhance the return of venous blood is well understood. This understanding promoted the development of IPC devices that could *mimic* or *artificially* activate these pumps (Delis, 2005).

B. MECHANICAL PRINCIPLE

All IPC devices work on the same principle, which is to mechanically squeeze, or compress, fluids (blood and lymph) from underlying veins, arteries, and lymphoid vessels to displace them proximally. This is achieved by intermittent cycles of mechanical energy, in the form of compression and decompression, created by inflating and deflating garments, cuffs, or bands filled with compressed air.

C. PRESSURE GRADIENT

IPC devices are designed to exert a compressive force, or pressure gradient, on the lower and upper extremities. Pressure (P) is defined as a force (F) applied over a surface area (A), where $P = F/A$. Pressure on IPC devices is commonly measured in millimeters of mercury (mm Hg), where 1 pound per square inch (psi) equals 51.8 mm Hg.

D. COMPRESSION MODES

IPC therapy is delivered using two compression modes: *uniform* and *sequential*. Each mode is characterized by the following parameters set by the clinician: pressure gradient, time to inflate, time held at set pressure, time to deflate, cycle ON time, cycle OFF time, cycle of intermittence, and time delay between inflation of chambers (when applicable).

1. Uniform Compression
Uniform, or nonsequential, compression refers to the use of single-chambered garments to compress the limb.

Number of chambers: 1

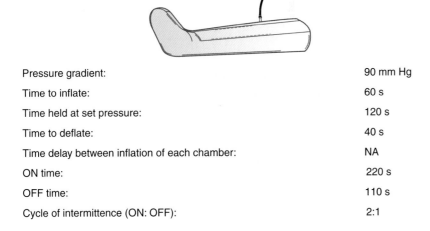

Pressure gradient: 90 mm Hg

Time to inflate: 60 s

Time held at set pressure: 120 s

Time to deflate: 40 s

Time delay between inflation of each chamber: NA

ON time: 220 s

OFF time: 110 s

Cycle of intermittence (ON: OFF):   2:1

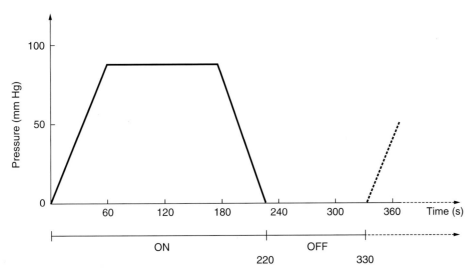

FIGURE 22-2 Uniform compression mode.

Uniform mode is illustrated in **Figure 22-2** using a single-chambered lower-limb garment or $IPC_{thigh-calf-foot}$. In the *example* presented, the pressure gradient, time to inflate, time held at set pressure, and time to deflate are kept constant for each cycle. The cycle ON and OFF times also remain the same for the entire treatment session.

2. Sequential Compression

Sequential compression refers to the use of multichambered garments and involves sequential inflation and deflation of each chamber, *always beginning with the distal chamber and ending with the proximal chamber.* The sequential-mode compression applied on the limb is similar to a milking action performed on the extremity. **Figure 22-3** illustrates the sequential mode using a three-chambered lower-limb garment. In this *example*, the sequential compression is said to be *graded* because the distal chamber inflates to the highest pressure and the proximal chamber inflates to the lowest pressure. *Nongraded* sequential compression is delivered when the magnitude of pressure in each chamber is the same.

IV. PHYSIOLOGICAL AND THERAPEUTIC EFFECTS

A. MECHANICAL/BIOCHEMICAL EFFECTS

The proposed physiological and therapeutic effects associated with IPC therapy are shown in **Figure 22-4**. The body of scientific literature suggests that this therapeutic agent exerts both *mechanical* and *biochemical* effects on the vascular systems of affected soft tissues (Gardner et al., 1983; Chouhan et al., 1999; Chen et al., 2001; Morris et al., 2004).

B. MECHANICAL EFFECTS

The increase in blood flow and emptying of venous and lymphatic vessels are primarily due to the mechanically compressive forces exerted on the walls of these vessels. The resulting therapeutic effects are used for the prevention of venous stasis and for the management of edema at the upper and lower extremities, lymphoedema, wounds, and vascular pain (**Fig 22-4**). For example, venous

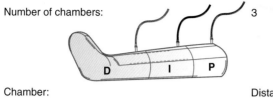

Number of chambers: 3

Chamber:	Distal (D)	Intermediate (I)	Proximal (P)
Pressure gradient:	100 mm Hg	80 mm Hg	50 mm Hg
Time to inflate:	60 s	60 s	60 s
Time held at set pressure:	140 s	80 s	20 s
Time to deflate:	40 s – simultaneously for all chambers		
Time delay between inflation of each chamber:	60 s		
ON time:	240 s		
OFF time:	100 s		
Cycle of intermittence (ON: OFF):	2.4:1		

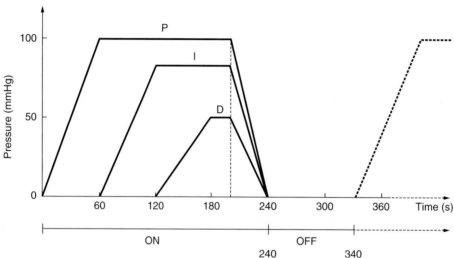

FIGURE 22-3 Sequential compression mode. The graded sequential mode is shown in this example.

stasis ulcers or wounds occur in the presence of incompetent venous valves that impair venous circulation. The backflow of venous blood causes venous congestion, tissue necrosis, and eventually ulceration. Another example is the vascular pain due to vascular intermittent claudication resulting from peripheral vascular diseases. The pain develops from walking because the arterial circulation is reduced and oxygen supply to muscles is insufficient.

C. BIOCHEMICAL EFFECTS

There is evidence to suggest that the mechanical effect of IPC triggers a biochemical effect that is responsible for the antithrombotic effect underlying the preventive treatment of DVT using such a therapeutic agent (Chouhan et al., 1999). This antithrombotic, or anticoagulation (see below), effect is attributed to increased shear stress imposed on the arterial endothelial cells by the compressive force. The initiating mechanism for

blood coagulation is the tissue factor–dependent pathway, which is affected by the tissue factor pathway inhibitor (Chouhan et al., 1999).

D. ANTICOAGULATION THERAPY

There is evidence to suggest that IPC therapy may be a *useful adjunct* to anticoagulation therapy for the prevention of DVT when pharmaceutical anticoagulation therapy (e.g., the use of warfarin [Coumadin] and heparin) is contraindicated because of the risk of increased bleeding (Hull et al., 1990; Fordyce et al., 1992; Woolson, 1996).

V. DOSIMETRY

A. PARAMETERS

The dosage associated with any IPC treatment consists of setting up the parameters listed below. Note that on

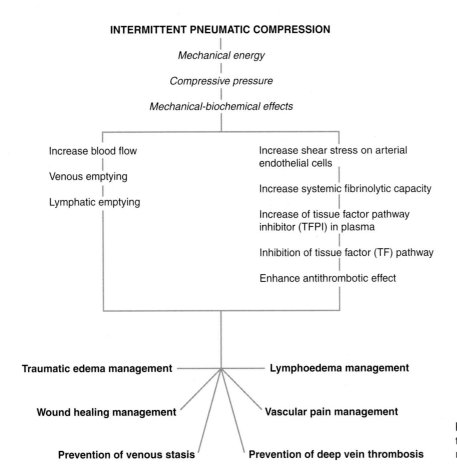

FIGURE 22-4 Proposed physiological and therapeutic effects of intermittent pneumatic compression therapy.

some devices some of these parameters may be preset. The range values shown below are provided as a *general guideline*; values will vary according to the types of IPC devices and types of pathologies under treatment.

1. Compression Mode

Select between the uniform or sequential mode. If the sequential mode is used, choose between graded or ungraded pressure gradients. No evidence could be found to suggest that one mode is therapeutically better than the other.

2. Pressure Gradient

Set the desired therapeutic pressure gradient. Pressure gradients may range from 30 to 140 mm Hg, depending on where they are applied (i.e., upper or lower extremities).

a. Upper Extremity Gradient

There is consensus in the scientific and corporate literature that pressure gradients used for the upper extremities should *range between 30 and 60 mm Hg*, and not exceed the patient's resting diastolic pressure, which should be about 80 mm Hg (Cameron, 2003; Lowe et al., 2005; Hecox et al., 2006).

b. Lower Extremity Gradient

Because venous pressure is usually higher in the lower extremities, there is also a consensus that pressure gra-dients used for the lower limb should be between 40 and 80 mm Hg, and as high as 140 mm Hg on some occa-sions (Cameron, 2003; Lowe et al., 2005; Hecox et al., 2006). There is evidence to suggest that the more dis-tal the compression (from foot, to calf, to thigh), the higher the pressure gradient should be. For example, it has been shown that foot compression needs signifi-cantly higher pressure than calf compression, typically 140 mm Hg or more, compared with approximately 40 mm Hg for the calf (Morris et al., 2004). Using an IPC_{foot} device can require pressure gradients as high as 100–140 mm Hg, and even greater pressure gradients may be needed to empty the plantar venous plexus (Morris et al., 2004; Starkey, 2004).

c. Pressure Gradients: Nongraded Versus Graded

In the uniform mode, the pressure gradient is always non-graded, that is, similar in all the garment's chambers. In the sequential mode, however, pressure gradients may be nongraded (similar in all chambers) or graded (different in each chamber).

3. Time to Inflate to Set Pressure

Select between 1 and 120 seconds. The longer the time is, the more comfortable the treatment.

4. Time Held at Set Pressure

Select between 1 and 60 seconds.

5. Time to Complete Deflation

Select between 1 and 60 seconds.

6. Time Delay Between Inflation of Each Chamber

Select between 1 and 60 seconds.

7. ON Time

The ON time is defined as the summation of the time to inflate, time held, and time to deflate. The ON time may be as short as 5 seconds and as long as 240 seconds.

8. OFF Time

The OFF time is defined as the time during which no pressure is exerted on the extremities. Select between 5 and 120 seconds.

9. Treatment Session Duration

This duration varies greatly according to the pathology under treatment. Durations may be as short as 45 minutes and may last as long as 4 hours; it may even be longer (up to 20 hours) when the therapeutic goal is to prevent DVT.

10. Number of Treatments per Day

The number of daily treatment may range between 1 and 3, depending again on the condition under treatment.

B. BLOOD PRESSURE MONITORING

IPC therapy may alter blood pressure. Monitor the patient's blood pressure before, during, and after treatment. If significant changes occur, consider modifying the dosage, and if significant changes persist, end the treatment.

VI. EVIDENCE FOR INDICATIONS

A. GUIDED BY EVIDENCE

Dictionaries generally define *evidence* as anything that establishes a fact or gives reason to believe something. The aim of this textbook is to present scientific evidence behind therapeutic EPAs. To be guided by evidence is the process of integrating the evidence from research, however imperfect or scarce this evidence may be, with clinical experience and patients' preferences. In other words, the *evidence-based practice* of EPA requires that practitioners consider the evidence from research, in addition to their own clinical experience and the patient's own preference and beliefs about a given EPA, when the time comes to justify, prescribe, and apply the therapeutic agent. To be guided by evidence is a process, not a search for the absolute truth. Finally, a lack of evidence from research behind any given EPA does not mean that this EPA should never be used. What it means is that no statement can be made about its therapeutic effectiveness and that until more evidence from research is presented, its routine use cannot be recommended.

B. EVIDENCE FROM HUMAN RESEARCH

Box 22-1 provides evidence for IPC therapy based on an exhaustive search of published English-language peer-reviewed studies on humans. The term *indication* is used in reference to a list of pathologies for which IPC therapy is employed. Ratings of clinical benefit (yes or no) and grading of strength of scientific evidence (I, II, or III), including the reference, are included for each pathological condition.

1. Rating Therapeutic Benefit

The rating, expressed as Yes or No, is based on the overall conclusion(s) reached on the issue of therapeutic effectiveness by the author(s) who conducted the peer-reviewed study.

2. Grading Strength of Evidence

The grading, numerically classified as I, II, and III, is based on the type of research methodology, or experimental design, used by the author(s). All those listed are studies on humans published in English-language peer-reviewed journals. It follows that studies graded I have stronger evidence than those graded II, whereas studies graded II have stronger evidence than those graded III.

a. Grade I

Evidence based on *controlled* studies on humans, regardless of their level of randomization and blindness.

b. Grade II

Evidence based on *noncontrolled* studies on humans, regardless of their level of randomization and blindness.

c. Grade III

Evidence based on *case* studies on humans, regardless of their level of randomization and blindness.

3. Strength of Evidence Behind the Agent

The strength of evidence behind the agent, as presented in the research-based indication box, is arbitrarily assessed in this textbook as *weak*, *moderate*, or *strong*. For example, the larger the number of studies graded I, regardless of therapeutic benefit, the stronger the scientific evidence behind the agent.

4. Evidence to Justify Usage of Agent

The strength of evidence to justify the usage of the agent for an individual pathology or groups of pathologies, as listed in the research-based indication box, is arbitrarily assessed in this textbook as *poor*, *fair*, *good*, or *conflicting*. For example, where a larger number of grade I studies show therapeutic benefit (Yes) than no benefit, for

Box 22-1	Research-Based Indications for Intermittent Pneumatic Compression Therapy

PATHOLOGY	BENEFIT	GRADE	REFERENCE
Prophylaxis for deep vein thrombosis (DVT)	Yes	I	Hull et al., 1990
	Yes	I	Skillman et al., 1978
	Yes	I	Coe et al., 1978
	Yes	I	Fisher et al., 1995
	Yes	I	Hartman et al., 1982
	Yes	I	Wilson et al., 1992
	Yes	II	Elliott et al., 1999
	Yes	II	Hass et al., 1990
	Yes	II	Ben-Galim et al., 2004
	Yes	II	Scurr et al., 1987
	Yes	II	Santori et al., 1994
	Yes	II	Bradley et al., 1993
	Yes	II	Fordyce et al., 1992
	Yes	II	Woolson, 1996
	Yes	II	Soderdahl et al., 1997
	Yes	II	Nicolaides et al., 1983
	Yes	II	Pidala et al., 1992
	Yes	II	Bailey et al., 1991
	Yes	II	Hooker et al., 1999
	Yes	II	Janssen et al., 1993
	Yes	II	Warwick et al., 1998
	Yes	II	Kamran et al., 1998
	Yes	II	Muhe, 1984
	Yes	II	Nicolaides et al., 1980
	Yes	III	Iwama et al., 2004
	Yes	II	Spain et al., 1998
	No	II	Muir et al., 2000
Lymphedema	Yes	II	Franzeck et al., 1997
	Yes	II	Swedborg, 1984
	Yes	II	Richmand et al., 1985
	Yes	II	Papas et al., 1992
	Yes	II	Zanolla et al., 1984
	Yes	III	Swedborg, 1977
	Yes	III	Klein et al., 1988
	Yes	III	Alexander et al., 1983
	Yes	III	Kim-Sing et al., 1987
	No	I	Dini et al., 1998
Venous ulcers	Yes	II	Nikolovska et al., 2005
	Yes	II	Samson, 1993
	Yes	II	Smith et al., 1990
	Yes	II	Rowland, 2000
	Yes	II	Kumar et al., 2002
	Yes	II	Alpagut et al., 2005
	Yes	II	Pfizenmaier et al., 2005
	Yes	II	McCulloch et al., 1994
	Yes	III	Hofman, 1995
	Yes	III	McCulloch, 1981
Vascular intermittent claudication	Yes	I	Delis et al., 2000c
	Yes	I	Delis et al., 2000d
	Yes	I	Delis et al., 2000e
	Yes	II	Delis et al., 2000b

(Continued)

Box 22-1	Continued

PATHOLOGY	BENEFIT	GRADE	REFERENCE
	Yes	II	Delis et al, 2005
	Yes	II	Ramaswani et al., 2005
	Yes	II	Kakkos et al., 2005
	Yes	II	Gaskel et al., 1978
Posttraumatic lower limb edema	Yes	I	Airaksinen, 1989
	Yes	I	Airaksinen et al., 1991
	Yes	I	Airaksinen et al., 1988
	Yes	II	Airaksinen et al., 1990
	Yes	II	Grieveson, 2003
	Yes	II	Thordarson et al., 1999
	Yes	II	Stockle et al., 1997
	Yes	II	Gardner et al., 1990
Limb ischemia—nonhealing wound	Yes	I	Kavros et al., 2008
	Yes	II	Montori et al., 2002
Delayed-onset muscle soreness	Yes	II	Chleboun et al., 1995
Infected foot wound	Yes	I	Armstrong et al., 2000
Dependent pregnancy edema	Yes	I	Jacobs et al., 1986
Poststroke hand edema	No	II	Roper et al., 1999
Diabetic wound	Yes	III	Wunderlich et al., 1998

a given pathology, the justification for usage of this agent for that pathology is assessed as *good*. *Conflicting* justification is reported when about an equal number of studies with similar grades show therapeutic benefit (Yes) and no benefit (No).

C. STRENGTH OF EVIDENCE AND JUSTIFICATION FOR USAGE

The results presented in **Box 22-1** show *strong* evidence for the use of IPC therapy, with the majority of studies graded II. These results also show *good* justification for the usage of this EPA for *prophylaxis* against DVT, as well as *moderate-to-good* justification for the treatment of lymphedema, venous ulcers, and vascular intermittent claudication. Until more evidence is provided, the *routine* use of IPC therapy for all of the other pathologies listed *cannot be recommended*.

VII. CONTRAINDICATIONS

Table 22-1 describes the contraindications associated with the practice of therapeutic IPC. Knowledge of the

patient's overall health status, particularly regarding his or her cardiac and respiratory condition, is essential.

VIII. RISKS, PRECAUTIONS, AND RECOMMENDATIONS

The practice of IPC therapy is not without risks for the patient. The main risks associated with this therapeutic agent, as well as some precautions and recommendations designed to improve safety and effectiveness, are listed in **Table 22-2**.

IX. CONSIDERATIONS FOR APPLICATION AND DOCUMENTATION

A. GENERAL CONSIDERATIONS

The application of IPC therapy may be relatively simple or complex, depending on the type of chambered IPC device used (IPC$_{thigh-calf-foot}$, IPC$_{calf-foot}$, IPC$_{foot.}$, IPC$_{arm-forearm-hand}$, or IPC$_{forearm-hand}$).

TABLE 22-1	CONTRAINDICATIONS TO INTERMITTENT PNEUMATIC COMPRESSION THERAPY
CONTRAINDICATIONS	**RATIONALE**
Over unstable extremity bone fracture	Risk of affecting adequate bone union because of bone movement caused by the compressive force (Cameron, 2003; Lowe et al., 2005).
In cases of acute pulmonary embolism and deep vein thrombosis (DVT) or thrombophlebitis	Risk of aggravation because the thrombus may dislodge or the embolus may travel under the compression force caused by the device to then block arteries to vital organs (Cameron, 2003; Lowe et al., 2005). For example an embolus to the pulmonary artery can impair lung function and may be life threatening. An embolus to a brain artery can cause a stroke.
In cases of severe peripheral arterial diseases	Risk of aggravation because the intermittent closing down of the damaged arteries may further impair circulation in the area (Cameron, 2003).
In cases of uncontrolled hypertension	Risk of increasing blood pressure to dangerous level by increasing vascular load on the heart.
In cases of congestive heart failure and pulmonary edema	Risk of increasing the vascular load on the failing organ system caused by the shifting of blood from the peripheral to the central circulation (Cameron, 2003; Lowe et al., 2005).
In cases of obstructed venous/lymphatic return	Risk of increased load (blood and lymph) on these systems because the obstruction to return flow does not allow adequate circulation (Cameron, 2003).

B. ILLUSTRATED APPLICATIONS

Figure 22-5 shows IPC therapy being applied to the lower extremity using a two-chambered device, IPC$_{calf-foot}$.

C. PROCEDURES

Safe, effective, and optimal application of IPC therapy requires that clinicians go through a systematic set of procedures for each and every application. The following is a list of such procedures.

1. Checklists

Before proceeding with treatment, always go through the list of contraindications (**Table 22-1**) and the list of risks, precautions, and recommendations (**Table 22-2**).

2. Patient Positioning

Ensure that the patient is comfortably positioned, and instruct him or her to relax the limb segment being treated.

TABLE 22-2	RISKS, PRECAUTIONS, AND RECOMMENDATIONS FOR INTERMITTENT PNEUMATIC COMPRESSION THERAPY
RISKS	**RATIONALE**
In cases of occult arterial diseases	Risk of developing a foot ulcer following IPC treatment, most likely caused by occult arterial disease (Oakley et al., 1998).
Malfunctioning of IPC device	Risk of developing an acute compartment due to malfunctioning of IPC devices (Werbel et al., 1986).
In cases of limb lymphedema	Risk of developing genital edema when IPC device is used for lower limb lymphedema (Boris et al., 1998).
Peroneal nerve compression	Risk of nerve compression at the level of the fibula head. Cases of peroneal nerve palsy have been documented (Pittman, 1989; Lachman et al., 1992; McGrory et al., 2000; Fukuda, 2006).

(Continued)

TABLE 22-2	CONTINUED

PRECAUTIONS	RATIONALE
Mentally impaired patients	Risk of improper dosimetry because patient is unable to report reliable information.
Patients with cancer	Risk of further growth of tumor from increase in blood circulation due to compression, which improves tissue nutrition (Cameron, 2003).
Numbness and tingling during therapy	Risk of peripheral nerve compression, caused by compressive force, may lead to nerve damage.
Improper device calibration	Risk of generating pressure far beyond the level indicated by the controller (Segers et al., 2002).

RECOMMENDATIONS	RATIONALE
Ensure correct application throughout treatment	Maintain correct application of the device and regular schedule of application for optimal results. IPC devices were found to be correctly applied only 60% of the time in a cohort of 1000 patients (Anglen et al., 1998). Fewer than 20% of patients at risk for DVT had the IPC devices on and functioning during the prescribed periods of treatment (Cornwell et al., 2002). The prescribed therapy was delivered on average only 78% of the time (Haddad et al., 2001).
Avoid simultaneous use of graduated compression stockings with IPC devices	No added benefit (Keith et al., 1992; Warwick et al., 2002).
Monitor patient's blood pressure during the course of therapy	To ensure that blood pressure stays within normal values or within the range established by the treating physician.
Use IPC$_{foot}$ devices for lower extremity fractures	Represents an effective alternative where the site of fracture precludes the use of calf and thigh devices (Spain et al., 1998).
Use recommended ON and OFF times	To prevent induced muscle ischemia, which may occur during inflation or ON times—if ON time is too long (Gilbart et al., 1995).
Use any limb position during therapy	Increased venous flow during IPC therapy occurs regardless of the limb positions used, i.e., elevated, horizontal, or dependent (Lurie et al., 2003).
Wash or discard stockinet after therapy	To ensure optimal hygiene.
Plug IPC devices into GFCI receptacles.	To eliminate the risk of electrical shock (see Chapter 27 for details).
Apply regular maintenance and calibration schedule	To ensure optimal functioning of devices and accessories. Follow manufacturer's recommendations and schedules.

3. Patient's Blood Pressure

Monitor and record blood pressure before, during, and at the end of treatment, to determine whether the treatment may be harmful.

4. Limb Preparation

Remove all jewelery and clothing. For sanitation purposes, cover the treated limb segment with a cylindrical cotton bandage, such as a stockinet. Make sure that the stockinet is free of wrinkles before sliding the garment over it.

5. Garment Application

Ensure that the garment is properly fitted to the limb segment before inflation. Regular monitoring is required to ensure that it stays properly adjusted.

6. Dosimetry

Select the dosimetric parameters (see Section V, Dosimetry) that will best meet the pathological condition and the desired therapeutic goal. Recall that the pressure gradients used for the upper and lower extremities may

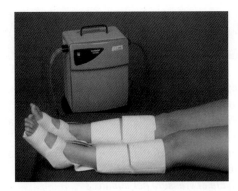

FIGURE 22-5 Application of IPC$_{foot}$ device. (Photo of VenAssist compression device used with permission of ACI Medical Management, Inc. © 1998 ACI Medical, Management, Inc. All rights reserved.)

vary between 30–60 mm Hg and 40–140 mm Hg, respectively.

7. End of Treatment

Inspect the exposed skin surface, and question the patient on the level of pressure perceived during treatment. Document any unusual sensation felt by the patient during treatment, in the patient's file.

D. DOCUMENTATION

Table 22-3 shows the key parameters that the clinician must document in the patient's file when using IPC therapy.

TABLE 22-3	KEY TREATMENT PARAMETERS TO BE DOCUMENTED IN PATIENT'S FILE AFTER INTERMITTENT PNEUMATIC COMPRESSION THERAPY

- *Patient's blood pressure at rest: diastolic/systolic:* mm Hg
- *IPC device:* I PC$_{thigh-calf-foot}$; IPC$_{calf-foot}$; IPC$_{foot}$; IPC$_{arm-forearm-hand}$; IPC$_{forearm-hand}$ or IPC$_{hand}$
- *Compression mode:* uniform or sequential
- *Pressure gradient:* mm Hg
- *Inflation–deflation time:* inflation : s; deflation; s
- *ON:OFF-time ratio:* s
- *Treatment session duration:* min
- *Number of treatments per day:* 1-2

Case Study 22-1 — Vascular Intermittent Claudication

A 63-year-old man suffering from peripheral arterial occlusive disease consults for treatment. His main complaint is decreasing ability to walk for relatively long periods of time and over relatively long distances. He also complains of leg pain when walking. Examination reveals an initial and absolute walking distance of only 100 and 250 m, respectively. This man has a 30-year history of smoking. Last month, a vascular surgeon declared him unfit for major vascular reconstructive surgery. He is under the regular care of his treating physician, who prescribes a daily dose of aspirin and recommends daily unsupervised exercise. The patient is increasingly worried because he has noticed a significant decrease in his quality of life his ability to walk freely and perform his regular daily living and leisure activities. His main goal is to improve his quality of life. He is looking for an effective home conservative treatment.

Evidence-Based Steps Toward the Resolution of This Case

1. List medical diagnosis.

  Stable vascular intermittent claudication

2. List key impairment(s).

- Leg pain during walking.

3. List key functional limitation(s).

- Difficulty walking for relatively long periods of time and over relatively long distances.
- Difficulty performing activities of daily living.

4. List key disability/disabilities.

- Difficulty with leisure activities

5. Justification for IPC therapy.

  Is there justification to use IPC therapy in this case? This chapter has established that there is *moderate-to-strong* evidence and *fair-to-good* justification for the use of IPC for intermittent claudication (see Section VI,). The selection of IPC is based on the body of evidence found in the following studies: Delis et al., 2000 b, c, d, e; Delis et al., 2005; Ramaswami et al., 2005. The use of IPC is expected to promote the development of collateral circulation in this patient, which would improve his ability to walk, for a longer time and over a greater distance, without leg pain. Because EPAs should not be used in isolation or as a sole intervention, this EPA

(Continued)

Case Study 22-1   Continued

is used here *concomitantly* with two other therapeutic procedures: a daily dose of aspirin and daily unsupervised exercise. The patient is also advised to reduce or, if possible, quit smoking.

6. **Search for contraindications.**

   None is found.

7. **Search for risks and precautions.**

   None is found.

8. **Outline the therapeutic goal(s) you and your patient wish to achieve.**

   - Decrease leg pain during walking
   - Improve ability to walk, in relation to time and distance
   - Improve leisure activity

9. **List the outcome measurement(s) used to assess treatment effectiveness.**

   - Walking
     - *Initial claudication distance,* that is, the distance (in meters) at which the patient feels pain or discomfort in the legs.
     - *Absolute claudication distance,* that is, the distance (in meters) at which the patient stops walking because the pain or discomfort becomes severe.

10. **Advise the patient about what he/she should experience, do, and not do during the SWD treatment.**

    - Sensation of intermittent pressure over the foot and calf

11. **Outline the prescription of IPC based on the evidence available.**

    The prescription given here is based on the following sources of evidence: Delis et al., 2000 b, c, d, e; Delis et al., 2005; Ramaswami et al., 2005. IPC is applied bilaterally over the foot and calf ($IPC_{foot-calf}$). This therapeutic regimen is initiated in the clinic and continued at home.

    - *IPC device:* two-chambered garment foot-and-calf device ($IPC_{foot-calf}$)
    - *Body position:* lying supine, lower extremities extended
    - *Application:* bilateral (right, then left side)

- *Mode:* sequential; foot garment inflation first followed, 1 s later, by calf garment inflation
- *Pressure gradient:* inflation: 120 mm Hg; deflation: 0 mm Hg
- *Inflation and deflation time:* inflation: 4 s; deflation: 16 s—cycle of pressure = 20 s
- *Cycle of pressure per minute:* 3
- *Treatment session duration:* 60 min for each extremity
- *Frequency of treatment per day:* 2
- *Total treatment duration:* 4 months

12. **Analyze outcome measurements.**

    Pre- and posttreatment comparison:

    - Initial claudication distance: gain of 200%; increased from 100 to 300 m.
    - Absolute claudication distance: gain of 400%; increased from 250 to 1250 m.

13. **Assess therapeutic effectiveness based on outcome measures.**

    The results show that daily bilateral applications of $IPC_{foot-calf}$ therapy, combined with a regimen of 1 aspirin daily and unsupervised exercise, for a period of 4 months, led to significant improvement in the walking ability of this patient, suffering from stable vascular intermittent claudication. The patient is very satisfied with the results because his pain-free walking distance has increased by 200% in addition to a 400% improvement in his total walking distance. He has now a much greater range of walking distance, which allows him to perform his daily activities and engage in more leisure activities, thus improving his quality of life. A follow-up at 12 months, revealed that the therapeutic gains are sustainable. Overall this treatment approach had a beneficial impact on the patient's disablement status created by the pathology, as illustrated in the **figure shown** on the next page.

14. **State the prognosis.**

    The prognostic is good if the patient complies with the following therapeutic recommendations: continue his daily regimen of aspirin and exercise, with emphasis on walking, and quit smoking. If his condition was to worsen, a new therapeutic regimen of home-based $IPC_{foot-calf}$ can be initiated once again.

THERAPEUTIC IMPACT on Disablement

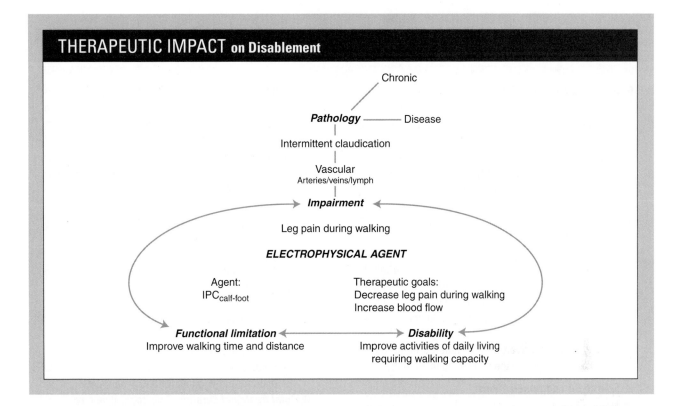

Chronic

Pathology ———— Disease

Intermittent claudication

Vascular
Arteries/veins/lymph

Impairment

Leg pain during walking

ELECTROPHYSICAL AGENT

Agent:
$IPC_{calf-foot}$

Therapeutic goals:
Decrease leg pain during walking
Increase blood flow

Functional limitation
Improve walking time and distance

Disability
Improve activities of daily living
requiring walking capacity

Case Study 22-2 — Deep Vein Thrombosis: Prevention After Total Hip Replacement

A 58-year-old male professional golfer is scheduled for a total replacement of his right hip because of severe osteoarthritis. His chief complaints are continuous hip pain and inability to play competitive golf on the senior professional tour. One of the most potentially lethal complications in the early postoperative period of hip arthroplasty is deep vein thrombosis (DVT), caused by venous stasis, which may lead to pulmonary embolism. DVT is the formation of a blood clot in a deep vein. Prevention of DVT is therefore essential in the management of this patient who is undergoing hip arthroplasty. This patient has a history of thromboembolism and hypertension. His hypertension problem is currently under control. The orthopedic surgeon is well aware that the prevention of DVT using drug anticoagulation therapy (such as warfarin [Coumadin] or heparin) is often associated with a major complication, namely, severe bleeding of soft tissue. The surgeon, considering this possible complication and the patient's history of thromboembolism, decides to manage the risk of DVT using IPC only, first applied intraoperatively and later postoperatively. The orthopedic surgeon handles the intraoperative portion of the IPC treatment and refers his patient to you for IPC for the postoperative period of treatment (day 2 to discharge from hospital). Contrary to all the other case studies presented in this textbook, the treatment goal here is the prevention of postsurgical DVT.

Evidence-Based Steps Toward the Resolution of This Case

1. **List medical diagnosis.**

   Severe right hip osteoarthritis leading to total hip replacement.

2. **List key impairment(s).**

   ■ Hip pain
   ■ Decrease hip range of motion

3. **List key functional limitation(s).**

   ■ Difficulty walking
   ■ Difficulty ascending and descending stairs

4. **List key disability/disabilities.**

   ■ Inability to play golf

(Continued)

Case Study 22-2   Continued

5. Justification for IPC therapy.

Is there justification to use IPC therapy in this case? This chapter has established that there is *strong* evidence and *good* justification for the use of IPC for prophylaxis against deep vein thrombosis following surgery (see Section VI). The selection of IPC is based on the body of evidence found in the following studies: Woolson, 1996; Spain et al., 1998; Hooker et al., 1999; Warwick et al., 1999. The orthopedic surgeon's goals are to prevent DVT and avoid the complication of bleeding in the soft tissues that is associated with oral anticoagulants. IPC is expected to discourage the development of venous stasis by exerting a pumping effect on the venous circulation. The use of IPC is highly recommended for cases in which patients are unable to bear weight for a few days after surgery. IPC therapy is used postoperatively, and graduated compressive stockings are worn by the patient, concomitantly.

6. Search for contraindications.

None is found.

7. Search for risks and precautions.

None is found. Note that although this patient has a history of hypertension, IPC therapy can be safely used in this case because his hypertensive condition is under control.

8. Outline the therapeutic goal(s) you and your patient wish to achieve.

■ Prevent DVT

9. List the outcome measurement(s) used to assess treatment effectiveness.

■ Monitoring signs for DVT: clinical examination
■ Monitoring soft-tissue bleeding: ultrasonography

10. Advise the patient about what he/she should experience, do, and not do during the IPC treatment.

■ Sensation of intermittent pressure over lower limbs

11. Outline the prescription of IPC based on the evidence available.

The prescription given here is based on the following publications: Woolson, 1996; Spain et al., 1998; Hooker

et al., 1999; Warwick et al., 1998. IPC is applied bilaterally over the foot, calf, and thighs. This postoperative therapeutic regimen is initiated in the recovery room and continued daily during the entire hospital stay (7 days). Practitioners are encouraged to read the excellent review article by Morris et al. (2004) on the prevention of DVT with IPC.

■ *IPC device:* $IPC_{thigh-calf-foot}$
■ *Sleeve type:* full limb sleeve with three chambers (one chamber each for the foot, calf, and thigh)
■ *Body position:* supine, lower limb elevated
■ *Mode:* sequential and graded inflation from distal to proximal chamber (foot, calf, thigh)
■ *Pressure (mm Hg):* 90 70 50
■ *Time to inflate (s):* 20 20 20
■ *Time held at set pressure (s):* 60 40 20
■ *Total time inflated (s):* 80 60 40
■ *Treatment time:* 18 hours a day; the sleeves were removed for bathing and for a few hours at night
■ *Total treatment duration:* 7 postoperative days

12. Analyze outcome measurements.

Pre- and posttreatment comparison:

■ Absence of DVT and soft-tissue bleeding as measured by ultrasonography

13. Assess therapeutic effectiveness based on outcome measures.

There was no evidence of DVT and soft-tissue bleeding during the 7-day treatment period while IPC was applied indicating total treatment success. The treatment was well tolerated by the patient. Overall, this preventive treatment approach had a beneficial impact on the patient's disablement status created by the pathology, as illustrated in the **figure shown** on the next page.

14. State the prognosis.

The prognosis is excellent if the patient continues to wear his graduated compression stockings at home for a few days and to gradually increase his weight-bearing duration and walking distance.

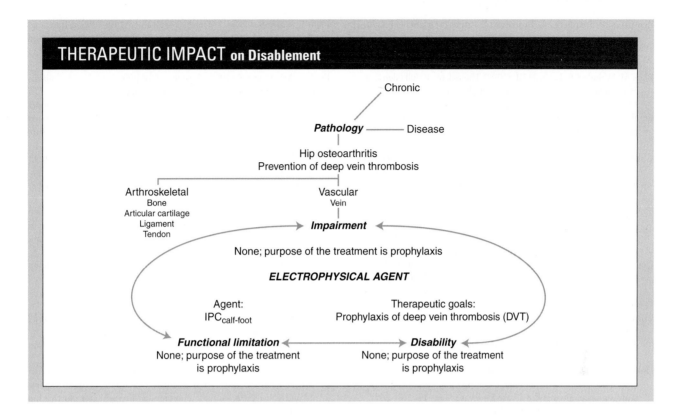

CRITICAL THINKING QUESTIONS

Clarification: What is meant by intermittent pneumatic compression (IPC) therapy?

Assumptions: You have assumed that the use of IPC therapy, as an alternative to drugs for the prevention of deep vein thrombosis (DVT), is well justified. How do you justify making that assumption?

Reasons and evidence: What led you to believe that IPC therapy can induce significant changes on the peripheral vascular system?

Viewpoints or perspectives: How would you respond to a colleague who says that there is no need for regular calibration of all IPC devices and that periodically checking the application during therapy is a waste of time?

Implications and consequences: What are the implications and possible consequences of a failure to record the patient's blood pressure before and during IPC treatment?

About the question: Can IPC therapy be beneficial for patients suffering from lymphedema, venous ulcers, and vascular intermittent claudication? Why do you think I ask this question?

References

Articles

Airaksinen O (1989) Changes in post traumatic ankle joint mobility, pain, and edema following intermittent pneumatic compression therapy. Arch Phys Med Rehab, 70: 341–344

Airaksinen O, Kolari PJ, Herve R, Holopainen R (1988) Treatment of post traumatic edema in lower legs using intermittent pneumatic compression. Scand J Rehab Med, 20: 25–28

Airaksinen O, Kolari PJ, Miettinen H (1990) Elastic bandages and intermittent pneumatic compression for treatment of acute ankle sprains. Arch Phys Med Rehab, 71: 380–383

Airaksinen O, Partanen K, Kolari PJ, Soimakallio S (1991) Intermittent pneumatic compression therapy in post traumatic lower limb edema: Computed tomography and clinical measurements. Arch Phys Med Rehab, 72: 667–670

Alexander M, Wright E, Wright J, Wright JB, Bikowski JB (1983) Lymphedema treated with linear pump: Pediatric case report. Arch Phys Med Rehab, 64: 132–133

Alpagut U, Davioglu E (2005) Importance and advantages of intermittent external pneumatic compression therapy in venous stasis ulceration. Angiology, 56: 19–23

Anglen JO, Goss K, Edwards J, Huckfeldt RE (1998) Foot pump prophylaxis for deep venous thrombosis: the rate of effective usage in trauma patients. Am J Orthop, 27: 580–582

Armstrong DG, Nguyen HC (2000) Intermittent pneumatic compression promoted healing in foot infections. Arch Surg, 135: 1405–1409

Bailey JP, Kruger MP, Solano FX, Zajko AB, Rubash HE (1991) Prospective randomized trial of sequential compression devices vs low-dose warfarin for deep venous thrombosis prophylaxis in total hip arthroplasty. J Arthroplasty, 6: 29–35

Ben-Galim P, Steinberg EL, Rosenblatt Y, Parnes N, Manehem A, Arbel R (2004) A miniature and mobile intermittent pneumatic compression device for the prevention of deep-vein thrombosis after joint replacement. Acta Orthop Scand, 75: 584–587

Boris M, Weindorf S, Lasinski BB (1998) The risk of genital edema after external pump compression for lower limb lymphedema. Lymphology, 31: 15–20

Bradley JG, Krugener GH, Jager HJ (1993) The effectiveness of intermittent plantar venous compression in prevention of deep venous thrombosis after total hip arthroplasty. J Arthroplasty, 1: 57–61

Chleboun GS, Howell JN, Baker HL, Ballard TN, Graham JL, Hallman HL, Perkins LE, Schauss JH, Conatser RR (1995) Intermittent pneumatic compression effect on eccentric exercise-induced swelling, stiffness, and strength loss. Arch Phys Med Rehab, 76: 744–749

Chouhan VD, Comerota AJ, Sun L, Harada R, Gaughan JP, Rao AK (1999) Inhibition of tissue factor pathway during intermittent pneumatic compression: A possible mechanism for antithrombotic effect. Arterioscler Thromb Vasc Biol, 19: 2812–2817

Coe NP, Collins Re, Klein LA, Bettmann MA, Skillman JJ, Shapiro RM, Salzman EW (1978) Prevention of deep vein thrombosis in urological patients: A controlled randomized trial of low-dose heparin and external pneumatic compression boots. Surgery, 83: 230–234

Cornwell EE, Chang D, Velmahos G, Jindal A, Baker D, Phillips J, Bonar J, Campbell K (2002) Compliance with sequential compression device prophylaxis in at-risk trauma patients: A prospective analysis. Am Surg, 68: 470–473

Delis KT, Azizi ZA, Stevens RJ, Wolfe JH, Nicolaides AN (2000a) Optimum intermittent pneumatic compression stimulus for lower-limb venous emptying. Eur J Vasc Endovasc Surg, 19: 261–269

Delis KT, Labropoulos N, Nicolaides AN, Glenville B, Stansby G (2000b) Effect of intermittent pneumatic compression on popliteal artery heamodynamics. Eur J Vasc Endovac Surg, 19: 270–277

Delis KT, Nicolaides AN (2005) Effects of intermittent pneumatic compression of foot and calf on walking distance, hemodynamics, and quality of life in patients with arterial claudication: A prospective randomized controlled study with 1-year follow-up. Ann Surg, 241: 431–441

Delis KT, Nicolaides AN, Labropoulos N, Stansby G (2000c) The acute effects of intermittent pneumatic foot versus calf versus simultaneous foot and calf compression on popliteal artery hemodynamics: A comparative study. J Vasc Surg, 32: 284–292

Delis KT, Nicolaides AN, Wolfe JH, Stansby G (2000d) Improving walking ability and ankle brachial pressure indices in symptomatic peripheral vascular disease with intermittent pneumatic foot compression: A prospective controlled study with a one-year follow-up. J Vasc Surg, 31: 650–651

Delis KT, Slimani G, Hafez HM, Nicolaides AN (2000e) Enhancing venous outflow in the lower limb with intermittent pneumatic compression: A comparative haemodynamic analysis on the effect of foot vs. calf vs. foot and calf compression. Eur J Vasc Endovasc Surg, 19: 250–260

Dini D, Del Mastro L, Gozza A, Lionetto O, Forno G, Vidili G, Bertelli G, Venturini M (1998) The role of pneumatic compression in the treatment of post mastectomy lymphedema: A randomized phase III study. Ann Oncol, 9: 187–190

Elliott CG, Dudney TM, Egger M, Orme JF, Clemmer TP, Horn SD, Waever L, Handrahan D, Thomas F, Merrell S, Kitterman N, Yeates S (1999) Calf-thigh sequential pneumatic compression compared with plantar venous pneumatic compression to prevent deep vein thrombosis after non-lower extremity trauma. J Trauma, 47: 25–32

Eze AR, Comerota AA, Cisek PL, Holland BS, Kerr RP, Veeramasuneri R, Camerota AJl (1996) Intermittent calf and foot compression increases lower extremity blood flow. Am J Surg, 172: 130–134

Fisher CG, Blachut PA, Salvian AJ, Meek RN, O'Brien PJ (1995) Effectiveness of pneumatic compression devices for the prevention of thromboembolic disease in orthopeadic trauma patients: A prospective, randomized study of compression alone versus no prophylaxis. J Orthop Trauma, 9: 1–7

Flam E, Berry S, Coyle A, Dardik H, Raab L (1996) Blood-flow augmentation of intermittent pneumatic compression system used for prevention of deep vein thrombosis prior to surgery. Am J Surg, 171: 312–315

Fordyce MJ, Ling RS (1992) A venous foot pump reduces thrombosis after total hip replacement. J Bone Joint Surg (B), 74: 45–49

Franzeck UK, Spiegel I, Fischer M, Bortzler C, Stahel HU, Bollinger A (1997) Combined physical therapy for lymphedema evaluated by fluorescence microlymphography and lymph capillary pressure measurements. J Vasc Res, 34: 306–311

Fukuda H (2006) Bilateral peroneal nerve palsy caused by intermittent pneumatic compression. Intern Med, 45: 93–94

Gardner AM, Fox RH (1983) The venous pump of the human foot—preliminary report. Bristol Med Chir J, 367: 109–112

Gardner AM, Fox RH, Lawrence C, Bunker TD, Ling RS, McEachen AG (1990) Reduction of posttraumatic swelling and compartment pressure by impulse compression of the foot. J Bone Joint Surg (B), 72: 810–815

Gaskell P, Parrott JC (1978) The effect of a mechanical venous pump on the circulation of the feet in the presence of arterial obstruction. Surg Gynecol Obst, 146; 583–592

Gilbart MK, Oglivie-Harris DJ, Broadhurst C, Clarfield M (1995) Anterior tibial compartment pressures during intermittent sequential pneumatic compression therapy. Am J Sports Med, 23: 769–772

Grieveson G (2003) Intermittent pneumatic compression pump settings for optimum reduction of oedema. J Tissue Viab, 13: 98–110

Haddad FS, Kerry RM, McEwen JA, Appleton L, Garbuz DS, Masri BA, Duncan CP (2001) Unanticipated variations between expected and delivered pneumatic compression therapy after elective hip surgery: A possible source of variation in reported patient outcomes. J Arthroplasty, 16: 37–46

Hartman JT, Pugh JL, Smith RD, Robertson WW, Yost RP, Janssen HF (1982) Cyclic sequential compression of the lower limb in prevention of deep venous thrombosis. J Bone Joint Surg (A), 64: 1059–1062

Hass SB, Insall JN, Scuderi GR, Windsor RE, Ghelman B (1990) Pneumatic sequential-compression boots compared with aspirin prophylaxis of deep-vein thrombosis after total knee arthroplasty. J Bone Joint Surg (A), 72: 27–31

Hofman D (1995) Intermittent compression treatment for venous leg ulcers. J Wound Care, 4: 163–165

Hooker JA, Lachiewicz PF, Kelley SS (1999) Efficacy of prophylaxis against thromboembolism with intermittent pneumatic compression after primary and revision of total hip arthroplasty. J Bone Joint Surg (A), 81: 690–696

Hull RD, Raskob GE, Gent M, McLoughlin D, Julian D, Smith FC, Dale NI, Reed-Davis R, Lofthouse RN, Anderson C (1990) Effectiveness of intermittent pneumatic leg compression for preventing deep vein thrombosis after total hip replacement. JAMA, 263: 2313–2317

Iwama H, Obara S, Ohmizo H (2004) Changes in femoral blood flow velocity by intermittent pneumatic compression: Calf compression device versus plantar-calf sequential compression device. J Aneasth, 18: 232–233

Iwama H, Suzuki M, Hojo M, Keneda M, Akutsu I (2000) Intermittent pneumatic compression on the calf improves peripheral circulation of the leg. J Crit Care, 15: 18–21

Jacobs M, McCance KL, Stewart ML (1986) Leg volume changes with EPIC and posturing in dependent pregnancy edema: External pneumatic intermittent compression. Nurs Res, 35: 86–89

Janssen H, Trevino C, Williams D (1993) Hemodynamic alterations in venous blood flow produced by external pneumatic compression. J Cardiovasc Surg, 34: 441–447

Kakkos SK, Geroulakos G, Nicolaides AN (2005) Improvement of the walking ability in intermittent claudication due to superficial femoral artery occlusion with supervised exercise and pneumatic foot and calf compression: A randomized controlled trial. Eur J Vasc Endovasc Surg, 30: 164–175

Kamran SI, Downey D, Ruff RL (1998) Pneumatic sequential compression reduces the risk of deep vein thrombosis in stroke patients. Neurology, 50: 1683–1688

Kavros SJ, Delis KT, Turner NS, Voll AE, Liedl DA, Gloviczki P, Rooke TW (2008) Improving limb salvage in critical ischemia with intermittent pneumatic compression: A controlled study with 18-month follow-up. J Vasc Surg, 47: 543–549

Keith SL, McLaughlin DJ, Anderson FA, Cardullo PA, Jones CE, Rohrer MJ, Cutler BS (1992) Do graduated compression stockings and pneumatic boots have an additive effect on the peak velocity of venous blood flow? Arch Surg, 127: 727–730

Kim-Sing C, Basco VE (1987) Post mastectomy lymphedema treated with the Wright linear pump. Can J Surg, 30: 368–370

Klein MJ, Alexander MA, Wright JM, Redmond CK, LeGasse AA (1988) Treatment of adult lower extremity lymphedema with the Wright linear pump: Statistical analysis of a clinical trial. Arch Phys Med Rehab, 69: 202–206

Kumar S, Samraj K, Nirujogi V, Budnik J, Walker M (2002) Intermittent pneumatic compression as an adjuvant therapy in venous ulcer disease. J Tissue Viability, 12: 42–50

Lachmann EA, Rook JL, Tunkel R, Nagler W (1992) Complications associated with intermittent pneumatic compression. Arch Phys Med Rehab, 73: 482–485

Landis EM (1935) The treatment of peripheral diseases by means of alternative negative and positive pressure. Penn Med J, 38: 579–583

Landis EM, Gibbon JH (1933) The effects of alternating suction and pressure on blood flow to the lower extremities. J Clin Invest, 12: 925–961

Lurie F, Awaya DJ, Kistner RL, Eklof B (2003) Hemodynamic effect of pneumatic compression and the position of the body. J Vasc Surg, 37: 137–142

Malone MD, Cisek PL, Comerota AJ, Holland B, Eid IG, Comerota AJ (1999) High-pressure, rapid inflation pneumatic compression improves venous hemodynamics in healthy volunteers and patients who are post-thrombotic. J Vasc Surg, 29: 593–599

Masri BA, Dunlop DJ, McEwen JA, Garbuz DS, Duncan CP (2004) Can new design pneumatic compression device reduce variations in delivery therapy for the mechanical prophylaxis of thromboembolic disease after total hip arthroplasty? Can J Surg, 47: 263–269

McCulloch JM (1981) Intermittent compression for the treatment of a chronic stasis ulceration: A case report. Phys Ther, 61: 1452–1453

McCulloch JM, Marler KC, Neal MB, Phifer TJ (1994) Intermittent pneumatic compression improves venous ulcer healing. Adv Wound Care, 7: 22–24, 26

McGrory BJ, Burke DW (2000) Peroneal nerve palsy following intermittent sequential pneumatic compression. Orthopedics, 23: 1103–1105

Montori VM, Kavros SJ, Walsh EE, Rooke TW (2002) Intermittent compression pump for nonhealing wounds in patients with limb ischemia: The Mayo Clinic experience (1998–2000). Int Angiol, 21: 360–366

Muhe E (1984) Intermittent sequential high-pressure compression of the leg: A new method of preventing deep vein thrombosis. Am J Surg, 147: 781–785

Muir KW, Watt A, Baxter G, Grosset DG, Lees KR (2000) Randomized trial of graded compression stockings for prevention of deep vein thrombosis after acute stroke. QJM, 93: 359–364

Nicolaides AN, Fernandes E, Fernandes J, Pollock AV (1980) Intermittent sequential pneumatic compression of the legs in the prevention of venous stasis and post operative deep venous thrombosis. Surgery, 87: 69–76

Nicolaides AN, Miles C, Hoare M, Jury P, Helmis E, Venniker R (1983) Intermittent sequential pneumatic compression of the legs and thromboembolism-deterrent stockings in the prevention of postoperative deep vein thrombosis. Surgery, 94: 21–25

Nikolovska S, Arsovski A, Damevska K, Gocev G, Pavlova L (2005) Evaluation of two different pneumatic compression cycle settings in the healing of venous ulcers: A randomized trial. Med Sci Monit, 7: 337–343

Oakley MJ, Wheelwright EF, James P (1998) Pneumatic compression boots for prophylaxis against deep vein thrombosis: Beware occult arterial disease. Br Med J, 316: 454–455

Pappas CH, O'Donnell TF (1992) Long-term results of compression treatment for lymphedema. J Vasc Surg, 16: 555–564

Pfizenmaier DH, Kavros SJ, Liedl DA, Cooper LT (2005) Use of intermittent pneumatic compression for treatment of upper extremity vascular ulcers. Angiology, 56: 417–422

Pidala MJ, Donovan DL, Kepley RF (1992) A prospective study on intermittent pneumatic compression in the prevention of deep vein thrombosis in patients undergoing total hip or total knee replacement. Surg Gynecol Obstet, 175: 47–51

Pittman GR (1989) Peroneal nerve palsy following sequential pneumatic compression. JAMA, 261: 2201–2202

Rasmaswami G, D'Ayala M, Hollier LH, Deutsch R, McElhinney AJ (2005) Rapid foot and calf compression increases walking distance in patients with intermittent claudication: Results of a randomized study. J Vasc Surg, 41: 794–801

Reid MR, Hermann LG (1934) Passive vascular exercises—treatment of vascular diseases by rhythmic alternation of environmental pressure. Arch Surg, 29: 697–704

Richmand DM, O'Donnell TF, Zelikovski A (1985) Sequential pneumatic compression for lymphedema: A controlled trial. Arch Surg 129: 1116–1119

Roper TA, Redford S, Tallis RC (1999) Intermittent compression for the treatment of the oedematous hand in hemiplegic stroke: A randomized control trial. Age Ageing, 28: 9–13

Rowland J (2000) Intermittent pump versus compression bandages in the treatment of venous leg ulcers. Aust NZ J Surg, 70: 110–113

Samson RH (1993) Compression stockings and non-continuous use of polyurethane foam dressings for the treatment of venous ulceration. A pilot study. J Dermatol Surg Oncol, 19: 68–72

Santori FS, Vitullo A, Stopponi M, Santori N, Ghera S (1994) Prophylaxis against deep-vein thrombosis in total hip replacement. Comparison of heparin and foot impulse pump. J Bone Joint Surg (B), 76: 579–583

Scurr JH, Coleridge-Smith PD, Hasty JH (1987) Regimen for improved effectiveness of intermittent pneumatic compression in deep venous thrombosis prophylaxis. Surgery, 102: 816–820

Segers P, Blegrado J, Leduc A, Leduc O, Verdonck P (2002) Excessive pressure in multichambered cuffs used for sequential compression therapy. Phys Ther, 82: 1000–1008

Skillman JJ, Collins RE, Coe RE, Goldstein BS, Shapiro RM, Zervas NT, Bettman MA, Salsman EW (1978) Prevention of deep vein thrombosis in neurosurgical patients: A controlled, randomized trial of external pneumatic compression boots. Surgery, 83: 354–358

Smith PC, Sarin S, Hasty J, Scurr JH (1990) Sequential gradient pneumatic compression enhances venous ulcer healing: A randomized trial. Surgery, 108: 871–875

Soderdahl DW, Henderson SR, Hansberry KL (1997) A comparison of intermittent pneumatic compression of the calf and whole leg in preventing deep venous thrombosis in urological surgery. J Urol, 157: 1774–1776

Spain DA, Bergamini TM, Hoffmann JF, Carrillo EH, Richardson JD (1998) Comparison of sequential compression devices and foot pumps for prophylaxis of deep venous thrombosis in high-risk trauma patients. Am Surg, 64: 522–525

Stockle U, Hoffmann R, Schutz M, Von Fournier C, Sudkamp NP, Haas N (1997) Fastest reduction of post traumatic edema: Continuous cryotherapy or intermittent impulse compression? Foot Ankle Int, 18: 432–438

Swedborg I (1977) Volumetric estimation of the degree of lymphedema and its therapy by pneumatic compression. Scand J Rehab Med, 9: 131–135

Swedborg I (1984) Effects of treatment with an elastic sleeve and intermittent pneumatic compression in post mastectomy patients with lymphoedema of the arm. Scand J Rehab Med, 16: 35–41

Thordarson DB, Greene N, Shepherd L, Perlman M (1999) Facilitating edema resolution with a foot pump after calcaneus fracture. J Orthop Trauma, 13: 43–46

Warwick D, Harrison J, Glew D, Mitchelmore A, Peters TJ, Donovan J (1998) Comparison of the use of a foot pump with the use of low-molecular-weight heparin for the prevention of deep-vein thrombosis after total hip replacement: A prospective randomized trial. J Bone Joint Surg (A), 80: 1158–1166

Warwick DJ, Pandit H, Shewale S, Shewale S, Sulkin T (2002) Venous impulse foot pumps: Should graduated compression stockings be used? J Arthroplasty, 17: 446–448

Werbel GB, Shybut GT (1986) Acute compartment syndrome caused by a malfunctioning pneumatic compression boot: A case report. J Bone Joint Surg (A), 68: 1445–1446

Westrich GH, Specht LM, Sharrock NE, Sculco TP, Salvati EA, Pellici PM, Treombley JF, Peterson M (2000) Pneumatic compression hemodynamic in total hip arthroplasty. Clin Orthop Relat Res, 372: 180–191

Westrich GH, Specht LM, Sharrock NE, Sharrock NE, Windsor RE, Sculco TP, Haas SB, Trombley JF, Peterson M (1998) Venous haemodynamics after total knee arthroplasty: Evaluation of active dorsal to plantar flexion and several mechanical compression devices. J Bone Joint Surg (B), 80: 1057–1066

Whitelaw GP, Oladipo OJ, Shah BP, DeMuth KA, Coffman J, Segal D (2001) Evaluation of intermittent pneumatic compression devices. Orthopedics, 24: 257–261

Wilson NV, Das SK, Kakkar VV, Maurice HD, Smibert JG, Thomas EM, Nixon JE (1992) Thrombo-embolic prophylaxis in total knee replacement. Evaluation of the A-V Impulse System. J Bone Joint Surg (B), 74: 50–52

Woolson ST (1996) Intermittent pneumatic compression prophylaxis for proximal deep vein thrombosis after total hip replacement. J Bone Joint Surg (A), 78: 1735–1740

Wunderlich RP, Armstrong DG, Harkless LB (1998) Is intermittent pulsatile pressure a valuable adjunct in healing the complicated diabetic wound? Ostomy Wound Manage, 44: 70–74, 76

Zanolla R, Mongeglio C, Balzarini A, Martino G (1984) Evaluation of the results of three different methods of postmastectomy lymphedema treatment. J Surg Oncol, 26: 210–213

Review Articles

Alguire PC, Mathes BM (1997) Chronic venous insufficiency and venous ulceration. J Gen Int Med, 12: 374–383

Berliner E, Ozbilgin B, Zarin DA (2003) A systematic review of pneumatic compression for treatment of chronic venous insufficiency and venous ulcers. J Vasc Surg, 37: 539–544

Boudouroglou D, Kakkos SK, Geroulakos (2004) Adjuvant medical therapy to deep venous reconstruction. Phlebology, 19: 4–6

Brennan M, Miller L (1998) Overview of treatment options and review of the current role and use of compression garments, intermittent pumps and exercise in the management of lymphedema. Cancer, 83: 2821–2827

Chen AH, Frangos SG, Kilaru S, Sumpio BE (2001) Intermittent pneumatic compression devices—physiological mechanisms of action. Eur J Vasc Endovasc Surg, 21: 383–392

Choucair M, Philips TJ (1998) Compression therapy. Phlebology, 24: 141–148

Delis KT (2005) The case for intermittent pneumatic compression of the lower extremity as a novel treatment in arterial claudication. Perspect Vasc Surg Endovasc Ther, 17: 29–42

Freedman KB, Brookenthal KR, Fitzgerald RH, Williams S, Lonner JH (2000) A meta-analysis of thromboembolic prophylaxis following elective total hip arthroplasty. J Bone Joint Surg (A), 82: 929–938

Hopkins A (2002) The use of intermittent pneumatic compression in venous leg ulcer management. LUF J, 16: 20–21

Kumar S, Walker MA (2002) The effects of intermittent pneumatic compression on the arterial and venous system of the lower limb: A review. J Tissue Viab, 12: 58–66

Illingworth C, Timmons S (2007) An audit of intermittent pneumatic compression (IPC) in the prophylaxis of asymptomatic deep vein thrombosis (DVT). J Perioper Pract, 17: 522–524; 526–528

Imperiale TF, Speroff T (1994) A meta-analysis of methods to prevent venous thromboembolism following total hip arthroplasty. JAMA, 271: 1780–1785

Kunimoto B, Cooling M, Gulliver W, Houghton P, Orsted H, Sibbald RG (2001) Best practices for the prevention and treatment of venous leg ulcers. Ostomy Wound Manage, 47: 34–46, 48–50

MacLellan DG, Fletcher JP (2007) Mechanical compression in the prophylaxis of venous thromboembolism. ANZ J Surg, 77: 418–423

Megens A, Harris SR (1998) Physical therapist management of lymphedema following treatment for breast cancer: A critical review of its effectiveness. Phys Ther, 78: 1302–1311

Morris RJ, Woodcock JP (2004) Evidence-based compression: Prevention of stasis and deep vein thrombosis. Ann Surg, 239: 162–171

O'Neil B (1997) A review of the role of sequential compression therapy in post-operative management of patients undergoing venous valve surgery. Physioth Can, 49: 109–122

Ramzi DW, Leeper KV (2004) DVT and pulmonary embolism: Part II. Treatment and prevention. Am Fam Physician, 69: 2841–2848

Roderick P, Ferris G, Wilson K, Halls H, Jackson D, Collins R, Baigent C (2005) Towards evidence-based guidelines for the prevention of venous thromboembolism: Systematic review of mechanical methods, oral anticoagulation, dextran and regional anaesthesia as thromboprolaxis. Health Technol Assess, 49: 1–78

Urbankova J, Quiroz R, Kucher N, Goldhaber SZ (2005) Intermittent pneumatic compression and deep vein thrombosis prevention. A meta-analysis in postoperative patients. Thromb Heamost, 94: 1181–1185

Vanek VW (1998) Meta-analysis of effectiveness of intermittent pneumatic compression devices with a comparison of thigh-high to knee-high sleeves. Am Surg, 64: 1050–1058

Vowden K (2001) The use of intermittent pneumatic compression in venous ulceration. Br J Nurs, 10: 491–509

Westrich GH, Haas SB, Mosca P, Peterson M (2000) Meta-analysis of thromboembolic prophylaxis after total knee arthroplasty. J Bone Joint Surg (B), 82: 795–800

Chapters of Textbooks

Cameron MH (2003) Compression. In: Physical Agents in Rehabilitation: From Research to Practice, 2nd ed. Saunders, St-Louis, pp 341–368

Hecox B, Jacobs LF (2006) External compression. In: Integrating Physical Agents in Rehabilitation, 2nd ed. Hecox B, Mehreteab TA, Weisberg J, Sanko J (Eds). Prentice Hall, Upper Saddle River, pp 387–396

Lowe E, Smith W, Nolan TP (2005) Mechanical modalities: Traction and intermittent pneumatic compression. In: Modalities for Therapeutic Intervention, 4th ed. Michlovitz SL, Nolan TP (Eds). FA Davis Co, Philadelphia, pp 165–181

Starkey C (2004) Intermittent compression. In: Therapeutic Modalities, 3rd ed. FA Davis Co., Philadelphia, pp 280–286

CHAPTER 23

Continuous Passive Motion Therapy

Chapter Outline

Learning Objectives

Knowledge: List the common technical features found in most continuous passive motion (CPM) devices.

Comprehension: Summarize the proposed physiological and therapeutic effects associated with CPM therapy.

Application: Outline the key parameters related to the dosimetry of CPM therapy.

Analysis: Explain the principle behind the use of CPM therapy.

Synthesis: Distinguish between CPM therapy and other therapies used to mobilize postsurgical joints.

Evaluation: Explain why CPM therapy should be initiated as soon as possible after joint surgery.

I. RATIONALE FOR USE

A. DEFINITION AND DESCRIPTION

The term *continuous passive motion*, known by the acronym CPM, is defined as a postoperative therapeutic agent that passively and continuously moves a joint through a prescribed range of motion (ROM) for an extended period of time. CPM therapy is a therapeutic intervention the key aim of which is to move human joints without the patient's assistance. In other words, CPM provides a motion substitute until the patient is able to actively move the affected joints in the desirable ROM. Practitioners can find, in the current market, commercial CPM devices designed to mobilize several joints, namely the *hip, knee, ankle, big toe, shoulder, elbow, wrist, thumb,* and *temporomandibular* joints.

B. CPM DEVICES

Figure 23-1 shows typical CPM devices used to mobilize some of the joints listed above. Considering the high prevalence and incidence of knee pathologies, the number of devices designed specifically for the knee joint far exceeds the number of devices for the other joints. As shown in **Figure 23-1**, a typical CPM device is made of three parts: (1) a carriage made of levers on which rests a body's

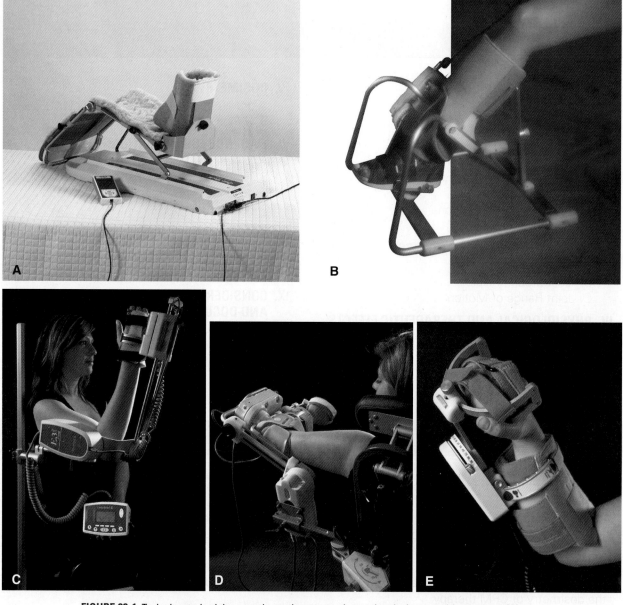

FIGURE 23-1 Typical motorized therapeutic continuous passive motion devices used for the knee (**A**), ankle (**B**), elbow (**C**), shoulder (**D**), and wrist (**E**). These devices present several bed- and chair-fitting features to accommodate different human segments and positions. (Courtesy of Otto Bock HealthCare.)

extremity support system, (2) an electrically powered motor-controller unit which moves the levers and may be programmed for ROM, speed of motion, and duration of treatment, and (3) a handheld control system used for programming and safety purposes. These devices can be used in hospital, clinical, and home settings.

C. RATIONALE FOR USE

Postsurgical joint management is very often associated with severe pain that prevents patients from actively mobilizing the affected joint in the hours and days after surgery. Research has shown that prolonged rest or immobilization of a joint after surgery significantly increases the risk of joint stiffness, which later may cause significant mobility and functional problems. The rationale behind the use of CPM therapy is thus to provide a substitute for the patient's temporary inability to actively move his or her affected joint, by providing controlled passive and continuous joint motion for an extended period of time. The main purpose of this therapeutic agent is to prevent postoperative joint stiffness, which in turn should enhance soft-tissue healing and accelerate the recovery of joint mobility and function.

II. HISTORICAL PERSPECTIVE

A. REST VERSUS MOVEMENT

Controversy between the use of rest or movement to treat soft-tissue pathologies dates back to Hippocrates and Aristotle, the former proposing that the best way to heal the body is to rest it, whereas the latter's viewpoint was that movement will best promote healing (McCarthy et al., 1992). The dilemma about using immobilization or motion to treat joint pathologies lasted until the 1960s, when evidence from scientific research began to document the ill effects of using rest or immobilization and the beneficial effects of using early mobilization to treat joint pathologies (Salter et al., 1960).

B. FOUNDATION

The use of CPM as a therapeutic agent for joint pathologies was originally proposed by Robert Salter, a Canadian physician, in the early 1970s (Salter et al., 1982, 1984, 1989, 1994, 1996). The principle underlying Salter's concept is that joint motion is necessary to maintain articular cartilages health. His concept was a blow to the time-honored but unproven dictum that joint pathologies must be rested or immobilized, just as with bones after fractures, to heal properly (Salter, 1989).

C. FIRST HUMAN APPLICATION

The first documented use of CPM therapy on human joints is that of Salter and colleagues in 1984. They reported on the therapeutic benefits of this treatment on nine individuals affected with various bone and joint pathologies (Salter et al., 1984). Since then, Salter's work has inspired a large body of basic and clinical research on the use and effects of this mechanical therapeutic agent for postoperative management of joint pathologies.

D. BODY OF LITERATURE

CPM therapy has been the subject of several *articles* (see Reference), *review articles* (Salter, 1982, 1989, 1994, 1996; McCarthy et al., 1992; Lawrence, 1996; Lachiewicz, 2000; O'Driscoll et al., 2000; Lenssen et al., 2003; Milne et al., 2003; Brosseau et al., 2004; Postel et al., 2007; Grella, 2008), and of a few *chapters in textbooks* (Turturro, 2003; Starkey, 2004).

III. BIOPHYSICAL CHARACTERISTICS

A. MECHANICAL PRINCIPLE

The biophysical principle underlying CPM therapy is mechanical. A mechanical torque, or moment of force about the affected joint axis of rotation, is generated by means of a programmable electrical motor embedded in the device, which moves metal or plastic levers, over which the affected limb rests, through various angles of the joint ROM (see **Fig 23-1**).

B. ILLUSTRATED PRINCIPLE

Figure 23-2 is a schematic illustration (side view) of this mechanical principle using a knee CPM device that passively moves the knee joint from full extension (**A**) through 120° flexion (**B**), and back to full extension (**C**). A full cycle of passive extension/flexion motion is thus created by the device in this example.

C. JOINT RANGE OF MOTION

The torque generated by the device passively moves the resting affected joint through a prescribed ROM, which is gradually increased over time until full ROM is achieved. For example, an initial ROM setting can be from 0° extension to 90° flexion, with increments of 5° every 2 days, until the full 0–120° range is obtained.

1. Passive Torque

The torque magnitude generated by some CPM devices can be set low or high. Torque setting (low or high) is dictated by the device's capacity to move the affected joint through its full ROM, meaning that a heavier limb, as opposed to a lighter limb, is most likely to require a high, rather than a low, torque setting.

2. Cycle of Motion

A cycle is defined as the total number of degrees a joint is moved by the device from the initial position to the target

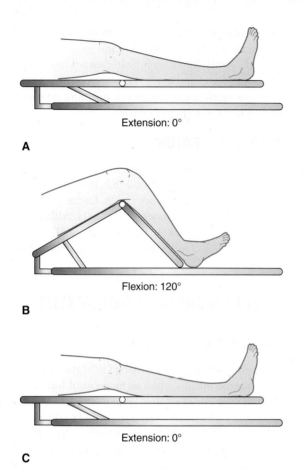

FIGURE 23-2 Schematic representation of the mechanical principle behind the use of CPM devices. Shown is a knee device mounted with its platform and moving metal levers, over which rests the affected lower limb. The cycle of motion is from 0° extension (**A**) to 120° flexion (**B**) and back to 0° extension (**C**).

position and back to the initial position. For example, if the ROM is set as shown in **Figure 23-2**, from 0° extension (E) to 120° flexion (F) and back to 0° extension (E), then the cycle will correspond to 0° E–120°F–0° E. The total ROM cycle will be 240°.

3. Speed of Motion

The device also moves the affected joint at a desired speed. For example, if the setting is 4°/s in the above example, then the total cycle of motion duration will be 60 seconds (240°/4°/s).

4. Application Duration per Day

CPM devices may be applied continuously, or intermittently, for periods of time ranging from one hour to several hours per day. For example, if the application duration is set at 8 hours per day, then the total number of joint motion cycles in the above example will be 480 (8 hours or 480 minutes or 28800 seconds / 60 seconds = 480 cycles).

IV. PHYSIOLOGICAL AND THERAPEUTIC EFFECTS

A. SPECIFIC MECHANICAL EFFECTS

Presented in **Figure 23-3** are the proposed physiological effects associated with CPM therapy. The immediate postsurgical passive and continuous cycling movements of the affected joint, over prolonged periods of time every day and over several consecutive days, are proposed to prevent joint stiffness by minimizing joint hemarthrosis and periarticular edema, and promoting or enhancing joint healing through increased cartilage nutrition (Salter, 1994; O'Driscoll et al., 2000, Grella, 2008).

B. OTHER THERAPEUTIC EFFECTS

In addition to the specific mechanical effects described, there is evidence from the literature cited in this chapter that CPM therapy may also provide related clinical benefits such as (1) reducing the frequency and dosage of postoperative analgesics, (2) decreasing the length of hospitalization stay, and (3) decreasing the requirement for surgical manipulation (see Grella, 2008).

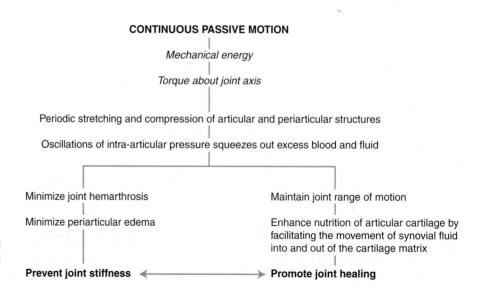

FIGURE 23-3 Proposed physiological and therapeutic effects of continuous passive motion therapy.

V. DOSIMETRY

A. PARAMETERS

CPM therapy dosimetry is achieved by setting the following parameters: range of motion (ROM), passive torque, speed of motion, ROM increment, application duration, and number of applications per day.

1. Range of Motion

Set the desired ROM, in degrees, through which the affected joint should be moved. This range should be as large as possible and within the patient's tolerance, for optimal results.

2. Torque Magnitude

Set the desired torque, in Nm (lbs-f), from low to high, according to the weight of the displaced body segments and the level of joint movement restriction.

3. Speed of Motion

Set the desired rate of motion, in degrees per second (°/s), from lower to higher speed.

4. Rate of Motion Increment

Program the device such as to increase, on a daily basis, the desired ROM until full ROM is achieved.

5. Other Features

Presented in **Box 23-1** are some other features, or parameters, found on CPM devices available on the market today. These features can be selected and pro-

grammed, simply by pushing buttons on a handheld digital motion controller. The reverse-on-load feature, as well as the patient's ON/OFF time switch, add to the safety of usage.

6. Application Duration

Set the duration of application, in minutes.

7. Number of Applications per Day

Set the number of application per day.

8. Progressive Dosage

The application duration is usually several hours per day during the in-hospital period. These periods are shortened over the postoperative days, and the number of applications is usually increased. For example, the application duration for the first 4 postoperative days may have been, on average, 14 hours per day (a single application interrupted for a few minutes only for hygiene care and for a few hours for sleep). For the next 4 days, the application duration would be 4 hours, repeated 3 times a day.

B. WHEN TO BEGIN TREATMENT

CPM therapy should be initiated *as soon as possible* after surgery, usually in the recovery room or on the morning of the first day after surgery (Grella, 2008). Recall that the key therapeutic purposes are to prevent joint stiffness, minimize joint hemarthrosis and periarticular edema, promote early weight bearing and enhance soft-tissue healing.

Box 23-1   Features of Continuous Passive Motion Devices

- *Programmable range of motion (ROM):* from neutral to full range of motion
- *Programmable speed of motion:* from a few to several degrees per second
- *Programmable torque:* from low to high torque (Nm or in-lb)
- *Programmable start and stop:* can be set for seconds, minutes, or hours
- *Programmable pause:* from 1 second to several minutes of hold motion at the end of ROM gains
- *ON/OFF switch:* manually controlled by patient for safety
- *Reverse on load:* reverse the direction of motion should the patient resist motion or if motion is restricted.
- *Warm-up:* increases the ROM from 50% of the programmed setting to the full setting over a certain number of cycles
- *Lockout:* allows the device to be programmed and locked, preventing patient tampering
- *Comfort zone:* reverses the direction and reduces the ROM by a few degrees allowing the patient time to recover by not taking the joint into the painful ROM.
- *Fast back:* increases the speed of motion in the non-therapeutic ROM (mid-range) leaving more time for the device to work, at the desired speed, in the therapeutic ROM (ends of range).
- *Oscillation zone:* reverses the direction of movement by a few degrees before returning to previous ROM; this reversal is repeated a few times (hence the word oscillation), with thus more time spent in the therapeutic zone (ends of ROM).
- *Progressive ROM:* automatic increases (increments) of ROM, by a certain number of degrees per day, until the final ROM is attained.
- *Compliance monitor:* allows treating clinicians to monitor patient compliance with treatment.
- *Handheld digital motion controller:* program and control over the above features,

VI. EVIDENCE FOR INDICATIONS

A. GUIDED BY EVIDENCE

Dictionaries generally define *evidence* as anything that establishes a fact or gives reason to believe something. The aim of this textbook is to present scientific evidence behind therapeutic EPAs. To be guided by the evidence is the process of integrating the evidence from research, however imperfect or scarce this evidence may be, with clinical experience and the patient's preferences. In other words, the *evidence-based practice* of EPA requires that practitioners consider the evidence from research, in addition to their own clinical experience and the patient's own preference and beliefs about a given EPA, when the time comes to justify, prescribe, and apply the therapeutic agent. To be guided by evidence is a process, not a search

for the absolute truth. Finally a lack of evidence from research behind any given EPA does not mean that this EPA should never be used. What it means is that no statement can be made about its therapeutic effectiveness and that until more evidence from research is presented its routine use cannot be recommended.

B. EVIDENCE FROM HUMAN RESEARCH

Box 23-2 provides evidence for CPM therapy based on an exhaustive search of published English-language, peer-reviewed literature on human research. The term *indication* is used in reference to a list of pathologies for which CPM therapy is employed. Ratings of therapeutic benefit (Yes or No) and the grading of scientific evidence (I, II, or III), including references, are included for each pathological condition.

| Box 23-2 | Research-Based Indications for the Use of Continuous Passive Motion Therapy |

PATHOLOGY	BENEFIT	GRADE	REFERENCE
Knee joint	Yes	I	Gose, 1987
	Yes	II	Lenssen et al., 2006
	Yes	II	Alfredson et al., 1999
	Yes	II	Colwell et al., 1992
	Yes	II	Freimert et al., 2006
	Yes	II	Johnson, 1990
	Yes	II	Johnson et al., 1992
	Yes	II	Lenssen et al., 2003
	Yes	II	London et al., 1999
	Yes	II	McInnes et al., 1992
	Yes	II	Mullaji et al., 1989
	Yes	II	Ververeli et al., 1995
	Yes	II	Vince et al., 1987
	Yes	II	Walker et al., 1991
	Yes	II	Wasilewski et al., 1990
	Yes	II	Witherow et al., 1993
	Yes	II	Maloney et al., 1990
	Yes	II	Worland et al., 1998
	Yes	II	Yashar et al., 1997
	Yes	II	Harms et al., 1991
	Yes	II	Basso et al., 1987
	Yes	II	May et al., 1999
	No	I	Bennett et al., 2005
	No	I	MacDonald et al., 2000
	No	I	Chiarello et al., 1997
	No	I	McCarthy et al., 1993
	No	II	Beaupre et al., 2001
	No	II	Chen et al., 2000
	No	II	Davies et al., 2003
	No	II	Denis et al., 2006
	No	II	Engstrom et al., 1995
	No	II	Kumar et al., 1996
	No	II	Lau et al., 2001

(Continued)

Box 23-2   **Continued**

PATHOLOGY	BENEFIT	GRADE	REFERENCE
	No	II	Leach et al., 2006
	No	II	Montgomery et al., 1996
	No	II	Nadler et al., 1993
	No	II	Nielsen et al., 1988
	No	II	Pope et al., 1997
	No	II	Richmond et al., 1991
	No	II	Ritter et al., 1989
	No	II	Rosen et al., 1992
Hand	Yes	III	Dirette et al., 1994
	Yes	III	Guidice, 1990
	No	II	Ring et al., 1998
Shoulder joint	Yes	II	Lastayo et al., 1998
	Yes	II	Lynch et al., 2005
	No	II	Raab et al., 1998
Ankle joint	Yes	III	Grumbine et al., 1990
	Yes	II	McNair et al., 2001
Foot: postsurgical clubfoot correction	Yes	II	Zeifang et al., 2005
	Yes	II	Kasten et al., 2007
Ankle hypertonia	Yes	II	Chang et al., 2007
Hip joint: osteoarthritis	Yes	II	Simkin et al., 1999
Wrist joint: carpal tunnel syndrome	Yes	III	Stevenson et al., 2005
Elbow joint	Yes	II	Gates et al., 1992
Low-back pain	Yes	I	Aota et al., 2007
Traumatic injury to the spine, pelvis, and lower limb: prevention of deep vein thrombosis	Yes	II	Fuchs et al., 2005

1. Rating Therapeutic Benefit

The rating, expressed as Yes or No, is based on the overall conclusion(s) reached on the issue of therapeutic effectiveness by the author(s) who conducted the peer-reviewed study.

2. Grading Strength of Evidence

The grading, numerically classified as I, II, and III, is based on the type of research methodology, or experimental design, used by the author(s). All those listed are studies on humans published in English-language, peer-reviewed journals. It follows that the evidence in studies graded I is stronger than in those graded II, and the evidence in studies graded II is stronger than in those graded III.

a. Grade I

Evidence based on *controlled* studies on humans, regardless of their level of randomization and blindness.

b. Grade II

Evidence based on *noncontrolled* studies on humans, regardless of their level of randomization and blindness.

TABLE 23-1	CONTRAINDICATIONS TO CONTINUOUS PASSIVE MOTION THERAPY
CONTRAINDICATIONS	**RATIONALE**
Unstable bone fractures related to the affected joint	Risk of bone displacement and bone union delay during passive motion.
Uncontrolled infection related to the affected joint	Risk of wound complications and delayed healing.
Muscle spasm and spasticity	Risk of triggering unwanted muscle contraction during passive motion.

c. Grade III

Evidence based on *case* studies on humans, regardless of their level of randomization and blindness.

3. Strength of Evidence Behind the Agent

The evidence behind an agent, as presented in the research-based indication box, is arbitrarily assessed in this textbook as *weak, moderate,* or *strong.* For example, the larger the number of studies graded I, regardless of therapeutic benefit, the stronger the scientific evidence behind the agent.

4. Evidence to Justify Usage of Agent

The evidence for the justification of usage of the agent for an individual pathology or groups of pathologies, as listed in each research-based indication box, is arbitrarily assessed in this textbook as *poor, fair, good,* or *conflicting.* For example, where a larger number of grade I studies show therapeutic benefit (Yes) than no benefit, for any given pathology, the justification for usage of the agent for that pathology is assessed as *good.* A *conflicting* justification is reported when about an equal number of studies, with similar grades, show therapeutic benefit (Yes) and no benefit (No).

C. STRENGTH OF EVIDENCE AND JUSTIFICATION FOR USAGE

The results presented in **Box 23-2** show *moderate strength* for the evidence behind use of CPM therapy, with the majority of studies graded II. These results also show *conflicting* justification for the usage of this EPA for all postsurgical joints, including the knee joints. They also show *poor* justification of usage for all the remaining pathologies listed. Until more evidence is provided, the *routine* use of CPM therapy for all of the other pathologies listed *cannot be recommended.*

VII. CONTRAINDICATIONS

Table 23-1 shows that CPM therapy is contraindicated for cases of unstable fracture, muscle spasticity, and infection related to the affected joint.

VIII. RISKS, PRECAUTIONS, AND RECOMMENDATIONS

Table 23-2 is presented with the purpose of increasing the safety and effectiveness of CPM therapy. Special attention should be given to postsurgical wound complications caused by skin stretching during joint mobilization.

IX. CONSIDERATIONS FOR APPLICATION AND DOCUMENTATION

A. PROCEDURES

Safe, effective, and optimal application of CPM therapy requires that clinicians go through a systematic set of

TABLE 23-2	RISKS, PRECAUTIONS, AND RECOMMENDATIONS FOR CONTINUOUS PASSIVE MOTION THERAPY	
RISK	**RATIONALE**	
Postsurgical wound	Risk of affecting wound healing by unduly pulling or tearing the wound edges (Johnson, 1990; Maloney et al., 1990; Drez et al., 1991).	
PRECAUTION	**RATIONALE**	
Combination of anticoagulant and CPM therapy	Risk of inducing an anterior compartment syndrome (Graham et al., 1985). No other articles can be found to substantiate this precaution.	

(Continued)

TABLE 23-2	CONTINUED

RECOMMENDATIONS	RATIONALE
Begin CPM therapy immediately after joint surgery	Although some have recommended that therapy be started the second day after surgery in order to minimize wound complications and blood loss (Maloney et al., 1990; Lotke et al., 1991, Pope et al., 1997), the general recommendation today is that therapy should begin as soon as possible after surgery (i.e., in the recovery room) for optimal results (Grella, 2008). Adequate prescription and monitoring during therapy should also minimize wound damage and blood loss.
Frequently check and adjust joint positioning in the CPM device	To minimize pressure-related problems (O'Driscoll et al., 2000).
Avoid circumferential wrapping of the treated limb during therapy	To prevent wound damage (O'Driscoll et al., 2000).
Plug line-powered CPM devices into GFCI receptacles	To eliminate the risk of electrical macroshock (see Chapter 27 for details).
Apply regular maintenance and calibration schedule	To ensure optimal functioning of devices. Follow the manufacturer's maintenance and calibration schedules.

procedures for each and every application. The following list of such procedures.

1. Checklists

Before proceeding with treatment, always go through the list of contraindications (**Table 23-1**) and list of risks, precautions, and recommendations (**Table 23-2**).

2. Patient's Positioning

Ensure that the patient is comfortably positioned and instruct him or her to relax the limb segment being treated.

3. Limb and Joint Preparation

Align the joint axis with the device's axis of motion. Secure the limb segments about the treated joint with the device's fixation system, such as Velcro straps.

4. Dosimetry

Select the dosimetric parameters and features (see Section V) that will best meet the pathological condition and the desired therapeutic goal.

5. End of Treatment

Inspect the surgical wounds on the joint and question the patient on the level of sensation perceived during treat-

ment. Document any unusual sensation felt by the patient during treatment in the patient's file.

B. DOCUMENTATION

Table 23-3 shows the key parameters to be documented in the patient's file after CPM therapy.

TABLE 23-3	KEY TREATMENT PARAMETERS TO BE DOCUMENTED IN PATIENT'S FILE AFTER CONTINUOUS PASSIVE MOTION THERAPY

- *CPM device:* description
- *Patient's position:* description
- *Range of motion:* degrees
- *Evoked torque:* Nm; lbs-f
- *Speed of motion:* degrees/s
- *Application duration:* min
- *Features used:* description
- *Number of applications per day:* number

Case Study 23-1   Total Knee Arthroplasty

A 59-year-old male electrician, who suffers from severe right-knee osteoarthritis, is referred by his treating orthopedic surgeon. You are asked to provide immediate postsurgical care and subsequent home care after hospital discharge following the patient's total right-knee arthroplasty. The patient has just undergone the surgery and is currently in the recovery room in the hospital. There was no complication during surgery, and the patient is slowly waking up. The short-term therapeutic goals for CPM treatment of this patient are to decrease knee pain, prevent knee-joint stiffness, increase knee ROM, and promote healing of the surgical wound. The longer-term goals are full weight bearing, normal walking over the next days, and return to work in the weeks to come.

Evidence-Based Steps Toward the Resolution of This Case

1. List medical diagnosis.

Total knee arthroplasty following severe right-knee osteoarthritis

2. List key impairment(s).

- Knee pain
- Decrease knee range of motion

3. List key functional limitation(s).

- Inability to walk

4. List key disabilities.

- Inability to work

5. Justification for CPM therapy.

Is there justification for the use of CPM therapy in this case? This chapter has established that the evidence for use of CPM therapy for postsurgical knee-joint pathologies is *moderate* in strength, and the justification *conflicting* (see Section VI,). The selection of this agent is based on the body of evidence found in several clinical studies (Colwell et al., 1989; McCarthy et al., 1993; Ververelli et al., 1995; Worland et al., 1998) and review articles (Lachiewicz, 2000; O'Driscoll et al., 2000; Grella, 2008). The use of CPM therapy immediately after surgery, and during the days that follow, is expected to prevent joint stiffness and decrease pain. Its use is also expected to promote early weight bearing and return to normal walking. Because EPAs should not be used in isolation or as a sole interaction, CPM therapy is used because the EPA's should not used into islotaion as a sole intervention here *concomitantly* with a full in-hospital care in addition to gradual weight-bearing exercises.

6. Search for contraindications.

None is found.

7. Search for risks and precautions.

None is found.

8. Outline the therapeutic goal(s) you and your patient wish to achieve.

- Decrease pain
- Prevent joint stiffness by maintaining full knee ROM
- Promote soft-tissue healing

9. List the outcome measurement(s) used to assess treatment effectiveness.

- Pain: Visual Analog Scale (VAS)
- Drug diary: total intake of analgesic tablets
- ROM: goniometry
- Weight bearing: weight scale

10. Educate the patient about what he/she should experience, do, and not do during the CPM treatment.

- Moderate soft-issue stretching
- Relax the affected knee joint; do not attempt to resist or facilitate joint movement.

11. Outline your therapeutic prescription based on the best sources of evidence available.

The following prescription is based on several clinical studies (Colwell et al., 1992; McCarthy et al., 1993; Ververelli et al., 1995; Worland et al., 1998) and review articles (Lachiewicz, 2000; O'Driscoll et al., 2000; Grella, 2008). The prescription is divided into three periods: recovery room, first day after surgery and subsequent in-hospital days, and home therapy:

Recovery room in hospital (Day 0):

- ***CPM type:*** knee device; line powered
- ***Patient position:*** lying supine in bed
- ***First application of CPM:*** in recovery room
- ***Initial ROM setting:*** 0° to 60°, up to patient's tolerance
- ***Initial torque setting:*** high
- ***Initial speed of motion:*** 0.5°/s
- ***Initial treatment session duration:*** 20 hours of continuous application
- ***Initial motion cycle duration:*** 4 minutes
  - 2 minutes from 0° extension to 60° flexion
  - 2 minutes from 60° flexion to 0° extension
- ***Initial number of motion cycles per hour:*** 15
- ***Device features setting:*** warm-up; reverse on load; lockout (see **Table 23-3**)

First postoperative day and subsequent days until discharge from hospital:

- ***ROM increment per day:*** increased by 6°, until full ROM is attained
- ***Speed of motion:*** 2°/s
- ***Treatment session duration:*** reduced by 2 hours a day over the first 3 postoperative days. From

the fourth day to discharge, 4 treatment sessions per day, each lasting 2 hours with 2-hour resting periods in between

- *Hospital discharge:* the discharge from hospital occurred on the seventh postoperative day.
- *Device features setting:* warm-up; reverse on load; lockout; pause, fast back (see **Table 23-3**)

Home therapy (next 10 days):

- *ROM setting:* progression from the maximum range obtained at discharge to full ROM.
- *Torque setting:* high
- *Rate of motion setting:* alternate between slow and fast rates
- *Number of treatment sessions:* 3 sessions a day lasting 2 hours each
- *Home therapy duration:* 10 consecutive days after hospital discharge
- *Device features setting:* warm-up; reverse on load; lockout; pause, fast back (see **Table 23-3**)

12. Collect outcome measurements.

Pre- and posttreatment comparison:

- Pain: VAS score reduced from 9 to 2
- Pain: total number of analgesic tablets reduced by 80%
- ROM: full range obtained (0° extension to 140° flexion)
- Weight bearing: gain of 90% in weight-bearing; safe walking with a cane achieved

13. Assess therapeutic effectiveness based on outcome measures.

The results show that the application of CPM therapy over 17 consecutive days (from the recovery room to home), in combination with full in-hospital care including progressive weight bearing, led to the full recovery of ROM in the operated knee in addition to a significant reduction in pain. The results also show that the patient is now capable of significant weight bearing on his prosthetic knee and of walking safely with a cane. The patient is more than happy with the progression of his knee condition and is even happier to finally recover his lost walking ability. He looks forward to continuing his rehabilitation program. Overall, the use of CPM therapy had a beneficial impact on the patient's disablement status created by the pathology, as illustrated in the **figure below**.

14. State the prognosis.

The prognosis is excellent because joint stiffness was totally prevented. The patient should be able to maintain full ROM on his operated knee through supervised daily strengthening and walking exercises. There is no knee edema and the surgical wound is healed. Over the next few weeks this patient should recover full knee mobility, including his walking ability over all surfaces. There is no reason that this patient should not resume full daily and leisure activities, including full-time return to work.

THERAPEUTIC IMPACT on Disablement

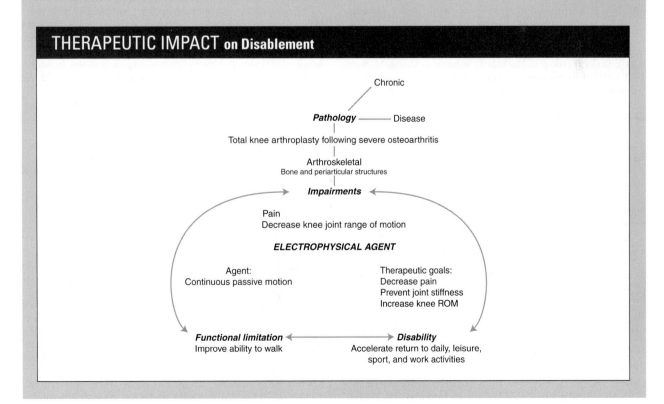

CRITICAL THINKING QUESTIONS

Clarification: What is meant by continuous passive motion (CPM) therapy?

Assumptions: You have assumed that motion is much better than rest or immobilization for the postsurgical treatment of joints. How do you justify making that assumption?

Reasons and evidence: Is there a difference between moving a joint using a CPM device and using your hand? If yes, what are the differences between these two therapeutic interventions?

Viewpoints or perspectives: How would you respond to a colleague who says that CPM therapy should not be used at home or after discharge from the hospital?

Implications and consequences: What are the implications and consequences if the patient involuntarily (e.g., a muscle spasm) or voluntarily offers resistance against the device during treatment?

About the question: What should the evidence-oriented clinician do in the face of strong conflicting evidence with regard to the use of a therapeutic agent for a given pathology? Why do you think I ask this question?

References

Articles

Alfredson H, Lorentzon R (1999) Superior results with continuous passive motion compared to active motion after periosteal transplantation. A retrospective study of human patella cartilage defect treatment. Knee Surg Sports Traumatol Arthrosc, 7: 232–238

Aota Y, Iizuka H, Ishige Y, Mochida T, Yoshihisa T, Uesugi M, Saito T (2007) Effectiveness of a lumbar support continuous passive motion device in the prevention of low back pain during prolonged sitting. Spine, 32: 674–677

Basso DM, Knapp L (1987) Comparison of two continuous passive motion protocols for patients with total knee implants. Phys Ther, 67: 360–363

Beaupre LA, Davies DM, Jones CA, Cinats JC (2001) Exercise combined with continuous passive motion or slider board therapy compared with exercise only: A randomized controlled trial of patients following total knee arthroplasty. Phys Ther 81: 1029–1037

Bennett LA, Brearley SC, Hart JA, Bailey MJ (2005) A comparison of two continuous passive motion protocols after total knee arthroplasty: A controlled and randomized study. J Arthroplasty, 20: 225–233

Chang YJ, Fang CY, Hsu MJ, Lien HY, Wong MK (2007) Decrease of hypertonia after continuous passive motion treatment in individuals with spinal cord injury. Clin Rehab, 21: 712–718

Chen B, Zimmerman JR, Soulen L, DeLisa JA (2000) Continuous passive motion after total knee arthroplasty: A prospective study. Am J Phys Med Rehab, 79: 421–426

Chiarello CM, Gunderson L, O'Halloran T (1997) The effect of continuous passive motion duration and increment on range of motion in total knee arthroplasty patients. J Orthop Sports Phys Ther, 25: 119–127

Colwell CW, Morris BA (1992) The influence of continuous passive motion on the results of total knee arthroplasty. Clin Orthop Relat Res, 276: 225–228

Davies DM, Johnston DW, Beaupre LA, Lier DA (2003) Effect of adjunctive range-of-motion therapy after primary total knee arthroplasty on the use of health services after hospital discharge. Can J Surg, 46: 30–36

Denis M, Moffet H, Caron F, Ouellet D, Paquet J, Nolet L (2006) Effectiveness of continuous passive motion and conventional physical therapy after total knee arthroplasty: A randomized clinical trial. Phys Ther, 86: 174–185

Dirette D, Hinojosa J (1994) Effects of continuous passive motion on the edematous hands of two persons with flaccid hemiplegia. Am J Occup Ther, 48: 403–409

Drez D, Paine RM, Neuschwander DC, Young JC (1991) In vivo measurement of anterior tibial translation using continuous passive motion devices. Am J Sports Med, 19: 381–383

Engstrom B, Sperber A, Wredmark T (1995) Continuous passive motion in rehabilitation after anterior cruciate ligament reconstruction. Knee Surg Sports Traumatol Arthrosc, 3: 18–20

Friemert B, Bach C, Schwarz W, Gerngross H, Schmidt R (2005) Benefits of active motion for joint position sense. Knee Surg Sports Traumatol Arthrosc, 14: 564–570

Fuchs S, Heyse T, Rudofsky G, Gosheger G, Chylarecki C (2005) Continuous passive motion in the prevention of deep-vein thrombosis: A randomized comparison in trauma patients. J Bone Joint Surg (B), 87: 1117–1122

Gates HS, Sullivan FL, Urbaniak JR (1992) Anterior capsulotomy and continuous passive motion in the treatment of post traumatic flexion contracture of the elbow: A prospective study. J Bone Joint Surg (A), 74: 1229–1234

Giudice ML (1990) Effects of continuous passive motion and elevation on hand edema. Am J Occup Ther, 44: 914–921

Gose JC (1987) Continuous passive motion in the postoperative treatment of patients with total knee replacement. Phy Ther, 67: 39–42

Graham G, Loomer RL (1985) Anterior compartment syndrome in a patient with fracture of the tibial plateau treated by continuous passive motion and anticoagulants: Report of a case. Clin Orthop Relat Res, 195: 197–199

Grumbine NA, Santoro JP, Chinn ES (1990) Continuous passive motion following partial ankle joint arthroplasty. J Foot Surg, 29: 557–566

Harms M, Engstrom B (1991) Continuous passive motion as an adjunct to treatment in the physical therapy management of the total knee arthroplasty patient. Physiotherapy, 77: 301–307

Johnson DP (1990) The effect of continuous passive motion on wound-healing mobility after knee arthroplasty. J Bone Joint Surg, 72 (A): 421–426

Johnson DP, Eastwood DM (1992) Beneficial effects of continuous passive motion after total condylar knee arthroplasty. Ann R Coll Surg Engl, 74: 412–416

Kasten P, Geiger F, Zeifang F, Weiss S, Thomsen M (2007) Compliance with continuous passive movement is low after surgical treatment of idiopathic club foot in infants: A prospective, double-blinded clinical trial. J Bone Joint Surg (B), 89: 375–377

Kumar PJ, McPherson EJ, Dorr LD, Wan Z, Baldwin K (1996) Rehabilitation after total knee arthroplasty: A comparison of two rehabilitation techniques. Clin Orthop Relat Res, 331: 93–101

Lau SK, Chiu KY (2001) Use of continuous passive motion after total knee arthroplasty. J Arthroplasty, 16: 336–339

Lastayo PC, Wright T, Jaffe R, Hartzel J (1998) Continuous passive motion after repair of the rotator cuff. A prospective outcome study. J Bone Joint Surg (A), 80: 1002–1111

Leach W, Reid J, Murphy F (2006) Continuous passive motion following total knee replacement: A prospective randomized trial with follow-up to 1 year. Knee Surg Sports Traumatol Arthrosc, 14: 922–926

Lenssen AF, De Bie RA, Bulstra SK, Van Steyn MJ (2003) Continuous passive motion (CPM) in rehabilitation following total knee arthroplasty: A randomized controlled trial. Phys Ther Rev, 8: 123–129

Lenssen AF, Crijns YH, Waltje EM, Roox GM, van Steyn MJ, Geesink RJ, van den Brandt PA, de Bie RA (2006) Effectiveness of prolonged use of continuous passive motion (CPM) as an adjunct to physiotherapy following total knee arthroplasty: Design of a randomized controlled trial. BMC Musculosket Disord, 23: 7–15

London NJ, Brown M, Newman RJ (1999) Continuous passive motion: Evaluation of a new portable low cost machine. Physiotherapy, 85: 610–612

Lotke PA, Faralli VJ, Orenstein EM, Ecker ML (1991) Blood loss after knee replacement. Effects of tourniquet release and continuous passive motion. J Bon Joint Surg (A), 73: 1037–1040

Lynch D, Ferraro M, Krol J, Trudell CM, Christos P, Volpe BT (2005) Continuous passive motion improves shoulder joint integrity following stroke. Clin Rehab, 19: 594–599

MacDonald SJ, Bourne RB, Rorabeck CH, McCalden RW, Kramer J, Vaz M (2000) Prospective randomized clinical trial of continuous passive motion after total knee arthroplasty. Clin Orthop Relat Res, 380: 30–35

Maloney WJ, Shurman DJ, Hangen D, Goodman SB, Edworthy S, Bloch DA (1990) The influence of continuous passive motion on outcome in total knee arthroplasty. Clin Orthop Relat Res, 256: 162–168

May LA, Buss W, Zayac D, Whitridge MR (1999) Comparison of continuous passive motion machines and lower limb mobility boards in the rehabilitation of patients with total knee arthroplasty. Can J Rehab, 12: 257–263

McCarthy MR, Yates CK, Anderson MA, Yates-McCarthy JL (1993) The effect of immediate continuous passive motion on pain during the inflammatory phase of soft tissue healing following anterior cruciate ligament reconstruction. J Orthop Sports Phys Ther, 17: 96–101

McInnes J, Larson MG, Daltroy LH, Brown T, Fossel AH, Eaton HM, Shulman-Kirwan B, Steindorf S, Poss R, Liang MH (1992) A controlled evaluation of continuous passive motion in patients undergoing total knee arthroplasty. JAMA, 268: 1423–1428

McNair PJ, Dombroski EW, Hewson DJ, Stanley SN (2001) Stretching at the ankle joint: Viscoelastic responses to holds and continuous passive motion. Med Sci Sports Exerc, 33: 354–358

Montgomery F, Eliasson M (1996) Continuous passive motion compared to active physical therapy after knee arthroplasty: Similar hospitalization times in a randomized study of 68 patients. Acta Orthop Scand, 67: 7–9

Mullaji AB, Shahane MN (1989) Continuous passive motion for prevention and rehabilitation of knee stiffness: A clinical evaluation. J Postgrad Med, 35: 204–208

Nadler SF, Malanga GA, Zimmerman JR (1993) Continuous passive motion in the rehabilitation setting: A retrospective study. J Phys Med Rehab, 72: 162–165

Neilsen PT, Rechnagel K, Nielsen S (1988) No effects of continuous passive motion after arthroplasty of the knee. Acta Orthop Scand, 59: 580–581

Pope RO, Corcoran S, McCaul K, Howie DW (1997) Continuous passive motion after primary total knee arthroplasty. Does it offer any benefits? J Bone Joint Surg (B), 79: 914–917

Rabb MG, Rzeszutko D, O'Conner W, Greatting MD (1996) Early results of continuous passive motion after rotator cuff repair. A prospective, randomized, blinded, controlled study. Am J Ortho, 25: 214–220

Richmond JC, Gladstone J, MacGillivray J (1991) Continuous passive motion after arthroscopically assisted anterior cruciate ligament reconstruction: Comparison of short- versus long-term use. Arthroscopy, 7: 39–44

Ring D, Simmons BP, Hayes M (1998) Continuous passive motion following metacarpophalangeal joint arthroplasty. J Hand Surg (A), 23: 505–511

Ritter MA, Gandolf VS, Holston KS (1989) Continuous passive motion versus physical therapy in total knee arthroplasty. Clin Ortho Relat Res, 244: 239–243

Rosen MA, Jackson DW, Atwell EA (1992) The efficacy of continuous passive motion in the rehabilitation of anterior cruciate ligament reconstructions. Am J Sports Med, 20: 122–127

Salter RB, Field P (1960) The effects of continuous compression on living articular cartilage. An experimental investigation. J Bone Joint Surg (A), 42: 31–49

Salter RB, Hamilton HW, Wedge JH, Tile M, Torode IP, O'Driscoll SW, Murnaghan JJ, Saringer JH (1984) Clinical application of basic research on continuous passive motion for disorders and injuries of synovial joints: A preliminary report of a feasibility study. J Orthop Res, 1: 325–342

Simkin PA, de Lateur BJ, Alquist AD, Questad KA, Beardsley RM, Esselman PC (1999) Continuous passive motion for osteoarthritis of the hip: A pilot study. J Rheumatol, 26: 1987–1991

Stevenson JR, Blake JM, Douglas TF, Kercheval DM (2005) Does continuous passive motion during keyboarding affects hand blood flow and wrist function? A prospective case report. Work, 24: 145–155

Ververeli PA, Sutton DC, Hearn SL, Booth RE, Hozack WJ, Rothman RR (1995) Continuous passive motion after total knee arthroplasty: Analysis of costs and benefits. Clin Orthop Relat Res, 321: 208–245

Vince K, Kelly MA, Beck J, Insall JN (1987) Continuous passive motion after total knee arthroplasty. J Arthroplasty, 2: 281–284

Walker RH, Morris BA, Angulo DL, Schneider J, Colwell CW (1991) Postoperative use of continuous passive motion, transcutaneous electrical nerve stimulation, and continuous cooling pad following total knee arthroplasty. J Arthroplasty, 6: 151–156

Wasilewski SA, Woods LC, Torgerson WR, Healy WL (1990) Value of continuous passive motion in total knee arthroplasty. Orthopedics, 13: 291–295

Witherow GE, Bollen SR, Pinczewski LA (1993) The use of continuous passive motion after arthroscopically assisted anterior cruciate ligament reconstruction: Help or hindrance? Knee Surg Sports Traumatol Arthrosc, 1: 68–70

Worland RL, Arredondo J, Angles F, Lopez-Jimenez FL, Jessup DE (1998) Home continuous passive motion machine versus professional physical therapy following total knee replacement. J Arthroplasty, 13: 784–788

Yashar AA, Venn-Watson E, Welsh T, Colwell CW, Lotke P (1997) Continuous passive motion with accelerated flexion after total knee arthroplasty. Clin Orthop Relat Res, 345: 38–43

Zeifang F, Carstens C, Schneider S, Thomsen M (2005) Continuous passive motion versus immobilisation in a cast after surgical treatment of idiopathic club foot in infants: A prospective, blinded, randomized, clinical study. J Bone Joint Surg (B), 87: 1663–1665

Review Articles

Brosseau L, Milne S, Wells G, Tugwell P, Robinson V, Casimiro L, Pelland L, Noel MJ, Davis J, Drouin H (2004) Efficacy of continuous passive motion following total knee arthroplasty: A meta analysis. J Rheumatol, 31: 2251–2264

Grella RJ (2008). Continous passive motion following total knee μ arthroplasty: a useful adjunct to early mobilization. Phys Ther Rev, 13: 269–279

Lachiewicz PF (2000) The role of continuous passive motion after total knee arthroplasty. Clin Orthop Relat Res, 380: 144–150

Lawrence BR (1996) The dose of continuous passive motion in postoperative rehabilitation of the first metatarsophalangeal joint. J Foot Ankle Surg, 35: 155–161

Lenssen AF, Koke AJ, DeBie RA, Geesink RG (2003) Continuous passive motion following primary total knee arthroplasty: Short-and long-term effects on range of motion. Phys Ther Rev, 8: 113–121

McCarthy MR, O'Donoghue PC, Yates CK, Yates-McCarthy JL (1992) The clinical use of continuous passive motion in physical therapy. J Orthop Sports Phys Ther, 15: 132–140

Milne S, Brosseau L, Robinson V, Noel MJ, Davis J, Drouin H, Wells G, Tugwell P (2003) Continuous passive motion following total knee arthroplasty. Cochrane Database Syst Rev, 2: CD004260

O'Driscoll SW, Giori NJ (2000) Continuous passive motion (CPM): Theory and principles of clinical application. J Rehab Res Dev, 37: 179–188

Postel JM, Thoumie P, Missaoui B, Biau D, Robinik P, Revel M, Rannou F (2007) Continuing passive motion compared with intermittent mobilization after total knee arthroplasty: Elaboration of French clinical guidelines. Ann Readap Med Phys, 50: 244–257

Salter RB (1982) Motion vs rest. Why immobilize joints? J Bone Joint Surg (B), 64: 251–254

Salter RB (1989) The biologic concept of continuous passive motion of synovial joints: The first 18 years of basic research. Clin Orthop, 242: 12–26

Salter RB (1994) The physiologic basis of continuous passive motion for articular healing and regeneration. Hand Clin, 10: 211–219

Salter RB (1996) History of rest and motion and the scientific basis for early passive motion. Hand Clin, 12: 1–11

Chapters of Textbooks

Starkey C (2004) Continuous passive motion. In: Therapeutic Modalities, 3rd ed. FA Davis Co, Philadelphia, pp 287–294

Turturro TC (2003) Continuous passive motion. In: DeLee & Drez's Orthopaedic Sports Medicine, Principles and Practice, 2nd ed. DeLee JC, Drez D (Eds). Saunders, St-Louis, pp 376–380

PART III

Practical
Clinical
Guidelines

Purchase of Therapeutic Electrophysical Agents

Chapter Outline

Learning Objectives

Knowledge: List each of the eight steps in purchasing electrophysical agents (EPAs).

Comprehension: Compare each step in relation to the whole process of purchasing.

Application: Show how each step contributes to the whole purchasing process.

Analysis: Explain the significance of each step.

Synthesis: Create a mock purchasing order based on the eight-step approach.

Evaluation: Discuss the benefit of purchasing EPAs using the eight-step approach presented in this chapter.

I. BACKGROUND AND PURPOSE

A. THE PURCHASING EXPERIENCE

The purchase of therapeutic electrophysical agents (EPAs) can be a pleasant experience or can easily turn into a frustrating exercise. Because a large variety of models and related accessories are available, educators and practitioners must learn how to navigate this market properly. To complicate matters further, they also must choose among a substantial number of manufacturers and distributors, and learn how to deal with sales representatives who, one after another, will display their best marketing efforts to sell their own line of equipment.

B. APTA ONLINE BUYER'S GUIDE

Every year, the American Physical Therapy Association (APTA) updates and publishes a comprehensive directory of companies and distributors located in the United States that supply rehabilitation products and services. This directory, available online (www.apta.org) and published yearly in APTA's *PT Magazine*, is an excellent buyer's guide for purchasing most of the EPAs discussed in this textbook.

C. PURPOSE OF CHAPTER

The purpose of this chapter is to further facilitate the process of purchasing EPAs by recommending a helpful *eight-step approach*. In other words, its purpose is to make the purchase of EPAs a pleasant, satisfactory, and cost-effective experience.

II. THE EIGHT-STEP APPROACH TO PURCHASING AN EPA

A. STEP 1: RESEARCH, GATHER, AND REVIEW TECHNICAL INFORMATION

The first step is to research, gather, and review all the necessary information related to the EPA you plan to purchase. For example, one needs to consider choice of models, prices, availability, warranty, and delivery terms, to mention only a few. As mentioned previously, one of the best tools available to research EPA equipment is the APTA's Online Buyer's Guide, in addition to the companies' own Web sites. The last thing you want to do is rely too heavily on the word of sales representatives who, logically, will do their best to convince you of the "merits" of their company's equipment.

B. STEP 2: MAKE SURE EVERYONE SPEAKS THE SAME TECHNICAL LANGUAGE

Now that your research information is completed, the second step is to contact some distributors through their head offices or sales representatives.

1. Technical Language
The field of therapeutic EPAs is highly technical, as exemplified by this textbook. Too often, major confusion arises because you, the users, and the sales representatives simply are not speaking the same language when discussing the technical features of the EPAs you are interested in purchasing.

2. Illustrated Glossary of Terms
One of the best ways to minimize such confusion is for both sides to use recommended terminology. The *Illustrated Glossary of Electrophysical Terminology*, presented in Chapter 5 of this textbook, provides you with a powerful tool that can be used to facilitate the discussion. The more standardized and accurate the technical terminology used, the better the verbal exchanges and written correspondence between you and sales representatives will be.

C. STEP 3: ASSESS YOUR NEED FOR PORTABLE VERSUS CABINET-TYPE DEVICES

The third step is to determine whether you need portable (battery-powered) or cabinet-type (line-powered) EPAs. This assessment should be based on your patient clientele.

1. Portable-Type EPAs
Portable devices are preferable when you need *greater mobility* in providing therapy to patients wherever they might be, whether that is in hospital wards, department rooms, outdoor fields, or at home. A key disadvantage with this type of equipment is the supply and maintenance of batteries. A key advantage is that they require minimal floor space and are easy to store after usage.

2. Cabinet-Type EPAs
Cabinet devices are preferable when a *large number* of patients need to be treated on a daily basis, which implies the frequent use of agents. A key advantage is that no battery is needed. A key disadvantage is that more floor space is needed.

D. STEP 4: INQUIRE ABOUT BUSINESS CREDENTIALS

The fourth step involves inquiring about the business credentials of manufacturers, distributors, and sales representatives. *Wise* consumers never make blind purchases; they want to know, before making a purchase, whether the product, the company, the distributor, and the sales representative all have solid credentials. Don't be afraid to ask questions about business credentials.

1. Manufacturers
The manufacturers' credentials are based on the *quality of the equipment* they manufacture as well as on the terms and duration of the *warranty* they provide. Keep in mind that manufacturers don't have the same quality control and warranty policies.

2. Distributors and Sales Representatives

The distributors' and sales representatives' credentials are based on the *quality of the services* they offer before, during, and—most importantly—after the purchase is made and the warranty has expired. Do not hesitate to draw on the experience of your colleagues, and that of colleagues working in other clinical settings, on this subject.

3. Repair Centers and Hourly Rates

Ask the sales representatives where their repair and parts centers are located and what their current hourly rate for a repair is. Also inquire about the terms related to the shipping of equipment to the repair centers.

4. Warranty and Service

Ask for *written* documents regarding the terms of the warranty, and the distributor's own policies and procedures for services offered, both during the warranty period and after the warranty expires.

E. STEP 5: ASK FOR AT LEAST TWO WRITTEN PRICE QUOTATIONS

This fifth step addresses the all-important issue of purchasing price. As is common in the field of health care, the cost of EPAs can vary greatly from one distributor to the next. So asking for at least two quotations can only guide you better toward a cost-effective purchase.

1. Written Quotation Only

Each quotation must be written and must include the price of each item, all taxes and shipping charges that apply, and other related costs such as customs fees, if you are buying from a foreign distributor. Beware of verbal quotes over the phone!

2. Quality and Service

Remember that quality and service have a price of their own. In the long run, you will *never regret* purchasing a quality piece of equipment from a reputable manufacturer, distributor, and sales representative.

F. STEP 6: CONSIDER PURCHASING THE EQUIPMENT ON A TRIAL BASIS

Purchasing equipment on a trial basis is preferable but, unfortunately, not always possible. Doing so will give you the opportunity to test it in your academic or clinical settings. It will also give you time to have a qualified technician inspect it for compliance with the manufacturer's listed specifications and safety standards.

G. STEP 7: CONSIDER PURCHASING A POST-WARRANTY MAINTENANCE AND/OR SERVICE CONTRACT

This seventh step addresses the all-important issue of post-warranty maintenance and service.

1. Contract

Some distributors may offer a post-warranty maintenance or service contract for 1 year or longer, at a fixed annual price, which may or may not include parts, labor, and shipping costs. Ask your sales representative for more details.

2. Maintenance

You may choose to give your maintenance business to local electronics repair shops. Remember, however, that these local shops may have a hard time obtaining replacement parts to make the necessary repairs, which may lead to a significant delay before you can use the equipment again.

H. STEP 8: ESTABLISH A DEADLINE FOR DELIVERY

This last step, if forgotten, can lead to a fair degree of frustration for you, the buyer. Before signing any purchase order, think of adding a clause regarding the delivery date that your distributor must meet for complete delivery, to your working site, of all the items purchased. This clause will likely prevent excessive delay in the delivery of your equipment. Discuss with your sales representative the consequences for the distributor if this deadline is not respected. To avoid any misunderstandings, put these delivery deadline terms in writing before putting your signature at the bottom of the purchase order.

CRITICAL THINKING QUESTIONS

Clarification: What is meant by having a pleasant, cost-effective, and satisfactory purchasing experience?

Assumptions: You have assumed that it is important to enquire about the business credentials of manufacturers, distributors, and sales representatives when purchasing EPAs. How do you justify making that assumption?

Reasons and evidence: The effective and cost-effective process of purchasing something requires preliminary research and processing of key information. Why are these precautions necessary?

Viewpoints or perspectives: You agree with the consensus that purchasing EPAs should include many, if not all, of the eight steps proposed in this chapter. What would someone who disagrees with you say?

Implications and consequences: You state that the effective purchase of EPAs is not as easy as one may think. What are you implying by that?

About the question: Does your clientele have anything to do with the types of EPAs you plan to purchase? Why do you think I ask this question?

Reference

PT Magazine Online Buyer's Guide: www.apta.org

CHAPTER 25

Skin Sensory Heat and Cold Discrimination Testing

Learning Objectives

Knowledge: List the five levels of heat and cold sensation and their related test-probe temperatures.

Comprehension: Compare the meaning of a normal versus a slightly, moderately, severely, and totally impaired skin sensory discrimination test result.

Application: Demonstrate how to conduct an objective skin sensory discrimination test.

Analysis: Explain the significance of each test score in relation to warnings (contraindications, risks, precautions) that practitioners must consider before using thermal agents.

Synthesis: Explain the distinctions between slightly, moderately, severely, and totally impaired test results when the time comes to decide if the thermal agent is contraindicated or not.

Evaluation: Discuss the importance of conducting an objective skin sensory heat and cold discrimination test before using thermal agents.

I. BACKGROUND AND PURPOSE

A. BACKGROUND

There is unanimity in the literature that *safe application* of thermal electrophysical agents (EPAs) *must always be preceded* by a skin sensory heat and cold discrimination test that assesses the patient's ability to normally perceive such stimuli. The rationale for such a test is to prevent thermal skin damages caused by the agents.

B. MANDATORY TESTING

Skin heat and cold sensory discrimination testing is recognized as being *mandatory* before application of all thermal EPAs because the best therapeutic guidance regarding thermal agents *always* begins with the patient's own sensory perception during treatment. Consequently, patients with impaired skin sensory discrimination abilities are at greater risk of not reporting accurately what their skin is really experiencing during the application of thermal agents.

C. SERIOUS CONSEQUENCES

An impaired ability to discriminate thermal stimuli may have serious consequences for patients, who could suffer effects ranging from a mild skin irritation to a severe skin burn, or from a frostnip to frostbite, during the application of thermo- and cryotherapeutic agents.

D. PURPOSE OF CHAPTER

Although all educators and practitioners know that to conduct such a test is mandatory before considering thermotherapy and cryotherapy, *nowhere* in current published textbooks on therapeutic EPAs can one find guidelines to help conduct such skin sensory discrimination tests. The purpose of this chapter is to fill that gap by offering a practical guide.

II. PRACTICAL GUIDE

A. SENSORY LEVELS

This guide recommends testing *five levels* of skin sensory heat and cold discrimination. It is important that testing discriminates between thermal stimuli that are normally perceived by healthy individuals, with intact skin, as either *very cold*, *cold*, *neutral*, *warm*, or *hot*.

B. SKIN SENSORY RECEPTORS

Human skin is composed of two distinct layers of cells: the epidermis and the dermis. Within the dermis are buried specialized sensory receptors, which allow an individual to sense and discriminate levels of pain (*nociceptors*), of heat and cold (*thermoreceptors*), and of touch and pressure (*mechanoreceptors*).

C. THERMONOCICEPTIVE TESTING

Testing skin discrimination of heat and cold allows practitioners to test both the patient's thermal and nociceptive capabilities to distinguish between hot and painfully hot, and very cold and painfully cold stimuli.

D. TESTING PROTOCOL

Described below are the tested probes needed and the testing procedures to be followed to adequately conduct skin sensory discrimination.

1. Test Probes

In order to test skin discrimination for levels perceived as very cold, cold, neutral (room temperature), warm and hot, five testing probes of different temperatures are needed, as shown in **Table 25-1**. This textbook recommends the use of the following custom-made probes. Test probes used in many clinical facilities are usually made of glass. Glass is an inexpensive material that can be easily and repeatedly exposed to high levels of cold and hot temperatures without losing its original shape. In addition, glass is an excellent thermal conductor.

a. Probe—Very Cold

Use a glass tube filled with water. Store it in the *freezer* compartment of a cold unit. The probe temperature should range between −5°C and 0°C (23°F and 32°F).

b. Probe—Cold

Use another glass tube filled with water. Store it in the *refrigerator* compartment of a cold unit. The probe temperature should range between 10°C and 13°C (50°F and 55°F).

TABLE 25-1	FIVE LEVELS OF THERMAL SENSATION AND RELATED TEST-PROBE TEMPERATURES
LEVEL OF SENSATION	**TEST-PROBE TEMPERATURE**
Very cold	−5°C to 0°C (23°F to 32°F)
Cold	10°C to 13°C (50°F to 55°F)
Neutral	20°C to 22°C (68°F to 71°F)
Warm	33°C to 35°C (91°F to 95°F)
Hot	51°C to 54°C (124°F to 130°F)

c. Probe—Neutral

Use a third glass tube filled with water. Store it in a small bucket of water left at room temperature. The probe temperature should range between 20°C and 22°C (68°F and 71°F). This tube is referred to as the neutral probe.

d. Probe—Warm

Use a fourth glass tube filled with water. Store it in a small bucket of water into which a custom thermal element is plunged to keep the bucket water warm. The probe temperature should range between 33°C and 35°C (91°F and 95°F).

e. Probe—Hot

Use a fifth glass tube filled with *paraffin wax*. Hook it to the wall of a thermoregulated paraffin bath unit. Keep the probe immersed in the paraffin mixture between uses. The probe temperature should range between 51°C and 54°C (124°F and 130°F).

2. Patient's Positioning

Position the patient in a comfortable manner while explaining the general purpose related to the skin testing session.

3. Skin Inspection

Expose the skin area to be treated, and visually inspect this area to determine the integrity of the skin (i.e., the absence of any skin damage).

4. Patient Blind to Testing

Cover the patient's eyes such that he or she cannot see which testing probes are being used. Discrimination must be perceived through the skin, not with the eyes.

5. Random Probe Application

Apply the five test probes *one at a time,* in a *random fashion,* and with *a constant, light pressure* over the designated area of skin. Keep the probe in contact with the skin for approximately 10–15 seconds, long enough for the patient to fully appreciate the thermal sensation. Wait 60 seconds between each application. Repeat applications until all five probes are used. The test should take less than 10 minutes.

6. Record the Patient's Response

After maintaining the test probe in place for 10–15 seconds, ask the patient if he or she perceives the probe as being very cold, cold, neutral, warm, or hot. Repeat for each probe.

7. Test Result

Determine whether the patient's response to each test probe is positive or negative. A *positive* response is recorded when the patient's response matches the probe used. For example, a test result would be *positive* if the patient answers *neutral* when the probe that was just applied over the skin was at *room temperature.* Conversely, the test will be recorded as *negative* if the patient answers *neutral* after the application of a *cold* test probe.

E. TEST SCORING AND INTERPRETATION

How do you score and interpret the test results? What are the restrictions to the use of thermal agents associated with each score? This chapter proposes the following arbitrary approach.

1. Test Scoring

The patient's score is established, as shown in **Table 25-2**, on the basis of the *number of test probe positively identified.* The maximum score is 5/5, and the minimum score 0/5.

2. Test Interpretation

Scores of 5/5 and 4/5, as shown in **Table 25-2**, are interpreted as normal and slightly impaired skin thermal sensation, respectively; both scores pose *no* restriction to, and identify as *safe,* the use of themo- and cryoagents. A score of 3/5 is interpreted as moderately impaired thermal skin discrimination; *precautions* are advised when using thermal agents with these patients. Scores of 2/5 and 1/5 are

TABLE 25-2	SKIN THERMAL DISCRIMINATION TEST SCORING	
SCALE	**NUMBER OF POSITIVE ANSWERS**	**USE OF THERMAL AGENTS**
Normal	5/5	Safe
Slightly impaired	4/5	Safe
Moderately impaired	3/5	Precaution
Severely impaired	2/5 and 1/5	Risk
Totally impaired	0/5	Contraindicated

interpreted as severely impaired and poses a *risk* if thermal agents are applied. Finally, a score of 0/5 is interpreted as totally impaired thermal skin discrimination and calls for *contraindication* to all thermal therapeutic EPAs.

CRITICAL THINKING QUESTIONS

Clarification: What is meant by a skin sensory heat and cold, or thermal, discrimination testing?

Assumptions: You have assumed that conducting such a discrimination test is mandatory before using thermal therapeutic agents. How do you justify making that assumption?

Reasons and evidence: The meaningful discrimination of thermal stimuli requires that testing be done with different levels of heat and cold stimuli in relation to room temperature, or neutral, stimuli. Why is this precaution necessary?

Viewpoints or perspectives: You agree with the consensus that skin sensory thermal discrimination testing must be scored not only qualitatively but also quantitatively. What would someone who disagrees with you say?

Implications and consequences: You state that it is important to discriminate between a slightly, moderately, severely, and totally impaired test result when considering the application of thermal agents. What are you implying by that?

About the question: Can therapeutic thermal agents be used with a patient who has an impaired skin sensory discrimination test? Why do you think I ask this question?

CHAPTER 26

Skin and Electrophysical Agent Temperature Measurements

Learning Objectives

Knowledge: Describe the qualitative and quantitative approach to temperature measurements in the field of therapeutic electrophysical agents (EPAs).

Comprehension: Explain the meaning of $T°_{ag-s}$ and $T°_{b-a}$.

Application: Demonstrate how to record $T°_{ag-s}$ and $T°_{b-a}$, using a noncontact portable thermometer.

Analysis: Contrast the qualitative and quantitative approaches to determining heat transfer between the agent and the skin after therapy.

Synthesis: Formulate a mock application of the quantitative approach using a thermal heat and cold application.

Evaluation: Discuss the benefit of using the quantitative approach over the qualitative approach.

I. BACKGROUND AND PURPOSE

A. BACKGROUND

The practice of evidence-based hot pack and paraffin bath therapy (Chapter 6), Fluidotherapy (Chapter 7), cryotherapy (Chapter 8), hydrotherapy (Chapter 9), shortwave diathermy therapy (Chapter 10), and ultrasound therapy (Chapter 20) requires that, after treatment, practitioners *assess the amount of heat* added to or subtracted (cryotherapy) from the exposed tissues by the various thermal EPAs used in the therapies listed above. To do this, practitioners can make use of two approaches: qualitative and quantitative.

B. QUALITATIVE APPROACH

The assessment approach used by the very large majority of practitioners is to simply question the patient, during or after treatment, about the thermal sensation felt, that is, whether the sensation felt was *light, moderate,* or *intense.* This qualitative approach is *subjective,* because it is based entirely on the *patient's perception* of heat and cold. The key advantage associated with this approach is that it is quick, in that it requires only one question and no actual temperature measurement. The key disadvantage, however, is that you, the practitioner, have *no idea* as to the thermal changes induced in the soft tissues under treatment. Moreover, because no temperature measurement is taken, you also have no idea as to the amount of heat delivered to, or extracted from, soft tissues by the thermal agents. The only thing you know, using this qualitative approach, is that the patient felt light, moderate, or intense heat or cold during therapy.

C. QUANTITATIVE APPROACH

Because this textbook rests on scientific evidence, its goal is to bring *objectivity* to the art and science of heat transfer between the thermal agent and the exposed skin after therapy. A quantitative approach is thus required, in which actual temperature measurements are made.

D. PURPOSE OF CHAPTER

The purpose of this chapter is to describe a quantitative approach to the surface measurement of heat transfer between the thermal agent and the exposed skin. This approach is meant to complement the traditional qualitative approach practiced by most practitioners.

II. QUANTITATIVE APPROACH

A. TEMPERATURE DIFFERENTIALS

The quantitative approach involves the use of a portable and accurate contact or noncontact *thermometer.* This approach is based on measuring two temperature differentials. The first temperature differential is the difference between the temperature of the agent (ag) and that of the skin surface to be treated before the application; this differential is designated as $T^{\circ}_{ag\text{-}s}$. The second temperature differential is that between the skin surface temperature before (b) and after (a) treatment, and is designated as $T^{\circ}_{b\text{-}a}$.

1. Potential Thermal Capacity: $T^{\circ}_{ag\text{-}s}$

$T^{\circ}_{ag\text{-}s}$ provides practitioners with a key objective measure to assess the agent's *potential* capacity to induce a thermal response in the soft tissues being treated. The larger the temperature difference between the agent and the skin surface before treatment, the greater the capacity of the agent to either increase or decrease the heat of soft tissues.

2. Actual Skin Temperature Change: $T^{\circ}_{b\text{-}a}$

$T^{\circ}_{b\text{-}a}$ provides practitioners with another key objective measure to assess the *actual* thermal skin change induced by the thermal agent, after treatment. What is the clinical significance of these two temperature differentials?

3. Clinical Example

Table 26-1 illustrates a hypothetical recording of these two temperature differentials before and after application of thermo- and cryoagents. As mentioned previously, this objective approach *complements* the subjective approach described above by assigning numbers (temperature scores) to the patient's qualitative assessment represented by words like mild, moderate, and intense heat or cold.

a. Thermotherapeutic Agent

This example shows that the agent had a *potential* heating ($\mathbf{T}^{\circ}_{ag\text{-}s}$) effect on the skin surface of 24°C (44°F) before treatment, which translated into an *actual* skin surface heating ($\mathbf{T}^{\circ}_{b\text{-}a}$) of +10°C (+18°F) after treatment (**Table 26-1**). In other words, the thermal agent *added* (hence the + sign) heat to the exposed soft tissues.

b. Cryotherapeutic Agent

This example shows that the agent had a *potential* cooling ($\mathbf{T}^{\circ}_{ag\text{-}s}$) effect on the skin surface of 26°C (47°F) before treatment, which translated into an *actual* skin surface cooling ($\mathbf{T}^{\circ}_{b\text{-}a}$) of −12°C (−22°F) after treatment (**Table 26-1**). In this case, the cryoagent *subtracted* (hence the − sign) heat from the exposed soft tissues.

B. TEMPERATURE RECORDING

A reliable and accurate *contact* or *noncontact* thermometer is required to measure the two temperature differentials described above.

TABLE 26-1	EXAMPLES OF TEMPERATURE DIFFERENTIAL MEASUREMENTS		
THERMOTHERAPEUTIC AGENT			
	T°_{ag}	T°_s	$T^\circ_{ag\text{-}s}$
Before treatment (b)	54°C (130°F)	30°C (86°F)	24°C (44°F)
After treatment (a)	—	40°C (104°F)	—
$T^\circ_{b\text{-}a}$	—	+10°C (+18°F)	—
CRYOTHERAPEUTIC AGENT			
	T°_{ag}	T°_s	$T^\circ_{ag\text{-}s}$
Before treatment (b)	4°C (39°F)	30°C (86°F)	26°C (47°F)
After treatment (a)	—	18°C (64°F)	—
$T^\circ_{b\text{-}a}$	—	−12°C (−22°F)	—

1. Contact Thermometer

As its name implies, a contact thermometer is characterized by its probe making *contact* with the material or biological tissue to record its temperature. Such thermometers have been used for decades in the industrial and clinical fields.

2. Noncontact Thermometer

Newer noncontact, portable, and low-cost infrared surface thermometers are now available on the market. A significant advantage of using noncontact as opposed to contact-type thermometers is that these thermometers quickly, accurately, and safely measure the surface temperature of materials and biological tissues *without contacting* their surfaces. Another key advantage is that noncontact thermometers eliminate the risk of damaging or contaminating the surface area being treated.

a. Typical Noncontact Thermometer

Figure 26-1 shows a typical handheld, infrared, noncontact surface thermometer equipped with a laser beam used for aiming purposes only. This textbook *strongly recommends* the use of noncontact thermometers, for the reasons presented above, to measure the temperature differentials discussed in this chapter.

b. Operating Mechanism

The thermometer's optic sensors emit, reflect, and transmit infrared energy, which is then collected and focused onto a deflector. The device then translates the optic information into a temperature reading, which is digitally displayed on its screen.

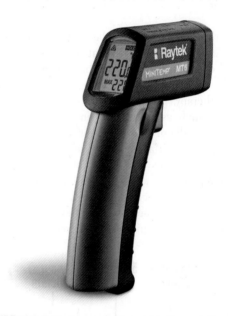

FIGURE 26-1 Typical noncontact, portable thermometer. (Courtesy of Raytek Corp.)

c. Thermometer's Laser Pointer

Because infrared rays are invisible, the thermometer is mounted with a class II laser pointer (see Chapter 11). The focused laser beam is used only for aiming or pointing purposes.

d. Easy Operation

These noncontact thermometers are very easy to use. Just aim, using the laser beam, at the surface of the agent or the skin, pull the trigger, and read its current surface temperature (°C or °F) in less than 1 second.

i. Distance-to-spot size ratio. When taking a measurement with such a noncontact thermometer, be sure to consider the distance-to-spot size ratio (D:S ratio) and the field of view. The type of infrared thermometer featured in **Figure 26-1** is intended for close-range targets with a D:S ratio of 10:1. This means that the thermometer measures a minimum target area of 2.5 cm (1 in.) in diameter from a distance of approximately 25 cm (10 in.), as illustrated in **Figure 26-2**, and has a 10-cm (4-in.) target measurement area at 100 cm (40 in.). So the farther away the thermometer from the surface of the agent or skin, the larger the agent and skin areas from which the temperature is taken.

ii. Intrasession and intersession recordings. To standardize the measurement of both $T^{\circ}_{ag\text{-}s}$ and $T^{\circ}_{b\text{-}a}$, keep the D:S ratio constant and aim the laser beam at the same spot during and between therapeutic sessions.

III. SURFACE VERSUS DEEP THERMAL TISSUE CHANGE

A. MEASURING DEEP-TISSUE TEMPERATURE CHANGE

Measuring the actual skin surface temperature change ($T^{\circ}_{b\text{-}a}$), as described above, does not reveal the extent of the thermal changes that occur in the deeper tissues. To quantify deeper-tissue thermal changes in patients following thermal therapy, practitioners must use *needle-probe thermometers,* such as those used in research settings. Each of these needle-probes is positioned in different layers of soft tissue, such as within muscles, tendons, ligaments, and joint capsules. This methodological approach to soft-tissue temperature measurement is, without a doubt, *unsuitable for clinical practice* because very few patients, if at all any, will volunteer to have these needle-probe thermometers inserted in their different tissue lay-

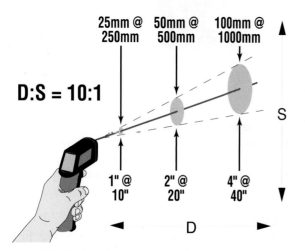

FIGURE 26-2 Noncontact infrared thermometer's optical thermal ranges and laser sighting. (Courtesy of Raytek Corp.)

ers after routine application of, for example, hot packs, cold packs, and shortwave diathermy. If can practitioners *estimate, or predict,* deep tissues thermal changes on the basis of the surface skin measurements taken and described above?

B. PREDICTING DEEP-TISSUE TEMPERATURE CHANGE

Results of experimental studies on humans using multi-needle thermometers implanted at various depths in soft tissues have revealed a general trend: *Keeping the duration of application identical, the greater the skin temperature differential between the agent and the skin area being treated* ($T^{\circ}_{ag\text{-}s}$)*, the greater the thermal changes in the deeper tissues* (see References in Chapters 6 to 10 and 20). The present quantitative approach, in keeping with this trend, *assumes that the skin temperature differential may be a reasonable clinical predictor* of the deeper-tissue thermal changes induced by the thermal agent.

IV. NEED FOR BOTH APPROACHES

A. QUALITATIVE PRACTICE

For practitioners to rely on their patients' thermal perception after the delivery of thermal therapy is fine. To rely *solely* on this source of information is, however, *questionable,* because there is no way for a practitioner to know, in the absence of temperature measurement, the exact thermal potential of the agent, and the actual skin thermal changes, induced by the agent following its application. For practitioners to base their dosage strictly on their patients' thermal perception is unacceptable in the present-day evidence-based world of health practice. There is no doubt that this qualitative practice of using words to describe thermal changes needs to *be validated* by an objective practice, which will put numbers on the patient's verbal thermal appreciation.

B. QUANTITATIVE PRACTICE

This chapter shows that the recording of temperature differentials by practitioners, during the course of their practice, can be done quickly and effectively using low-cost, accurate, portable, noncontact-type thermometers. This quantitative practice is needed to establish the therapeutic foundation of thermal therapy. It is fine to record in the patient's file, for example, that a given cryoagent was perceived as *moderately* cold by the patient. It is better, if one's practice of therapeutic EPAs is guided by the evidence, to quantify this moderately cold sensation by recording, for this example, that the cryoagent has a potential cooling effect of 12 degrees ($T^{\circ}_{ag\text{-}s}$), which led to an actual skin cooling ($T^{\circ}_{b\text{-}a}$) of 5 degrees.

C. DUAL APPROACHES

This textbook *urges* practitioners to use *both*, the qualitative and quantitative approaches, in their daily practice of thermal therapy. Measuring temperature differentials puts a meaning to words such as light, moderate, or intense thermal perception. Measuring temperature differentials is also most valuable when the time comes to determine therapeutic dosages and evaluate treatment effectiveness. It is no longer acceptable for practitioners to document in the patient's file that the thermal sensation felt by the patient was light, moderate, or intense. It is the duty and responsibility of the evidence-based practitioners to quantify how light, moderate, or intense this sensation was. This can only be done if temperature measurements are taken.

CRITICAL THINKING QUESTIONS

Clarification: Describe the meaning of $T^{\circ}_{ag\text{-}s}$ and $T^{\circ}_{b\text{-}a}$ temperature differentials.

Assumptions: You have assumed that it is important to measure $T^{\circ}_{ag\text{-}s}$ and $T^{\circ}_{b\text{-}a}$. How do you justify making that assumption?

Reasons and evidence: A colleague tells you that the hot pack treatment he just gave was perceived by his patient as moderately hot at the end of treatment. A few minutes later another colleague tells you that the cold pack he just gave was felt as intensely cold by his patient. He also adds that his cryoagent had a cooling potential of 25°C and induced an actual skin temperature drop (cooling) of 18°C after 14 minutes of application. Which of these two verbal reports is more meaningful clinically, and why?

Viewpoints or perspectives: How would you respond to a colleague who says that taking these two temperature differential measurements ($T^{\circ}_{ag\text{-}s}$ and $T^{\circ}_{b\text{-}a}$) is a waste of time, and that simply asking the patient if he or she perceived the thermal treatment just received as mild, moderate, or intense is just as good an approach to assessing soft-tissue temperature changes after treatment?

Implications and consequences: You tend to agree with the assumption that one can reasonably predict the temperature changes in the deeper tissues if one knows the temperature changes at the skin surface. What are you implying by that?

About the question: Is it true that recording temperature measurements from the thermal agent and the treated skin surface requires a sophisticated and expensive thermometer and that the recording protocol is complicated and lengthy? Why do you think I ask this question?

Electrical Shocks, Safety Measures, and Maintenance of Line-Powered Devices

Chapter Outline

Learning Objectives

Knowledge: Describe the genesis and nature of a micro and macro electrical shock.

Comprehension: Explain the operating mechanism behind a ground-fault circuit interrupter (GFCI) receptacle.

Application: Show how a macroshock can be prevented when line-powered devices are used.

Analysis: Distinguish between standard three-wire and ground-fault circuit interrupter (GFCI) electrical receptacles.

Synthesis: Formulate all the possible physiological consequences resulting from the flow of a 1-ampere AC leakage current through the thoracic area of a patient via his or her two hands.

Evaluation: Elaborate a rescue plan in case of occurrence of a severe macroshock and electrocution in your clinical setting.

I. BACKGROUND AND PURPOSE

A. ELECTRICAL SHOCK

Electricity is a ubiquitous source of energy that can be fatal for human beings. Electrical shocks, although rare in the field of health care, represent a serious occupational hazard for both patients and clinicians operating line-powered electrophysical agents (EPAs). To *be unaware of, or to overlook*, the dangers associated with electrical shocks increases one's vulnerability to, and the risk of one's becoming a victim of, electrical shock (Greenwald, 1991, 1993; Myklebust et al., 1992; Ritter, 1996).

B. LINE- VERSUS BATTERY-POWERED DEVICES

A *line-powered* device is one that is powered by a building's conventional power-line voltage, which in North America is characterized by a 60-Hz alternating current (AC), delivered between 110 and 125 V. A *battery-powered* device is one that is powered by a battery source, characterized by the delivery of a continuous 0-Hz direct current (DC) at relatively low voltage, such as 9 V.

C. DANGERS OF LINE-POWERED DEVICES

The flow of an *unwanted* 60-Hz AC current in the body, referred to as a leakage current, can cause severe to lethal physiological responses, depending on its amplitude, duration, and path of flow (see below). Electrical shocks are caused by leakage currents flowing in the body.

1. Leakage Current

A leakage current can be *defined* as any loss of current from a line-powered device, usually resulting from breaks in the insulation system (chassis and power cord). In other words, a leakage current is an *unwanted* current that *leaks out* from the intended pathway as a result of defective insulation, often caused by excessive wear and tear and misuse.

2. Danger

Using line-powered devices is *dangerous* because passage of this 60-Hz AC leakage current in the body, if of sufficient amplitude and duration, can depolarize motor nerves, thus inducing light-to-strong involuntary muscle contractions. Because fused tetanus (i.e., maximum tetanic muscle contraction) occurs in most human muscles at frequencies between 40 and 60 Hz, the passage of this 60-Hz AC leakage current can cause such fused muscle tetanus.

3. Battery-Powered Devices

Is leakage current from a battery-powered (DC current) device as dangerous as that originating from a line-powered device? The answer is *no*. Battery-powered devices are *safe* because the continuous 0-Hz DC leakage current, regardless of its amplitude and duration, is incapable of causing nerve depolarization and, thus, unable to induce electrically evoked muscle contraction.

D. PHYSIOLOGICAL DAMAGE

When a 60-Hz AC leakage current *larger than* 5 mA passes through the body (see below), the individual is exposed to a variety of unwanted physiological responses, such as tetanic muscle contraction and tissue burn, which may cause minor-to-severe body injury, including death.

1. Tetanic Muscle Contraction

The victim may display *minimal-to-extremely violent tetanic muscle contractions*, ranging from the classic "*can't let go*" *contraction* (forearm muscles) to *respiratory arrest* (intercostal muscles) to *cardiac arrest* (ventricle/heart fibrillation) to, at worst, *death* by electrocution.

2. Tissue Burn

This 60-Hz AC current passing through the body can also cause light-to-severe *burn injuries*, because heat is produced when the current flows through the resistance offered by the tissues. Burn injuries caused by an electrical shock are located primarily at the skin surface (external) level rather than in the deeper tissues (internal), because skin tissue offers much greater resistance to current flow than deeper, moist tissues. Internal burn injuries are likely to be more substantial if the skin, in contact with the live, faulty electrical source, is wet. Wet skin presents much less resistance to current than dry skin and, as a result, decreases the natural protection that dry skin offers against internal burn injuries. Note that even if the victim survives cardiorespiratory failure, the damages caused by internal burn injuries to the neurovascular system are often the cause of death following an electrical shock.

3. Extent of Body Injury

The extent of body injury caused by an electrical shock depends on three key factors: the *leakage current's amplitude, duration of flow within the body*, and *path of flow through the body*.

a. Leakage Current Amplitude

The *maximum* 60-Hz leakage AC current amplitude that can *safely* flow though the human chest area is **5 mA** (Ritter, 1996). Leakage currents will cause microshocks, and possibly lethal macroshocks, depending of their amplitudes.

i. Microshock. Leakage currents lower than 5 mA produce *microshocks*, which are harmless to humans.

ii. Macroshock. Leakage currents higher than 5 mA produce macroshocks, which trigger a cascade of harmful physiological responses. Thus, the higher the leakage current amplitudes, the larger the macroshocks, and the more damaging and deadly the body injuries will be.

b. Duration of Current Flow

For body injuries to occur, the *duration of flow* of the leakage current must also be sufficiently long. It is common sense that the longer the duration of current flow into the body (from seconds to minutes), the more severe the body damages will be.

c. Path of Flow Through the Body

The path of leakage current flow through the thoracic region, via both arms, is potentially much more dangerous and deadly (i.e., current passes through vital tissues such as the vagus and phrenic nerves) than a path of flow from one arm to the trunk and leg, and finally to earth. This is why touching with two hands, as opposed to one hand, the chassis or power cord of a live line-powered EPA device always represents a greater risk of suffering from a potentially deadly macroshock.

d. Recap

First, always remember that it is the magnitude of the leakage current amplitude (greater than 5 mA), not the magnitude of voltage (e.g., 120 V) or current amplitude (e.g., 1 A) powering the device, that is responsible for the body damages. Second, remember that a large leakage current (for example 400 mA) flowing for only 2 seconds causes much less tissue damages and is much less dangerous than a weaker leakage current (e.g., 25 mA) flowing for 45 seconds. Third, always recall that the danger of a leakage current is determined by the path of flow it takes in the body, meaning a leakage current flowing through a sensitive area, such as the thorax, may interfere with the functioning of life-sustaining organs (heart and respiratory muscles) in addition to inducing muscle contractions and tissue burns.

E. PURPOSE OF CHAPTER

The purpose of this chapter is threefold: (1) to describe the conditions that can generate an electrical shock, (2) to facilitate the safe use of line-powered EPAs by providing a list of safety measures, and (3) to provide practitioners with a list of immediate steps and procedures to follow in case an electrical shock occurs during treatment.

II. GENESIS OF AN ELECTRICAL SHOCK

A. GROUND-FAULT PATHWAY

An electrical shock occurs when the victim's hand(s) or other body parts contact a leakage source of electrical current, thus providing a path for this current to go to the ground. For this to occur, a *ground-fault pathway* must be present. A ground fault is described as an unintentional electrical path between a source of current and a grounded surface. It occurs when current leaks to the ground from the line-powered device's hardware, in other words, when the AC line-powered current escapes from the device to travel through the victim's body to earth. The leakage

current that results from the ground fault is what causes a microshock or a macroshock.

B. DEVICE ELECTRICAL INSULATION

The main cause of a leakage current is a *break* or *failure* in the device's hardware electrical insulation, often due to abuse of the device and a lack of regular electrical maintenance. Faulty insulation of the live wire within the power cord is a common example that results from abusive or careless use (e.g., pulling on and walking over the cable). Another example is a live chassis caused by a break in the internal device's electrical insulation system due to repeated mechanical vibrations and shocks sustained by the device over time.

C. BODY AS PATHWAY

If the patient's or operator's body provides the path for this leakage current to flow to the ground, one or both will be the victims of an electrical shock that can cause burn injuries, respiratory/cardiac arrest, and, potentially, death by electrocution, as discussed above.

III. PROTECTION AGAINST ELECTRICAL SHOCKS

A. GROUND-FAULT CIRCUIT INTERRUPTER RECEPTACLE

One of the best and easiest ways to protect against a macroshock is to plug each line-powered EPA device into a *ground-fault circuit interrupter* (GFCI) receptacle or outlet, as opposed to the standard *three-wire receptacles* found practically everywhere in clinics, hospitals, and homes. **Figure 27-1** shows the most common type of *GFIC*

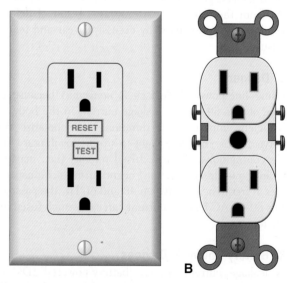

FIGURE 27-1 Ground-fault circuit interrupter (**A**) and standard three-wire electrical (**B**) receptacles.

receptacle (**A**), which is characterized by its TEST and RESEST buttons , as well as the *standard three-wire receptacle* (**B**), which is used in practically all homes and buildings.

B. OPERATING MECHANISM

The GFCI receptacle is designed to protect both the patient and operator from severe-to-fatal electric shocks. It does it by constantly monitoring the flow of the 60-Hz AC current from the device to the circuit interrupter, and back, thus detecting any loss or leakage of the current. Its purpose is to detect ground faults. GFCIs are designed to cut off electrical power to the device, within a fraction of a second, if a leakage current *greater than 5 mA* (the safe limit for the human thoracic region) is present, thus preventing any harmful or deadly injuries (Miklebust et al., 1992; Ritter, 1996). In other words, doing so prevents the operator and patient from being exposed to a potentially lethal leakage current.

C. TESTING GFCI RECEPTACLE

All GFCIs are mounted with a TEST and RESEST button, as shown in **Figure 27-1A.** These buttons are used to quickly test the receptacle to see if it is working properly.

1. Procedure

To test a GFCI, plug a regular lamp into the receptacle and turn the light ON. Now press the TEST button; the RESET button should immediately pop out, and the light should go out. This indicates that the GFCI is working properly. Press the RESET button to restore power to the outlet.

2. Troubleshooting

If the RESET button pops out but the light is still on, the GFCI is incorrectly wired. If the RESET button does not pop out, the GFCI receptacle is defective and should be replaced immediately.

3. Periodic Testing

It is recommended that all GFCIs be tested once a month.

IV. PREVENTION, OPERATIONAL SAFETY, AND MAINTENANCE

A. OVERALL MEASURES

The adoption of *preventive*, *operational safety*, and *maintenance* measures is the best way to prevent the genesis of electrical shocks when working with line-powered EPAs.

B. PREVENTIVE MEASURES

As a first step in the prevention of electrical shocks, two measures need to be considered: safe wall electrical receptacle and line-powered device's electrical certification.

1. Wall Receptacle

Replace all wall standard three-wire receptacles (**Fig 27-1B**) with GFCI receptacles (**Fig 27-1A**). Three-wire receptacles provide a true ground connection to the earth, but they offer *no protection* against harmful leakage currents passing through the body. Their purpose is to protect the equipment, not the users, against a sudden flow of large leakage currents. The U.S. National Electric Code requires that, in all health facilities, electrically line-powered devices and accessories be plugged into GFCI receptacles or outlets to ensure their safe use in areas where water is omnipresent (Ritter, 1996). Wet skin, as opposed to dry skin, presents less resistance to current flow, thus overexposing the person to macroshocks when working in a wet environment, such as in a hydrotherapy unit. This textbook *urges* all operators of line-powered EPAs to **always** plug their devices into GFCI outlets to assure maximum protection against electrical shocks.

2. Device's Electrical Certification

Assure that the seal of a reputable testing laboratory, such as the Underwriter Laboratories (UL), is on the device's chassis before using it. This seal certifies that the device has a maximum leakage current of less than 1 mA, which is considered to be absolutely safe to humans. If any of your older devices do not have this seal, take them to a qualified technician for a complete inspection and upgrade, in order to bring all your line-powered EPA devices into compliance with currently recognized electrical safety standards.

C. OPERATIONAL SAFETY MEASURES

Adopting proper operational safety measures is another good way to prevent an electrical shock.

1. Manufacturer's Brochure

Always read the manufacturer's brochure regarding safety measures and manipulation of the line-powered device before using it for the first time.

2. Plug, Power Cord, and Extension Cords

Always disconnect the device by gripping and pulling its plug, not its power cord. Make sure the plug remains firmly seated in the socket and that the tines of the plug are not visible. Never use extension cords.

3. Instruction to Patients

Instruct all patients never to touch a line-powered device, including its knobs, power cord, cables, and electrodes. Instruct each of them on how to shut off the device himself or herself in case of an emergency or major discomfort during treatment sessions. Instruct all patients on how to call for help when needed during treatment sessions.

4. Visible Warning Signs

Post visible signs, either on the entry door or the walls adjacent to the treatment areas, to warn patients, visitors, and staff that they are entering an area in which electrical, electromagnetic, and acoustic fields of radiation are being generated. Also post a visible sign on the same entry door to alert those persons wearing electronic implants, such as a cardiac pacemaker, or carrying electronic devices, such as a cellular phone, not to enter this area without receiving full authorization by an attending clinician.

5. Home Therapy

Battery-powered devices are highly recommended over line-powered devices for home therapy because a leakage DC current is harmless (no motor nerve depolarization is possible) compared with a 60-Hz leakage AC current. Before recommending the use of a line-powered device for home therapy, make sure the patient's home is equipped with at least one GFCI receptacle, and instruct the patient to plug the device into *that receptacle only*.

D. MAINTENANCE MEASURES

Adopting regular maintenance measures can only help minimizing the occurrence of an electrical shock.

1. Visual Inspection

Do weekly visual inspections to check the integrity of the device's basic components and accessories such as knobs, power cords, plugs, cables, and electrodes.

2. Technical Support and Log

Have a qualified technician inspect, repair, and calibrate all line-powered EPAs used in the facility at least once a year or whenever a problem is suspected. Ask the repair technician to place a sticker on the chassis of each line-powered device that shows the date of its last inspection, repair, and calibration. Keep an inspection/repair/calibration log for each EPA used in your facility.

3. Designated Clinician in Charge

Designate one clinician, from among those practicing with line-powered EPAs, as the *clinician in charge* for all matters relating to the functioning and maintenance of these devices. This person's role is one of prevention and central information gathering to ensure proper and timely communication between users and maintenance technicians about safety and maintenance issues for all line-powered equipment. His or her role is *not* to be held fully responsible in case an electrical hazard occurs.

V. PROCEDURES IMMEDIATELY FOLLOWING A MACROSHOCK

A. RECOMMENDATIONS

The procedures outlined below serve only as *recommendations* from the author. Therefore, users of line-powered EPAs are reminded to always apply the procedures *ap-*

proved in their own facility in case an electrical macroshock occurs before applying those described below. Only when no such procedures are stipulated should the users adopt and expand on those listed below.

1. Legal Consequences

Practitioners should always remember that the occurrence of any macroshock involving patients, colleagues, and staff might have *serious legal consequences;* hence the necessity to draft, adopt, and follow standardized procedures in the case of an electrical shock.

2. Author's Disclaimer

The following procedures must not be interpreted in any way, shape, or form as containing any legal statement or advice. Readers must refer to legal counsel in their own country for any legal advice relating to this subject.

B. SCENARIO AND PROCEDURES

Consider the following *hypothetic scenario*. Your line-powered ultrasound device, plugged into a *standard three-wire receptacle*, is ready to be used. Your patient, in a courteous effort to help you move the device closer to the treatment table, grabs with *both hands* the device's power cord. An unfortunate break of insulation in this power cord causes the patient to be victim of a major electrical shock, manifested by violent "can't let go" forearm muscle contractions. The patient falls on the floor, unable to let go the faulty power cord. What should you do to rescue this patient?

1. Stop the Current Flow First

Before touching the victim, the rescuer must stop the origin of the leakage current, that is, the 60-Hz AC current powering the device. This is achieved by *pulling the power cord plug* (safe insulation through its thick rubber coating), *not the cord* (faulty insulation), out of the wall electrical receptacle or outlet. If the rescuer fails to disconnect the device from the electrical outlet before touching or attending to the victim, he or she will be exposed to the same electrical shock, thus becoming the second victim.

2. Attend to the Victim Second

The rescuer should then immediately attend to the victim by checking his or her vital signs —measuring carotid pulse and monitoring respiratory rate. If the vital signs are absent or very weak, the rescuer must call immediately for emergency help and begin cardiopulmonary resuscitation (CPR) maneuvers. All clinicians using line-powered EPA devices **must** be knowledgeable in both the theory and practice of cardiopulmonary resuscitation.

3. Arrange the Victim's Transfer Third

When vital signs are reestablished to the point at which the victim can breathe regularly on his or her own, the rescuer should plan for the victim's immediate transfer to the nearest hospital for a full medical examination. If the electrical shock occurs at the hospital, the rescuer should arrange for the victim to be taken immediately to the emergency department. In this case, the victim should be attended to according to the standardized guidelines of the hospital. The rescuer should plan for such a transfer even if the victim's vital signs were maintained after the electrical shock. Because of the possible legal and/or fatal consequences of an electrical shock, it is in the best interests of both the victim and the rescuer that a physician conducts a complete physical examination of the victim immediately or within hours after an electrical shock.

4. Secure the Faulty Equipment and Accessories Fourth

After the victim's departure from the scene, the rescuer should immediately secure all the faulty equipment related to this event so that no one else can access them. Instruct all colleagues not to touch or use this equipment until further notice from the facility's administrative authorities.

5. File an Incident Report Fifth

The rescuer should report, in writing, to the administrative authorities the nature of the incident and all the circumstances surrounding it. Either the rescuer or another person directly involved with the incident should create a device incident file. Because the rescuer involved in the incident may be asked to testify in court if a lawsuit is launched by the victim, he or she should be kept informed about the evolution of the case. The person can help ensure a proper resolution of the incident by working in collaboration with facility administrative authorities.

C. LESSON TO BE LEARNED

The unfortunate incident (severe macroshock) narrated in the above scenario could have been prevented if the EPA device had been plugged into a GFCI receptacle. In such a case, no current would have flown into the power cord because the GFCI outlet would have detected the ground-fault pathway (leakage current) caused by the break in the power cord electrical insulation, thus switching off the electrical power supply to the device. The operator would have realized that something was wrong because he or she would not have been able to switch on the device. A quick look at the GFCI would have indicated that the RESET button had popped out.

CRITICAL THINKING QUESTIONS

Clarification: What is meant by an electrical shock, and what is the difference between a micro- and macroshock?

Assumption: You have assumed that the genesis of an electrical shock can be prevented if users of line-powered EPAs take adequate measures. How do you justify making that assumption?

Reasons and evidence: Ground-fault circuit interrupter (GFCI) receptacles are designed to prevent the flow of a leakage current capable of generating a macroshock. How does this happen?

Viewpoints or perspectives: You agree with the viewpoint that users of line-powered EPAs should take and apply regular preventive, operational, and maintenance measures even though death by electrocution using such EPAs is extremely rare. What would someone who disagrees with you say?

Implications and consequences: You state that the first thing to do before attending to the victim of a macroshock is to unplug the device from the wall receptacle. What are the possible consequences if the rescuer fails to do this first?

About the question: Why is it important for the rescuer to follow all the procedures described in this chapter if some day his or her patient received a severe macroshock during the application of a line-powered EPA? Why do you think I ask this question?

References

Chapters of Textbooks

Myklebust BM, Kloth LC (1992) Electrodiagnostic and electrotherapeutic instrumentation: Characteristics of recording and stimulation systems and the principles of safety. In: Electrotherapy in Rehabilitation. Gersh MR (Ed). FA Davis, Philadelphia, pp 87–100.

Ritter HT (1996) Instrumentation considerations: Operating principles, purchases, management and safety. In: Thermal Agents in Rehabilitation, 3rd ed. Michlovitz SL (Ed). FA Davis, Philadelphia, pp 61–77.

Textbooks

Greenwald EK (1991) Electrical Hazards and Accidents: Their Cause and Prevention. John Wiley & Sons, New York, NY.

Greenwald EK (1993) An Illustrated Guide to Electrical Safety. American Society of Safety Engineering, Des Plaines, IL.

Equivalency Between Metric and U.S. Units of Measure

METRIC PREFIXES

Nano	0.000000001	10^{-9}
Micro	0.000001	10^{-6}
Milli	0.001	10^{-3}
Centi	0.01	10^{-2}
Deci	0.1	10^{-1}
Deca	10	10^{1}
Hecto	100	10^{2}
Kilo	1,000	10^{3}
Mega	1,000,000	10^{6}
Giga	1,000,000,000	10^{9}

UNIT EQUIVALENCY

DISTANCE

1 inch = 2.54 centimeters

1 foot = 30.5 centimeters

1 yard = 91.5 centimeters

1 mile = 1.61 kilometers

1 meter = 3.28 feet

1 angstrom = 10^{-4} microns = 10^{-10} meter

MASS

1 kilogram = 0.07 slug

1 slug = 14.59 kilograms

WEIGHT

1 gram = 0.0353 ounce

1 ounce = 28.35 grams

1 pound = 16 ounces = 0.454 kilograms

1 kilogram = 2.2 pounds

FORCE

1 pound = 4.45 newtons

1 kilogram = 2.2 pounds

CAPACITY

1 milliliter = 0.0338 fluid ounce

1 liter = 0.2642 gallon

1 pint = 2 cups

1 quart = 2 pints

1 gallon = 4 quarts = 3.785 liters

VOLUME

1 cubic meter = 35.31 cubic feet

AREA

1 square centimeter = 0.16 square inch

VELOCITY

Speed of light (C) = 3×10^8 meters/second = 186,000 miles/second

PRESSURE

1 atmosphere = 14.7 pounds/square inch (psi)

1 pound/square inch = 51.8 millimeters of mercury (mmHg)

ENERGY

1 calorie = 4.18 joules

1 kilocalorie = 4,180 joules or 3.97 British thermal units

GRAVITATIONAL ACCELERATION

9.8 meters/second^2 = 32.2 feet/second^2

U.S. METRIC ASSOCIATION

The U.S. Metric Association (USMA) is a national non-profit organization that *advocates* U.S. *conversion* to the International System of Units, known by the abbreviation SI and also called the modern metric system. The process of changing measurement units to the metric system is called metric transition or metrication. The USMA offers a selection of books, charts, posters, rulers, measuring tapes, bumper stickers, and thermometers specifically for learning the metric system (www.metric.org).

Temperature Equivalency Table

°F	°C
212	100
194	90
176	80
158	70
140	60
122	50
104	40
86	30
68	20
50	10
32	0
0	-18

CONVERTING DEGREES CELSIUS (°C) TO DEGREES FAHRENHEIT (°F)

Multiply by 1.8, and then add 32°C

Formula: $°F = (°C \times 1.8) + 32°F$
Example: $45°C = 45.0° \times 1.8 = 81.0° + 32.0° = 113.0°F$
Example: $5°C = 5.0° \times 1.8 = 9.0° + 32.0° = 41.0°F$
Example: $26°C = 26.0° \times 1.8 = 46.8° + 32.0° = 78.8°F$

CONVERTING DEGREES FAHRENHEIT (°F) TO DEGREES CELSIUS (°C)

Subtract 32°, and then divide by 1.8

Formula: $°C = (°F - 32°)/1.8$
Example: $70°F = 70.0° - 32.0° = 38.0°/1.8 = 21.1°C$
Example: $10°F = 10.0° - 32.0° = -22.0°/1.8 = -12.2°C$
Example: $24°F = 24.0° - 32.0° = -80.0°/1.8 = -4.4°C$

Water freezing point: 0°C, 32°F
Water boiling point: 100°C, 212°F

CELSIUS TO FAHRENHEIT CONVERSION

	10	20	30	40	50	60	70	80	90	100
0	32.0	50.0	68.0	86.0	104.0	122.0	140.0	158.0	176.0	194.0	212.0
1	33.8	51.8	69.8	87.8	105.8	123.8	141.8	159.8	177.8	195.8
2	35.6	53.6	71.6	89.6	107.6	125.6	143.6	161.6	179.6	197.6
3	37.4	55.4	73.4	91.4	109.4	127.4	145.4	163.4	181.4	199.4
4	39.2	57.2	75.2	93.2	111.2	129.2	147.2	165.2	183.2	201.2
5	41.0	59.0	77.0	95.0	113.0	131.0	149.0	167.0	185.0	203.0
6	42.8	60.8	78.8	96.8	114.8	132.8	150.8	168.8	186.8	204.8
7	44.6	62.6	80.5	98.6	116.6	134.6	152.6	170.6	188.6	206.6
8	46.4	64.4	82.4	100.4	118.4	136.4	154.4	172.4	190.4	208.4
9	48.2	66.2	84.2	102.2	120.2	138.2	156.2	174.2	192.2	210.2

Celsius degrees in bold type.

FAHRENHEIT TO CELSIUS CONVERSION

	10	20	30	40	50	60	70	80	90	100	110	120	130	140	150	160	170	180	190	200	210
0	−12.2	−6.7	−1.1	4.4	10.0	15.6	21.1	26.7	32.2	37.8	43.3	48.9	54.4	60.0	65.6	71.1	76.7	82.2	87.8	93.3	98.9
1	−11.7	−6.1	−0.6	5.0	10.6	16.1	21.7	27.2	32.8	38.3	43.9	49.4	55.0	60.6	66.1	71.7	77.2	82.8	88.3	93.9	99.4
2	−11.1	−5.6	0.0	5.6	11.1	16.7	22.2	27.8	33.3	38.9	44.4	50.0	55.6	61.1	66.7	72.2	77.8	83.3	88.9	94.4	100.0
3	−10.6	−5.0	0.6	6.1	11.7	17.2	22.8	28.3	33.9	39.4	45.0	50.6	56.1	61.7	67.2	72.8	78.3	83.9	89.4	95.0	
4	−10.0	−4.4	1.1	6.7	12.2	17.8	23.3	28.9	34.4	40.0	45.6	51.1	56.7	62.2	67.8	73.3	78.9	84.4	90.0	95.6	
5	−9.4	−3.9	1.7	7.2	12.8	18.3	23.9	29.4	35.0	40.6	46.1	51.7	57.2	62.8	68.3	73.9	79.4	85.0	90.6	96.1	
6	−8.9	−3.3	2.2	7.8	13.3	18.9	24.2	30.0	35.6	41.1	46.7	52.2	57.8	63.3	68.9	74.4	80.0	85.6	91.1	96.7	
7	−8.3	−2.8	2.8	8.3	13.9	19.4	25.0	30.6	36.1	41.7	47.2	52.8	58.3	63.9	69.4	75.0	80.6	86.1	91.7	97.2	
8	−7.8	−2.2	3.3	8.9	14.4	20.0	25.6	31.1	36.7	42.2	47.8	53.3	58.9	64.4	70.0	75.6	81.1	86.7	92.2	97.8	
9	−7.2	−1.7	3.9	9.4	15.0	20.6	26.1	31.7	37.2	42.8	48.3	53.9	59.4	65.0	70.6	76.1	81.7	87.2	92.8	98.3	

Fahrenheit degrees in bold type.

Note: Page numbers in *italics* denote figures; those followed by b or t denote boxes and tables, respectively.